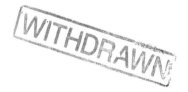
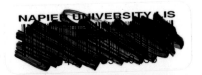
Differential Diagnosis in Physical Therapy

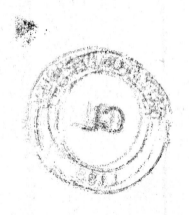

Differential Diagnosis in Physical Therapy

CATHERINE CAVALLARO GOODMAN, MBA, PT

Faculty Affiliate
University of Montana
Missoula, Montana

TERESA E. KELLY SNYDER, MN, RN, CS

(Clinical Specialist in Medical-Surgical Nursing)
Associate Professor of Nursing
Montana State University
Bozeman, Montana

THIRD EDITION

W.B. SAUNDERS COMPANY
A Harcourt Health Sciences Company
Philadelphia   London   Montreal   Sydney   Tokyo   Toronto

W.B. SAUNDERS COMPANY

A Harcourt Health Sciences Company

The Curtis Center
Independence Square West
Philadelphia, Pennsylvania 19106

DIFFERENTIAL DIAGNOSIS IN PHYSICAL THERAPY   ISBN 0–7216–8184–0

Printed in the United States of America.

Last digit is the print number: 9   8   7   6   5   4   3   2

To Cliff, Ben, and Guy, all of my true loves.
C.C.G.

To my husband, R.C.; my son, Jim; and my daughter,
Deann, who fill my life with laughter and unending
adventures.
T.E.K.S.

Foreword

Goodman and Snyder have once again provided an invaluable resource to all physical therapists by updating this book. As expected by recent trends in health care, there is a growing interest in physical therapists being highly trained in differentiating conditions that require medical intervention from conditions that require physical therapy intervention. The trend toward direct access to physical therapy has grown substantially with only five states remaining that require a physician's referral to access physical therapy. Furthermore, a large HMO has recently developed and implemented a program using physical therapists for the initial screening of patients with musculoskeletal symptoms. Appropriate recognition of the patient's problem and immediate recommendations for treatment are the keys to meeting demands for cost containment and the need for patient satisfaction. Physical therapists' ability to screen for medical conditions is also important as we become even more involved in developing fitness and wellness programs for patients with special needs and for the general public.

But it would be a mistake to believe that only therapists who are practicing as direct contact practitioners will benefit from a thorough knowledge of the information provided in this book. The reduced length of hospital stays means that therapists are treating patients in subacute facilities, nursing homes, in the patients' homes, and in outpatient settings who are more seriously ill than was the situation 10 or 15 years ago. Thus a thorough knowledge of medical conditions that mimic musculoskeletal problems is as essential to therapists treating patients who have been referred by a physician as by those without a referral.

The authors' experience as direct-contact practitioners, responsible for medical screening, explains the appropriateness of the text to the needs of physical therapists. The purpose of this text is not to have physical therapists make a differential medical diagnosis; that is beyond their scope of practice. Rather, the intention is to describe the medical conditions whose symptoms mimic musculoskeletal problems; knowing these conditions is critical for safe practice. Goodman and Snyder have written a well-organized and timely book. I also believe this book provides a good model of how therapists can structure their diagnostic decision-making thought processes. Therapists must practice as diagnosticians, and our resource material should reinforce this role. This book serves that purpose and contains vital information physical therapists need for responsible patient care and should be a welcome resource for many other nonphysician clinicians.

Shirley A. Sahrmann, PhD, PT, FAPTA
Professor of Physical Therapy/Cell Biology
Associate Professor of Neurology
Director, Program in Movement Science
Washington University School of Medicine
St. Louis, Missouri

Preface

Since publication of the first edition of *Differential Diagnosis in Physical Therapy,* the need for medical screening of all physical therapy clients has become readily apparent. Increased specialization in the health care delivery system combined with new and more virulent diseases has resulted in both a "sicker" client base and an increased possibility that systemic conditions will mimic musculoskeletal signs and symptoms.

At the time of the first edition of this publication, we recognized the need for a pathophysiology textbook written for physical therapists by physical therapists. The second edition was a step toward that goal as we included much more information about disease etiology, risk factors, pathogenesis, prognosis, and treatment. Since that time, in collaboration with other health care professionals, the dream of a pathology text for physical therapists is now a reality in *Pathology: Implications for the Physical Therapist* (Goodman and Boissonnault, 1998).

This third edition of *Differential Diagnosis in Physical Therapy* reflects the availability of a complete pathology textbook for physical therapists and has been revised to accomplish its original purpose: to provide a guide for the physical therapist to use in screening for medical disease. This material has been incorporated into the curriculum of many physical therapy programs in Canada and the United States. Our design in this third edition is to provide a synthesis text that can be used throughout the student's education, in the newly developing synthesis courses presented as seminars in the final coursework, as well as into clinical practice.

One final note: The Guide to Physical Therapist Practice (1997) defines *patients* as "individuals who are the recipients of physical therapy care and direct intervention" and *clients* as "individuals who are not necessarily sick or injured but who can benefit from a physical therapist's consultation, professional advice, or prevention services." We differ from those definitions in this text. Our philosophical viewpoint is that consumers of health care services are no longer to be viewed as passive recipients of treatment, referred to as *patients,* but rather encouraged as *clients* to participate in their own health care plan whenever possible. We believe our use of the term *client* for most consumers of health care more accurately reflects current clinical practice.

Catherine Cavallaro Goodman

Acknowledgments

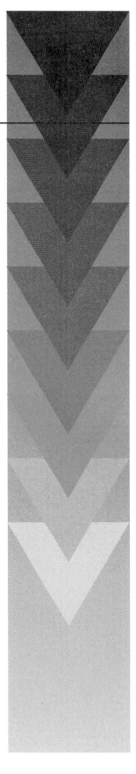

Differential Diagnosis in Physical Therapy is a direct result of experience in the military as an independent practitioner. To the numerous men and women of the United States Army who have assisted in bringing this book to publication, we say thank you. In addition, special thanks go to the staff of W. B. Saunders Company and to the many other family members, friends, and colleagues who remain unnamed.

Your support and encouragement have made possible this third edition of *Differential Diagnosis in Physical Therapy.*

Catherine Cavallaro Goodman
Teresa E. Kelly Snyder

Contents

3

OVERVIEW OF CARDIOVASCULAR SIGNS AND SYMPTOMS 88

4

OVERVIEW OF PULMONARY SIGNS AND SYMPTOMS 145

5

OVERVIEW OF HEMATOLOGIC SIGNS AND SYMPTOMS..........................181

6

OVERVIEW OF GASTROINTESTINAL SIGNS AND SYMPTOMS..........................197

7

OVERVIEW OF RENAL AND UROLOGIC SIGNS AND SYMPTOMS..........................234

8

OVERVIEW OF HEPATIC AND BILIARY SIGNS AND SYMPTOMS.............................260

9

OVERVIEW OF ENDOCRINE AND METABOLIC SIGNS AND SYMPTOMS.........................287

10

OVERVIEW OF ONCOLOGIC SIGNS AND SYMPTOMS......334

11

OVERVIEW OF IMMUNOLOGIC SIGNS AND SYMPTOMS......390

12

SYSTEMIC ORIGINS OF MUSCULOSKELETAL PAIN..................................434

Introduction to Differential Screening in Physical Therapy

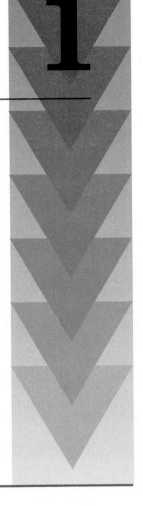

1

Whether following the model of independent practice under the increasingly prevalent direct access laws or practicing by physician referral, physical therapists must know how to recognize systemic disease masquerading as neuromusculoskeletal dysfunction.

Under direct access, the physical therapist may have primary responsibility or become the first contact for some clients in the health care delivery system. On the other hand, clients may obtain a signed prescription for physical therapy from their primary care physician, based on similar past complaints of musculoskeletal symptoms, without actually seeing that physician (see Case Example A).

Additionally, with the increasing specialization of medicine, more and more clients are being evaluated for the first time by a medical specialist who may not recognize the underlying systemic disease (see Case Example B). Early signs and symptoms of systemic disease may be difficult or impossible to recognize until the disease has progressed (see Case Example C). In such cases the alert physical therapist may be the first to ask the client pertinent questions to elicit underlying symptoms requiring medical referral.

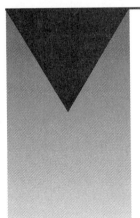

CASE EXAMPLE A*

A 60-year-old man retired from his job as the president of a large vocational technical school and called his physician the next day for a long put-off referral to physical therapy. This client had a history of three previous total hip replacements (anterior approach, lateral approach, posterior approach) on the right side performed over the last 10 years. Based on previous rehabilitation experience, he felt certain that his current symptoms of right anterior hip and groin pain could be alleviated by physical therapy.

The client arrived at the physical therapy clinic with a signed prescription in hand, but when asked if he had actually seen the physician, he explained that he received this prescription after a telephone conversation with his physician.

*All case examples and case studies presented in this text are based on actual clinical experiences in a variety of inpatient and outpatient physical therapy practices.

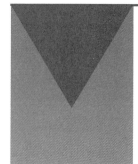

Physical examination revealed a mass of scar tissue in the right flank quadrant with a centralized core of thick, rigid scar tissue over the right greater trochanter. There was a severe right hip flexion contracture and positive right Trendelenburg present.

Bilateral pitting edema of the ankles (evident on the right side more than the left) signaled to the therapist that this edema was probably a chronic condition, and this prompted some additional questions about past medical history. This client had open heart surgery 5 years ago and reported a history of congestive heart failure. He was taking antihypertensive medication but could not name or describe the prescription.

Vital signs taken in the clinic were recorded as:
Temperature: 98.0° F
Pulse: 98 BPM*
Blood pressure: 182/98 mm Hg

Clinical Decision: An appropriate physical therapy program of soft tissue mobilization, stretching, and home exercise was initiated. However, the client was returned to his physician for a follow-up appointment. A brief report from the therapist stated the key objective findings and outlined the proposed physical therapy plan. The letter included a short paragraph with the following remarks:

Given Mr. Y's sedentary lifestyle, previous history of heart disease, and blood pressure reading today, I would like to recommend a physical conditioning program. Would you please let me know if he is medically stable? Based on your findings, we will begin him in a preaerobic training program here and progress him to a home-based or fitness center program.

CASE EXAMPLE B

A 45-year-old long-haul truck driver with bilateral carpal tunnel syndrome was referred for physical therapy by an orthopedic physician specializing in hand injuries. During the course of treatment the client mentioned that he was also seeing an acupuncturist for wrist and hand pain. The acupuncturist told the client that, based on his assessment, acupuncture treatment was indicated for liver disease.†

Result: The therapist continued to treat this client, but knowing that the referring specialist did not routinely screen for systemic causes of carpal tunnel syndrome (or even screen for cervical involvement) combined with the acupuncturist's information, raised a red flag for possible systemic origin

---

*The pulse measurement is difficult to evaluate given the fact that this client is taking hypertensive medications. Beta-blockers, for example, reduce the heart rate so that the body's normal compensatory mechanisms (e.g., increased stroke volume and therefore increased heart rate) are unable to function in response to the onset of congestive heart failure.

†Protein (from food sources or from a gastrointestinal bleed) is normally taken up and detoxified by the liver. Ammonia is produced as a by-product of protein breakdown and then transformed by the liver to urea, glutamine, and asparagine before being excreted by the renal system. When liver dysfunction results in increased serum ammonia and urea levels, peripheral nerve function can be impaired. (See detailed explanation in Chapter 8.)

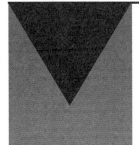

of symptoms. A phone call was made to the physician with the following approach*:

Say, Mr. Y was in for therapy today. He happened to mention that he is seeing an acupuncturist who told him that his wrist and hand pain is from a liver problem. I recalled seeing some information here at the office about the effect of liver disease on the peripheral nervous system. Since Mr. Y has not improved with our carpal tunnel protocol, would you like to have him come back in for a reevaluation?

CASE EXAMPLE C

A 44-year-old woman was referred to the physical therapist with a complaint of right paraspinal/low thoracic back pain. There was no reported history of trauma or assault and no history of repetitive movement. The past medical history was significant for a kidney infection treated 3 weeks ago with antibiotics. The client stated that her follow-up urinalysis was "clear" and the infection resolved.

The physical therapy examination revealed true paraspinal muscle spasm with an acute presentation of limited movement and exquisite pain in the posterior right middle to low back. Spinal accessory motions were tested following application of a cold modality and were found to be mildly restricted in right sidebending and left rotation of the T8-T12 segments. It was the therapist's assessment that this joint motion deficit was still the result of muscle spasm and guarding and not true joint involvement.

Result: After three sessions with the physical therapist in which modalities were used for the acute symptoms, the client was not making observable, reportable, or measurable improvement. Her fourth scheduled appointment was cancelled because of the "flu." Given the recent history of kidney infection, the lack of expected improvement, and the onset of constitutional symptoms (see "Constitutional Symptoms" box on p. 8), the therapist contacted the client by telephone and suggested that she make a follow-up appointment as soon as possible.

As it turned out, this woman's kidney infection had recurred, and she recovered from her back sequelae within 24 hours of initiating a second antibiotic treatment. This is not the typical medical picture for a urologically compromised person. Sometimes it is not until the disease progresses that the systemic disorder (masquerading as a musculoskeletal problem) can be clearly differentiated.

Last, sometimes clients do not relay all the necessary or pertinent medical information to their physicians but will confide in the physical therapist. They may feel intimidated, forget, become unwilling or embarrassed, or fail to recognize the significance of the symptoms and neglect to mention important medical details (see "Reasons for Medical Screening" box on p. 8).

---

*How to respond to each situation will require a certain amount of diplomacy, with consideration given to the individual therapist's relationship with the physician and the physician's openness to direct communication. It is the physical therapist's responsibility to recognize when a client's presentation falls outside the parameters of a true neuromusculoskeletal condition. Unless prompted by the physician, it is not the therapist's role to suggest specific medical testing procedures.

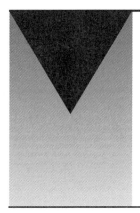

Knowing that systemic diseases can mimic neuromusculoskeletal dysfunction, the therapist is responsible for identifying as closely as possible what neuromusculoskeletal pathologic condition is present. The final result should be to treat as specifically as possible. This is done by closely identifying the underlying neuromusculoskeletal pathological condition and the accompanying movement dysfunction, while at the same time investigating the possibility of systemic disease.

This text will help the clinician quickly recognize problems that are beyond the expertise of the physical therapist. The therapist who recognizes hallmark signs and symptoms of systemic disease will know when to refer clients to the appropriate health care practitioner.

By the end of your course of study of this material, you will know what questions to ask clients so that you can identify the need for medical referral, and you will know what medical conditions can cause shoulder, back, thorax, pelvic, hip, sacroiliac, and groin pain.

This text provides students, physical therapist assistants, and physical therapy clinicians alike with a step-by-step approach to client evaluation, which follows the standards for competency established by the American Physical Therapy Association (APTA) related to conducting a screening examination.

With the physical therapy interview as a foundation for subjectively evaluating each client, each organ system is reviewed with regard to the most common disorders encountered, particularly those that may mimic primary musculoskeletal lesions.

To assist the physical therapist in making a treatment-versus-referral decision, specific pain patterns corresponding to systemic diseases are presented. Special follow-up questions are listed in the subjective examination to help the physical therapist determine when these pain patterns are accompanied by associated signs and symptoms that indicate visceral involvement.

Throughout the text, guidelines for when and how to refer a client to a physician (or other health care provider) for further evaluation or medical follow-up are provided. Each individual case must be reviewed carefully. The client's history, presenting pain patterns, and possible associated signs and symptoms must be reviewed along with results from the objective evaluation in making a treatment-versus-referral decision.

PHYSICAL THERAPY DIAGNOSIS

Medical diagnosis is traditionally defined as the recognition of disease. It is the determination of the cause and nature of pathologic conditions. Medical differential diagnosis is the comparison of symptoms of similar diseases and medical diagnostics (laboratory and test procedures performed) so that a correct assessment of the client's actual problem can be made. A physical therapy differential diagnosis is the comparison of neuromusculoskeletal signs and symptoms to identify the underlying movement dysfunction so that treatment can be planned as specifically as possible (see Case Example D).

Historical Perspective

Physical therapy diagnosis was first described in the literature by Sahrmann (1988) as the name given to a collection of relevant signs and symptoms associated

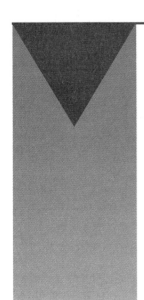

CASE EXAMPLE D

A 31-year-old man was referred to physical therapy by an orthopedic physician. The diagnosis was "shoulder-hand syndrome." This client had been evaluated for this same problem by three other physicians and two physical therapists before arriving at our clinic. Treatment to date had been unsuccessful in alleviating symptoms.

The medical diagnosis itself provided some useful information about the referring physician. "Shoulder-hand syndrome" is an outdated nomenclature previously used to describe reflex sympathetic dystrophy syndrome (RSDS, but usually referred to as RSD), also known as complex regional pain syndrome (CRPS).*

Shoulder-hand syndrome was a condition that occurred following a myocardial infarct, or MI (heart attack), usually after prolonged bedrest. This condition has been significantly reduced in incidence by more up-to-date and aggressive cardiac rehabilitation programs. Today RSDS or CRPS, primarily affecting the limbs, develops after injury or surgery, but it can still occur as a result of a cerebrovascular accident (CVA) or heart attack.

This client's clinical presentation included none of the typical signs and symptoms expected with RSD, such as skin changes (smooth, shiny, red skin), hair growth pattern (increased dark hair patches or loss of hair), temperature changes (increased or decreased), hyperhidrosis (excessive perspiration), restricted joint motion, and severe pain. The clinical picture appeared consistent with a trigger point of the latissimus dorsi muscle, and, in fact, treatment of the trigger point completely eliminated all symptoms.

Conducting a thorough physical therapy examination to identify the specific underlying cause of symptomatic presentation was essential to the treatment of this case. Treatment approaches for a trigger point differ greatly from standard protocols for RSD. Accepting the medical diagnosis without performing a physical therapy diagnostic evaluation would have resulted in wasted time and unnecessary charges for this client.

*The International Association for the Study of Pain replaced the term *RSDS* with *CPRS I* in 1995 (Raj, 1996). Other names given to RSD include neurovascular dystrophy, sympathetic neurovascular dystrophy, algodystrophy, "red-hand disease," Sudeck's atrophy, and mimocausalgia. It should be noted that causalgia is not RSD but a similar syndrome involving trauma to a peripheral nerve with burning pain along the distribution of the nerve (Fealy and Ladd, 1996).

with the primary dysfunction toward which the physical therapist directs treatment. The dysfunction is identified by the physical therapist based on the information obtained from the history, signs, symptoms, examination, and tests the therapist performs or requests. The function of a diagnosis is to provide information that can guide treatment (Sahrmann, 1988).

In 1990, teaching and learning content and the skills necessary to determine a diagnosis became a required part of the curriculum standards established by the Standards for Accreditation for Physical Therapist Educational Program. These standards have been updated. As of January 1, 1998, evaluative criteria for accreditation lists diagnosis as (APTA, 1998, pp 29-30):

Diagnosis

3.8.3.18   Engage in the diagnostic process in an efficient manner consistent with the policies and procedures of the practice setting.

3.8.3.19   Engage in the diagnostic process to establish differential diagnoses for patients across the lifespan based on evaluation of results of examinations and medical and psychosocial information.

3.8.3.20   Take responsibility for communication or discussion of diagnoses or clinical impressions with other practitioners.

In 1995 the APTA house of delegates amended the 1984 policy *Diagnosis by Physical Therapists* to make the definition of *diagnosis* consistent with current use of the term as reflected in the "Guide to Physical Therapist Practice" (1997) (Fosnaught, 1996). The policy defines diagnosis as "a label encompassing a cluster of signs and symptoms commonly associated with a disorder or syndrome or category of impairment, functional limitation, or disability."

Classification System

According to Rothstein (1993), in many fields of medicine when a medical diagnosis is made, the pathologic condition is determined and stages and classifications that guide treatment are also named. This model is a good one to follow. Although we recognize that the term *diagnosis* relates to a pathologic process, we know that pathologic evidence alone is inadequate to guide the physical therapist.

Thus far there is agreement that physical therapists do not diagnose disease in the sense of identifying a specific organic pathologic condition. However, identified clusters of signs, symptoms, symptom-related behavior, and other data from the client history and other testing can be used to confirm or rule out the presence of a physical therapy problem. These diagnostic clusters can be labeled as impairment classifications or movement dysfunctions by physical therapists and can guide efficient and effective management of the client (Delitto and Snyder-Mackler, 1995).

Within the profession of physical therapy, diagnostic classification systems that direct treatment interventions are being developed based on client prognosis and definable outcomes demonstrated in the literature (Guccione, 1997). The "Guide to Physical Therapist Practice" (1997) groups diagnostic patterns into four categories of conditions: musculoskeletal, neuromuscular, cardiopulmonary, and integumentary. An individual may belong to one or more of these diagnostic groups or patterns.*

Scope of Practice

According to the "Guide to Physical Therapy," the diagnostic-based practice requires

---

*See also *Diagnosis and Treatment of Movement Impairment Syndromes* (Sahrmann, 1999) for the first classification model for physical therapists.

ELEMENTS OF PATIENT/CLIENT MANAGEMENT

Examination:	History, systems review, and tests and measures
Evaluation:	Assessment or judgment of the data
Diagnosis:	Determined within the scope of practice
Prognosis:	Projected outcome
Intervention:	Coordination, communication, and documentation of an appropriate treatment plan for the diagnosis based on the previous four elements

From Guide to physical therapist practice. Phys Ther 77(11):1-5, 1997.

the physical therapist to integrate five elements of patient/client management (see the box on p. 6) in a manner designed to maximize outcomes (Fig. 1-1). The diagnostic process* requires evaluation of information obtained from the client examination, including the history, systems review, administration of tests, and interpretation of data.

The key phrase in these standards is "within the scope of physical therapist practice." This process usually involves the determination of location, severity, and pattern of a neuromusculoskeletal abnormality. Identification of causative factors or etiology by the physical therapist is limited primarily to those pathokinesiologic problems associated with faulty biomechanical or neuromuscular action. When no apparent movement dysfunction, causative factors, or syndrome can be identified, the physical therapist may treat symptoms as part of an ongoing diagnostic process.† If, however, the findings are not consistent with a musculoskeletal or neuromuscular dysfunction, referral to an appropriate medical professional may be required.

*There has been some discussion that evaluation is a process with diagnosis as the end result (Fosnaught, 1996). The concepts around the "diagnostic process" remain part of an evolving definition that will continue to be discussed and clarified by physical therapists.

†Sometimes even physicians use physical therapy as a diagnostic tool, observing the client's response during treatment to confirm or rule out medical suspicions.

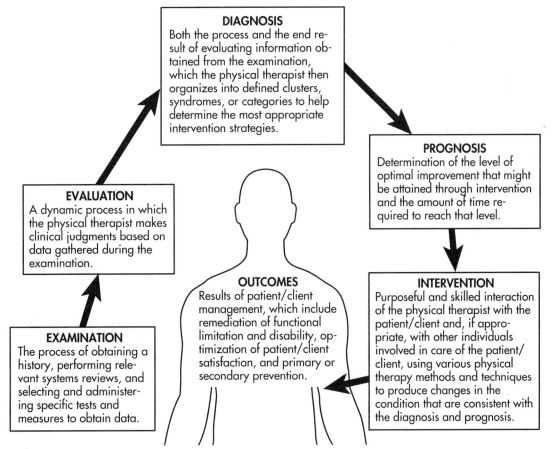

FIGURE 1-1 • The elements of patient/client management leading to optimal outcomes. Reprinted with permission from Guide to physical therapist practice. Phys Ther 77(11):1-4, 1997.

Practicing within the scope of physical therapist practice, we communicate with physicians and other health care practitioners to request or recommend further medical evaluation. Whether in a private practice, home health, acute care hospital, or rehabilitation setting, physical therapists may observe important findings outside the realm of neuromusculoskeletal disorders requiring additional medical evaluation and treatment.

Direct Access

Direct access is the right of any individual to obtain evaluation and/or treatment from a licensed physical therapist. Before 1968 a physician referral was necessary for a client to be treated by a physical therapist. Now all but five states in the United States permit direct access to physical therapy.

The Physical Therapy Practice Act is being changed in many more states to provide for the independent practice of physical therapists. Thus a consumer (i.e., the patient or client) can be evaluated or evaluated and treated by a physical therapist without previous examination by a physician or other practitioner.*

For the reasons outlined in the accompanying box, physical therapy practice in all

*The reality is that many insurance companies and most managed care organizations do not reimburse for physical therapy services without a physician's referral. Additional, large deductibles have resulted in a trend toward cash-based business, also referred to as direct consumer services or direct fee-for-service. In such circumstances consumers are willing to pay out-of-pocket for physical therapy services, bypassing the need for a medical evaluation unless requested by the physical therapist. This scenario can take place only where direct access has been passed and within the legal parameters of the state's practice act.

REASONS FOR MEDICAL SCREENING

- Direct access: Therapist has primary responsibility or first contact.
- Clients may obtain a signed prescription for physical/occupational therapy based on similar past complaints of musculoskeletal symptoms without direct physician contact.
- Medical specialization: Medical specialists may fail to recognize underlying systemic disease.
- Disease progression: Early signs and symptoms are difficult to recognize, or symptoms may not be present at the time of medical examination.
- Client does not report symptoms or concerns to the physician because of forgetfulness, fear, or embarrassment.

CONSTITUTIONAL SYMPTOMS

- Fever
- Diaphoresis (unexplained perspiration)
- Night sweats (can occur during the day)
- Nausea
- Vomiting
- Diarrhea
- Pallor
- Dizziness/syncope (fainting)
- Fatigue
- Weight loss

settings now requires that the physical therapist be able to evaluate a client's complaint knowledgeably and determine whether there are signs and symptoms of a systemic disease or a medical condition that should be evaluated by a more appropriate health care provider (See "Constitutional Symptoms" on p. 8). This text endeavors to provide the necessary information that will assist the physical therapist in making these decisions.

The purpose and the scope of this text are not to teach physical therapists to be all-purpose diagnosticians. The concern for physical therapists in relation to direct access to clients is in the differentiation of clients who need an appropriate referral. The purpose of this text is to provide a method for physical therapists to recognize readily (in a step-by-step problem-solving manner) areas that are beyond their expertise.

▼ DECISION-MAKING PROCESS

This text is designed to help physical therapists screen for medical disease when it is appropriate to do so. Four parameters are used in evaluating each client:

- Client History
- Pain Patterns/Pain Types
- Associated Signs and Symptoms of Systemic Diseases
- Systems Review

Client history, also referred to as *diagnostic physical therapy interviewing,* is the key feature of these four decision-making guidelines. *Pain patterns/pain types* include drawings of primary and referred pain patterns for quick reference in each chapter. *Associated signs and symptoms of systemic diseases* are the red flag signs and symptoms accompanying musculoskeletal dysfunction that will assist the therapist in recognizing the presence of an underlying systemic condition. Finally, when the therapist looks at the associated signs and symptoms, there

may be a cluster of signs and symptoms characteristic of a particular body system. The *systems review* process is a useful tool in recognizing these clusters and the need for medical referral.

Medical referral must be preceded by a thorough physical therapy examination, including screening techniques for systemic disease. The knowledge base required to accomplish this screening process comes from the APTA competencies (APTA, 1985)* for conducting a screening examination:

Describe the clinical manifestations of the more common disorders of organ systems other than neuromuscular system(s).

Describe the etiology and clinical manifestations of disorders that mimic dysfunction of the neuromuscular system.

Describe normal and abnormal reactions to common drugs; drugs that may affect the neuromusculoskeletal system(s); drug reactions that mimic disorders of these systems, and drug interactions.

Interpret information from the client's history, including a history that includes the client's description and perception of the chief complaint, an accurate and comprehensive medical and family/social history, and a comprehensive and appropriately focused review of organ systems.

Interpretation of the client's history must be accurate, identify noncontributory information, identify chief and secondary problems, identify information that is inconsistent with the presenting complaint, generate a working hypothesis regarding possible causes of complaints, and determine whether referral or consultation is indicated.

Client History (Diagnostic Interviewing)

The interview with the client is very important because it helps the physical therapist

---

*Although this particular document has been replaced by *A Normative Model of Physical Therapist Professional Education: Version 97* and "Guide to Physical Therapist Practice" (1997), the information as presented in the 1985 competencies has never been more clearly delineated for the purposes of this text.

distinguish between problems that he or she can treat and problems that should be referred to a physician for diagnosis and treatment. This information establishes a solid basis for the physical therapy objective evaluation, assessment, and therefore treatment.

This material is intended to serve as a reference guide for the skilled clinician and as a teaching text for use with physical therapy students. The student of physical therapy can use the book to develop necessary skills for clinical work, and the experienced clinician can refer to it as a guide for addressing specific clinical issues.

For example, a student can use the detailed step-by-step breakdown of the interview with the client to understand and practice each part of the process. The experienced clinician can refer to chapters on systemic problems and can have quick access to information about what specific questions to ask each client, depending on the presenting chief complaint. For example, the person with neck, back, chest, hip, groin, sacral, or sacroiliac pain should be asked specifically about both systemic and musculoskeletal origins of the present pain and symptoms.

An interviewing process is described that includes concrete and structured tools and techniques for conducting a thorough and informative interview. The use of follow-up questions is discussed because these questions help structure the interview.

Illiteracy

Throughout the interviewing process and even throughout the treatment period, the therapist must keep in mind that 44 million American adults are illiterate and an additional 35 million read only at a functional level for survival.*

These figures can be broken down for the total population of adults who are nonliterate in English as follows:

41% are English-speaking whites

22% are English-speaking African Americans

22% are Spanish speaking

15% are non–English-speaking people

More than 14 million people age 5 and older in the United States speak English poorly or not at all. Up to 86% of non–English speakers who are illiterate in English are also illiterate in their native language. In addition, 19.8 million immigrants enter U.S. communities every year. Of these people, 1.7 million who are age 25 and older have less than a fifth-grade education. There is a heavy concentration of persons with low literacy skills among the poor and those who are dependent on public financial support.

Finally, although the percentages of illiterate African-American and Hispanic adults are much higher than those of white adults, the actual number of white nonreaders is twice that of African-American and Hispanic nonreaders, a fact that dispels the myth that literacy is not a problem among whites.

People who are illiterate cannot read instructions on bottles of prescription medicine or over-the-counter medications. They cannot know when a medicine is past the year of safe consumption; nor can they read about allergic risks, warnings to diabetics, or the potential sedative effect of medications. They cannot read about "the seven warning signs" of cancer or the indications of blood sugar fluctuations (Kozol, 1988).

They cannot understand the written details on a health insurance form, accurately complete a personal/family history form (see example, Chapter 2), or read the details of exercise programs provided by physical therapists. For this reason the therapist is encouraged to complete any intake forms for or with the client and to provide pictures of only prescribed exercises with space made available for the client to make notes. Several companies make such custom exercise programs available.*

---

*This means that although these individuals can read at a fourth-grade level, they need higher levels of literacy to function effectively in society, to find employment, or to be trained for new jobs as the workplace changes.

---

*Two such companies are VHI Exercise and Rehabilitation (1-800-356-0709) and Saunders Group (1-800-588-0602).

Case Studies

Case examples and case studies are provided with each chapter to provide the physical therapist with a working understanding of how to recognize the need for additional questions. In addition, information is given concerning the type of questions to ask and how to correlate the results with the objec-tive findings. Whenever possible, information about when and how to refer a client to the physician is presented. Each case study is based on actual case histories to provide reasonable examples of what to expect when the physical therapist is functioning under any of the circumstances listed in the "Reasons for Medical Screening" box on p. 8.

Pain Patterns/Pain Types

Pain is often the primary symptom in many physical therapy practices. Recognizing pain patterns that are characteristic of systemic disease is an important step. Therefore this chapter includes a detailed overview of pain patterns that can be used as a foundation for all the organ systems presented.

Each section discusses specific pain patterns characteristic of disease entities that can mimic pain from musculoskeletal disorders. Detailed information regarding the location, referral pattern, description, intensity, and duration of systemic pain is augmented by facts about associated symptoms and relieving and aggravating factors. This information is then compared with presenting features of primary musculoskeletal lesions that have similar patterns of presentation.

Pain patterns of the chest, back, shoulder, scapula, pelvis, hip, groin, and sacroiliac joint are included because these are the most common sites of referred pain from a systemic disease process.

Physical therapists are often called on to wear many different hats, representing a multitude of trades and professions. Although ideally physical therapy clients would have access to all the services necessary for recovery or rehabilitation from their injury or medical condition, the fact is that the physical therapist is often their counselor, friend, support person, priest, rabbi, and so on. For this reason a section has been included that addresses the psychologic factors associated with pain.

This inclusion does not endorse physical therapists' practicing outside the scope of their expertise and experience. It merely recognizes that, in treating the whole client, not only the physical but also the psychologic, emotional, and spiritual needs of that person will be represented in his or her magnitude of symptoms, length of recovery time, response to pain, and responsibility for recovery.

Assessment of Pain and Symptoms*

There are many possible *sources* of pain and many *types* of pain. Physical therapists frequently see clients whose primary complaint is pain, which often leads to a loss of function. However, focusing on sources of pain does not always help us to identify the causes of tissue irritation. The most effective physical therapy diagnosis will define the syndrome and address the causes of pain rather than just identifying the sources of pain (Sahrmann, 1997). Usually, a careful assessment of pain behavior is invaluable in determining the nature and extent of the underlying pathology.

The interviewing techniques and specific questions outlined in Chapter 2 provide a description of the client that is clear, accurate, and comprehensive. The portion of the core interview regarding a client's perception of pain is a critical factor in the evaluation of signs and symptoms. Questions must be understood by the client and should be presented in a nonjudgmental manner.

---

*It is beyond the scope of the text to describe or discuss the physiologic mechanisms of pain or the many factors affecting perception of pain (e.g., age, personality, ethnic or cultural background, behavioral needs, previous pain experiences). The reader is referred to other text sources that address these issues. See especially these references listed at the end of this chapter: "Management of the Individual With Pain" (Parts 1 and 2); Wells et al, 1994; and Cailliet, 1996.

To elicit a complete description of symptoms from the client, the physical therapist may wish to use a term other than *pain*. For example, referring to the client's *symptoms* or using descriptors such as *hurt* or *sore* may be more helpful with some individuals. If the client has completed the McGill Pain Questionnaire (Melzack, 1975) (Chapter 2), the physical therapist may choose the most appropriate alternative word selected by the client from the list to refer to the symptoms.

The use of alternative words to describe a client's symptoms may also aid in refocusing attention away from pain and toward improvement of functional abilities.

SOURCES OF PAIN

In listening to the client's description of pain, four general sources of pain must be considered (Table 1-1):

Cutaneous Pain (related to the skin). This source of pain includes superficial somatic structures located in the skin and subcutaneous tissue. The pain is well localized because the client can point directly to the area that "hurts." Cutaneous (skin) tenderness may occur with both referred and deep somatic pain.

Somatic Pain (emotional, musculoskeletal, or visceral). Somatic pain is labeled according to its source—as deep somatic, somatovisceral, somatoemotional (also referred to as psychosomatic), or viscerosomatic.

Deep somatic pain comes from pathologic conditions of the periosteum and cancellous (spongy) bone, nerve, muscle, tendon, ligaments, and arteries. *Somatovisceral* pain occurs when a myalgic condition causes functional disturbance of the underlying viscera, such as the trigger points of the abdominal muscles causing diarrhea, vomiting, or excessive burping.

Somatoemotional or *psychosomatic* sources of pain occur when emotional or psychologic distress produces physical symptoms either for a relatively brief period or with recurrent and multiple physical manifestations spanning many months or years. The person affected by the latter may be referred to as a somatizer, and the condition is called a somatization disorder.

Alternately, there are *viscerosomatic* sources of pain when visceral structures affect the somatic musculature, such as the reflex spasm and rigidity of the abdominal muscles in response to the inflammation of acute appendicitis or the pectoral trigger point associated with an acute myocardial infarction. These visible and palpable changes in the tension of skin and subcutaneous and other connective tissues that are segmentally related to visceral pathologic processes are referred to as connective tissue zones or reflex zones (Wells et al, 1994).

Parietal pain (related to the wall of the chest or abdominal cavity) is also considered deep somatic. The visceral pleura (the membrane enveloping the organs) is insensitive to pain, but the parietal pleura is well supplied with pain nerve endings. For this reason it is possible for a client to have extensive disease without pain until the disease

---

TABLE 1-1 ▼ Pain Types/Pain Patterns

Sources	Types	Characteristics
Cutaneous	Myofascial pain	Location/onset
Deep somatic	Joint pain	Description
Visceral	Radicular pain	Intensity
Referred	Arterial, pleural, tracheal pain	Duration
	Gastrointestinal pain	Frequency
	Pain at rest	Pattern
	Pain with activity	• Vascular
	Diffuse pain	• Neurogenic
	Chronic pain	• Musculoskeletal/spondylotic
		• Visceral
		• Emotional

progresses enough to involve the parietal pleura.*

Deep somatic pain is poorly localized and may be referred to the body surface, becoming cutaneous pain. It can be associated with an autonomic phenomenon, such as sweating, pallor, or changes in blood pressure, and is commonly accompanied by a subjective feeling of nausea and faintness.

Pain associated with deep somatic lesions follows patterns that relate to the embryologic development of the musculoskeletal system. This explains why such pain may not be perceived directly over the involved organ. The human brain has no felt image for internal organs. Rather, pain is referred to a site where the organ was located in fetal development. Although the organ migrates during fetal development, referred sensations persist from the former location.

Visceral Pain (related to internal organs). This source of pain includes all body organs located in the trunk or abdomen, such as those of the respiratory, digestive, urogenital, and endocrine systems, as well as the spleen, the heart, and the great vessels.

Visceral pain is not well localized for two reasons. First, innervation of the viscera is multisegmental with few nerve endings (Fig. 1-2). For example, cardiac pain can extend from C3 to T4. This accounts for the many and varied clinical pictures of myocardial infarction (see Fig. 3-8).

Second, the site of visceral pain corresponds to dermatomes from which the diseased organ receives its innervation. For example, the pericardium (sac around the entire heart) is adjacent to the diaphragm. Pain of cardiac and diaphragmatic origin is often experienced in the shoulder because the C5-6 spinal segment (innervation for the shoulder) also supplies the heart and the diaphragm.

When diseases of internal organs are accompanied by cutaneous hypersensitivity to

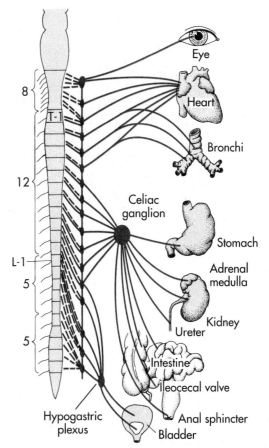

FIG. 1-2 • Diagram of the autonomic nervous system. The visceral afferent fibers mediating pain travel with the sympathetic nerves, except for those from the pelvic organs, which follow the parasympathetics of the pelvic nerve.
(From Guyton AC, Hall JE: *Textbook of medical physiology*, ed 9, Philadelphia, 1996, WB Saunders.)

touch, pressure, and temperature, this viscerocutaneous reflex occurs during the acute phase of the disease and disappears with its recovery. The skin areas affected are innervated by the same cord segments as for the involved viscera, and they are referred to as Head's zones (Wells et al, 1994).

Visceral disease of the abdomen and pelvis is more likely to refer pain to the back, whereas intrathoracic disease refers pain to the shoulder(s). Visceral pain rarely occurs without associated signs and symptoms, although the client may not recognize the correlation. Careful questioning will usually elicit a systemic pattern of symptoms.

---

*There are two exceptions to this: (1) inflammation and ischemia of the gut can cause steady visceral (gastrointestinal) pain, and (2) visceral pain fibers in the gut are sensitive to stretching or tension from rapid distension or forceful contractions (e.g., secondary to large pockets of gas, bowel obstruction, or spasm). Gradual distension of the gut is not painful until ulceration occurs.

Back or shoulder range of motion is usually full and painless in the presence of visceral pain, especially in the early stages of disease. When the painful stimulus increases or persists over time, muscle splinting and guarding can result in subsequent changes in biomechanical patterns, making it more difficult to recognize the systemic origin of musculoskeletal dysfunction.

Referred Pain (related to irritation of deep somatic or visceral structures). Referred pain is experienced at a site other than the actual anatomic area where it is stimulated. It occurs in tissues supplied by the same or adjacent neural segments that supply the diseased organ (this occurs by way of shared central pathways for afferent neurons). Referred pain does not follow normal anatomic pathways and is perceived in an area far removed from the site of the lesion.

This source of pain includes all cutaneous, deep somatic, and visceral structures. Examples include shoulder pain caused by a perforated posterior duodenal ulcer or midthoracic back pain from esophageal obstruction or perforation.

Referred pain may occur alone or with accompanying deep somatic or visceral pain. When caused by an underlying visceral or systemic disease, visceral pain usually precedes the development of referred musculoskeletal pain. However, the client may not remember or mention this previous pain pattern.

Referred pain is well localized (i.e., the person can point directly to the area that hurts), but it does not have sharply defined borders. Local tenderness is present in the tissue of the referred pain area, but there is no objective sensory deficit. Referred pain is often accompanied by muscle hypertonus over the referred area of pain.

TYPES OF PAIN

Although there are four sources of most physiologic pain, many types of pain exist within these categories (see Table 1-1). When orienting to pain from these four sources, it may be helpful to consider some specific types of pain patterns. Not all pain types can be discussed here, but some of the most commonly encountered are included.

Additionally, body activities and physiologic processes serve to modify pain by increasing or decreasing afferent activity. These relationships are helpful in identifying the site and nature (i.e., musculoskeletal or potentially systemic) of the pathologic process responsible for the pain.

Myofascial Pain. Myofascial pain affecting the muscles and/or the fascia covering the muscles can be categorized into five types: (1) muscle tension, (2) muscle spasm, (3) muscle trauma, (4) muscle deficiency, and (5) trigger points (Kraus, 1994).

Muscle tension, or sustained muscle tone, occurs when prolonged muscular contraction or co-contraction results in local ischemia, increased cellular metabolites, and subsequent pain.* Muscle tension and the subsequent ischemia may occur as a result of faulty ergonomics, prolonged work positions (e.g., as with computer or telephone operators), or repetitive motion.

Muscle spasm is a sudden involuntary contraction of a muscle or group of muscles, occurring as a result of overuse or injury of the adjoining neuromusculoskeletal or musculotendinous attachments. A person with a painful musculoskeletal problem may also have a varying degree of reflex muscle spasm to protect the joint(s) involved. Spasm pain cannot be attributed to increased muscle tension because the intramuscular pressure is insufficiently elevated. Pain may occur from contraction under an ischemic situation because an increase in the partial pressure of oxygen has been documented inside the muscle in spasm (Emre and Mathies, 1988).

Muscle trauma can be considered as unaccustomed intensity or duration of muscle contraction, especially eccentric contractions. Muscle pain occurs as broken fibers leak potassium into the interstitial fluid and blood extravasation results from damaged blood vessels, setting off a cascade of chemical reactions within the muscle (Cailliet, 1995).

---

*Ischemia as a factor in muscle pain remains controversial. Interruption of blood flow in a resting extremity does not cause pain unless the muscle contracts during the ischemic condition (Cailliet, 1995).

Muscle deficiency is muscular pain caused by weakness and stiffness. It is often ameliorated by increased activity and exercise. For example, when muscular stiffness occurs as a result of aging,* increased physical activity and movement can reduce associated muscular pain.

Trigger points are hyperirritable spots within a taut band of skeletal muscle or in the fascia. When trigger points are compressed, local tenderness with possible referred pain result. The referred pain pattern is characteristic and specific for every muscle. Pain and dysfunction of myofascial tissues is the subject of two extensive volumes to which the reader is referred for more information (Travell and Simons, 1983; Travell and Simons, 1992).

Joint Pain. Joint pain that awakens the client at night is often due to bone disease or neoplasm. The pain of systemic joint disease is most often deep, aching, and throbbing; it may be reduced by pressure. This type of pain may be constant or occur in waves or spasms, and it may be sharp or dull.

On the other hand, the pain of joint dysfunction is invariably sharp; it usually ceases immediately when the stressful action that produces it ceases; it is invariably relieved or is at least greatly improved by rest and is aggravated by activity. The client's answers to questions regarding what aggravates and what improves the pain may be very significant.

Pain from primary joint dysfunction is characterized by sudden onset, having occurred after some unguarded joint movement, and is unassociated with marked swelling or warmth. The pain is limited to one joint, is reduced by rest (which is not followed by stiffness), and is aggravated by activity (Mennell, 1964).

Allergic reactions to medication may manifest as intermittent hydrarthrosis (fluid in a joint), possibly with joint pain. Allergic reactions can be delayed by as long as 6 weeks. The client with joint pain should be questioned about a history of allergies, use of prescription medication in the last 6 weeks, and recent change in prescription medications.

The development of characteristic features of systemic involvement, such as jaundice in cases of infectious hepatitis, migratory nature of the pain (moving from joint to joint), presence or recent history of skin rash, fatigue, weight loss, low-grade fever, muscular weakness, or cyclical and progressive nature of symptoms should help the physical therapist identify joint pain of a systemic nature (Table 1-2).

TABLE 1-2 ▼ Comparison of Systemic and Musculoskeletal Joint Pain

Systemic	Musculoskeletal
Awakens at night	Decreases with rest
Deep aching, throbbing	Sharp
Reduced by pressure	Ceases when stressful action is stopped
Constant or waves/spasm	Associated signs and symptoms:
History of infection (hepatitis, streptococcosis, mononucleosis, measles, urinary tract infection, upper respiratory infection)	Usually none
	Trigger points may be accompanied by nausea, sweating
Recent medications	
Associated signs and symptoms:	
Jaundice	
Migratory arthralgias	
Skin rash	
Nodules (extensor surfaces)	
Oral/nasal ulcers	
Enlarged, rubbery, pain-free lymph nodes	
Fatigue	
Weight loss	
Low-grade fever	
Muscular weakness	
Cyclic, progressive symptoms	

---

*Connective tissue changes may occur as small amounts of fibrinogen (produced in the liver and normally converted to fibrin to serve as a clotting factor) leak from the vasculature into the intracellular spaces, adhering to cellular structures. The resulting microfibrinous adhesions among the cells of muscle and fascia cause increased muscular stiffness. Activity and movement normally break these adhesions; however, with the aging process, production of fewer and less efficient macrophages combined with immobility for any reason result in reduced lysis of these adhesions (Sinnott, 1993). Other possible causes of aggravated stiffness include increased collagen fibers, increased cross-links of aged collagen fibers, changes in the mechanical properties of connective tissues, and structural and functional changes in the collagen protein.

Radicular Pain. Radicular (radiating) pain is experienced in the musculoskeletal system in a dermatome, sclerotome, or myotome because of direct irritation or involvement of a spinal nerve.

In systemic disease radiating pain occurs because of dysfunction of the autonomic innervation of the body (see Fig. 1-2).

Radicular pain of the viscera is generally within the segmental innervation of the affected organ.

For example, cardiac pain may be described as beginning retrosternally (behind the sternum) and radiating to the left shoulder and down the inner side of the left arm; gallbladder pain may be felt to originate in the right upper abdomen and to radiate to the angle of the scapula.

Physical disease will localize pain in dermatomal or myotomal patterns, but the client who describes radicular pain that does not match a dermatomal or myotomal pattern (e.g., whole leg pain or whole leg numbness) may be experiencing *inappropriate illness behavior.*

Inappropriate illness behavior is recognized clinically as illness behavior that is out of proportion to the underlying physical disease and is related more to associated psychologic disturbances than to actual physical disease (Waddell et al, 1984). This behavioral component to pain is discussed in the next section (Psychologic Factors in Pain Assessment).

Arterial, Pleural, and Tracheal Pain. Pain arising from arteries, as with arteritis (inflammation of an artery), migraine, and vascular headaches, increases with systolic impulse so that any process associated with increased systolic pressure, such as exercise, fever, alcohol consumption, or bending over, may intensify the already throbbing pain. Pain from the pleura, as well as from the trachea, correlates with respiratory movements.

Gastrointestinal Pain. Pain arising from the gastrointestinal tract tends to increase with peristaltic activity, particularly if there is any obstruction to forward progress. The pain increases with ingestion and may lessen with fasting or after emptying the involved segment (vomiting or bowel movement). When hollow viscera, such as the liver, kidneys, spleen, and pancreas, are distended, body positions or movements that increase intraabdominal pressure may intensify the pain, whereas positions that reduce pressure or support the structure may ease the pain.

For example, the client with an acutely distended gallbladder may slightly flex the trunk. With pain arising from a tense, swollen kidney (or distended renal pelvis), the client flexes the trunk and tilts toward the involved side; with pancreatic pain, the client may sit up and lean forward or lie down with the knees drawn up to the chest.

Pain may occur secondary to the effect of gastric acid on the esophagus, stomach, or duodenum. This pain is relieved by the presence of food or by other neutralizing material in the stomach, and the pain is intensified when the stomach is empty and secreting acid. In these cases it is important to ask the client about the effect of eating on musculoskeletal pain: whether the pain increases, decreases, or stays the same immediately after eating and 1 to 3 hours later.

Pain at Rest. Pain at rest may arise from ischemia of a wide variety of tissue (e.g., vascular disease or tumor growth). The acute onset of severe unilateral extremity involvement accompanied by the "five Ps"—pain, pallor, pulselessness, paresthesia, and paralysis—signifies acute arterial occlusion (peripheral vascular disease [PVD]). Pain in this situation is usually described by the client as burning or shooting and may be accompanied by paresthesia.

Pain related to ischemia of the skin and subcutaneous tissues is characterized by the client as burning and boring. All these occlusive causes of pain are usually worse at night and are relieved to some degree by dangling the affected leg over the side of the bed and by frequent massaging of the extremity.

Pain at rest secondary to neoplasm occurs usually at night. Although neoplasms are highly vascularized (a process called angiogenesis), the host organ's vascular supply and nutrients may be compromised simultaneously, causing ischemia of the local tissue. The pain awakens the client from sleep and prevents the person from going back to sleep, despite all efforts to do so.

The client may describe pain noted on weight-bearing or bone pain that may be mild and intermittent in the initial stages, becoming progressively more severe and more constant. A series of questions to identify the underlying cause of night pain is presented in Chapter 2.

Activity pain. When pain is caused by vascular compromise, as with intermittent vascular claudication or angina, it is referred to as activity pain. Pain from an ischemic muscle (including heart muscle) builds up with the use of the muscle and subsides with rest. Thus there is a direct relationship between the degree of circulatory insufficiency and muscle work. In other words, the interval between the beginning of muscle contraction and the onset of pain depends on how long it takes for hypoxic products of muscle metabolism to accumulate and exceed the threshold of receptor response.*

The client complains that a certain distance walked, a certain level of increased physical activity, or a fixed amount of usage of the extremity brings on the pain. When a vascular pathologic condition causes ischemic muscular pain, the location of the pain depends on the location of the vascular pathologic source. This is discussed in greater detail later in this text (see Arterial Disease, Chapter 3).

Diffuse Pain. Diffuse pain that characterizes some diseases of the nervous system and viscera may be difficult to distinguish from the equally diffuse pain so often caused by lesions of the moving parts. Most clients in this category are those with obscure pain in the trunk, especially when the symptoms are felt only anteriorly (Cyriax, 1982). The distinction between visceral pain and pain caused by lesions of the vertebral column may be difficult to make and will require a medical diagnosis.

Chronic Pain. Chronic pain persists past the expected physiologic time of healing. This may be less than 1 month or, more often, longer than 6 months. The International Association for the Study of Pain has fixed 3 months as the most convenient point of division between acute and chronic pain (Merskey and Bogduk, 1994).†

In some cases of chronic pain, a diagnosis is finally made (e.g., spinal stenosis or thyroiditis) and the treatment is specific, not merely pain management. More often, identifying the cause of chronic pain is unsuccessful.‡ Instead, the approach is to assess how the pain has affected the person.

Chronic pain syndrome is characterized by a constellation of life changes that produce altered behavior in the individual and persist even after the cause of the pain has been eradicated. This syndrome is a complex multidimensional phenomenon that requires a focus toward maximizing functional abilities rather than treatment of pain (see later discussion of Illness Behavior).

In acute pain the pain is proportional and appropriate to the problem and is treated as a symptom. In the chronic pain syndrome the pain may be inappropriate and exaggerated for the existing problem; the pain *is* the disease. The person's description of chronic pain is less well defined and poorly localized; objective findings are not identified. The person's verbal description of the pain may contain words associated with emotional overlay (see Table 2-4). This is in contrast to the predominance of sensory descriptors associated with acute

---

*In the case of chest pain associated with increased activity, the onset of pain is not immediate. It occurs 5 to 10 minutes after activity begins. This is referred to as the "lag time" and is a diagnostic tool used by the physical therapist to determine when chest pain is caused by musculoskeletal dysfunction (immediate chest pain occurs with use) or by vascular compromise (chest pain occurs 5 to 10 minutes after activity begins).

†There are many different types of chronic pain. An in-depth discussion of this topic is beyond the scope of this text. The reader is referred to a text that describes these in detail (Merskey and Bogduk, 1994). (See also Chronic Pain and the Paradox of Managed Care, 1996.)
‡The therapist should be aware that chronic pain is often associated with physical and/or sexual abuse in both men and women. (See discussion of Assault, Chapter 2.)

pain (Management of the Individual With Pain, 1996).

However, painful symptoms that are out of proportion to the injury or that are not consistent with the objective findings may be a red flag indicating systemic disease. A chronic pain syndrome can be differentiated from a systemic disease because the chronic pain syndrome is characterized by multiple complaints, excessive preoccupation with pain, and, frequently, excessive drug use. Systemic disease is usually accompanied by a cluster of associated signs and symptoms characteristic of a particular organ or body system (see later discussion of Systems Review).

The client with a chronic pain syndrome may live in a socially narrow world and exhibit altered behavior patterns, such as depression, neurosis, and anxiety. The amount of pain behaviors and the intensity of pain perceived changes with alterations in environmental reinforcers (e.g., increasing as the time to return to work draws near, decreasing when no one is watching).

Secondary gain may be a factor in perpetuating the problem. This may be primarily financial, but social and family benefits, such as increased attention or avoidance of unpleasant activities or work situations, may be factors (see later discussion of behavior responses to injury/illness).

It may be helpful to ask the client or caregiver to maintain a pain log (see Figs. 2-2 and 2-3). This should include entries for pain intensity and its relationship to activities or treatments given. Clients can be reevaluated regularly for improvement, deterioration, or complications, using the same scales that were used for the initial evaluation.

To address the special needs of older adults, the American Geriatrics Society (AGS) has developed specific recommendations for assessment and management of chronic pain that is not related to cancer (AGS, 1998).

PSYCHOLOGIC FACTORS IN PAIN ASSESSMENT

Psychologic factors such as emotional stress and conflicts leading to anxiety, depression, and panic disorder play an important role in the client's experience of physical symptoms. In the past, physical symptoms caused or exacerbated by psychologic variables were labeled psychosomatic. Today the interconnections between the mind, the immune system, the hormonal system, the nervous system, and the physical body have led us to view psychosomatic disorders as psychophysiologic disorders.

Psychophysiologic disorders are generally characterized by subjective complaints that exceed objective findings, symptom development in the presence of psychosocial stresses, and physical symptoms involving one or more organ systems. It is the last variable that can confuse the therapist when trying to screen for medical disease.

It is impossible to discuss the broad range of psychophysiologic disorders that comprise a large portion of the physical therapy caseload in a screening text of this kind. The therapist is strongly encouraged to become familiar with the *Diagnostic and Statistical Manual-IV* (1994) to better understand the psychologic factors affecting the successful outcome of rehabilitation.

However, at minimum, recognizing clusters of signs and symptoms characteristic of the psychologic component of illness is very important in the screening process. Likewise, the therapist will want to become familiar with nonorganic signs indicative of psychologic factors (Scalzitti, 1997; Teasell and Shapiro, 1994; Waddell et al, 1980).

Anxiety. Musculoskeletal complaints such as sore muscles, back pain, headache, or fatigue can result from anxiety-caused tension or heightened sensitivity to pain. Anxiety increases muscle tension, thereby reducing blood flow and oxygen to the tissues, resulting in a buildup of cellular metabolites. In fact, somatic symptoms are diagnostic for several anxiety disorders, including panic disorder, agoraphobia (fear of open places, especially fear of being alone or of being in public places) and other phobias (irrational fears), obsessive-compulsive disorder (OCD), post-traumatic stress disorder (PTSD), and generalized anxiety disorders.

Anxious persons have a reduced ability to tolerate painful stimulation, noticing it more or interpreting it as more significant than do nonanxious persons. This leads to further complaining about pain and to more disability and pain behavior such as limping, grimacing, or medication-seeking. To complicate matters more, persons with an organic illness sometimes develop anxiety known as *adjustment disorder with anxious mood*. Additionally, the advent of a known organic condition, such as a pulmonary embolus or chronic obstructive pulmonary disease (COPD), can cause an agoraphobia-like syndrome in older persons, especially if the client views the condition as unpredictable, variable, and disabling.

According to C. Everett Koop, the former U.S. Surgeon General, 80 to 90 percent of all people seen in a family practice clinic are suffering from illnesses caused by anxiety and stress. Emotional problems amplify physical symptoms such as ulcerative colitis, peptic ulcers, or allergies. Although allergies may be inherited, anxiety amplifies or exaggerates the symptoms. Symptoms may appear as physical, behavioral, cognitive, or psychologic (Table 1-3).

Panic Disorder. Persons with panic disorder have episodes of sudden, unprovoked feelings of terror or impending doom with associated physical symptoms, such as racing or pounding heartbeat, breathlessness, nausea, sweating, and dizziness. During an attack people may fear that they are gravely ill, going to die, or going crazy. The fear of another attack can itself become debilitating so that these individuals avoid situations and places that they believe will trigger the episodes, thus affecting their work, their relationships, and their ability to take care of everyday tasks.

Initial panic attacks may occur when people are under considerable stress, for example, an overload of work or from loss of a family member or close friend. The attacks may follow surgery, a serious accident, illness, or childbirth. Excessive consumption of caffeine or use of cocaine, other stimulant drugs, or medicines containing caffeine or stimulants used in treating asthma can also trigger panic attacks (Hendrix, 1993).

The symptoms of a panic attack can mimic those of other medical conditions, such as respiratory or heart problems. Residual sore muscles are a consistent finding after the panic attack and can also occur in individuals with social phobias. People suffering from these attacks may be afraid or embarrassed to report their symptoms to the physician.

TABLE 1-3 ▼ Symptoms of Anxiety

Physical	Behavioral	Cognitive	Psychologic
Increased sighing respirations	Hyperalertness	Fear of losing mind	Phobias
Increased blood pressure	Irritability	Fear of losing control	Obsessive-compulsive behavior
Tachycardia	Uncertainty		
Shortness of breath	Apprehension		
Dizziness	Difficulty with memory or concentration		
Lump in throat	Sleep disturbance		
Muscle tension			
Dry mouth			
Diarrhea			
Nausea			
Clammy hands			
Sweating			
Pacing			
Chest pain*			

*Chest pain associated with anxiety accounts for more than half of all emergency department admissions for chest pain. The pain is substernal, a dull ache that does not radiate and is not aggravated by respiratory movements but is associated with hyperventilation and claustrophobia.

▼ *Clinical Signs and Symptoms of*
Panic Disorder

- Racing or pounding heartbeat
- Chest pains
- Dizziness, lightheadedness, nausea
- Difficulty in breathing
- Bilateral numbness or tingling in nose, cheeks, lips, fingers, toes
- Sweats or chills
- Hand wringing
- Dreamlike sensations or perceptual distortions
- Sense of terror
- Extreme fear of losing control
- Fear of dying

Modified from Hendrix ML: Understanding panic disorder. Washington, DC, U.S. Department of Health and Human Services, National Institutes of Health, 1993. For more information, contact the National Institute of Mental Health: 1-800-64-PANIC.

▼ *Clinical Signs and Symptoms of*
Depression

- Persistent sadness or feelings of emptiness
- Frequent or unexplained crying spells
- A sense of hopelessness
- Feelings of guilt or worthlessness
- Problems in sleeping
- Loss of interest or pleasure in ordinary activities or loss of libido
- Fatigue or decreased energy
- Appetite loss (or overeating)
- Difficulty in concentrating, remembering, and making decisions
- Irritability
- Persistent aches and pains
- Thoughts of death or suicide
- Pacing and fidgeting

Modified from Hendrix ML: Understanding panic disorder. Washington, DC, U.S. Department of Health and Human Services, National Institutes of Health, January 1993.

The alert therapist may recognize the need for a medical referral. A combination of antidepressants known as selective serotonin reuptake inhibitors (SSRIs) combined with cognitive behavioral therapy (CBT) has been proven effective in controlling symptoms.

Depression. Once defined as a deep and unrelenting sadness lasting 2 weeks or more, depression is no longer viewed in such simplistic terms. As an understanding of this condition has evolved, scientists have come to speak of *the depressive illnesses*. This term gives a better idea of the breadth of the disorder, encompassing several conditions including depression, dysthymia, bipolar disorder, and seasonal affective disorders (SAD).

Although these conditions can differ from individual to individual, each includes some of the symptoms listed. Often the classic signs of depression are not as easy to recognize in people older than 65, and many people attribute such symptoms simply to "getting older" and ignore them.

Although anyone can be affected by depression at any time, women are more often affected than men. A medical diagnosis is necessary because several known physical causes of depression are reversible if treated (e.g., thyroid disorders, vitamin B_{12} deficiency, medications [especially sedatives], some hypertensives, and H_2 blockers for stomach problems*). About half of clients with panic disorder will have an episode of clinical depression during their lives.

Depression is not a normal part of the aging process, but it is a normal response to pain or disability and may influence the client's ability to cope. Whereas anxiety is more apparent in acute pain episodes, depression occurs more often in clients with chronic pain. The therapist may want to

---

*There are, in fact, many underlying physical and medical causes of depression. The therapist should be familiar with these. For an in-depth discussion of depression, the reader is referred to more appropriate texts (*DSM-IV*, 1994; Goodman and Boissonnault, 1998; Lyness et al, 1996).

screen for psychosocial factors, such as depression that influences physical rehabilitation outcomes, especially when a client demonstrates acute pain that persists for more than 6 to 8 weeks.

Tests such as the Beck Depression Index (BDI) (Beck et al, 1961; C de C Williams and Richardson, 1993) or the Geriatric Depression Scale (Yesavage, 1983) can be administered by a physical therapist to obtain baseline information that may be useful in determining the need for a medical referral. These tests do not require interpretation that is out of the scope of physical therapist practice. For example, the BDI consists of 20 questions that are noninvasive and straightforward in presentation. If the resultant score suggests clinical depression, the therapist may want to review this outcome with the client and ask for permission to communicate this information to the physician.

Depression can be treated effectively with a combination of therapies, including exercise, proper nutrition, antidepressants, and psychotherapy.

Nonorganic Signs. Waddell et al. (1980) identified five nonorganic signs, each identifiable by one or two tests to assess a client's pain behavior (Table 1-4). A person with three or more positive nonorganic signs is said to have a clinical pattern of nonmechanical, pain-focused behavior.

A positive finding for nonorganic signs does not suggest an absence of pain but rather a behavioral response to pain (see discussion of symptom magnification syndrome). Waddell et al, have given us a tool that can help us identify early in the rehabilitation process those who need counseling as an adjunct to physical therapy (Rothstein, 1997).*

Illness Behavior. Pain in the absence of an identified source of disease or pathologic condition may elicit a behavioral response from the client that is now labeled *illness behavior syndrome*. This syndrome has been identified most often in people with chronic pain. Components of this syndrome include (1) dramatization of complaints, leading to

---

*Recently, the value of these nonorganic signs as predictors for return to work for clients with low back pain was investigated (Karas et al., 1997). The results of how this study might affect practice is available (Rothstein et al, 1997).

TABLE 1-4 ▼ Waddell's Nonorganic Signs

Test	Signs
Tenderness	Superficial—the patient's skin is tender to light pinch over a wide area of lumbar skin
	Nonanatomic—deep tenderness felt over a wide area, not localized to one structure
Simulation tests	Axial loading—light vertical loading over client's skull in the standing position causes typical lumbar pain
	Acetabular rotation—back pain is reported when the pelvis and shoulders are passively rotated in the same plane as the client stands; this is considered to be a positive test if pain is reported within the first 30 degrees
Distraction tests	Straight-leg-raise discrepancy—marked improvement of straight leg raising on distraction as compared with formal testing
	Double leg raise—when both legs are raised after straight leg raising, the organic response would be a greater degree of double leg raising; clients with a nonorganic component demonstrate less double leg raise as compared with the single leg raise
Regional disturbances	Weakness—cogwheeling or giving way of many muscle groups that cannot be explained on a neurologic basis
	Sensory disturbance—diminished sensation fitting a "stocking" rather than a dermatomal pattern
Overreaction	Disproportionate verbalization, facial expression, muscle tension and tremor, collapsing, or sweating

From Karas R, McIntosh G, Hall H, et al: The relationship between nonorganic signs and centralization of symptoms in the prediction of return to work for patients with low back pain. Phys Ther 77(4):354-360, 1997.

overtreatment and overmedication; (2) progressive dysfunction, leading to decreased physical activity and often compounding preexisting musculoskeletal or circulatory dysfunction; (3) drug misuse; (4) progressive dependency on others, including health care professionals, leading to overuse of the health care system; and (5) income disability, in which the person's illness behavior is perpetuated by financial gain (Management of the Individual With Pain, 1996a).

Symptom magnification syndrome (SMS) is another term used to describe the phenomenon of illness behavior.* It was first coined by Leonard N. Matheson in 1977 to describe clients whose symptoms have reinforced their behavior; that is, the symptoms have become the predominant force in the client's function rather than the physiologic phenomenon of the injury determining the outcome. By definition, SMA is a self-destructive, socially reinforced behavioral response pattern consisting of reports or displays of symptoms that function to control the life of the sufferer (Matheson, 1986; Matheson, 1987; Matheson, 1991).

The affected person acts as if the future cannot be controlled because of the presence of symptoms. All present limitations are blamed on the symptoms: "My (back) pain won't let me . . . ." The client may exaggerate limitations beyond those that seem reasonable in relation to the injury, apply minimal effort on maximal-performance tasks, and overreact to physical loading during objective examination.

It is important for physical therapists to recognize that we often contribute to SMS by focusing on the relief of symptoms, especially pain, as the goal of therapy. Reducing pain is an acceptable goal for some types of clients, but for those who experience pain after their injuries have healed, the focus should be restoration, or at least improvement, of function.

In these situations, instead of asking whether the client's symptoms are "better,

the same, or worse," it may be more appropriate to inquire about functional outcomes: for example, what can the client accomplish at home that she or he was unable to attempt at the beginning of treatment, last week, or even yesterday.

Conversion Symptoms. Whereas SMS is a behavioral, learned, inappropriate *behavior,* conversion is a psychodynamic phenomenon and quite rare in the chronically disabled population.

Conversion is a physical expression of an unconscious psychologic conflict, such as an event (e.g., loss of a loved one) or a problem in the person's work or personal life. The conversion may provide a solution to the conflict or a way to express "forbidden" feelings. It may be a means of enacting the sick role to avoid responsibilities, or it may be a reflection of behaviors learned in childhood (Maestri, 1996).

Diagnosis of a conversion syndrome is difficult and often requires the diagnostic and evaluative input of the physical therapist. Presentation always includes a motor and/or sensory component that cannot be explained by a known medical or neuromusculoskeletal condition. The clinical presentation is often mistaken for an organic disorder such as multiple sclerosis, systemic lupus erythematosus, myasthenia gravis, or idiopathic dystonias.

At presentation, when a client has an unusual limp or bizarre gait pattern that cannot be explained by functional anatomy, family members may be interviewed to assess changes in the client's gait and whether this alteration in movement pattern is consistently present. The physical therapist can look for a change in the wear pattern of the client's shoes to decide if this alteration in gait has been long-standing.

During manual muscle testing, true weakness results in smooth "giving way" of a muscle group; in hysterical weakness the muscle "breaks" in a series of jerks. Often the results of muscle testing are not consistent with functional abilities observed. For example, the person cannot raise the arm overhead during testing but has no difficulty dressing, or the lower extremity appears flaccid during

---

*Conscious symptom magnification is referred to as *malingering,* whereas unconscious symptom magnification is labeled *illness behavior.*

▼ Clinical Signs and Symptoms of Conversion

- Sudden, acute onset
- Lack of concern about the symptoms
- Unexplainable motor or sensory function impairment
  Motor:
  - Impaired coordination or balance and/or bizarre gait pattern
  - Paralysis or localized weakness
  - Loss of voice, difficulty swallowing, or sensation of a lump in the throat
  - Urinary retention
  Sensory:
  - Altered touch or pain sensation (paresthesia or dysesthesia)
  - Visual changes (double vision, blindness, black spots in visual field)
  - Hearing loss (mild to profound deafness)
- Hallucinations
- Seizures or convulsions
- Absence of significant laboratory findings
- Electrodiagnostic testing within normal limits
- Deep tendon reflexes within normal limits

recumbency but the person can walk on the heels and toes when standing.

The physical therapist should carefully evaluate and document all sensory and motor changes. Conversion symptoms are less likely to follow any dermatome, myotome, or sclerotome patterns.

Associated Signs and Symptoms of Systemic Diseases

The major focus of this text is the recognition of signs and symptoms either reported by the client subjectively or observed objectively by the physical therapist. *Signs* are observable findings detected by the physical therapist in an objective examination (e.g.,

unusual skin color, clubbing of the fingers [swelling of the terminal phalanges of the fingers or toes], hematoma [local collection of blood], effusion [fluid]).

Symptoms are reported indications of disease that are perceived by the client but cannot be observed by someone else. Pain, discomfort, or other complaints such as numbness, tingling, or "creeping" sensations are symptoms that are difficult to quantify but are most often reported as the chief complaint.

Because physical therapists spend a considerable amount of time investigating pain, it is easy to remain focused exclusively on this symptom when clients might otherwise bring to the forefront other important problems. Thus the physical therapist is encouraged to become accustomed to using the word *symptoms* instead of *pain* when interviewing the client. It is likewise prudent for the physical therapist to refer to symptoms when talking to clients with chronic pain in order to move the focus away from pain.

Systemic signs and symptoms that are listed for each condition should serve as a warning to alert the informed physical therapist of the need for further questioning and possible medical referral.

Nail and Skin Assessment

Changes in the skin and nail beds indicate systemic disease and can occur with involvement of a variety of organs. Nail and skin assessment is an example of signs that should raise a red flag for the therapist.

The hands, arms, feet, and legs should be assessed for *skin changes* (texture, color, temperature), vascular changes, clubbing, capillary filling, and edema. Texture changes include shiny, stiff, coarse, dry, or scaly skin. Skin mobility and turgor are affected by the fluid status of the client. Dehydration and aging reduce skin turgor, and edema decreases skin mobility.

Vascular changes of an affected extremity may include paresthesia, muscle fatigue and discomfort, numbness, pain, coolness (poikilothermy), and loss of hair from a reduced blood supply. Clubbing of the fingers and toes usually results from chronic oxygen deprivation in these tissue beds but can occur within 10 days in someone with paraneoplastic syndrome associated with cancer (see Paraneoplastic Syndromes, Chapter 10). Clubbing is most often observed in clients with advanced chronic obstructive pulmonary disease, congenital heart defects, and cor pulmonale. Clubbing can be assessed by the Schamrath method (see Fig. 1-3, *A*).

Capillary filling of the fingers and toes is an indicator of peripheral circulation. Pressing or blanching the nail bed of a finger or toe produces a whitening effect; when pressure is released, a return of color should occur within 3 seconds. If the capillary refill time exceeds 3 seconds, the lack of circulation may be due to arterial insufficiency from atherosclerosis or spasm.

Edema is an accumulation of fluid in the interstitial spaces. The location of edema helps identify the potential cause. Bilateral edema of the legs may be seen in clients with heart failure or with chronic venous insufficiency. Abdominal and leg edema can be seen

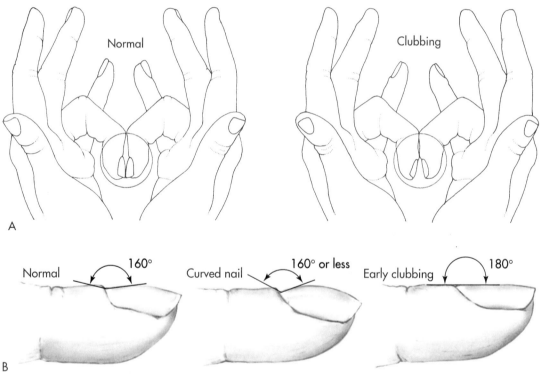

FIG. 1-3 • **A,** Assessment of clubbing by the Schamrath method. The client places the fingernails of opposite fingers together and holds them up to a light. If the examiner can see a diamond shape between the nails, there is no clubbing. Clubbing is identified by the absence of the diamond shape. It occurs first in the thumb and index finger. (From Ignatavicius DD, Bayne MV: Assessment of the cardiovascular system. In: Ignatavicius DD, Bayne MV[eds]: Medical-Surgical Nursing. Philadelphia, WB Saunders Company, 1993.) **B,** The index finger is viewed at its profile, and the angle of the nail base is noted (it should be about 160 degrees). The nail base is firm to palpation. Curved nails are a variation of normal with a convex profile. They may look like clubbed nails, but the angle between the nail base and the nail is normal (i.e., 160 degrees or less). Clubbing of nails occurs with congenital chronic cyanotic heart disease, emphysema, and chronic bronchitis. In early clubbing the angle straightens out to 180 degrees, and the nail base feels spongy to palpation. (From Jarvis C: *Physical examination and health assessment*, Philadelphia, 1992, WB Saunders.)

in clients with heart disease and cirrhosis of the liver. Edema may also be noted in dependent areas, such as the sacrum, when a person is confined to bed. Localized edema in one extremity may be the result of venous obstruction (thrombosis) or lymphatic blockage of the extremity (lymphedema).

Nail beds (fingers and toes) should be evaluated for color, shape, thickness, texture, and the presence of lesions (see Figs. 1-3 and 1-4). Many individual variations in color, texture, and grooming of the nails are influenced by factors unrelated to disease, such as occupation, chronic use of nail polish, or exposure to chemical dyes and detergents. In assessment of the elderly client, minor variations associated with the aging process may be observed (e.g., gradual thickening of the nail plate, appearance of longitudinal ridges, yellowish-gray discoloration).

Any positive findings in the nail beds should be viewed in light of the entire clinical presentation. For example, a positive Schamrath test without observable clinical changes in skin color, capillary refill time, or shape of the fingertips may not signify systemic disease but rather a normal anatomic variation of nail curvature.

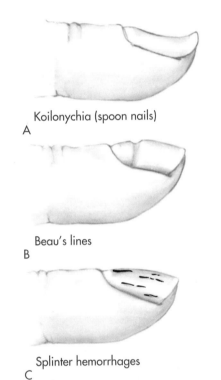

Koilonychia (spoon nails)
A

Beau's lines
B

Splinter hemorrhages
C

FIG. 1-4 • **A,** Koilonychia (spoon nails). These are thin, depressed nails with lateral edges tilted upward, forming a concave profile. They may be a congenital characteristic or a hereditary trait, occasionally a result of hypochromic anemia, iron deficiency (with or without anemia), poorly controlled diabetes of more than 15 years duration, chemical irritants, local injury, developmental abnormality, or psoriasis. **B,** Beau's lines or grooves. These are transverse furrows or grooves. A depression across the nail extends down to the nail bed. This occurs with any trauma that temporarily impairs nail formation, such as acute illness, prolonged fever, toxic reaction, or local trauma. A dent appears first at the cuticle and moves forward as the nail grows. All nails can be involved. **C,** Splinter hemorrhages. These red-brown streaks, embolic lesions, occur with subacute bacterial endocarditis; also, they may be a nonspecific sign. (From Jarvis C: *Physical examination and health assessment,* Philadelphia, 1992, WB Saunders.)

Systems Review

When a physician conducts a systems review, the examination is a routine physical assessment of each system—starting with ear, nose, and throat, followed by chest auscultation for pulmonary and cardiac function, palpation of lymph nodes, and so on.

A systems review of this type is not a part of the physical therapy examination. Rather, after conducting an interview and assessment of pain type/pain patterns, if there are characteristics of systemic disease in the history or clinical presentation (see box on p. 26), the identified cluster(s) of associated signs and symptoms are reviewed to search for a potential pattern that will identify the underlying cause.

For example, cutaneous (skin) manifestations and joint pain may be the presenting features of systemic disease such as Crohn's disease (regional enteritis), psoriatic arthritis, or a delayed reaction to medications. Hair and nail changes, temperature intolerance, and unexplained excessive fatigue are cluster signs and symptoms associated with the endocrine system. Changes in urinary frequency, flow of urine, or color of urine point to urologic involvement. Other

▼ **When to Screen for**
Systemic Disease

History
- Age over 40
- Personal or family history of cancer
- No known cause, unknown etiologic basis, or insidious onset

Pain Pattern/Pain Type
- Gradual, progressive, or cyclic presentation of symptoms (worse/better/worse)
- Pain unrelieved by rest or change in position; no position is comfortable
- If pain relieved by rest, positional change, application of heat or other relieving factors, even these relieving factors in time no longer reduce symptoms
- Symptoms that persist beyond the expected time for recovery
- Symptoms out of proportion to the injury
- Inability to alter (provoke, reproduce, alleviate, eliminate, aggravate) the symptoms during the examination
- Not fitting the expected mechanical or neuromusculoskeletal pattern
- No discernible patterns of symptoms (see Table 2-4)
- Physical therapy treatment does not change the clinical picture
- Night pain (see qualifiers in text as to the specific pattern of night pain)
- Symptoms (especially pain) are constant and intense
- Pain described as knifelike, boring, deep, colicky, deep aching
- Pattern of pain coming and going as spasms

▼ **When to Screen for**
Systemic Disease, cont'd

Associated Signs and Symptoms
- Presence of constitutional symptoms:
  Fever
  Diaphoresis (unexplained perspiration)
  Night sweats (can occur during the day)
  Nausea
  Vomiting
  Diarrhea
  Pallor
  Dizziness/syncope (fainting)
  Fatigue
  Weight loss
- Presence of bilateral symptoms (clubbing, paresthesias, numbness/tingling, nail bed changes, skin pigmentation or other skin changes, skin rash, weakness, edema)
- Proximal muscle weakness accompanied by change in one or more deep tendon reflexes
- Change in muscle tone or joint range of motion for individuals with cerebral palsy, spinal cord injury, or other neurologic condition with altered muscle tone (e.g., multiple sclerosis, stroke)
- Joint pain associated with skin rashes, nodules
- Any cluster of signs and symptoms observed during the systems review that is characteristic of a particular organ system

groupings of signs and symptoms associated with each system are listed (see box on p. 27).

The physical therapist is not responsible for identifying the specific pathologic disease underlying the clinical signs and symptoms present. However, the alert therapist who classifies groups of signs and symptoms in a systems review will be more likely to identify a problem outside the scope of physical therapy practice and make the appropriate referral.

SYSTEMS REVIEW

GENERAL QUESTIONS

- Fever, chills, sweating
- Excessive, unexplained weight gain or loss
- Appetite loss, nausea, vomiting
- Vital signs: blood pressure, temperature, pulse
- Insomnia
- Fatigue, weakness
- Irritability

RHEUMATOLOGIC

- Presence/location of joint swelling
- Muscle pain, weakness
- Skin rashes
- Reaction to sunlight
- Raynaud's phenomenon
- Nail bed changes

NEUROLOGIC

- Headaches
- Vision changes
- Vertigo
- Paresthesias
- Weakness; atrophy
- Involuntary movements; tremors
- Radicular pain
- Seizures or loss of consciousness

CARDIOVASCULAR

- Chest pain or discomfort
- Palpitations
- Claudication (leg pain, cramps, limping)
- Peripheral edema; nocturia
- Persistent cough
- Fatigue, dyspnea, syncope
- High or low blood pressure
- Differences in blood pressure from side to side with position change (10 mm Hg or more; increase or decrease/diastolic or systolic; associated symptoms: dizziness, headache, nausea, vomiting, diaphoresis, heart palpitations, increased primary pain or symptoms)

PSYCHOLOGIC*

- Sleep disturbance
- Stress levels
- Fatigue, psychomotor agitation
- Changes in personal habits, appetite
- Depression, confusion, anxiety

GASTROINTESTINAL

- Abdominal pain
- Indigestion; heartburn
- Difficulty in swallowing
- Nausea/vomiting
- Diarrhea or constipation
- Change in bowel habits
- Rectal bleeding; blood in stool
- Skin rash followed by joint pain

HEMATOLOGIC

- Skin color or nail bed changes
- Bleeding: nose, gums, easy bruising, melena
- Hemarthrosis, muscle hemorrhage, hematoma
- Fatigue, dyspnea, weakness
- Confusion, irritability
- Headache

GENITOURINARY

- Reduced stream, decreased output
- Burning, bleeding, change in urine color
- Incontinence
- Impotence, pain with intercourse
- Hesitation, urgency
- Nocturia, frequency
- Dysuria (painful or difficult urination)
- Testicular pain or swelling

ENDOCRINE

- Hair and nail changes
- Temperature intolerance

---

*Cluster of three to four or more lasting longer than 1 month.

continued

SYSTEMS REVIEW—cont'd

ENDOCRINE—cont'd

- Cramps
- Edema, polyuria, polydipsia
- Unexplained weakness, fatigue, paresthesia
- Carpal tunnel syndrome
- Periarthritis, adhesive capsulitis

PULMONARY

- Cough, hoarseness
- Sputum, hemoptysis
- Shortness of breath; wheezing
- Night sweats
- Pleural pain
- Clubbing

GYNECOLOGIC

- Irregular menses, menopause
- Pain with menses, intercourse
- Vaginal discharge
- Surgical procedures
- Birth/abortion histories
- Spotting, bleeding—especially for the postmenopausal woman >12 months after last period (without hormone replacement therapy)

▼ PHYSICIAN REFERRAL

The hallmark of professionalism in any health care practitioner is the ability to understand the limits of his or her professional knowledge. The physical therapist, either on reaching the limit of his or her knowledge or on reaching the limits prescribed by the client's condition, should refer the patient to the physician. In this way the physical therapist will work within the scope of his or her level of skill, knowledge, and practical experience.

Guidelines for appropriate referral to a physician (or other health care practitioner) have been outlined in the *APTA Code of Ethics and Guide for Professional Conduct and Standards for Physical Therapy Services* (APTA, 1990):

If symptoms are present for which physical therapy is contraindicated or which are indicative of conditions for which treatment is outside the scope of his knowledge, the physical therapist must refer [clients] to a licensed practitioner of medicine.

In the event that a medical diagnosis is required and has not been established prior to treatment, then the physical therapist must refer to a licensed practitioner of medicine, dentistry, or podiatry.

Knowing how to refer the client or how to notify the physician of important findings is not always clear. It may be appropriate to make a summary statement regarding the objective findings with a follow-up question for the physician. This may be filed in the client's chart in the hospital or sent in a letter to the outpatient's physician (or dentist).

For example, after treatment of a person who has not responded to physical therapy, a report to the physician may include additional information: "Miss Jones reported a rash skin over the backs of her knees 2 weeks before the onset of joint pain and experiences recurrent bouts of sore throat and fever when her knees flare up. These features are not consistent with an athletic injury. Would you please take a look?" (For an additional sample letter, see Fig. 1-5).

Other useful wording may include "Please advise" or "What do you think?" At no time should the therapist suggest a possible cause or attempt to diagnose the findings

Referral. A 32-year-old female university student was referred for physical therapy through the health service 2 weeks ago. The physician's referral reads: "Possible right oblique abdominis tear/possible right iliopsoas tear." This woman was screened initially by a faculty member, and the diagnosis was confirmed as being a right oblique abdominal strain.

History. Two months ago, while the client was running her third mile, she felt "severe pain" in the right side of her stomach, which caused her to double over. She felt immediate nausea and had abdominal distension. She could not change the position of her leg to relieve the pain at the time. Currently, she still cannot run without pain.

Presenting Symptoms. Pain increases during sit-ups, walking fast, reaching, turning, and bending. Pain is eased by heat and is reduced by activity. Pain in the morning versus evening depends on body position. Once the pain starts, it is intermittent and aches. The client describes the pain as being severe, depending on her body position. She is currently taking aspirin when necessary.

SAMPLE LETTER

Date

John Smith, M.D.
University of Montana Health Service
Eddy Street
Missoula, MT 59812

Re: Jane Doe

Dear Dr. Smith,
Your client, Jane Doe, was evaluated in our clinic on 5/2/99 with the following pertinent findings:

<u>Subjective.</u> She has severe pain in the right lower abdominal quadrant associated with nausea and abdominal distension. Although the onset of symptoms started while the client was running, she denies any precipitating trauma. She describes the course of symptoms as having begun 2 months ago with temporary resolution and now with exacerbation of earlier symptoms. Additionally, she has chronic fatigue and frequent night sweats.

<u>Objective.</u> Presenting pain is reproduced by resisted hip or trunk flexion with accompanying tenderness/tightness on palpation of the right iliopsoas muscle (compared with the left iliopsoas muscle). There are no implicating neurologic signs or symptoms.

<u>Assessment.</u> A musculoskeletal screening examination is consistent with your diagnosis of a possible iliopsoas or abdominal oblique tear. Jane appears to have a combination of musculoskeletal and systemic symptoms, such as those outlined earlier. Of particular concern are the symptoms of fatigue, night sweats, abdominal distension, nausea, repeated episodes of exacerbation and remission, and severe quality of pain and location (right lower abdominal quadrant). These symptoms appear to be of a systemic nature rather than caused by a musculoskeletal lesion.

<u>Recommendations.</u> I suggest that the client return to you for further medical follow-up to rule out any systemic involvement before the initiation of physical therapy services. I am concerned that my proposed treatment plan of ultrasound, soft tissue mobilization, and stretching may aggravate an underlying disease process.

I will contact you directly by telephone by the end of the week to discuss these findings and to answer any questions that you may have. Thank you for this interesting referral.

Sincerely,

Catherine C. Goodman, M.B.A., P.T.

Result. This client returned to the physician, who then ordered laboratory tests. After an acute recurrence of the symptoms described earlier, she had exploratory surgery. A diagnosis of a ruptured appendix and peritonitis was determined at surgery. In retrospect, the proposed treatment of ultrasound and soft tissue mobilization would have been contraindicated in this situation.

FIG. 1-5 • Sample letter of the physical therapist's findings that is sent to the referring physician.

medically. Making a report and stating that the clinical presentation does not follow a typical neuromuscular or musculoskeletal patterns should be sufficient.

When the client has come to physical therapy without a medical referral (i.e., self-referred) and the physical therapist recommends medical follow-up, the client should be referred to the primary care physician.

Occasionally, the client indicates that he or she has not contacted a physician or was treated by a physician (whose name cannot be recalled) a long time ago or that he or she has just moved to the area and does not have a physician.

In these situations the client can be provided with a list of recommended physicians. It is not necessary to list every physician in the area, but the physical therapist should provide several appropriate choices. Whether or not the client makes an appointment with a medical practitioner, the physical therapist is urged to document subjective and objective findings carefully, as well as the recommendation made for medical follow-up. The client should make these physical therapy records available to the consulting physician.

PHYSICIAN REFERRAL

IMMEDIATE MEDICAL ATTENTION

- Client with anginal pain not relieved in 20 minutes
- Client with angina who has nausea, vomiting, profuse sweating
- Client with bowel/bladder incontinence and/or saddle anesthesia secondary to cauda equina lesion or cervical spine pain concomitant with urinary incontinence
- Client in anaphylactic shock (see Chapter 11)
- Client with symptoms of inadequate ventilation or CO_2 retention (see Respiratory Acidosis, Chapter 4)
- Client with diabetes who appears confused or lethargic or who exhibits changes in mental function; perform fingerstick glucose testing and report findings
- Client with positive McBurney's point (appendicitis) or rebound tenderness (inflamed peritoneum) (see Chapter 6)
- Sudden worsening of intermittent claudication may be due to thromboembolism and must be reported to the physician immediately
- Throbbing chest, back, or abdominal pain that increases with exertion accompanied by a sensation of a heartbeat when lying down and palpable pulsating abdominal mass may indicate an aneurysm

MEDICAL ATTENTION NECESSARY
General Systemic

- Unknown cause
- Lack of significant objective neuromusculoskeletal signs and symptoms
- Lack of expected progress with physical therapy treatment
- Development of constitutional symptoms or associated signs and symptoms over the course of treatment
- Discovery of significant past medical history (PMH) unknown to physician
- Changes in health status that persist 7 to 10 days beyond expected time period
- Client who is jaundiced and has not been diagnosed or treated
- Changes in size, shape, tenderness, and consistency of lymph nodes in more than one area that persist more than 4 weeks; painless, enlarged lymph nodes

continued

PHYSICIAN REFERRAL—cont'd

For Women

- Low back, hip, pelvic, groin, or sacroiliac symptoms without known etiologic basis and in the presence of constitutional symptoms
- Symptoms correlated with menses
- Any spontaneous uterine bleeding after menopause
- For pregnant women:
  Vaginal bleeding
  Elevated blood pressure
  Increased Braxton-Hicks contractions during exercise

Vital Signs (Report these findings)

- Persistent rise or fall of blood pressure
- Blood pressure elevation in any woman taking birth control pills (should be closely monitored by her physician)
- Pulse amplitude that fades with inspiration and strengthens with expiration
- Pulse increase over 20 BPM lasting more than 3 minutes after rest or changing position
- Difference in pulse pressure (between systolic and diastolic measurements) of more than 40 mm Hg
- Persistent low-grade (or higher) fever, especially associated with constitutional symptoms, most commonly sweats
- Any unexplained fever without other systemic symptoms, especially in the person taking corticosteroids

Cardiac

- Angina at rest
- Anginal pain not relieved by rest or use of nitroglycerin in 20 minutes
- More than three sublingual nitroglycerin tablets required to gain relief
- Angina continues to increase in intensity after stimulus (e.g., cold, stress, exertion) has been eliminated
- Changes in pattern of angina
- Abnormally severe chest pain
- Client with angina or chest pain has nausea, vomiting
- Anginal pain radiates to jaw/left arm
- Upper back feels abnormally cool, sweaty, or moist to touch
- Client has any doubts about his or her condition
- Palpitation in any person with a history of unexplained sudden death in the family requires medical evaluation; more than six episodes of palpitation in 1 hour or palpitations lasting for hours or occurring in association with pain, shortness of breath, fainting, or severe lightheadedness requires medical evaluation
- Clients who are neurologically unstable as a result of a recent CVA, head trauma, spinal cord injury, or other central nervous system insult often exhibit new arrhythmias during the period of instability; when the client's pulse is monitored, any new arrhythmias noted should be reported to the nursing staff or physician

continued

PHYSICIAN REFERRAL—cont'd

- Anyone who cannot climb a single flight of stairs without feeling moderately to severely winded or who awakens at night or experiences shortness of breath when lying down should be evaluated by a physician
- Anyone with known cardiac involvement who develops progressively worse dyspnea should notify the physician of these findings
- Fainting (syncope) without any warning period of lightheadedness, dizziness, or nausea may be a sign of heart valve or arrhythmia problems; unexplained syncope in the presence of heart or circulatory problems (or risk factors for heart attack or stroke) should be evaluated by a physician

Cancer

- Early warning sign(s) of cancer:

  Seven early warning signs plus two additional signs pertinent to the physical therapy examination: proximal muscle weakness and change in deep tendon reflexes
- All soft tissue lumps that persist or grow, whether painful or painless
- Any woman presenting with chest, breast, axillary, or shoulder pain of unknown etiologic basis, especially in the presence of a positive medical history (self or family) of cancer
- Any man with pelvic, groin, sacroiliac, or low back pain accompanied by sciatica and a history of prostate cancer
- Bone pain, especially on weight-bearing, that persists more than 1 week and is worse at night
- Any unexplained bleeding from any area

Pulmonary

- Shoulder pain aggravated by respiratory movements; have the client hold his or her breath and reassess symptoms; any reduction or elimination of symptoms with breath holding or the Valsalva maneuver suggests pulmonary or cardiac source of symptoms
- Shoulder pain that is aggravated by supine positioning; pain that is worse when lying down and improves when sitting up or leaning forward is often pleuritic in origin (abdominal contents push up against diaphragm and in turn against parietal pleura; see Figs. 4-5 and 12-6)
- Shoulder, chest (thorax) pain that subsides with autosplinting (lying on painful side)
- For the client with asthma: Signs of asthma or bronchial activity during exercise
- Weak and rapid pulse accompanied by fall in blood pressure (pneumothorax)
- Presence of associated signs and symptoms, such as persistent cough, dyspnea (rest or exertional), or constitutional symptoms (see boxes on pp. 26-28).

Genitourinary

- Abnormal urinary constituents—for example, change in color, odor, amount, flow of urine
- Any amount of blood in urine
- Cervical spine pain accompanied by urinary incontinence (unless cervical disk protrusion already has been medically diagnosed)

Gastrointestinal

- Back pain and abdominal pain at the same level, especially when accompanied by constitutional symptoms
- Back pain of unknown cause in a person with a history of cancer

continued

PHYSICIAN REFERRAL—cont'd

- Back pain or shoulder pain in a person taking nonsteroidal antiinflammatory drugs, especially when accompanied by gastrointestinal upset or blood in the stools
- Back pain associated with meals or relieved by a bowel movement

Musculoskeletal

- Symptoms that seem out of proportion to the injury or symptoms persisting beyond the expected time for the nature of the injury
- Severe or progressive back pain accompanied by constitutional symptoms, especially fever
- New onset of joint pain following surgery with inflammatory signs (warmth, redness, tenderness, swelling)

PRECAUTIONS/CONTRAINDICATIONS TO THERAPY

- Uncontrolled chronic heart failure or pulmonary edema
- Active myocarditis
- Resting heart rate >120 or 130 BPM*
- Resting systolic rate >180 to 200 mm Hg*
- Resting diastolic rate >105 to 110 mm Hg*
- Moderate dizziness, near-syncope
- Marked dyspnea
- Unusual fatigue
- Unsteadiness
- Loss of palpable pulse
- Postoperative posterior calf pain
- For the client with diabetes: Chronically unstable blood sugar levels must be stabilized (fasting target glucose range: 70 to 110 mg/dl; precaution: <100 or >250 mg/dl)

---

*Unexplained or poorly tolerated by client.

 KEY POINTS TO REMEMBER

▶ Systemic diseases can mimic neuromusculoskeletal dysfunction.

▶ There are many reasons for medical screening of the physical therapy client (see "Reasons for Medical Screening" box on p. 8).

▶ Screening for medical disease is an ongoing process and does not occur only during the initial evaluation.

▶ The therapist uses four parameters in making the screening decision: client history, pain patterns/pain types, associated signs and symptoms, and systems review. Any red flags in the first three parameters will alert the therapist to the need for a screening examination. A systems review consists of identifying clusters of signs and symptoms that may be characteristic of a particular organ system.

▶ The two body parts most commonly affected by visceral pain patterns are the back and the shoulder, although the thorax, pelvis, hip, sacroiliac, and groin can be involved.

▶ The physical therapist is qualified to make a physical therapy diagnosis regarding primary neuromusculoskeletal conditions.

▶ The purpose of the physical therapy diagnosis, established through the subjective and objective examinations, is to identify as closely as possible the underlying neuromusculoskeletal pathologic condition. In this way screening for medical disease, ruling out the need for medical referral, and treating the physical therapy problem as specifically as possible are possible.

▶ Sometimes in the diagnostic process the symptoms are treated because the client's condition is too acute to evaluate thoroughly. Usually even medically diagnosed problems (e.g., "shoulder pain" or "back pain") are evaluated.

▶ Careful, objective, detailed evaluation of the client with pain is critical for accurate identification of the sources and types of pain (underlying pathologic process) and for accurate assessment of treatment effectiveness (Management of the Individual With Pain, 1996).

▶ Painful symptoms that are out of proportion to the injury or that are not consistent with objective findings may be a red flag indicating systemic disease. Other key red flags are listed in the box on p. 26.

▶ If the client or the physical therapist is in doubt, communication with the physician, dentist, family member, or referral source is indicated.

PRACTICE QUESTIONS

1. The primary purpose of a physical therapy diagnosis is

   a. to obtain reimbursement

   b. to guide treatment

   c. to practice within the scope of physical therapy

   d. to meet the established standards for accreditation

2. Pain described as knifelike, stabbing, and boring is characteristic of a

   a. cutaneous source of pain

   b. visceral source of pain

   c. somatic source of pain

   d. referred source of pain

3. Gradual onset of tender, stiff, aching muscles is characteristic of a

   a. cutaneous source of pain

   b. visceral source of pain

   c. somatic source of pain

   d. referred source of pain

4. The client with joint pain of unknown cause should be questioned about

   a. history of allergies

   b. use of prescription drugs

   c. presence of skin rash

   d. all of the above

   e. (b) and (c) only

5. When someone has symptoms that have persisted beyond the expected time for physiologic healing, how do you differentiate between emotional content and medical disease?

References

AGS Panel on Chronic Pain in Older Persons, *J Am Geriatr Soc* 46:635-651, 1998.

American Physical Therapy Association: *Competencies in physical therapy—an analysis of practice,* Alexandria, Virginia, March, 1985, The Association.

American Physical Therapy Association: Direct access to physical therapy—Information Packet. Alexandria, Virginia, Government Affairs Department, 1990.

American Physical Therapy Association: *Evaluative criteria for accreditation of education programs for the preparation of physical therapists,* Alexandria, Virginia, January, 1998, The Association.

American Physical Therapy Association: *House of delegates policies,* Alexandria, Virginia, 1984, p. 19, The Association.

Beck AT, Ward CH, Mendelson M et al: An inventory for measuring depression, *Arch Gen Psychiatry* 4:561-571, 1961.

Cailliet R: *Low back pain syndrome,* ed 5, Philadelphia, 1995, F A Davis.

Cailliet R: *Soft tissue pain and disability,* ed 3, Philadelphia, 1996, F A Davis.

C de C Williams A, Richardson PH: What does the BDI measure in chronic pain? *Pain* 55:259-266, 1993.

Chronic pain and the paradox of managed care, *PT Magazine* 4(9):40-47, 77, 1996.

Cyriax J: *Textbook of orthopaedic medicine,* ed 8, vol 1, London, 1982, Baillière Tindall.

Delitto A, Snyder-Mackler L: The diagnostic process: examples in orthopedic physical therapy, *Phys Ther* 75(3):203-211, 1995.

Diagnostic and Statistical Manual of Mental Disorders, ed 4 [DSM-IV], Washington, DC, 1994, American Psychiatric Association.

Emre M, Mathies H: *Muscle spasms and pain,* Park Ridge, Illinois, 1988, Parthenon.

Fealy MJ, Ladd AL: Reflex sympathetic dystrophy: early diagnosis and active treatment, *J Musculoskel Med* 13(3):29-36, March 1996.

Fosnaught M: A critical look at diagnosis, *PT Magazine* 4(6):48-54, 1996.

Goodman CC, Boissonnault WG: *Pathology: implications for the physical therapist,* Philadelphia, 1998, WB Saunders.

Guccione A: *Diagnosis and diagnosticians: the future in physical therapy.* Combined sections meeting, Dallas, February 13-16, 1997.

Guide to Physical Therapist Practice, *Phys Ther* 77(11), November 1997.

Hendrix ML: *Understanding panic disorder,* Washington, DC, 1993, National Institutes of Health.

Karas R, McIntosh G, Hall H et al: The relationship between nonorganic signs and centralization of symptoms in the prediction of return to work for patients with low back pain, *Phys Ther* 77(4):354-360, April 1997.

Koop CE: Incidence of anxiety-based medical problems, Personal communication, 1992.

Kozol J: *Illiterate America,* New York, 1988, New American Library—Putnam.

Kraus H: Muscle deficiency. In Rachlin ES, editor: *Myofascial pain and fibromyalgia,* St Louis, 1994, Mosby.

Lyness JM, Bruce ML, Koenig HG et al: Depression and medical illness in late life: report of a symposium, *J Am Geriatr Soc (JAGS)* 44(2):198-203, 1996.

Maestri A: PT for patients with psychiatric disorders, *PT Magazine* 4(7):54-57, 1996.

Management of the individual with pain. I. Physiology and evaluation, *PT Magazine* 4(11):54-63, November 1996.

Management of the individual with pain. II. Treatment, *PT Magazine* 4(12):58-65, December 1996.

Matheson LN: *Work capacity evaluation: systematic approach to industrial rehabilitation,* Anaheim, Calif, 1986, Employment and Rehabilitation Institute of California.

Matheson LN: *Symptom magnification casebook,* Anaheim, Calif, 1987, Employment and Rehabilitation Institute of California.

Matheson LN: Symptom magnification syndrome structured interview: rationale and procedure, *J Occup Rehab* 1(1):43-56, 1991.

Melzack R: The McGill Pain Questionnaire: major properties and scoring methods, *Pain* 1:277, 1975.

Mennell JM: *Joint pain: diagnosis and treatment using manipulative techniques,* Boston, 1964, Little Brown.

Merskey H, Bogduk N: *Classification of chronic pain,* ed 2, Seattle, 1994, International Association for the Study of Pain.

Raj PP: *Pain medicine: a comprehensive review,* St Louis, 1996, Mosby.

Rothstein JM: Patient classification, *Phys Ther* 73(4):214-215, April 1993.

Rothstein JM: Unnecessary adversaries (editorial), *Phys Ther* 77(4):352, April 1997.

Rothstein JM, Erhard RE, Nicholson GG et al: Conference, *Phys Ther* 77(4):361-369, April 1997.

Sahrmann S: *Diagnosis and diagnosticians: the future in physical therapy.* Combined sections meeting, Dallas, February 13-16, 1997.

Sahrmann S: *Diagnosis and treatment of movement impairment syndromes,* St Louis, 1999, Mosby.

Sahrmann S: Diagnosis by the physical therapist—a prerequisite for treatment. A special communication, *Phys Ther* 68:1703-1706, 1988.

Scalzitti DA: Screening for psychological factors in patients with low back problems: Waddell's nonorganic signs, *Phys Ther* 77(3):306-312, 261-369, March 1997.

Sinnott M: *Assessing musculoskeletal changes in the geriatric population,* American Physical Therapy Association Combined Sections Meeting, February 3-7, 1993.

Teasell RW, Shapiro AP: Strategic-behavioral intervention in the treatment of chronic nonorganic motor disorders, *Am J Phys Med Rehabil* 73(1):44-50, 1994.

Travell JG, Simons DG: *Myofascial pain and dysfunction: the trigger point manual,* vol 1, Baltimore, 1993, Williams & Wilkins.

Travell JG, Simons DG: *Myofascial pain and dysfunction: the trigger point manual,* vol 2, Baltimore, 1993, Williams & Wilkins.

Waddell G et al: Symptoms and signs: physical disease or illness behavior? *Br Med J* 289:739-741, 1984.

Waddell G, McCulloch JA, Kummer E et al: Nonorganic physical signs in low back pain, *Spine* 5(2):117-125, March/April 1980.

Wells PE, Frampton V, Bowsher D: *Pain management by physical therapy,* ed 2, Oxford, 1994, Butterworth-Heinemann.

Yesavage JA: The geriatric depression scale, *J Psychiatr Res* 17(1):37-49, 1983.

Bibliography

Diagnosis in physical therapy (A Roundtable Discussion), *PT Magazine* 1(6):58-65, 1993.

Guccione AA: Physical therapy diagnosis and the relationship between impairments and function, *Phys Ther* 71:499-504, 1991.

Jette AM: Diagnosis and classification by physical therapists: special communication, *Phys Ther* 69: 967-969, 1989.

Rose SJ: Musing on diagnosis (editorial), *Phys Ther* 68(11), November 1988.

Rose SJ: Physical therapy diagnosis: role and function, *Phys Ther* 69:535-537, 1989.

Introduction to the Interviewing Process

2

Y ou are interviewing a client for the first time, and she tells you, "The pain in my hip started 12 years ago, when I was a waitress standing on my feet 10 hours a day. It seems to bother me most when I am having premenstrual symptoms. My left leg is longer than my right leg, and my hip hurts when the scars from my bunionectomy ache. This pain occurs with any changes in the weather. I have a bleeding ulcer that bothers me, and the pain keeps me awake at night. I dislocated my shoulder 2 years ago, but I can lift weights now without any problems." She continues her monolog, and you feel out of control and unsure of how to proceed.

This scenario was taken directly from a clinical experience and represents what we call "an organ recital." In this situation the client provides detailed information regarding all previously experienced illnesses and symptoms, which may or may not be related to the current problem.

Interviewing is an important skill for the clinician to learn. It is generally agreed that 80 percent of the information needed to clarify the cause of symptoms is given by the client during the interview. This chapter is designed to provide the physical therapist with interviewing guidelines and important questions to ask the client. The materials presented are not intended to teach the therapist how to interview a client. Other more appropriate texts that emphasize interviewing for the health care professional are available (Bates, 1995; Coulehan and Block, 1997).

Medical practitioners (including nurses, physicians, and therapists) begin the interview by determining the client's chief complaint. The **chief complaint** is usually a symptomatic description by the client (i.e., symptoms reported for which the person is seeking care or advice). The **present illness**, including the chief complaint and other current symptoms, gives a broad, clear account of the symptoms—how they developed and events related to them.

Questioning the client may also assist the physical therapist in determining whether an injury is in the acute, subacute, or chronic stage. This information guides the clinician in providing

37

symptomatic relief for the acute injury, more aggressive treatment for the chronic problem, and a combination of both methods of treatment for the subacute lesion.

The interviewing techniques, interviewing tools, core interview, and review of the inpatient hospital chart in this chapter will help the therapist determine the location and potential significance of any symptom (including pain).

The interview format provides detailed information regarding the frequency, duration, intensity, length, breadth, depth, and anatomic location as these relate to the client's chief complaint. The physical therapist will later correlate this information with objective findings from the examination to rule out possible systemic origin of symptoms.

The subjective examination may also reveal any contraindications to physical therapy treatment or indications for the kind of treatment that is most likely to be effective.

The information obtained from the interview guides the physical therapist in either referring the client to a physician or planning physical therapy treatment.

▼ INTERVIEWING TECHNIQUES

An organized interview format assists the physical therapist in obtaining a complete and accurate database. Using the same outline with each client ensures that all pertinent information related to previous medical history and current medical problem(s) is included. This information is especially important when correlating the subjective data with objective findings from the physical examination.

The most basic skills required for a physical therapy interview include:

- Open-ended questions
- Closed-ended questions
- Funnel sequence or technique
- Paraphrasing technique

Open-Ended and Closed-Ended Questions

Beginning an interview with an *open-ended question* (i.e., questions that elicit more than a one-word response) is advised, even though this gives the client the opportunity to control and direct the interview. Initiating an interview with the open-ended directive, "Tell me why you are here" can potentially elicit more information in a relatively short (5- to 15-minute) period than a steady stream of *closed-ended questions* requiring a "yes" or "no" type of answer (Table 2-1).

A client who takes control of the interview by telling the therapist about every ache and pain of every friend and neighbor can be rechanneled effectively by interrupting the client with a polite statement such as, "I'm beginning to get an idea of the nature of your problem. Now I would like to obtain some more specific information" (Hertling and Kessler, 1990). At this point the interviewer may begin to use closed-ended questions (i.e., questions requiring the answer to be "yes" or "no") in order to characterize the symptoms more clearly. Moving from the open-ended line of questions to the closed-ended questions is referred to as the *funnel technique* or *funnel sequence*.

TABLE 2-1 ▼ Interviewing Techniques

Open-Ended Questions	Closed-Ended Questions
1. How does bed rest affect your back pain?	1. Do you have any pain after lying in bed all night?
2. Tell me how you cope with stress and what kinds of stressors you encounter on a daily basis.	2. Are you under any stress?
3. What makes the pain (better) worse?	3. Is the pain relieved by food?
4. How did you sleep last night?	4. Did you sleep well last night?

Each question format has advantages and limitations. The use of open-ended ques-tions to initiate the interview may allow the client to control the interview, but it can also prevent a false-positive or false-negative response that would otherwise be elicited by starting with closed-ended (yes or no) questions. False responses elicited by closed-ended questions may develop from the client's attempt to please the health care provider or to comply with what the client believes is the correct response or expectation.

Closed-ended questions tend to be more impersonal and may set an impersonal tone for the relationship between the client and the physical therapist. These questions are limited by the restrictive nature of the information received so that the client may respond only to the category in question and may omit vital, but seemingly unrelated, information.

Use of the funnel sequence to obtain as much information as possible through the open-ended format first (before moving on to the more restrictive but clarifying "yes" or "no" type of questions at the end) can establish an effective forum for trust between the client and the physical therapist.

Follow-up Questions

The funnel sequence is aided by the use of *follow-up* questions, referred to as *FUPs* in the text. Beginning with one or two open-ended questions in each section, the interviewer may follow up with a series of closed-ended questions, which are listed in the core interview presented later in this chapter. For example, starting with an open-ended question such as: "How does rest affect the pain or symptoms?" The therapist can follow up with clarifying questions such as:

- Are your symptoms aggravated or relieved by any activities? If yes, what?

- How has this problem affected your daily life at work or at home?

- How has it affected your ability to care for yourself without assistance (e.g., dress, bathe, cook, drive)?

Paraphrasing Technique

A useful interviewing skill that can assist in synthesizing and integrating the information obtained during questioning is the *paraphrasing technique*. When using this technique, the interviewer repeats information presented by the client. This technique can assist in fostering effective, accurate communication between the health care recipient and the health care provider.

For example, once a client has responded to the question, "What makes you feel better?" The physical therapist can paraphrase the reply by saying, "You've told me that the pain is relieved by such and such, is that right? What other activities or treatment brings you relief from your pain or symptoms?" If you cannot paraphrase what the client has said, or if you are unclear about the meaning of the client's response, ask for clarification by requesting an example of what the person is saying.

▼ INTERVIEWING TOOLS

With the changing requirements of hospital accreditation and payment sources, physical therapists are required more and more to identify problems, to quantify symptoms (e.g., pain), and to demonstrate the effectiveness of treatment.

Documenting the effectiveness of treatment is called *outcomes management*. Using standardized tests, functional tools, or questionnaires to relate pain, strength, or range of motion to a quantifiable scale is defined as *outcome measures*. The information obtained from such measures is then compared with the functional outcomes of treatment to assess the effectiveness of those interventions.

In this way physical therapists are gathering information about the most appropriate treatment progression for a specific diagnosis. Such a database shows the efficacy of physical therapy treatment and provides data for use with insurance companies in requesting reimbursement for service.

No single instrument or method of pain measurement can be considered the best under all circumstances. However, for the clinician interested in quantifying pain, some form of assessment is necessary. There are numerous pain assessment scales designed to assess the quality and location of pain and the percentage of impairment or functional levels associated with pain.* Presenting and explaining each scale is beyond the scope of this text. There are courses and texts for the physical therapist that will provide knowledge and experience of these measures.

▼ **SUBJECTIVE EXAMINATION**

The subjective examination is usually thought of as the "client interview." It is intended to provide a database of information that is important in determining the need for medical referral or the direction for physical therapy treatment. The subjective examination must be conducted in a complete and organized manner. It includes several components, all gathered through the interview process (Fig. 2-1):

- Family/Personal History
  - Age and aging
  - Past medical history
  - General health
  - Medical testing/previous surgery
  - Work environment
  - Vital signs
- Core Interview
  - History of present illness
  - Assessment of pain and symptoms
  - Medical treatment and medications

- Current level of fitness
- Sleep-related history
- Stress
- Special questions for women and men

The family/personal history is usually obtained by using a written form or questionnaire. The therapist uses this information to ask any further questions during the interview. The interview that follows the administration of the Family/Personal History form is referred to in this text as the Core Interview.

Family/Personal History

It is unnecessary and probably impossible to complete the entire subjective examination on the first day. Most clinics or health care facilities use what is called an initial intake form before the client's first visit with the physical therapist. The Family/Personal History form is one example of an initial intake form.†

This component of the subjective examination can elicit valuable data regarding the client's family history of disease and personal lifestyle, including working environment and health habits. Once the client has completed the Family/Personal History intake form, the clinician can then follow up with appropriate questions based on any "yes" selections made by the client.

For example, a client who circles "yes" on the Family/Personal History form indicating a history of ulcers or stomach problems lists a chief complaint of back pain during the History of Present Illness. Obtaining further information at the first appointment with the client by using Special Questions to Ask (see Chapter 6) is necessary so that a decision

---

*Each test has a specific focus—whether to assess pain levels, level of balance, risk for falls, functional status, and so on. Examples of specific tests include the Visual Analogue Scale (VAS), Pain Estimate (PE), McGill Pain Questionnaire, Pain Impairment Rating Scale (PAIRS), Oswestry Back Pain Disability Questionnaire, Likert Scale, and Alzheimer's Discomfort Rating Scale.

†Given the potential for illiteracy (see discussion, Chapter 1), it is suggested that questionnaires such as the Family/Personal History form be completed by the physical therapist or a trained member of the health care staff. The client is asked each question as part of the intake interview. Appropriate follow-up questions can be asked by the physical therapist at the time of the interview (or after reviewing the form when someone else conducts the intake interview).

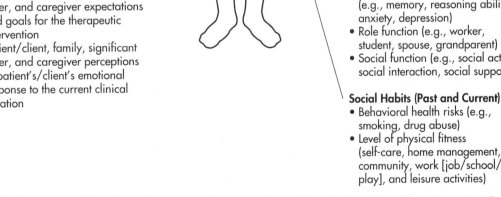

General Demographics
- Age
- Primary language
- Race/ethnicity
- Sex

Social History
- Cultural beliefs and behaviors
- Family and caregiver resources
- Social interactions, social activities, and support systems

Occupation/Employment
- Current or prior community and work (job/school) activities

Growth and Development
- Hand and foot dominance
- Developmental history

Living Environment
- Living environment and community characteristics
- Projected discharge destinations

History of Current Condition
- Concerns that led the individual to seek the services of a physical therapist
- Concerns or needs of patient/client who requires the services of a physical therapist
- Current therapeutic interventions
- Mechanisms of injury or disease, including date of onset and course of events
- Onset and pattern of symptoms
- Patient/client, family, significant other, and caregiver expectations and goals for the therapeutic intervention
- Patient/client, family, significant other, and caregiver perceptions of patient's/client's emotional response to the current clinical situation

Functional Status and Activity Level
- Current and prior functional status in self-care and home management, including activities of daily living (ADL) and instrumental activities of daily living (IADL)

Medications
- Medications for current condition for which patient/client is seeking the services of a physical therapist
- Medications for other conditions

Other Tests and Measures
- Laboratory and diagnostic tests
- Review of available records
- Review of nutrition and hydration

Past History of Current Condition
- Prior therapeutic interventions
- Prior medications

Past Medical/Surgical History
- Endocrine/metabolic
- Cardiopulmonary
- Gastrointestinal
- Genitourinary
- Integumentary
- Musculoskeletal
- Neuromuscular
- Pregnancy, delivery, and postpartum
- Prior hospitalizations, surgeries, and preexisting medical and other health-related conditions

Family History
- Familial health risks

Health Status (Self-Report, Family Report, Caregiver Report)
- General health perception
- Physical function (e.g., mobility, sleep patterns, energy, fatigue)
- Psychological function (e.g., memory, reasoning ability, anxiety, depression)
- Role function (e.g., worker, student, spouse, grandparent)
- Social function (e.g., social activity social interaction, social support)

Social Habits (Past and Current)
- Behavioral health risks (e.g., smoking, drug abuse)
- Level of physical fitness (self-care, home management, community, work [job/school/play], and leisure activities)

FIGURE 2-1 • Types of data that may be generated from a client history. (From Guide to physical therapist practice. *Phys Ther* 77(11):1182, 1997.)

regarding treatment or referral can be made immediately.

This treatment-versus-referral decision is further clarified as the interview and other objective evaluation procedures continue. Thus if further questioning fails to show any association of back pain with gastrointestinal symptoms and the objective findings from the back evaluation point to a true musculoskeletal lesion, medical referral is unnecessary and treatment with physical therapy can begin.

Each clinical situation requires slight adaptations or alterations to the interview. These modifications, in turn, affect the depth and range of questioning. For example, a client who has pain associated with an anterior shoulder dislocation and who has no history of other disease is unlikely to require in-depth questioning to rule out systemic origins of pain. Conversely, a woman with no history of trauma but with a previous history of breast cancer who is self-referred to the physical therapist without a previous medical examination and who complains of shoulder pain should be interviewed more thoroughly. The simple question "How will the answers to the questions I am asking permit me to help the client?" can serve as a guide to you (Wolf, 1977).

Continued questioning may occur both during the objective examination and during treatment. In fact, the physical therapist is encouraged to carry on a continuous dialogue during the objective examination, both as an educational tool (i.e., reporting findings and mentioning possible treatment alternatives) and as a method of reducing any apprehension on the part of the client. This open communication may bring to light other important information.

The client may wonder about the extensiveness of the interview, thinking, for example, "Why is the therapist asking questions about bowel function when my primary concern relates to back pain?" The physical therapist may need to make a qualifying statement to the client regarding the need for such detailed information. For example, questions about bowel function to rule out gallbladder involvement (which can refer pain to the back) may seem to be unrelated to the client but make sense when the physical therapist explains the possible connection between back pain and systemic disease.

Throughout the questioning, record both positive and negative findings in the subjective and objective reports in order to correlate information when making an initial assessment of the client's problem. Efforts should be made to quantify all information by frequency, intensity, duration, and exact location (including length, breadth, depth, and anatomic location).

This Family/Personal History form may be set up in a variety of ways. One type is outlined in the sample on pp. 43-45. More detailed information and follow-up questions can be found in subsequent chapters under each system heading.

Physical therapists may modify the information required depending on individual differences in client base and specialty areas served. For example, an orthopedic-based facility or a sports medicine center may want to include questions on the intake form concerning current level of fitness and orthopedic devices used, such as orthotics, splints, or braces. Physical therapists working with the geriatric population may want more information regarding current medications prescribed or levels of independence in activities of daily living.

Age and Aging

The age of a client is an important variable to consider when evaluating the underlying neuromusculoskeletal pathologic condition and when screening for medical disease. Table 2-2 provides some of the age-related systemic and neuromusculoskeletal pathologic conditions.

Of all the people who have ever lived to age 65 years, more than half are currently alive. Shortly after the year 2020, there will be more Americans older than age 65 than younger than age 13. Enrollment in Medicaid/Medicare has increased steadily since 1993, with the number of home health care visits financed by Medicare reaching 280 million in 1996. Although the implications of these startling statistics are usually viewed

FAMILY/PERSONAL HISTORY

DATE: _____

Client's Name: _____ DOB:_____ Age: _____

Diagnosis: _____ Date of onset: _____

Physician: _____ Date of surgery (if any): _____ Therapist: _____

Past Medical History

Have you or any immediate family member ever been told you have:

Circle one:

(Do **NOT** complete) **For the therapist:**

		Relation to Client	Date of Onset	Current Status
• Cancer	Yes No			
• Diabetes	Yes No			
• Hypoglycemia	Yes No			
• Hypertension or high blood pressure	Yes No			
• Heart disease	Yes No			
• Angina or chest pain	Yes No			
• Shortness of breath	Yes No			
• Stroke	Yes No			
• Kidney disease/stones	Yes No			
• Urinary tract infection	Yes No			
• Allergies	Yes No			
• Asthma, hay fever	Yes No			
• Rheumatic/scarlet fever	Yes No			
• Hepatitis/jaundice	Yes No			
• Cirrhosis/liver disease	Yes No			
• Polio	Yes No			
• Chronic bronchitis	Yes No			
• Pneumonia	Yes No			
• Emphysema	Yes No			
• Migraine headaches	Yes No			
• Anemia	Yes No			
• Ulcers/stomach problems	Yes No			
• Depression	Yes No			
• Chemical dependency (alcohol/drugs)	Yes No			

Therapists: Use this space to record baseline information. This is important in case something changes in the client's status. You are advised to record the date and initial this form for documentation and liability purposes, indicating that you have reviewed this form with the client.

continued

Circle one:

		(Do **NOT** complete) **For the therapist:**		
		Relation to Client	Date of Onset	Current Status
• Arthritis/gout	Yes No			
• Hemophilia/slow healing	Yes No			
• Guillain-Barré syndrome	Yes No			
• Epilepsy	Yes No			
• Thyroid problems	Yes No			
• Multiple sclerosis	Yes No			
• Tuberculosis	Yes No			
• Fibromyalgia/myofascial pain syndrome	Yes No			
• Other (please describe)	Yes No			

General Health

1. Are you taking any prescription or over-the-counter medications?   Yes   No
   If yes, please list:
2. Have you had any illnesses within the last 3 weeks (e.g., colds, influenza,   Yes   No
   bladder or kidney infection)?
3. Have you noticed any lumps or thickening of skin or muscle anywhere on
   your body?   Yes   No
4. Do you have any sores that have not healed or any changes in size, shape,
   or color of a wart or mole?   Yes   No
5. Have you had any unexplained weight gain or loss in the last month?   Yes   No
6. Do you smoke or chew tobacco?   Yes   No
   If yes, how many packs a day? _____ For how many
   months or years? _____
7. How much alcohol do you drink in the course of a week?

   _____
8. Do you use recreational drugs (marijuana, cocaine, crack, amphetamines,   Yes   No
   etc.)? If yes, what, how much, how often? _____

   _____
9. How much caffeine do you consume daily (including soft drinks, coffee,
   tea, or chocolate)? _____
10. Are you on any special diet prescribed by a physician?   Yes   No
11. Do you have a pacemaker, transplanted organ, joint replacements, or   Yes   No
    metal implants?

continued

Medical Testing

1. Have you had any x-rays, sonograms, computed tomography (CT) scans,   Yes   No
   or magnetic resonance imaging (MRI) done recently?
   If yes, when?   Where?   Results?
2. Have you had any laboratory work done recently (urinalysis or blood tests)?   Yes   No
   If yes, when?   Where?   Results (if known)?
3. Please list any operations that you have ever had and the date(s):
   Operation   Date

Work Environment

Occupation:
Does your job involve: [ ] prolonged sitting (e.g., desk, computer, driving)
                                [ ] prolonged standing (e.g., equipment operator, sales clerk)
                                [ ] prolonged walking (e.g., mill worker, delivery service)
                                [ ] use of large or small equipment (e.g., telephone, forklift,
                                     typewriter, drill press, cash register)
                                [ ] lifting, bending, twisting, climbing, turning
                                [ ] exposure to chemicals, pesticides, toxins, or gases
                                [ ] other: please describe

Do you use any special supports: [ ] back cushion, neck cushion
                                  [ ] back brace, corset
                                  [ ] other kind of brace or support for any body part

History of falls: [ ] I have had no falls.
                                [ ] I have just started to lose my balance/fall.
                                [ ] I fall occasionally.
                                [ ] I fall frequently (more than two times during the past 6 months).
                                [ ] Certain factors make me cautious (e.g., curbs, ice, stairs, getting
                                     in and out of the tub).

For the physical therapist:

Vital Signs

Resting pulse rate:
Oral temperature:
Blood pressure: 1st reading _____   2nd reading _____
                        Position: Extremity:

TABLE 2-2 ▼ Some Age-Related Medical Conditions

Diagnosis	Sex	Age in (Years)
Neuromusculoskeletal		
Guillain-Barré syndrome		Any age; history of infection/alcoholism
Multiple sclerosis		15–50
Rotator cuff degeneration		30+
Spinal stenosis	Men > women	60+
Tietze's syndrome		Before 40, including children
Costochondritis	Women > men	40+
Neurogenic claudication		40–60+
Systemic		
AIDS/HIV	Men > women	20–49
Buerger's disease	Men > women	20–40 (smokers)
Abdominal aortic aneurysm	(Hypertensive) Men > women	40–70
Cancer		See Table 10–3
Breast cancer	Women > men	45–70 (peak incidence)
Hodgkin's disease	Men > women	20–40; 50–60
Osteoid osteoma (benign)	Men > women	10–20
Pancreatic carcinoma	Men > women	50–70
Skin cancer	Men = women	Rarely before puberty
Gallstones	Women > men	40+
Gout	Men > women	40–59
Gynecologic conditions	Women	20–45 (peak incidence)
Prostatitis	Men	40+
Primary biliary cirrhosis	Women > men	40–60
Reiter's syndrome	Men > women	20–40
Renal tuberculosis	Men > women	20–40
Rheumatic fever	Girls > boys	4–9; 18–30
Shingles		60+
Spontaneous pneumothorax	Men> women	20–40
Systemic backache		45+
Thyroiditis	Women > men	30–50
Vascular claudication		40–60+

in demographic and economic terms, the impact of age on medical care is also substantial and requires significant alterations in the approach to the older client.

Human aging is best characterized as the progressive constriction of each organ system's homeostatic reserve. This decline, often referred to as "homeo-stenosis," begins in the third decade and is gradual, linear, and variable among individuals. Each organ system's decline is independent of changes in other organ systems and is influenced by diet, environment, and personal habits.

An abrupt change or sudden decline in any system or function is always due to disease and not to "normal aging." In the absence of disease the decline in homeostatic reserve should cause no symptoms and impose no restrictions on activities of daily living regardless of age. In short, "old people are sick because they are sick, not because they are old."

The onset of a new disease in older people generally affects the most vulnerable organ system, which often is different from the newly diseased organ system and explains why disease presentation is so atypical in this population. For example, at presentation, less than one fourth of older clients with hyperthyroidism have the classic triad of goiter, tremor, and exophthalmos; more likely symptoms are atrial fibrillation, confusion, depression, syncope, and weakness.

Because the "weakest link" is so often the brain, lower urinary tract, or cardiovascular or musculoskeletal system, a limited number of presenting symptoms predominate no matter what the underlying disease. These include:

- Acute confusion
- Depression
- Falling
- Incontinence
- Syncope

The corollary is equally important: The organ system usually associated with a particular symptom is less likely to be the cause of that symptom in older individuals than in younger ones. For example, acute confusion in older patients is less often due to a new brain lesion, incontinence is less often due to a bladder disorder; falling, to a neuropathy; or syncope, to heart disease.

For women, gender-linked protection against coronary artery disease ends with menopause. At age 45 years, one in nine women develops heart disease. By age 65 years, this statistic changes to one in three women. Women who have heart attacks are twice as likely as men to die within the first 2 weeks. Whether this is due to discriminatory medicine, natural physiologic differences between men and women, or some other factor is under investigation at this time.

Past Medical History

The initial Family/Personal History form also provides the physical therapist with some idea of the client's previous medical history, medical testing, and current general health status. It is important to take time with these questions and to ensure that the client understands what is being asked. As stated earlier, the interviewer may follow up on any "yes" response on the intake form. For example, a "yes" response to questions on this form directed toward *allergies, asthma,* and *hay fever* should be followed up by asking the client to list the allergies and to list the symptoms that may indicate a manifestation of allergies, asthma, or hay fever. The physical therapist can then be alert for any signs of respiratory distress or allergic reactions during exercise or with the use of topical agents.

Likewise, clients may indicate the presence of *shortness of breath* with only mild exertion or without exertion, possibly even after waking at night. This condition of breathlessness can be associated with one of many conditions, including heart disease, bronchitis, asthma, obesity, emphysema, dietary deficiencies, pneumonia, and lung cancer. A "yes" response to any question in this section would require further questioning, correlation to objective findings, and consideration of referral to the client's physician.

General Health

Medications. Although the Family/Personal History form includes a question about prescription or over-the-counter (OTC) medications, the follow-up questions come later in the Core Interview under Medical Treatment and Medications. Further discussion about this topic can be found in that section of this chapter.

Recent Infections. Recent infections such as mononucleosis, hepatitis, or upper respiratory infections may precede the onset of Guillain-Barré syndrome. Recent colds, influenza, or upper respiratory infections may also be an extension of a chronic health pattern of systemic illness. Further questioning may reveal recurrent influenza-like symptoms associated with headaches and musculoskeletal complaints. These complaints could originate with medical problems, such as endocarditis (a bacterial infection of the heart) or pleuropulmonary disorders, which should be ruled out by a physician.

Knowing that the client has had a recent bladder, vaginal, uterine, or kidney infection, or that the client is likely to have such infections, may help explain back pain in the absence of any musculoskeletal findings. The client may or may not confirm previous back pain associated with previous infections. If there is any doubt, a medical referral is recommended. On the other hand, chest or sacroiliac pain may be caused by repeated coughing after a recent upper respiratory infection.

Screening for Cancer. Any "yes" responses to early screening questions for cancer (General Health questions 3, 4, and 5) must be followed up by a physician. Changes in appetite and unexplained weight loss can be associated with cancer, onset of diabetes, hyperthyroidism, depression, or pathologic anorexia (loss of appetite). Weight loss significant for neoplasm would be a 10 percent loss of total body weight over a 4-week period unrelated to any intentional diet or fasting.

A significant, unexplained weight gain can be caused by congestive heart failure, hypothyroidism, or cancer. A key "red flag" symptom is demonstrated by the person with back pain who, despite reduced work levels and decreased activity, experiences unexplained weight loss. Weight gain/loss does not always correlate with appetite. For example, weight gain associated with neoplasm may be accompanied by appetite loss, whereas weight gain associated with hyperthyroidism may be accompanied by increased appetite. An in-depth discussion of screening for cancer is presented in Chapter 10.

Substance Abuse. According to the National Institute on Drug Abuse, if every worker between ages 18 and 40 were tested for drugs on any given day, between 14 percent and 25 percent would test positive. Looking at a broader perspective of substances and including older adults would increase the percentage dramatically. *Substance* refers to all mood-affecting chemicals. Among the substances most commonly used that cause druglike reactions but are not usually thought of as drugs are alcohol, tobacco, coffee, black tea, and caffeinated carbonated beverages.

Other substances commonly abused include *depressants* such as alcohol, barbiturates (barbs, downers, pink ladies, rainbows, reds, yellows, sleeping pills), *stimulants* such as amphetamines and cocaine (crack, coke, snow, white, lady, blow, rock), *opiates* (heroin), *cannabis derivatives* (marijuana, hashish), and *hallucinogens* (LSD or acid, mescaline, magic mushroom, PCP, angel dust).

Behavioral and physiologic responses to any of these substances depend on the characteristics of the chemical itself, the route of administration, and the adequacy of the client's circulatory system (Table 2-3).

Questions designed to screen for the presence of chemical substance abuse need to become part of the physical therapy assessment. Clients who depend on alcohol and/or other substances require lifestyle intervention. However, direct questions may be offensive to some people and identifying a person as an alcohol abuser often results in referral to professionals who treat alcoholics, a label that is not accepted in the early stage of this condition.

Because of the controversial nature of interviewing the alcohol- or drug-dependent client, the questions in this section of the Family/Personal History form are suggested as a guideline for interviewing. After (or possibly instead of) asking questions about use of alcohol, tobacco, caffeine, and other chemical substances, the therapist may want to use a new screening approach that makes no mention of alcohol but asks about previous trauma. Follow-up questions include (Israel et al, 1996):

- Have you had any fractures or dislocations to your bones or joint?
- Have you been injured in a road traffic accident?
- Have you injured your head?
- Have you been in a fight or assault?

These questions are based on the established correlation between trauma and alcohol use. "Yes" answers to two or more of these questions should be reported to the physician. Depending on how the interview has proceeded thus far, the therapist may want to conclude with one final question: "Are there any drugs or substances you take that you haven't mentioned?" Other screening tools for assessing alcohol abuse are available, as are more complete guidelines for interviewing this population (see Coulehan and Block, 1997; Goodman and Boissonnault, 1998).

TABLE 2-3 ▼ Specific Effects and Adverse Reactions to Substances

Caffeine	Cannabis	Depressants*	Narcotics	Stimulants	Tobacco
Nervousnes	Short-term memory loss	Vasodilation	Euphoria	Increased alertness	Increased heart rate
Irritability	Sedation	Fatigue	Drowsiness	Excitation	Vasoconstriction
Agitation	Tachycardia	Depression	Respiratory depression	Euphoria	Decreased oxygen to heart
Sensory disturbances	Euphoria	Altered pain perception		Increased pulse rate	Increased risk of thrombosis
Tachypnea	Increased appetite	Slurred speech		Increased blood pressure	Loss of appetite
Urinary frequency	Relaxed inhibitions	Altered behavior		Insomnia	Poor wound healing
Sleep disturbances	Fatigue	Slow, shallow breathing		Loss of appetite	
Fatigue	Paranoia	Clammy skin		Agitation, increased body temperature, hallucinations, convulsions, death (overdose)	
Muscle tension	Psychosis	Coma (overdose)			
Headaches	Ataxia, tremor				
Intestinal disorders	Paresthesias				
Enhances pain perception					
Heart palpitation					
Vasoconstriction					

From Goodman CC, Boissonnault WG: *Pathology: implications for the physical therapist,* Philadelphia, 1998, WB Saunders, p 14.
*Includes alcohol.

Tobacco. In 1996 the American Physical Therapy Association (APTA) endorsed Agency for Health Care Policy and Research (AHCPR) Clinical Practice Guideline No. 18 on smoking cessation.* As primary care providers, we have an important obligation to assess tobacco use and incorporate smoking cessation education into the physical therapy plan.

Nicotine in tobacco, whether in the form of chewing tobacco or pipe or cigarette smoking, acts directly on the heart, blood vessels, digestive tract, kidneys, and nervous system. For the client with respiratory or cardiac problems, nicotine stimulates the already compensated heart to beat faster, narrows the blood vessels, reduces the supply of oxygen to the heart and other organs, and increases the chances of developing blood clots.

The combination of coffee ingestion and smoking raises the blood pressure of hypertensive clients about 15/30 mm Hg for as long as 2 hours. All these effects have a direct impact on the client's ability to exercise and must be considered when the client is starting an exercise program.

Smoking markedly increases the need for vitamin C, which is poorly stored in the body. One cigarette can consume 25 mg of vitamin C (one pack would consume 500 mg/day). The capillary fragility associated with low ascorbic acid levels greatly increases the tendency for tissue bleeding, especially at injection sites (Travell and Simons, 1983). The detrimental effects of cigarette smoking on wound healing and peripheral circulation are well known.

Smoking has been linked with acute lumbar and cervical intervertebral disk herniation (Frymoyer et al, 1983; Heliövaara et al, 1987; Holm and Nachemson, 1988).

*Single copies of *Helping smokers quit: a guide for primary care clinicians, Smoking cessation: information for specialists,* and *You can quit smoking* (Consumer Guide) can be obtained from AHCPR Publications Clearinghouse, P.O. Box 8547, Silver Spring, MD 20907, 800-358-9295. Electronic versions of these publications are available through the Internet (http://www.ahcpr.gov/clinic/).

Alcohol. The National Institute on Alcohol Abuse and Alcoholism reports that 2 to 10 percent of individuals aged 65 years or older are alcoholics. That percentage translates into about 3 million older Americans and is likely a gross underestimate. As the graying of America continues, this figure may escalate, especially as "baby boomers" (people born between 1945 and 1960), having grown up in an age of alcohol and substance abuse, carry that practice into old age.

Alcohol is a toxic drug that is harmful to all body tissues. It has both vasodilatory and depressant effects that may produce fatigue and mental depression or alter the client's perception of pain or symptoms.

Besides deleterious effects on the gastrointestinal, hepatic, cardiovascular, hematopoietic, genitourinary, and neuromuscular systems, prolonged use of excessive alcohol may affect bone metabolism, resulting in reduced bone formation, disruption of the balance between bone formation and resorption, and incomplete mineralization (Schapira, 1990). Alcoholics are often malnourished, which exacerbates the direct effects of alcohol on bones. Alcohol-induced osteoporosis (the predominant bone condition in most people with cirrhosis) may progress for years without any obvious symptoms.

Regular consumption of alcohol may indirectly perpetuate trigger points through reduced serum and tissue folate levels. Ingestion of alcohol reduces the absorption of folic acid, while increasing the body's need for it (Travell and Simons, 1983). Of additional interest to physical therapists is the fact that alcohol diminishes the accumulation of neutrophils necessary for "clean-up" of all foreign material present in inflamed areas. This phenomenon results in delayed wound healing and recovery from inflammatory processes involving tendons, bursae, and joint structures.

Alcohol may interact with prescribed medications to produce various effects, including death. Unless the client has a chemical dependency on alcohol, appropriate education may be sufficient for the client experiencing negative effects of alcohol use during physical therapy treatment.

If the client's breath smells of alcohol, you may want to say more directly:

- I can smell alcohol on your breath right now. How many drinks have you had today?

As a follow-up to such direct questions, you may want to say:

- Alcohol, tobacco, and caffeine often increase our perception of pain, mask or even increase other symptoms, and delay healing. I would like to ask you to limit as much as possible your use of any of these stimulants. At the very least, it would be better if you didn't drink alcohol before our therapy sessions, so I can accurately assess your symptoms and progress and move along quickly through our treatment plan.

Caffeine. Caffeine is a known stimulant drug. Caffeine ingested in toxic amounts (more than 250 mg/day, or three cups of caffeinated coffee) has many effects, including nervousness, irritability, agitation, sensory disturbances, tachypnea (rapid breathing), heart palpitations (strong, fast, or irregular heartbeat), nausea, urinary frequency, diarrhea, and fatigue.

People who drink 8 to 15 cups of caffeinated beverages per day have been known to have problems with sleep, dizziness, restlessness, headaches, muscle tension, and intestinal disorders. Caffeine may enhance the client's perception of pain. Pain levels can be reduced dramatically by reducing the daily intake of caffeine.

In large doses caffeine is a stressor, but the withdrawal from caffeine can be equally stressful. Withdrawal from caffeine induces a withdrawal syndrome of headaches, lethargy, fatigue, poor concentration, nausea, impaired psychomotor performance, and emotional instability, which begins within 12 to 24 hours and lasts about 1 week (Hughes et al, 1993; Hughes et al, 1998). Other sources of caffeine are tea (black and

Case Example. A 44-year-old man previously seen in the physical therapy clinic for a fractured calcaneus returns to the same therapist 3 years later because of new onset of midthoracic back pain. There was no known cause or injury associated with the presenting pain. This man had been in the construction business for 30 years and attributed his symptoms to "general wear and tear."

Although there were objective findings to support a musculoskeletal cause of pain, the client also mentioned symptoms of fatigue, stomach upset, insomnia, hand tremors, and headaches. From the previous treatment period, the therapist recalled a history of substantial use of alcohol, tobacco, and caffeine (3 six-packs of beer after work each evening, 2 pack/day cigarette habit, 18+ cups of caffeinated coffee during work hours).

The therapist pointed out the potential connection between the client's symptoms and the level of substance use, and the client agreed to "pay more attention to cutting back." After 3 weeks the client returned to work with a reduction of back pain from a level of 8 to a level of 0-3 (intermittent symptoms), depending on the work assignment.

Six weeks later this client returned again with the same symptomatic and clinical presentation. At that time, given the client's age, the insidious onset, the cyclic nature of the symptoms, and significant substance abuse, the therapist recommended a complete physical with a primary care physician. Medical treatment with antiinflammatories caused considerable gastrointestinal upset, which persisted after the client stopped taking the nonsteroidal antiinflammatory drugs. Further medical diagnostic testing determined the presence of pancreatic carcinoma. The prognosis was poor, and the client died 6 months later, after extensive medical intervention.

In this case it could be argued that the therapist should have referred the client to a physician immediately because of the history of substance abuse and the presence of additional symptoms. A more thorough screening examination during the first treatment for back pain may have elicited additional red-flag gastrointestinal symptoms (e.g., melena or bloody diarrhea in addition to the stomach upset). Earlier referral for a physical examination may have resulted in earlier diagnosis and treatment for the cancer. Unfortunately, these clinical situations occur often and are very complex, requiring ongoing screening (as happened here).

green), cocoa, chocolate, caffeinated carbonated beverages, and some drugs, including many over-the-counter medications.

Cocaine and Amphetamines. Cocaine and amphetamines affect the cardiovascular system in the same manner as does stress (Majid et al, 1992). The drugs stimulate the sympathetic nervous system to increase its production of adrenaline. Surging adrenaline causes severe constriction of the arteries, a sharp rise in blood pressure, rapid and irregular heartbeats, and seizures (Christan et al, 1990). Heart rate can accelerate by as much as 60 to 70 beats per minute. In otherwise healthy and fit people, this overload can cause death in minutes, even to first-time cocaine users. In addition, cocaine can cause the aorta to rupture, the lungs to fill with fluid, the heart muscle and its lining to become inflamed, blood clots to form in the veins, and strokes to occur as a result of cerebral hemorrhage.

Medical Testing

Tests contributing information to the physical therapy assessment may include radiography (x-rays, sonograms), computed tomography (CT) scans, magnetic resonance imaging (MRI), lumbar puncture analysis, urinalysis, and blood tests. The client's medical records may contain information regarding which tests have been performed and the results of the test. It may be helpful to question the client directly by asking:

• What medical test have you had for this condition?

After giving the client time to respond, you may need to probe further by asking:

• Have you had any x-ray films, sonograms, CT scans, or MRIs in the last 2 years?

• Do you recall having any blood tests or urinalyses done?

If the response is affirmative, the physical therapist will want to know when and where these tests were performed and the results (if known to the client). Knowledge of where the test took place provides the therapist with access to the results (with the client's written permission for disclosure).

As often as possible, the physical therapist will want to examine the available test results either with a radiologist or with the client's physician or assistant. Familiarity with the results of these tests, combined with an understanding of the clinical presentation, can assist physical therapists in knowing what to look for clinically with future clients and to offer some guidelines for knowing when to suggest or recommend additional testing for clients who have not had a radiologic workup or other potentially appropriate medical testing.

Laboratory values of interest to physical therapists are displayed on the inside covers of this book.

Previous Surgery. Previous surgery or surgery related to the client's current symptoms may be indicated on the Family/ Personal History form. Whenever treating a client postoperatively, the physical therapist should try to read the surgical report and should look for notes on complications, blood transfusions, and the position of the client during the surgery and the length of time in that position.

Clients in an early postoperative stage (within 3 weeks of surgery) may have stiffness, aching, and musculoskeletal pain unrelated to the diagnosis, which may be attributed to position during the surgery. Postoperative infections can lie dormant for months. Accompanying constitutional symptoms may be minimal with no sweats, fever, or chills until the infection progresses with worsening of symptoms or significant change in symptoms.

Specific follow-up questions differ from one client to another depending on the type of surgery, age of client, accompanying medical history, and so forth, but it is always helpful to assess how quickly the client recovered from surgery to determine an appropriate pace for a therapy treatment program.

Work Environment

Questions related to the client's daily work activities and work environments are included in the Family/Personal History to assist the physical therapist in planning a program of client education that is consistent with the objective findings and proposed treatment plan.

For example, the physical therapist is alerted to the need for follow-up with a client complaining of back pain who sits for prolonged periods without a back support or cushion. Likewise, a worker involved in bending and twisting who complains of lateral thoracic pain may be describing a muscular strain from repetitive overuse. These work-related questions may help the client report significant data contributing to symptoms that may otherwise have been undetected.

Occupation. Questions related to occupation and exposure to toxins such as chemicals or gases are included because well-defined physical (e.g., cumulative trauma disorder) and health problems occur in people engaging in specific occupations (Newman, 1995).

For example, military service at various periods has potential association with known diseases. Seven diseases (asthma, laryngitis, chronic bronchitis, emphysema, and three eye ailments) have been identified by the Department of Veterans Affairs as associated with soldiers' exposure to toxic chemicals during World War II (P.T. Bulletin, 1993).

Similarly, survivors of the Vietnam War who have been exposed to the defoliant Agent Orange are at risk for developing soft tissue sarcoma, non-Hodgkin's lymphoma, Hodgkin's disease, and a skin-blistering disease called chloracne.

The cause of the Gulf War syndrome, with its multiple clusters of signs and symptoms (e.g., chronic fatigue, memory loss, joint pain and inflammation, and other musculoskeletal disorders), remains undetermined at this time. Research has investigated chemical agents, sandfly-borne parasites, nerve gas, and other possible biologic and chemical weapons attacks.

After determining the client's occupation and depending on the client's chief complaint and accompanying associated signs and symptoms, the therapist may want to ask (Newman, 1995):

- Do you think your health problems are related to your work?

- Are your symptoms better or worse when you are at home or at work?

- Are you now or have you previously been exposed to dusts, fumes, chemicals, radiation, loud noise, tools that vibrate, or a new building/office space?

- Do others at work have similar problems?

History of Falls. This question may help the therapist to assess balance and function of the aging population. Well older adults have no falling patterns but may have a fear of falling in specific instances (e.g., getting out of the bath or shower; walking on ice, curbs, or uneven terrain). Elderly clients who have just started to fall or who fall frequently may be fearful of losing their independence by revealing this information even to a physical therapist. Even if the client indicates no difficulty with falling, the therapist is encouraged to review this part of the form carefully with each older client.

During the Core Interview, the physical therapist will have an opportunity to ask further questions about the client's Current Level of Fitness (see discussion later in this chapter). With careful questioning, any potential problems with balance may come to light. Such information will alert the therapist to the need for testing static and dynamic balance and to look for potential systemic or medical causes of falls (see accompanying box, next page).*

Other examples include pesticide exposure among agricultural workers, asthma and sick building syndrome among office workers, lung disease in miners, silicosis in those who must work near silica, and tuberculosis in health care workers.

Each geographic area has its own specific environmental/occupational concerns but overall, the chronic exposure to chemically based products and pesticides has escalated the incidence of environmental allergies and cases of multiple chemical sensitivity. Frequently, these conditions present in a physical therapy setting with nonspecific neuromusculoskeletal manifestations (Radetsky, 1997).

---

*The subject of balance impairment and falls as it relates to medications and medical conditions exceeds the scope of this text but is very important in the diagnostic and screening process. As an example, orthostatic hypotension as a risk factor for falls may occur as a result of volume depletion (e.g., diabetes mellitus, sodium or potassium depletion), venous pooling (e.g., pregnancy, varicosities of the legs, immobility following a motor vehicle or cerebrovascular accident), side effects of medications such as antihypertensives, starvation associated with anorexia or cachexia, and sluggish normal regulatory mechanisms associated with anatomic variations or secondary to other conditions such as metabolic disorders or diseases of the central nervous system. The therapist must remain alert to such details and is referred to more appropriate texts for more information (see Goodman and Boissonnault, 1998).

CAUSES OF FALLS

AGE CHANGES

Muscle weakness
Decreased balance
Impaired proprioception or sensation
Delayed muscle response time/increased reaction time

ENVIRONMENTAL

Poor lighting
Throw rugs, loose carpet, complex carpet designs
Cluster of electric wires or cords
Stairs without handrails
Bathrooms without grab bars
Slippery floors (water, urine, floor surface)
Restraints
Footwear, especially slippers
Use of alcohol

PATHOLOGIC CONDITIONS

Vestibular disorders
Orthostatic hypotension (especially before breakfast)
Neuropathies
Osteoarthritis
Osteoporosis
Visual or hearing impairment
Cardiovascular disease
Urinary incontinence
Central nervous system disorders (e.g., stroke, Parkinson's disease, multiple sclerosis)

MEDICATIONS

Antihypertensives
Sedative-hypnotics
Antidepressants
Antipsychotics
Diuretics
Narcotics
Use of more than four medications

OTHER

Elder abuse/assault
Nonambulatory status (requiring transfers)
Gait changes (decreased stride length or speed)
Postural instability
Fear of falling

Vital Signs

Assessment of baseline vital signs, including resting pulse, blood pressure, and temperature should be a part of the initial data collected so that correlations and comparisons with the baseline are available when necessary. Support staff can be trained to perform these simple tests. Normal ranges of values for the vital signs are provided for your convenience. However, these ranges can be exceeded by a client and still represent normality for that person. It is the unusual vital sign in combination with other signs and symptoms, medications, and medical status that gives clinical meaning to the pulse rate, blood pressure, and temperature.

Pulse Rate. A resting pulse rate (normal range: 60 to 100 beats/min), taken at the carotid artery or radial artery pulse point, should be available for comparison with the pulse rate taken during treatment or after exercise.* A rate above 100 beats per minute indicates tachycardia; below 60 beats per minute indicates bradycardia.

Pulse amplitude (weak or bounding quality of the pulse) that fades with inspiration and strengthens with expiration is *paradoxic* and should be reported to the physician. A pulse increase with activity of more than 20 beats per minute lasting for more than 3 minutes after rest or changing position should also be reported.

The resting pulse may be higher than normal with fever, anemia, infections, some medications, hyperthyroidism, anxiety, or pain. Other medications, such as beta-blockers and calcium channel blockers may prevent the normal rise in pulse rate that occurs during exercise.

Blood Pressure. Blood pressure is the measurement of pressure in an artery at the peak of systole (contraction of the left ventricle) and during diastole (when the heart is at rest after closure of the aortic valve, which prevents blood from flowing back to the heart chambers). The measurement (in mm Hg) is listed as systolic (contraction phase)/diastolic (relaxation phase).

The normal range differs slightly with age and varies greatly among individuals. Normal systolic pressure ranges from 100 to 140 mm Hg, and diastolic pressure ranges from 60 to 90 mm Hg. It is more accurate to evaluate consecutive blood pressure readings over time rather than to make an isolated measurement for reporting blood pressure abnormalities. Blood pressure also should be correlated with any related diet or medication.

The blood pressure should be taken in the same arm and in the same position (supine or sitting) each time it is measured. This information should be recorded with the initial reading (see Family/Personal History form). Blood pressure depends on many factors, including age, vessel, size, blood viscosity, force of contraction, current medications, diet, time of last meal (systolic drops after eating, especially among older adults), amount of caffeine or alcohol ingested, and presence or perceived degree of pain.

Hypotension is a systolic pressure below 95 mm Hg or a diastolic pressure below 60 mm Hg. *Hypertension* is a systolic pressure above 140 mm Hg or a diastolic pressure above 90 mm Hg. The difference between the systolic and diastolic pressure readings is called *pulse pressure*. A difference of more than 40 mm Hg is abnormal and should be reported. The overall goal of treating clients with hypertension is to prevent morbidity and mortality associated with high blood pressure. The specific objective is to achieve and maintain arterial blood pressure below 140/80 mm Hg, if possible† (Frohlich, 1997).

---

*It is recommended that the pulse always be checked in two places in older adults and in anyone with diabetes.

†In recent years an unexpected increase in illness and death caused by hypertension has prompted the National Institutes of Health to issue new treatment guidelines to reflect the need for more effective blood pressure control. The ideal blood pressure level of lower than 120/80 mm Hg has been recommended (see discussion, Chapter 3). Achieving this level through lifestyle changes (e.g., losing weight; regular aerobic exercise; limiting salt, alcohol, and dietary fat; and increasing intake of fruits and vegetables) is the first treatment approach for anyone without other health conditions.

Postural hypotension is defined as a blood pressure fall of more than 10 to 15 mm Hg of the systolic pressure or more than 10 mm Hg of the diastolic pressure *and* a 10 to 20 percent increase in heart rate; changes must be noted in *both* the blood pressure and the heart rate.

Gravitational effects on the circulator system can cause a 10 mm Hg drop in systolic blood pressure when a person changes position from supine to sitting to standing. This drop usually occurs without symptoms as the body quickly compensates to ensure no reduction in cardiac output. In clients on prolonged bed rest or on antihypertensive drug therapy, there may be either no reflexive increase in heart rate or a sluggish vasomotor response. These clients may experience larger drops in blood pressure and often experience lightheadedness.

A difference of 10 mm Hg in either systolic or diastolic measurements from one extremity to the other may be an indication of vascular problems (look for associated symptoms). With a change in position (supine to sitting), the normal fluctuation of blood pressure and heart rate increases slightly (about 5 mm Hg for systolic and diastolic pressures and 5 to 10 beats per minute in heart rate).

A slightly elevated blood pressure may be considered a normal finding in older adults as a protective mechanism to maintain adequate blood flow to the brain and essential organs. Blood pressure values greater than 180 mm Hg (systolic) and 100 mm Hg (diastolic) are treated in older clients toward a target value of 160/90 mm Hg.

Systolic pressure increases with age and with exertion in a linear progression. If systolic pressure does not rise as workload increases, or if this pressure falls, it may be an indication that the functional reserve capacity of the heart has been exceeded. For any person, exercise or activity should be reduced or stopped if the systolic pressure exceeds 225 mm Hg. Diastolic blood pressure increases during upper extremity exercise or isometric exercise involving any muscle group. Activity or exercise should be decreased or halted if the diastolic pres-

sure exceeds 130 mm Hg (Hillegass and Sadowsky, 1999).

Before reporting abnormal blood pressure readings, measure both sides for comparison, remeasure both sides, have another health professional check the readings, correlate blood pressure measurements with other vital signs, and screen for associated signs and symptoms such as pallor, fatigue, perspiration, and/or palpitations. A persistent rise or fall in blood pressure requires medical attention and possible intervention.

Temperature. Normal body temperature is not a specific number but a range of values that depends on factors such as the time of day, age, medical status, or presence of infection. Oral body temperature ranges from 36° to 37.5° C (96.8° to 99.5° F), with an average of 37° C (98.6° F).

There is a tendency among the aging population to develop an increase in temperature on hospital admission or in response to any change in homeostasis.

However, some persons with infectious disease remain afebrile, especially the immunocompromised, those with chronic renal disease, alcoholics, and older adults. Unexplained fever in adolescents may be a manifestation of drug abuse or endocarditis.

In the home health setting abscess formation 3 to 4 days postoperatively may appear as a hectic fever pattern with increases and declines of body temperature but no return to baseline (normal). Such a situation would warrant telephone consultation with the physician's office nurse.

Any client who has back, shoulder, hip, sacroiliac, or groin pain of unknown cause must have a temperature reading taken. Temperature should also be assessed for any client who has constitutional symptoms, especially night sweats (gradual increase followed by a sudden drop in body temperature), pain, or symptoms of unknown etiologic basis and for clients who have not been medically screened by a physician.

When measuring body temperature, the physical therapist should ask if the person's normal temperature differs from 37° C (98.6° F). It is also important to ask whether the client has taken aspirin or acetaminophen (Tylenol) to reduce the fever, which might mask an underlying problem.

The therapist should use discretionary caution with any client who has a fever. Exercise with a fever stresses the cardiopulmonary system, which may be further complicated by dehydration.

Core Interview

History of Present Illness

The history of present illness (often referred to as the chief complaint and other current symptoms) may best be obtained through the use of open-ended questions. This section of the interview is designed to gather information related to the client's reason(s) for seeking clinical treatment.

The following open-ended statements may be appropriate to start an interview:

- Tell me why you are here today.
- Tell me about your injury.
- (Alternatively) What do you think is causing your problem or pain?

During this initial phase of the interview, allow the client to carefully describe his or her current situation. Follow-up questions and paraphrasing can now be used in conduction with the primary, open-ended questions (see Core Interview on pp. 69-73).

Insidious Onset. When the client describes an insidious onset or unknown cause, it is important to ask further questions. Did the symptoms develop after a fall, trauma (including assault), or some repetitive activity (such as painting, cleaning, gardening, filing, or driving long distances)? The alert therapist may recognize causative factors requiring medical screening.

Likewise, the client may wrongly attribute the onset of symptoms to a particular activity that is really unrelated to the current symptoms. *When the symptoms seem out of proportion to the injury, or when the symptoms persist beyond the expected time for that condition, a red flag should be raised in the therapist's mind.*

Twenty-five percent of clients with primary malignant tumors of the musculoskeletal system report a prior traumatic episode. Often the trauma or injury brings attention to a preexisting malignant or benign tumor. Whenever a fracture occurs with minimal trauma or involves a transverse fracture line, the physician considers the possibility of a tumor. The presence of night pain or lack of change with activity or position is a red flag. A growing mass, whether painless or painful, is assumed to be a tumor unless diagnosed otherwise by a physician. A hematoma should decrease in size over time, not increase (Lane, 1990).

Finally, extrinsic trauma from a motor vehicle accident, assault, fall, or known accident or injury may result in intrinsic trauma to another part of the musculoskeletal system or other organ system. Such intrinsic trauma may be masked by the more critical injury and may become more symptomatic as the primary injury resolves.

Assault. In the move toward becoming primary service providers, physical therapists must be aware of the signs of assault associated with domestic violence and know how to respond appropriately. Domestic violence is a serious public health concern that often goes undetected by clinicians. Women (especially those who are pregnant or disabled), children, and older adults are at greatest risk, regardless of race, religion, or socioeconomic status. Early intervention may reduce the risk of future abuse.

Although some interviewing guidelines are presented here, questioning clients about abuse is a complex issue with important effects on the outcome of rehabilitation. All therapists are encouraged to familiarize themselves with the information available for screening and intervening in this area of clinical practice (APTA Guidelines for Recognizing and Providing Care for Victims of Domestic Violence, 1997*; Clark et al, 1996; Johnson, 1997).

Assault is defined as a physical or verbal attack. Domestic violence, according to the

---

*To order this document, call APTA's Service Center at 800-999-2782, ext. 3395.

APTA, is a pattern of coercive behaviors perpetrated by a current or former intimate partner that may include physical, sexual, and/or psychologic assaults (Ketter, 1997). Many people who have been physically struck, pushed, or kicked do not consider the

Clinical Signs and Symptoms of Domestic Violence

Physical Cues
- Bruises, black eyes, malnutrition, fractures
- Skin problems (e.g., eczema, sores that do not heal, burns)
- Chronic or migraine headaches
- Diffuse pain, vague or nonspecific symptoms
- Chronic injuries
- Vision and hearing loss
- Chronic low back, sacral, or pelvic pain
- Temporomandibular joint (TMJ) pain
- Dysphagia (difficulty swallowing) and easy gagging
- Gastrointestinal disorders

Social Cues
- Continually missing appointments
- Bringing all the children to a clinic appointment
- Spouse, companion, or partner always accompanying client
- Changing physicians often
- Multiple trips to the emergency department
- Multiple car accidents

Psychologic Cues
- Anorexia/bulimia
- Panic attacks, nightmares, phobias
- Hypervigilance, tendency to startle easily or be very guarded
- Substance abuse
- Depression, anxiety, insomnia
- Self-mutilation or suicide attempts
- Multiple personality disorders
- Mistrust of authority figures
- Demanding, angry, distrustful of health care provider

action assault, especially if it is inflicted by someone they know. Therefore it may be necessary to use some other word besides *assault* or *assaulted*. For example:

- Were you (or have you been) hit, kicked, or pushed?

Addressing the possibility of sexual or physical assault/abuse during the interview may not take place until the therapist has established a working relationship with the client. Each question must be presented in a sensitive, respectful manner with observation for nonverbal cues. It may be helpful to use lead-in statements such as: "We are required to ask everyone we see about domestic violence. Many of the people I treat tell me they are in difficult, hurtful, sometimes even violent relationships. Is this your situation?"

Follow-up questions will depend on the client's initial response. The following may be helpful:

- May I ask you a few more questions?

  If yes, has anyone ever touched you against your will?

  How old were you when it started? When it stopped?

  Have you ever told anyone about this?

On the other hand, although physical therapists should not turn away from signs of physical or sexual abuse, in attempting to address such a sensitive issue, the therapist must make sure that the client will not be endangered by intervention. Physical therapists who are not trained to be counselors should be careful about offering advice to those believed to have sustained abuse (or even those who have admitted abuse).

The best course of action may be to document all observations and, when necessary or appropriate, to communicate those documented observations to the referring or family physician, without offering any conclusions (Hulme, 1997). When an abused individual asks for help or direction, always be prepared to provide information about available community resources.

CLINICAL SIGNS AND SYMPTOMS

Physical injuries caused by battering are most likely to occur in a central pattern (i.e., head, neck, chest/breast, abdomen). Injuries to these areas are easily hidden by clothes, hats, or hair, but they are frequently observable by the therapist in a clinical setting that requires changing into a gown or similar treatment attire.

Assessment of Pain and Symptoms

Characteristics of Pain. It is very important to identify how the client's description of pain as a symptom relates to sources and types of pain discussed in Chapter 1. Many characteristics of pain can be elicited from the client during the Core Interview to help define the source or type of pain in question. These characteristics include:

- Location
- Description of sensation
- Pattern
- Frequency
- Intensity or duration

Other additional components are related to factors that aggravate the pain, factors that relieve the pain, and other symptoms that may occur in association with the pain. Specific questions are included for each descriptive component. Keep in mind that an increase in frequency, intensity, or duration of symptoms over time can indicate systemic disease.

Location of Pain. Questions related to the location of pain focus the client's description as precisely as possible. An opening statement might be:

- Show me exactly where your pain is located.

Follow-up questions may include:

- Do you have any other pain or symptoms anywhere else?
  - If yes, what causes the pain or symptoms to occur in this other area?

If the client points to a small localized area and the pain does not spread, the cause is likely to be a superficial lesion and is probably not severe. If the client points to a small localized area but the

pain does spread, this is more likely to be a diffuse, segmental, referred pain that may originate in the viscera or deep somatic structure.

Description of Pain. To assist the physical therapist in obtaining a clear description of pain sensation, pose the question:

- What does it feel like?

Allow the client some choices in potential descriptors. Some common words might include:

Knifelike	Dull
Boring	Burning
Throbbing	Prickly
Deep aching	Sharp

Follow-up questions may include:

- Has the pain changed in quality since it first began?
- Changed in intensity?
- Changed in duration (how long it lasts)?

When a client describes the pain as knifelike, boring, colicky, coming in waves, or a deep aching feeling, this description should be a signal to the physical therapist to consider the possibility of a systemic origin of symptoms. Dull, somatic pain of an aching nature can be differentiated from the aching pain of a muscular lesion by squeezing or by pressing the muscle overlying the area of pain. This reproduces aching of muscular origin with no connection to deep somatic aching.

Pattern of Pain. After listening to the client describe the pain or symptoms, the therapist may recognize a vascular, neurogenic, musculoskeletal (including spondylogenic), emotional, or visceral pattern (Table 2-4). The following sequence of questions may be helpful in further assessing the pattern of pain, especially how the symptoms may change with time:

- Tell me about the pattern of your pain/symptoms.
- *Alternative question:* When does your back/shoulder (name the involved body part) hurt?
- *Alternative question:* Describe your pain/symptoms from first waking up in the

TABLE 2-4 ▼ Recognizing Pain Patterns

Vascular	Neurogenic	Musculoskeletal	Emotional
Throbbing	Stabbing	Aching	Tiring
Pounding	Crushing	Sore	Miserable
Pulsing	Pinching	Heavy	Vicious
Beating	Burning	Hurting	Agonizing
	Hot	Dull	Nauseating
	Searing		Frightful
	Itchy		Piercing
	Stinging		Dreadful
	Pulling		Punishing
	Jumping		Torturing
	Shooting		Killing
	Pricking		Unbearable
	Gnawing		Annoying

From Melzack R: The McGill Pain Questionnaire: major properties and scoring methods. *Pain* 1:277, 1975.

morning to going to bed at night. (See special sleep-related questions that follow.)

Follow-up questions may include:

- Have you ever experienced anything like this before?
  - If yes, do these episodes occur more or less often than at first?
- How does your pain/symptom(s) change with time?
- Are your symptoms worse in the morning or evening?

The pattern of pain associated with systemic disease is often a progressive pattern with a cyclical onset (i.e., the client describes symptoms as being alternately worse, better, and worse over a period of months). This pattern differs from the sudden sequestration of a discogenic lesion that appears with a pattern of increasingly worse symptoms followed by a sudden cessation of all symptoms. Such involvement of the disk occurs without the cyclical return of symptoms weeks or months later, which is more typical of a systemic disorder.

If the client appears to be unsure of the pattern of symptoms or has "avoided paying any attention" to this component of pain description, it may be useful to keep a record at home assisting the client to take note of the symptoms for 24 hours. A chart such as the McGill

Home Recording Card (Melzack, 1975) (Fig. 2-2) may help the client outline the existing pattern of the pain and can be used later in treatment to assist the therapist in detecting any change in symptoms or function.

A client frequently will comment that the pain or symptoms have not changed despite 2 or 3 weeks of treatment with physical therapy. This information can be discouraging to both client and therapist; however, when the symptoms are reviewed, a decrease in pain, increase in function, reduced need for medications, or other significant improvement in the pattern of symptoms may be seen. The improvement is usually gradual and is best documented through the use of a baseline of pain activity established at an early stage in treatment by using a record such as the Home Recording Card.

However, if no improvement in symptoms or function can be demonstrated, the therapist must again consider a systemic origin of symptoms. Repeating screening questions for medical disease is encouraged throughout the treatment process even if such questions were included in the intake interview. Because of the progressive nature of systemic involvement, the client may not have noticed any constitutional symptoms at the start of physical therapy treatment that may now be present. Constitutional symptoms (see box on p. 8) affect the whole body

---

McGill Home Recording Card

Name:_____   Date started: _____

	Morning	Noon	Dinner	Bedtime
M				
Tu				
W				
Th				
F				
Sa				
Su				

Please record:

1. Pain intensity #:
   0 = No pain
   1 = Mild
   2 = Discomforting
   3 = Distressing
   4 = Horrible
   5 = Excruciating

2. # analgesics taken

3. Note any unusual pain, symptoms, or activities on back of card.

4. Record # hours slept in morning column.

Please note: If the client previously rated the pain on a scale from 0–10, substitute the 0–10 scale in place of the 0–5 scale used to describe pain intensity.

FIGURE 2-2 • McGill Home Recording Card. (From Melzack R: The McGill Pain Questionnaire: major properties and scoring methods. *Pain* 1:298, 1975.)

and are characteristic of systemic disease or illness.

Frequency and Duration of Pain. The frequency of occurrence is related closely to the pattern of the pain, and the client should be asked how often the symptoms occur and whether the pain is constant or intermittent. Duration of pain is a part of this description.

• How long do the symptoms last?

For example, pain related to systemic disease has been shown to be a *constant* rather than an *intermittent* type of pain experience. Clients who indicate that the pain is constant should be asked:

• Do you have this pain right now?
• Did you notice these symptoms this morning immediately when you woke up?

Further responses may reveal that the pain is perceived as being constant but in fact is not actually present hourly and/or can be reduced with rest or position change, which is more characteristic of pain of musculoskeletal origin.

Intensity of Pain. The level or intensity of the pain is an extremely important, but difficult, component to assess in the overall pain profile. Assist the client with this evaluation by providing a rating scale. For example, the physical therapist might ask the client to rate the pain on a scale from 0 (no pain) to 10 (worst pain experienced with this condition).

An alternative method provides a scale of 1 to 5 with word descriptions for each number (Melzack, 1975) and asks:

• How strong is your pain?

1 = Mild
2 = Discomforting
3 = Distressing
4 = Horrible
5 = Excruciating

As with the Home Recording Card, this scale for measuring the intensity of pain can be used to establish a baseline measure of pain for future reference. A client who describes the pain as "excruciating" (or a 5 on the scale) during the initial interview may question the value of therapy when several weeks later there is no subjective report of improvement. A quick check of intensity by using this scale often reveals a decrease in the number assigned to pain levels. This can be compared with the initial rating, providing the client with assurance and encouragement in the rehabilitation process. A quick assessment using this method can be made by asking:

• How strong is your pain?

1 = Mild
2 = Moderate
3 = Severe

The description of intensity is highly subjective. What might be described as "mild" for one person could be "horrible" for another person. Careful assessment of the person's nonverbal behavior (e.g., ease of movement, facial grimacing, guarding movements) and correlation of the person's personality with his or her perception of the pain may help to clarify the description of the intensity of the pain. Pain of an intense, unrelenting (constant) nature is often associated with systemic disease.

Associated Symptoms. These symptoms may occur alone or in conjunction with the pain of systemic disease. The client may or may not associate these additional symptoms with the chief complaint. The physical therapist may ask:

• What other symptoms have you had that you can associate with this problem?

If the client denies any additional symptoms, follow up this question with a series of possibilities such as:

Burning
Difficulty in breathing
Difficulty in swallowing
Dizziness
Heart palpitations
Hoarseness
Nausea
Night sweats
Numbness
Problems with vision
Tingling
Vomiting
Weakness

Whenever the client says "yes" to such associated symptoms, check for the presence of these symptoms bilaterally. Also, bilateral weakness, either proximally or distally, should serve as an indicator of more than a musculoskeletal lesion.

Blurred vision, double vision, scotomas (black spots before the eyes), or temporary blindness may indicate early symptoms of multiple sclerosis or may possibly be warning signs of an impending cerebrovascular accident. The presence of any associated symptoms, such as those mentioned here, would require contact with the physician to confirm the physician's knowledge of these symptoms.

Aggravating/Relieving Factors. Finally, a series of questions addressing aggravating and relieving factors must be included. The McGill Pain Questionnaire provides a chart, shown in Fig. 2-3, that may be useful in determining the presence of relieving or aggravating factors (Melzack, 1975). A question related to aggravating factors could be:

	Indicate a plus (+) for aggravating factors or a minus (−) for relieving factors.		
	Liquor		Sleep/rest
	Stimulants (e.g., caffeine)		Lying down
	Eating		Distraction (e.g., television)
	Heat		Urination/defecation
	Cold		Tension/stress
	Weather changes		Loud noises
	Massage		Going to work
	Pressure		Intercourse
	No movement		Mild exercise
	Movement		Fatigue
	Sitting		Standing

FIGURE 2-3 ● Factors aggravating and relieving pain. (From Melzack R: The McGill Pain Questionnaire: major properties and scoring methods. *Pain* 1:277, 1975.)

- What kinds of things make your pain or symptoms worse (e.g., eating, exercise, rest, specific positions, excitement, stress)?

To assess relieving factors, ask:

- What makes the pain better?

Follow-up questions include:

- How does rest affect the pain/symptoms?
- Are your symptoms aggravated or relieved by any activities?
  - If yes, what?
- How has this problem affected your daily life at work or at home?
- How has this problem affected your ability to care for yourself without assistance (e.g., dress, bathe, cook, drive)?

Systemic pain tends to be relieved minimally, relieved only temporarily, or unrelieved by change in position or by rest. However, musculoskeletal pain is *often* relieved both by a change of position and by rest.

In summary, careful, sensitive, and thorough questioning regarding the multifaceted experience of pain can elicit essential information necessary when making a decision regarding treatment or referral. The use of pain assessment tools may facilitate clear and accurate descriptions of this critical symptom.

Medical Treatment and Medications

Medical Treatment. Medical treatment includes any intervention performed by a physician (family practitioner or specialist), dentist, physician's assistant, nurse, nurse practitioner, physical therapist, or occupational therapist. The client may also include

▼ *Clinical Signs and Symptoms of*
Systemic Pain

Onset
- Recent, sudden
- Does not present as chronically observed for several years intermittently

Description
- Knifelike quality of stabbing from the inside out, boring, deep aching
- Cutting, gnawing
- Throbbing
- Bone pain
- Unilateral or bilateral

Intensity (related to the degree of noxious stimuli; usually unrelated to presence of anxiety)
- Dull to severe
- Mild to severe

Duration
- Constant, no change, awakens the person at night

Pattern
- Although constant, may come in waves
- Gradually progressive, cyclic
- Night pain
- Symptoms unrelieved by rest or change in position
- Migratory arthralgias: Pain/symptoms last for 1 week in one joint, then resolve and appear in another joint

▼ *Clinical Signs and Symptoms of*
Musculoskeletal Pain

Onset (may be sudden or gradual, depending on the history)
- Sudden: Usually associated with acute overload stress, traumatic event, repetitive motion
- Gradual: Secondary to chronic overload of the affected part; may be present off and on for years

Description
- Local tenderness to pressure is present
- Achy, cramping pain
- May be stiff after prolonged rest, but pain level decreases
- Usually unilateral

Intensity (related to presence of anxiety)
- May be mild to severe
- May depend on the person's anxiety level—the level of pain may increase in a client fearful of a "serious" condition

Duration
- May be constant but is more likely to be intermittent, depending on the activity or the position

Pattern
- Restriction of active/passive/accessory movement observed
- One or more particular movements "catch" the client and aggravate the pain

▼ *Clinical Signs and Symptoms of*
Systemic Pain—cont'd

Aggravating Factors
- Depends on the organ involved (see specific chapters)
  Examples: Esophagus: Swallowing
  GI: Peristalsis (eating)
  Heart: Cold, exertion, stress

Relieving Factors
- Usually none (some exceptions: gallbladder— lean forward; kidney—lean to involved side; pancreas—lean forward/sit upright)
- If rest or change in position relieves the pain, there is usually a cyclic progression of increasing frequency, intensity, or duration of pain until rest or change in position is no longer a relieving factor

Associated Signs and Symptoms
- Fever, chills
- Night sweats
- Unusual vital signs
- Warning signs of cancer (see Chapter 10)
- GI symptoms: Nausea, vomiting, anorexia, unexplained weight loss, diarrhea, constipation
- Early satiety (feeling full after eating)
- Bilateral symptoms (e.g., paresthesias, weakness, edema, nail bed changes, skin rash)
- Painless weakness of muscles: More often proximal but may occur distally
- Dyspnea (breathlessness at rest or after mild exertion)
- Diaphoresis (excessive perspiration)
- Headaches, dizziness, fainting
- Visual disturbances
- Skin lesions, rashes, or itching that the client may not associate with the musculoskeletal symptoms
- Bowel/bladder symptoms
  - Hematuria (blood in the urine)
  - Nocturia
  - Urgency (sudden need to urinate)
  - Frequency
  - Melena (blood in feces)
  - Fecal or urinary incontinence
  - Bowel smears

▼ *Clinical Signs and Symptoms of*
Musculoskeletal Pain—cont'd

Aggravating Factors
- Altered by movement; pain may become worse with movement or some myalgia decreases with movement

Relieving Factors
- Muscle pain is relieved by short periods of rest without resulting stiffness, except in the case of fibromyalgia; stiffness may be present in older adults
- Stretching

Associated Signs and Symptoms
- Usually none, although stimulation of trigger points may cause sweating, nausea, blanching

chiropractic treatment when answering the question:

- What medical treatment have you had for this condition?

In addition to eliciting information regarding specific treatment performed by the medical community, follow-up questions relate to previous physical therapy treatment:

- Have you been treated by a physical therapist for this condition before?
  - If yes, when, where, and for how long?
- What helped and what didn't help?
- Was there any treatment that made your symptoms worse? If yes, please elaborate.

Knowing the client's response to previous types of treatment techniques may assist the therapist in determining an appropriate treatment protocol for the current chief complaint. For example, previously successful treatment techniques described may provide a basis for initial treatment until the therapist can fully assess the objective data and consider all potential types of treatments.

Medications. Medications (either prescription or over-the-counter) may or may not be listed on the Family/Personal History form. Often, it is necessary to probe further regarding the use of aspirin, acetaminophen (Tylenol), laxatives, or other drugs that can alter the client's symptoms.

Seventy-five percent of all older clients take OTC medications that may cause confusion, cause or contribute to additional symptoms, and interact with other medications. Sometimes the client is receiving the same drug under different brand names, increasing the likelihood of drug-induced confusion.

Watch for the four *D*s: dizziness, drowsiness, depression, and visual disturbance. Because many older people do not consider these "drugs" worth mentioning, it is important to ask specifically about OTC drug use. Additionally, drug abuse and alcoholism are more common in older people than is generally recognized, especially in depressed clients.

Medications can mask signs and symptoms or produce signs and symptoms that are seemingly unrelated to the client's current medical problem. For example, long-term use of steroids resulting in side effects such as proximal muscle weakness, tissue edema, and increased pain threshold may alter objective findings during the examination of the client. A detailed description of gastrointestinal (GI) disturbances and other side effects caused by nonsteroidal antiinflammatory drugs (NSAIDs) resulting in back, shoulder, or scapular pain is presented in Chapter 6. Every therapist should be very familiar with these.

In the aging population, drug side effects can occur even with low doses that usually produce no side effects in younger populations. Older people are two or three times more likely than young to middle-aged adults to have adverse drug reactions.

Many people who take prescribed medications cannot recall the name of the drug or tell you why they are taking it. It is essential to know whether the client has taken OTC or prescription medication before the physical therapy examination or treatment because the symptomatic relief or possible side effects may alter the objective findings. Similarly, when appropriate, treatment can be scheduled to correspond with the time of day when clients obtain maximal relief from their medications.

For every client the therapist is strongly encouraged to take the time to look up indications for use and possible side effects of prescribed medications. Drug reference guidebooks that are updated and published every year are available in hospital and clinic libraries or pharmacies. Pharmacists are also invaluable sources of drug information. (See also Medications and the PT's Role, 1995, and Ciccone, 1996.)

Distinguishing drug-related signs and symptoms from disease-related symptoms may require careful observation and consultation with family members or other health professionals to see whether these signs tend to increase following each dose (Ciccone, 1993). This information may come to light by asking the question:

- Do you notice any increase in symptoms, or perhaps the start of symptoms, after taking your medications? [This may occur 30 minutes to 2 hours after taking the drug.]

The physical therapist is often in the role of educator and may find it necessary to reeducate the client regarding the importance of taking medications as prescribed, whether on a daily or other regular basis. In the case of hypertension medication, the therapist should ask whether the client has taken the medication today as prescribed. It is not unusual to hear a client report, "I take my blood pressure pills when I feel my heart starting to pound." The same situation may occur with clients taking antiinflammatory drugs, antibiotics, or any other medications that must be taken consistently for a specified period to be effective.

Appropriate FUPs include the following:

• Why are you taking these medications?
• When was the last time that you took these medications?
• Have you taken these drugs today?
• Do the medications relieve your pain or symptoms?
    • If yes, how soon after you take the medications do you notice an improvement?
• If prescription drugs, who prescribed this medication for you?
• How long have you been taking these medications?
• When did your physician last review these medications?

Current Level of Fitness

An assessment of current physical activity and level of fitness (or level just before the onset of the current problem) can provide additional necessary information relating to the origin of the client's symptom complex. The level of fitness can be a valuable indicator of potential response to treatment based on the client's motivation (i.e., those who are more physically active and healthy seem to be more motivated to return to that level of fitness through disciplined self-rehabilitation).

It is important to know what type of exercise or sports activity the client participates in, the number of times per week (frequency) that this activity is performed, the length (duration) of each exercise or sports session, as well as how long the client has been exercising (weeks, months, years), and the level of difficulty of each exercise session (intensity). It is very important to ask:

• Since the onset of symptoms, are there any activities that you can no longer accomplish?

The client should give a description of these activities, including how physical activities have been affected by the symptoms. Follow-up questions include:

• Do you ever experience shortness of breath or lack of air during any activities (e.g., walking, climbing stairs)?
• Are you ever short of breath without exercising?
• Are you ever awakened at night breathless?
    • If yes, how often and when does this occur?

If the Family/Personal History form is not completed, it may be helpful to ask some of the questions under Work Environment. For example, assessing the history of falls with older people is essential. One third of community-dwelling older adults and a higher proportion of institutionalized older people fall annually. Aside from the serious injuries that may result, a debilitating "fear of falling" may cause many older adults to reduce their activity level and restrict their social life. This is one area that is often treatable and even preventable with physical therapy.

Older persons who are in bed for prolonged periods are at risk for secondary complications, including pressure ulcers, urinary tract infections, pulmonary infections and/or infarcts, congestive heart failure, osteoporosis, and compression fractures.

Sleep-Related History

Sleep patterns are valuable indicators of underlying physiologic and psychologic disease processes. The primary function of sleep is believed to be the restoration of body function. When the quality of this restorative sleep is decreased, the body and mind cannot perform at optimal levels.

Physical problems that result in pain, increased urination, shortness of breath, changes in body temperature, perspiration, or side effects of medications are just a few causes of sleep disruption. Any factor precipitating sleep deprivation can contribute to an increase in the frequency, intensity, or duration of a client's symptoms.

For example, fevers and night sweats are characteristic signs of systemic disease. Night sweats occur as a result of a gradual increase followed by a sudden drop in body temperature. This change in body temperature can be related to pathologic changes in immunologic, neurologic, and endocrine function.*

Certain neurologic lesions may produce local changes in sweating associated with nerve distribution. For example, a client with a spinal cord tumor may report changes in skin temperature above and below the level of the tumor. At presentation, any client with a history of either night sweats or fevers should be referred to the primary physician. This is especially true for clients with back pain or multiple joint pain without traumatic origin.

Pain is usually perceived as being more intense during the night because of the lack of outside distraction when the person lies quietly without activity. The sudden quiet surroundings and lack of external activity create an increased perception of pain that is a major disrupter of sleep. It is very important to ask the client about pain during the night. Is the person able to get to sleep? If not, the pain may be a primary focus and may become continuously intense so that falling asleep is a problem.

---

*Be aware that many people, especially women, experience night sweats associated with menopause, poor room ventilation, or too many clothes and covers used at night. Anyone reporting night sweats of a systemic origin often also experiences the same phenomenon during the waking hours, a more definitive clue than an isolated nocturnal experience.

• Does a change in body position affect the level of pain?

If a change in position can increase or decrease the level of pain, it is likely to be a musculoskeletal problem. If, however, the client is awakened from a deep sleep by pain in any location that is unrelated to physical trauma and is unaffected by a change in position, this may be an ominous sign of serious systemic disease, particularly cancer. FUPs include:

• If you wake up because of pain, is it because you rolled onto that side?
• Can you get back to sleep?
    • If yes, what do you have to do (if anything) to get back to sleep? (This answer may provide clues for treatment.)

Many other factors (primarily environmental and psychologic) are associated with sleep disturbance, but a good, basic assessment of the main characteristics of physically related disturbances in sleep pattern can provide valuable information related to treatment or referral decisions.

Stress
(See also Psychologic Factors in Pain Assessment, Chapter 1)

By using the interviewing tools and techniques described in this chapter, the physical therapist can communicate a willingness to consider all aspects of illness, whether biologic or psychologic. Client self-disclosure is unlikely if there is no trust in the health professional, if there is fear of a lack of confidentiality, or if a sense of disinterest is noted.

Most symptoms (pain included) are aggravated by unresolved emotional or psychologic stress. Prolonged stress may gradually lead to physiologic changes. Stress may result in depression, anxiety disorders, and behavioral consequences (e.g., smoking, alcohol and substance abuse, and accident proneness).

The effects of emotional stress may be increased by physiologic changes brought on by the use of medications or poor diet and health habits (e.g., cigarette smoking or ingestion of caffeine in any form).

As part of the Core Interview, the physical therapist may assess the client's subjective report of stress by asking:

- What major life changes or stresses have you encountered that you would associate with your injury/illness?

or

- What situations in your life are "stressors" for you?

It may be helpful to quantify the stress by asking the client:

- On a scale from 0 to 10, with 0 being no stress and 10 being the most extreme stress you have ever experienced, what number rating would you give your stress in general at this time in your life?
- What number would you give your stress level today?

Emotions such as fear and anxiety are common reactions to illness and treatment and may increase the client's awareness of pain and symptoms. These emotions may cause autonomic (branch of nervous system not subject to voluntary control) distress manifested in such symptoms as pallor, restlessness, muscular tension, perspiration, stomach pain, diarrhea or constipation, or headaches.

It may be helpful to screen for anxiety-provoked hyperventilation by asking:

- Do you ever get short of breath or dizzy or lose coordination when you are fatigued?

After the objective evaluation has been completed, the physical therapist can often provide some relief of emotionally based symptoms by explaining the cause of pain, but outlining a treatment plan, and by providing a realistic prognosis for improvement. This may not be possible if the client demonstrates signs of hysterical symptoms or conversion symptoms.

Whether the client's symptoms are systemic or caused by an emotional/psychologic overlay, if the client does not respond to treatment, it may be necessary to notify the physician that you are unable to find a satisfactory explanation for the client's complaints. Further medical evaluation may be indicated at that time.

THE CORE INTERVIEW

HISTORY OF PRESENT ILLNESS

Chief Complaint (Onset)

- Tell me why you are here today.
- Tell me about your injury.

    Alternative question: What do you think is causing your problem/pain?

    FUPs: How did this injury or illness begin?

    Was your injury or illness associated with a fall, trauma, assault, or repetitive activity (e.g., painting, cleaning, gardening, filing papers, driving)?

    Have you been hit, kicked, or pushed? [For the therapist: See text (Assault) before asking this question.]

    When did the present problem arise and did it occur gradually or suddenly?

    Systemic disease: Gradual onset without known cause.

FUPs, Follow-up Questions

continued

THE CORE INTERVIEW—cont'd

Have you ever had anything like this before? If yes, when did it occur? Describe the situation and the circumstances.

How many times has this illness occurred? Tell me about each occasion.

Is there any difference this time from the last episode?

How much time elapses between episodes?

Do these episodes occur more or less often than at first?

Systemic disease: May present in a gradual, progressive, cyclical onset: worse, better, worse.

PAIN/SYMPTOM ASSESSMENT

• Do you have any pain associated with your injury or illness? If yes, tell me about it.

Location

• Show me exactly where your pain is located.

FUPs: Do you have this same pain anywhere else?

Do you have any other pain or symptoms anywhere else?

If yes, what causes the pain or symptoms to occur in this other area?

Description

• What does it feel like?

FUPs: Has the pain changed in quality, intensity, frequency, or duration (how long it lasts) since it first began?

Pattern

• Tell me about the pattern of your pain or symptoms.

Alternative question: When does your back/shoulder [name the body part] hurt?

Alternative question: Describe your pain/symptoms from first waking up in the morning to going to bed at night. (See special sleep-related questions that follow.)

FUPs: Have you ever experienced anything like this before?

If yes, do these episodes occur more or less often than at first?

How does your pain/symptom(s) change with time?

Are your symptoms worse in the morning or in the evening?

Frequency

• How often does the pain/symptom(s) occur?

FUPs: Is your pain constant, or does it come and go (intermittent)?

Are you having this pain now?

Did you notice these symptoms this morning immediately after awakening?

Duration

• How long does the pain/symptom(s) last?

Systemic disease: Constant.

THE CORE INTERVIEW—cont'd

Intensity

- On a scale from 0 to 10, with 0 being no pain and 10 being the worst pain you have experienced with this condition, what level of pain do you have right now?

  Alternative question: How strong is your pain?

  1 = Mild
  2 = Moderate
  3 = Severe

  FUPs: Which word describes your pain right now?_____

  Which word describes the pain at its worst?_____

  Which word describes the least amount of pain?_____

  Systemic disease: Pain tends to be intense.

Associated Symptoms

- What other symptoms have you had that you can associate with this problem?

  FUPs: Have you experienced any of the following?

Burning	Hoarseness	Problems with vision
Difficulty in breathing	Nausea	Tingling
Difficulty in swallowing	Night sweats	Vomiting
Dizziness	Numbness	Weakness
Heart palpitations		

  Systemic disease: Presence of symptoms bilaterally (e.g., edema, nail bed changes, bilateral weakness, paresthesia, tingling, burning). Determine the frequency, duration, intensity, and pattern of symptoms. Blurred vision, double vision, scotomas (black spots before the eyes), or temporary blindness may indicate early symptoms of multiple sclerosis (MS), cerebral vascular accident (CVA), or other neurologic disorders.

Aggravating Factors

- What kinds of things affect the pain?

  FUPs: What makes your pain/symptoms worse (e.g., eating, exercise, rest, specific positions, excitement, stress)?

Relieving Factors

- What makes it better?

  Systemic disease: Unrelieved by change in position or by rest.

- How does rest affect the pain/symptoms?

  FUPs: Are your symptoms aggravated or relieved by any activities? If yes, what?

  How has this problem affected your daily life at work or at home?

  How has it affected your ability to care for yourself without assistance (e.g., dress, bathe, cook, drive)?

continued

THE CORE INTERVIEW—cont'd

MEDICAL TREATMENT AND MEDICATIONS

Treatment

- What medical treatment have you had for this condition?

  FUPs: Have you been treated by a physical therapist for this condition before? If yes:

    When?

    Where?

    How long?

    What helped?

    What didn't help?

    Was there any treatment that made your symptoms worse? If yes, please elaborate.

Medications

- Are you taking any prescription or over-the-counter medications?

  FUPs: If no, you may have to probe further regarding use of laxatives, aspirin, acetaminophen (Tylenol), and so forth. If yes:

    What medication do you take?

    How often?

    What dose do you take?

    Why are you taking these medications?

    When was the last time that you took these medications? Have you taken these drugs today?

    Do the medications relieve your pain or symptoms?

    If yes, how soon after you take the medications do you notice an improvement?

    Do you notice any increase in symptoms or perhaps the start of symptoms after taking your medication(s)? (This may occur 30 minutes to 2 hours after ingestion.)

    If prescription drugs, who prescribed them for you?

    How long have you been taking these medications?

    When did your physician last review these medications?

CURRENT LEVEL OF FITNESS

- What is your present exercise level?

  FUPs: What type of exercise or sports do you participate in?

    How many times do you participate each week (frequency)?

    When did you start this exercise program (duration)?

    How many minutes do you exercise during each session (intensity)?

    Are there any activities that you could do before your injury or illness that you cannot do now? If yes, please describe.

  Dyspnea: do you ever experience any shortness of breath (SOB) or lack of air during any activities (e.g., walking, climbing stairs)?

    FUPs: Are you ever short of breath without exercising?

    If yes, how often?

    When does this occur?

THE CORE INTERVIEW—cont'd

Do you ever wake up at night and feel breathless?

If yes, how often?

When does this occur?

SLEEP-RELATED

- Can you get to sleep at night? If no, try to determine whether the reason is due to the sudden decrease in activity and quiet, which causes you to focus on your symptoms.
- Are you able to lie or sleep on the painful side? If yes, the condition may be considered to be chronic, and treatment would be more vigorous than if no, indicating a more acute condition that requires more conservative treatment.
- Are you ever wakened from a deep sleep by pain?

  FUPs: If yes, do you awaken because you have rolled onto that side? Yes may indicate a subacute condition requiring a combination of treatment approaches, depending on objective findings.

  Can you get back to sleep?

  FUPs: If yes, what do you have to do (if anything) to get back to sleep? (The answer may provide clues for treatment.)
- Have you had any unexplained fevers, night sweats, or unexplained perspiration?

  Systemic disease: Fevers and night sweats are characteristic signs of systemic disease.

STRESS

- What major life changes or stresses have you encountered that you would associate with your injury/illness?

  Alternative question: What situations in your life are "stressors" for you?
- On a scale from 0 to 10, with 0 being no stress and 10 being the most extreme stress you have ever experienced, in general, what number rating would you give to your stress at this time in your life?
- What number would you assign to your level of stress today?
- Do you ever get short of breath or dizzy or lose coordination with fatigue (anxiety-produced hyperventilation)?

FINAL QUESTION

- Do you wish to tell me anything else about your injury, your health, or your present symptoms that we have not discussed yet?

  Alternative question: Is there anything else you think is important about your condition that I haven't asked yet?

Special Questions for Women

Gynecologic disorders can refer pain to the low back, hip, pelvis, groin, or sacroiliac joint. Any woman having pain or symptoms in any one or more of these areas should be screened for possible systemic diseases. The need to screen for systemic disease is essential when there is no known cause of the symptoms or pain.

Any woman with a positive personal/family history of cancer should be screened for medical disease even if the current symptoms can be attributed to a known neuromusculoskeletal cause.

The therapist will not need to ask every woman each question listed but should take into consideration the data from the Family/Personal History form, Core Interview, and clinical presentation when choosing appropriate FUPs.

Menopause. Like menarche, menopause (cessation of menstruation) is an important developmental event in a woman's life. Menopause is not a disease but rather a complex sequence of biologic aging events during which the body makes the transition from fertility to a nonreproductive status. The usual age of menopause is between 48 and 54 years, although it may occur as early as age 35 years, and early undetected physiologic changes have often begun in women's mid-30s.

The pattern of menstrual cessation varies. It may be abrupt, but more often it occurs over 1 to 2 years. Periodic menstrual flow gradually occurs less frequently, becoming irregular and less in amount. Occasional episodes of profuse bleeding may be inter-spersed with episodes of scant bleeding. Menopause is said to have occurred when there have been no menstrual periods for 12 consecutive months. *Any spontaneous uterine bleeding after this time is abnormal and requires medical evaluation.*

Within the past decade, removal of the uterus (hysterectomy) has become a common major surgery in the United States. In fact, more than one third of women in the United States have hysterectomies. The majority of these women have this operation between the ages of 25 and 44 years. Removal of the uterus and cervix, even without removal of the ovaries, usually brings on an early meno-

SPECIAL QUESTIONS FOR WOMEN EXPERIENCING BACK, HIP, PELVIC, GROIN, OR SACROILIAC PAIN*

MENSTRUAL HISTORY

- Is there any connection between your (back, hip, sacroiliac) pain/symptoms and your menstrual cycle (related to either ovulation, midcycle, or menses)?
- Since your back/sacroiliac (or other) pain/symptoms started, have you seen a gynecologist to rule out any gynecologic cause of this problem?
- Where were you in your menstrual cycle when your injury or illness occurred?
- Where are you in your menstrual cycle today (premenstrual/midmenstrual/postmenstrual)? **(Appropriate question for shoulder or back pain of unknown cause)**
- Are you taking birth control pills? (If yes, check blood pressure.)
- Do you have an intrauterine coil or loop contraceptive device (IUD or IUCD)? **(Appropriate question for abdominal, pelvic, low back, or sacral pain; pelvic inflammatory disease and ectopic pregnancy can occur)**
- Have you recently had a baby? **(Birth trauma)**
  If yes:
  - Did you have an epidural (anesthesia)? **(Postpartum back pain)**
  - Did you have any significant medical problems during your pregnancy or delivery?
  - Have you ever had a tubal or ectopic pregnancy? Is it possible that you may be pregnant now?
- How many pregnancies have you had?
- How many live births have you had?
- Do you ever experience a "falling out" feeling or pelvic heaviness after standing for a long time? **(Uterine prolapse; pelvic floor weakness; incontinence)**
  - If yes to incontinence: Ask several additional questions to determine the frequency, the amount of protection needed (as measured by the number and type of pads used daily), and how much this problem interferes with daily activities and lifestyle.

*NOTE: Bold type indicates possible significance of the client's response.

pause, within 2 years of the operation. Oophorectomy (removal of the ovaries) brings on menopause immediately, regardless of the age of the woman, and early surgical removal of the ovaries (before age 30) doubles the risk of osteoporosis.

Past Medical History. Detailed questions about past labors and methods of delivery, past surgical procedures, incontinence, history of sexually transmitted or pelvic inflammatory disease(s), and history of osteoporosis and/or compression fractures are important for women.

For example, pregnancy and birth history are important because the hormone relaxin, secreted by the corpus luteum, is elevated in a woman's system during pregnancy and 7 to 10 days before menstruation begins. Women who have had multiple pregnancies or births may have sacroiliac or low back pain associated with poor abdominal tone and ligamentous laxity. Relaxin increases elongation of ligaments by placing them at the end-range, and it has a relaxation effect on joints, thus increasing the chances for injury.

The symptomatic sacroiliac problem may be aggravated by intercourse in the supine position. Change in position can alter painful intercourse when the cause of pain is musculoskeletal.

SPECIAL QUESTIONS FOR WOMEN EXPERIENCING BACK, HIP, PELVIC, GROIN, OR SACROILIAC PAIN—cont'd

- If no: Do you ever leak urine with coughing, laughing, lifting, exercising, or sneezing? **(Stress incontinence; tension myalgia of pelvic floor)**
- How many miscarriages or abortions have you had? **(Weakness secondary to blood loss, infection, scarring; blood in peritoneum irritating diaphragm causing lumbar and/or shoulder pain)**
- Do you have an unusual amount of vaginal discharge or vaginal discharge with an obvious odor? **(Referred back pain)**
- Is there any connection between when the discharge started and when you first noticed your back/sacroiliac (or other) symptoms?
- For the postmenopausal woman: Are you taking hormone replacement therapy (HRT)?
  - Have you ever been told you have "brittle bones" or osteoporosis?
  - Have you ever had a compression fracture of your back?

PAST MEDICAL HISTORY

- Have you ever been told that you have:
  - Retroversion of the uterus (tipped back)
  - Ovarian cysts
  - Fibroids or tumors
  - Endometriosis
  - Cystocele (sagging bladder)
  - Rectocele (sagging rectum)
- Have you ever had pelvic inflammatory disease?
- Do you have any known sexually transmitted diseases? **(Cause of pelvic inflammatory disease)**
- Have you had vaginal surgery or a hysterectomy? **(Hysterectomy: joint pain and myalgias may occur; vaginal surgery: incontinence)**
- Have you had a recent history of bladder or kidney infections? **(Referred back pain)**

The risk of developing chronic postpartum back pain may be doubled among women who received epidural anesthesia during labor (Pauls, 1993). Additionally, women who have had an abortion may seek health care months to years later with a variety of physical and psychologic symptoms referred to as postabortion syndrome or postabortion survivors syndrome, a subset of posttraumatic stress disorders. This new syndrome has not been classified in the *Diagnostic and Statistical Manual.*

Physician Referral. Women who have a history of hip, sacroiliac, pelvic, groin, or low back pain without traumatic cause should be referred for a gynecologic evaluation if there is a history of fever or night sweats or an indication of correlation between menses and symptoms.

Any woman with a positive family or personal history of breast cancer who has chest or shoulder pain of unknown cause should make an appointment with her physician.

Any woman whose blood pressure is elevated and who is currently taking birth control pills should be monitored closely by her physician.*

Any spontaneous uterine bleeding after menopause is abnormal and requires medical evaluation.

▼
Clinical Signs and Symptoms of
Menopause

- Fatigue and malaise
- Depression, mood swings
- Headache
- Altered sleep pattern (insomnia)
- Hot flashes
- Irregular menses, cessation of menses
- Vaginal dryness, pain during intercourse
- Atrophy of breasts and vaginal tissue
- Pelvic floor relaxation (cystocele/rectocele)
- Urge incontinence

Special Questions for Men

Men describing symptoms related to the groin, low back, hip, or sacroiliac joint may have some urologic involvement. The screening questions presented on the intake form assess the need for further medical follow-up.

A positive response to any or all of these questions may be evaluated further following the format provided. Additional Special Questions to Ask may assist the physical therapist in making an appropriate referral for a possible urologic evaluation (see accompanying box).

*Originally, birth-control pills contained as much as 20 percent more estrogen than the amount that is present in these pills today. Women taking the newer pills have a slightly increased risk of high blood pressure, which returns to normal shortly after the pill is discontinued.

SPECIAL QUESTIONS FOR MEN EXPERIENCING BACK, HIP, PELVIC, GROIN, OR SACROILIAC PAIN

- Do you ever have difficulty with urination (e.g., difficulty starting or continuing flow or a very slow flow of urination)?
- Do you ever have blood in your urine?
- Do you ever have pain, burning, or discomfort on urination?
- Do you urinate often, especially during the night?
- Does it feel like your bladder is not emptying completely?
- Have you ever been treated for prostate problems (prostate cancer, prostatitis)?
- Have you recently had kidney stones, bladder or kidney infections?
- Have you ever been told that you have a hernia, or do you think you have a hernia?

▼ HOSPITAL INPATIENT INFORMATION

Medical Chart

Treatment of hospital or nursing home inpatients requires a slightly different interview (or information-gathering) format. Reviewing the patient's chart* thoroughly for information will assist the physical therapist in developing a safe and effective treatment plan.

Important information to look for might include:

- Age
- Diagnosis
- Surgery report
- Physician's notes
- Associated or additional problems relevant to physical therapy
- Medications
- Restrictions
- Laboratory results
- Vital signs

An evaluation of the patient's medical status in conjunction with age and diagnosis can provide valuable guidelines for treatment.

If the patient has had recent surgery, the physician's report should be scanned for preoperative and postoperative orders (in some cases there is a separate physician's orders book). For example:

- Was the patient treated preoperatively with physical therapy for gait, strength, range of motion, or other objective assessments?
- Were there any unrelated preoperative conditions?
- How long was the procedure?
- How much fluid and/or blood products were given?

- What position was the patient placed in during the procedure?

Fluid received during surgery may affect arterial oxygenation, leaving the person breathless with minimal exertion and experiencing early muscle fatigue. Prolonged time in the lithotomy position (supine, legs flexed on thighs, flexed on abdomen and abducted) often results in residual musculoskeletal complaints.

This surgical position for men and for women during laparoscopy (examination of the peritoneal cavity) may place patients at increased risk for thrombophlebitis because of the decreased blood flow to the legs during surgery.

Other valuable information that may be contained in the physician's report may include:

- What are the current short-term and long-term medical treatment plans?
- Are there any known or listed contraindications to physical therapy treatment?
- Does the patient have any weight-bearing limitations?

Associated or additional problems to the primary diagnosis may be found within the chart contents (e.g., diabetes, heart disease, peripheral vascular disease, or respiratory involvement). The physical therapist should look for any of these conditions in order to modify exercise accordingly and to watch for any related signs and symptoms that might affect the exercise program:

- Are there complaints of any kind that may affect exercise (e.g., shortness of breath [dyspnea], heart palpitations, rapid heart rate [tachycardia], fatigue, fever, or anemia)?

If the patient is diabetic, the therapist should ask:

- What are the current blood glucose levels?
- When is insulin administered?

Avoiding peak insulin levels in planning exercise schedules is discussed more

---

*Clients are still more likely to be referred to as patients in a hospital setting.

completely in Chapter 9. Other questions related to medications can follow the Core Interview outline with appropriate follow-up questions:

- Is the patient receiving oxygen or receiving fluids/medications through an intravenous line?
  - If the patient is receiving oxygen, will he or she need increased oxygen levels before, during, or following physical therapy? What level(s)?
- Are there any dietary or fluid restrictions?
  - If so, check with the nursing staff to determine the full limitations. For example:
    - Are ice chips or wet washcloths permissible?
    - How many ounces or milliliters of fluid are allowed during therapy?
    - Where should this amount be recorded?

Laboratory values and vital signs should be reviewed. For example:

- Is the patient anemic?
- Is the patient's blood pressure stable?

Anemic patients may demonstrate an increased normal resting pulse rate that should be monitored during exercise. Patients with unstable blood pressure may require initial standing with a tilt table or monitoring of the blood pressure before, during, and after treatment. Check the nursing record for pulse rate at rest and blood pressure to use as a guide when taking vital signs in the clinic or at the patient's bedside.

Nursing Assessment

After reading the patient's chart, check with the nursing staff to determine the nursing assessment of the individual patient. The essential components of the nursing assessment that are of value to the physical therapist may include:

- Medical status

- Pain
- Physical status
- Patient orientation
- Discharge plans

The nursing staff are usually intimately aware of the patient's current medical and physical status. If pain is a factor:

- What is the nursing assessment of this patient's pain level and pain tolerance?

Pain tolerance is relative to the medications received by the patient, the number of days after surgery or after injury, fatigue, and the patient's personality.

To assess the patient's physical status, ask the nursing staff:

- Has the patient been up at all yet?
- If yes, how long has the patient been sitting, standing, or walking?
- How far has the patient walked?
- How much assistance does the patient require?

Ask about the patient's orientation:

- Is the patient oriented to time, place, and person?

In other words, does the patient know the date and the approximate time, where he or she is, and who he or she is? Treatment plans may be altered by the patient's awareness; for example, a home program may be impossible without family compliance.

- Are there any known or expected discharge plans?
- If yes, what are these plans and when is the target date for discharge?

Cooperation between nurses and the physical therapist is an important part of the multidisciplinary approach to planning the patient's treatment. The questions to ask and factors to consider provide the physical therapist with the basic information related to the hospital or nursing home that is necessary to carry out an objective examination and to plan a treatment protocol. Each individual patient's situation may require that the physical therapist obtain additional pertinent information.

HOSPITAL INPATIENT INFORMATION

MEDICAL CHART

- **Patient age**
- **Diagnosis**
- **Surgery:** Did the patient have surgery?
  FUPs:
  - Was the patient seen by a physical therapist preoperatively?
  - Were there any unrelated preoperative conditions?
  - How long was the procedure? Were there any surgical complications?
  - How much fluid and/or blood products were given?
  - What position was the patient placed in and for how long?
- Physician's report
  - What are the short-term and long-term medical treatment plans?
  - Are there precautions or contraindications for treatment?
  - Are there weight-bearing limitations?
- **Associated or additional problems,** such as diabetes, heart disease, peripheral vascular disease, respiratory involvement
  FUPs: Are there precautions or contraindications of any kind that may affect exercise?
  - If diabetic, what are the current blood glucose levels (normal range: 70 to 110 mg/dl)?
  - When is insulin administered? (Use this to avoid the peak insulin levels in planning an exercise schedule.)
- **Medications** (what, when received, what for, potential side effects)
  FUPs: Is the patient receiving oxygen or receiving fluids/medications through an intravenous line?
- **Restrictions:** Are there any dietary or fluid restrictions?
  FUPs: If yes, check with the nursing staff to determine the patient's full limitation.
  - Are ice chips or a wet washcloth permissible?
  - How many ounces or milliliters of fluid are allowed during therapy?
- **Laboratory values:** Hematocrit/hemoglobin level (see inside cover for normal values and significance of these tests); exercise tolerance test results if available for cardiac patients; pulmonary function test (PFT) to determine severity of pulmonary problem; arterial blood gas (ABG) levels to determine the need for supplemental oxygen during exercise
- **Vital signs:** Is the blood pressure stable?
  FUPs: If no, consider initiating standing with a tilt table or monitoring the blood pressure before, during, and after treatment.

NURSING ASSESSMENT

- **Medical status:** What is the patient's current medical status?
- **Pain:** What is the nursing assessment of this patient's pain level and pain tolerance?
- **Physical status:** Has the patient been up at all yet?
  FUPs: If yes, is the patient sitting, standing, or walking? How long and (if walking) what distance, and how much assistance is required?
- **Patient orientation:** Is the patient oriented to time, place, and person? (Does the patient know the date and the approximate time, where he or she is, and who he or she is?)

continued

HOSPITAL INPATIENT INFORMATION—cont'd

- **Discharge plans:** Are there any known or expected discharge plans?
  FUPs: If yes, what are these plans and when will the patient be discharged?
- **Final question:** Is there anything else that I should know before exercising the patient?

INTERVIEWING DOs AND DON'Ts

DOs

Do use a sequence of questions that begins with open-ended questions.

Do leave closed-ended questions for the end as clarifying questions.

Do select a private location where confidentiality can be maintained.

Do listen attentively and show it both in your body language and by occasionally making reassuring verbal prompts, such as "I see" or "Go on."

Do ask one question at a time and allow the client to answer the question completely before continuing with the next question.

Do encourage the client to ask questions throughout the interview.

Do listen with the intention of assessing the client's current level of understanding and knowledge of his or her current medical condition.

Do eliminate unnecessary information and speak to the client at his or her level of understanding.

Do correlate signs and symptoms with medical history and objective findings to rule out systemic disease.

Do provide several choices or selections to questions that require a descriptive response.

DON'Ts

Don't jump to premature conclusions based on the answers to one or two questions. (Correlate all subjective and objective information before consulting with a physician.)

Don't interrupt or take over the conversation when the client is speaking.

Don't destroy helpful open-ended questions with closed-ended follow-up questions before the person has a chance to respond (e.g., How do you feel this morning? Has your pain gone?).

Don't use professional or medical jargon when it is possible to use common language (e.g., don't use the term *myocardial infarct* instead of heart attack).

Don't overreact to information presented. Common overreactions include raised eyebrows, puzzled facial expressions, gasps, or other verbal exclamations such as "Oh, really?" or "Wow!" Less dramatic reactions may include facial expressions or gestures that indicate approval or disapproval, surprise, or sudden interest. These responses may influence what the client does or does not tell you.

Don't use leading questions. Pain is difficult to describe, and it may be easier for the client to agree with a partially correct statement than to attempt to clarify points of discrepancy between your statement and his or her pain experience.

Leading Questions	**Better Presentation of Same Questions**
Where is your pain?	Do you have any pain associated with your injury? If yes, tell me about it.
Does it hurt when you first get out of bed?	When does your back hurt?
Does the pain radiate down your leg?	Do you have this pain anywhere else?
Do you have pain in your lower back?	Point to the exact location of your pain.

▼ PHYSICIAN REFERRAL

The physical therapist may be able to determine detailed and specific information regarding symptoms of possible systemic origin by using the questions presented in this chapter. Then, by correlating the client's answers with family/personal history, vital signs, and objective findings from the physical examination, the therapist can screen for medical disease and decide whether a referral to the physician is indicated (Table 2-5).

This information is not designed to be used to provide the client with a medical diagnosis but rather to perform an accurate assessment of pain and systemic symptoms that may mimic or occur simultaneously with a musculoskeletal problem.

Some of the specific indications for physician referral mentioned in this chapter include the following:

- Spontaneous postmenopausal bleeding

- A growing mass, whether painful or painless
- Persistent rise or fall in blood pressure
- Hip, sacroiliac, pelvic, groin, or low back pain in a woman without traumatic etiologic complex who reports fever, night sweats, or an association between menses and symptoms
- A positive family/personal history of breast cancer in a woman with chest, back, or shoulder pain of unknown cause
- Elevated blood pressure in any woman taking birth control pills; this should be closely monitored by her physician

Table 2-5 lists systemic signs and symptoms evaluated as part of the client's subjective examination. In each chapter a list of possible signs or symptoms is provided for your consideration when making an evaluation and referral. As always, correlate *history* with *patterns of pain* and any *unusual findings* that may indicate *systemic disease.*

TABLE 2-5 ▼ Systemic Signs and Symptoms Requiring Physician Referral

Constitutional Symptoms	Pattern of Symptoms	Associated Signs/Symptoms
Fever	Constant pain/night pain	Pain on urination
Diaphoresis	Cyclic pattern	Blood in urine
Night sweats	Pain description:	Tachycardia
Nausea	Boring	Bradycardia
Vomiting	Knifelike	Difficulty in swallowing
Diarrhea	Deep ache	Dyspnea
Pallor	Colicky	Vision changes
Dizziness/syncope	Bilateral symptoms:	Hoarseness
Fatigue	Edema	Heart palpitations
Weight loss	Clubbing	
	Numbness	
	Tingling	
	Nail bed changes	
	Skin pigmentation changes	
	Skin rash	
	Unusual menstrual history	
	Association between menses and symptoms	
	Temporary relief/no relief with rest or change in position	

KEY POINTS TO REMEMBER

▶ Most of the information needed to determine the cause of symptoms is contained within the subjective assessment (interview process).

▶ The Family/Personal History form can be used as the first tool to screen clients for medical disease. Any "yes" responses should be followed up with appropriate questions. The therapist is strongly encouraged to review the form with the client, entering the date and his or her own initials. This form can be used as a document of baseline information.

▶ Medical screening examinations (interview and vital signs) should be completed for any person experiencing back, shoulder, scapular, hip, groin, or sacroiliac symptoms of unknown cause. The presence of constitutional symptoms will almost always warrant a physician's referral but definitely requires further follow-up questions in making that determination.

▶ It may be necessary to explain the need to ask such detailed questions about organ systems seemingly unrelated to the musculoskeletal symptoms.

▶ With the older client, a limited number of presenting symptoms predominate—no matter what the underlying disease is—including acute confusion, depression, falling, incontinence, and syncope.

▶ A recent history of any infection (bladder, uterine, kidney, vaginal, upper respiratory), mononucleosis, influenza, or colds may be an extension of a chronic health pattern of systemic illness.

▶ Special Questions for Women and Special Questions for Men are provided to screen for gynecologic or urologic involvement for any woman or man with back, shoulder, hip, groin, or sacroiliac symptoms of unknown origin at presentation.

▶ Other red flags: Symptoms that seem out of proportion to the injury, symptoms that persist beyond the expected time for the condition, presence of night pain, or no change in symptoms with change in activity or position.

▶ Consider the possibility of physical/sexual assault or abuse in anyone with an unknown cause of symptoms, clients who take much longer to heal than expected, or any combination of physical, social, or psychologic cues listed.

▶ In screening for systemic origin of symptoms, review the subjective information in light of the objective findings. Compare the client's *history* with *clinical presentation* and look for any *associated signs and symptoms*.

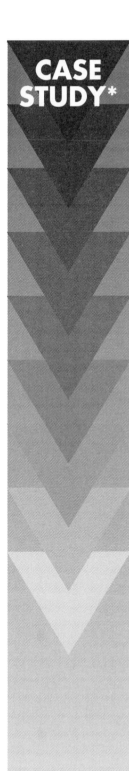

CASE STUDY*

REFERRAL

Your latest referral is a 28-year-old white man who has had a diagnosed progressive idiopathic Raynaud's syndrome of the bilateral upper extremities for the last 4 years. The client has been examined by numerous physicians, including an orthopedic specialist. The client has complete numbness and cyanosis of the right second, third, fourth, and fifth digits on contact with even a mild decrease in temperature. He says that his symptoms have progressed to the extent that they appear within seconds if he picks up a glass of cold water.

This man works almost entirely outside, often in cold weather, and uses saws and other power equipment. The numbness has created a very unsafe job situation.

The client received a gunshot wound in a hunting accident 6 years ago. The bullet entered the posterior left thoracic region, lateral to the lateral border of the scapula, and came out through the anterior lateral superior chest wall. He says that he feels as if his shoulders are constantly rolled forward. He reports no cervical, shoulder, or elbow pain or injury.

PHYSICAL THERAPY INTERVIEW

Note that not all of these questions would necessarily be presented to the client because his answers may determine the next question and may eliminate some questions.

Tell me why you are here today. (Open-ended question)

Pain

Do you have any pain associated with your past gunshot wound? If yes, describe your pain.

FUPs: Give the client a chance to answer and prompt only if necessary with suggested adjectives such as "Is you pain sharp, dull, boring, or burning?" or "Show me on your body where you have pain."

To pursue this line of questioning, if appropriate:

FUPs: What makes your pain better or worse?

What is your pain like when you first get up in the morning, during the day, and in the evening?

Is your pain constant or does it come and go?

On a scale from 0 to 10, with zero being no pain and 10 being the worst pain you have ever experienced with this problem, what level of pain would you say that you have right now?

Do you have any other pain or symptoms that are not related to your old injury?

If yes, pursue as above to find out about the onset of pain, etc.

You indicated that you have numbness in your right hand. How long does this last?

---

*This case study was adapted and used with permission from the primary physical therapist.

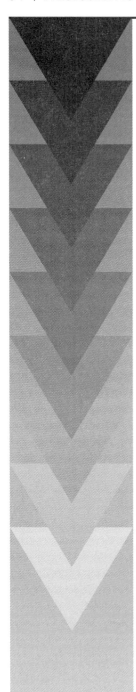

FUPs: Besides picking up a glass of cold water, what else brings it on?

How long have you had this problem?

You indicated that this numbness has progressed over time. How quickly has this progression occurred?

Do you ever have similar symptoms in your left hand?

Associated Symptoms

Even though this person has been seen by numerous physicians, it is important to ask appropriate questions to rule out a systemic origin of current symptoms, especially if there has been a recent change in the symptoms or presentation of symptoms bilaterally. For example:

What other symptoms have you had that you can associate with this problem?

In addition to the numbness, have you had any of the following?

- Tingling
- Burning
- Weakness
- Vomiting
- Hoarseness
- Difficulty with breathing

- Nausea
- Dizziness
- Difficulty with swallowing
- Heart palpitations or fluttering
- Unexplained sweating or night sweats
- Problems with your vision

How well do you sleep at night? (Open-ended question)

Do you have trouble sleeping at night? (Closed-ended question)

Does the pain awaken you out of a sound sleep? Can you sleep on either side comfortably?

Medications

Are you taking any medications? If yes, and the person does not volunteer the information, probe further:

What medications?

Why are you taking this medication?

When did you last take the medication?

Do you think the medication is easing the symptoms or helping in any way?

Have you noticed any side effects? If yes, what are these effects?

Previous Medical Treatment

Have you had any recent medical tests, such as x-ray examination, MRI, or CT scan? If yes, find out the results.

Tell me about your gunshot wound. Were you treated immediately?

Did you have any surgery at that time or since then? If yes, pursue details with regard to what type of surgery and where and when it occurred.

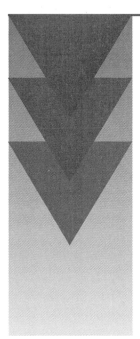

Did you have physical therapy treatment at any time after your accident? If yes, relate when, for how long, with whom, what was done, did it help?

Have you had any other kind of treatment for this injury (e.g., acupuncture, chiropractic, osteopathic, naturopathic, and so on)?

Activities of Daily Living (ADLs)

Are you right-handed?

How do your symptoms affect your ability to do your job or work around the house?

How do your symptoms affect caring for yourself (e.g., showering, shaving, other ADLs such as eating or writing)?

Final Question

Is there anything else you feel that I should know concerning your injury, your health, or your present situation that I have not asked about?

NOTE: If this client had been a woman, the interview would have included questions about breast pain and the date when she was last screened for cancer (cervical and breast) by a physician.

PRACTICE QUESTIONS

1. What is the effect of NSAIDs (e.g., naprosyn, motrin, anaprox, ibuprofen) on blood pressure?

   a. No effect

   b. Increases blood pressure

   c. Decreases blood pressure

2. Most of the information needed to determine the cause of symptoms is contained in the:

   a. Subjective examination

   b. Family/personal history form

   c. Objective information

   d. All of the above

   e. a and c

3. With what final question should you always end your interview?

4. What are constitutional symptoms? Name five.

5. After interviewing a new client, you summarize what she has told you by saying, "You told me you are here because of right neck and shoulder pain that began 5 years ago as a result of a car accident. You also have a "pins and needles" sensation in your third and fourth fingers but no other symptoms at this time. You have noticed a considerable decrease in your grip strength, and you would like to be able to pick up a pot of coffee without fear of spilling it."

   This is an example of:

   a. An open-ended question

   b. A funnel technique

   c. A paraphrasing technique

   d. None of the above

6. What is the best follow-up question for someone who tells you that the pain is constant?

7. A 52-year-old woman with shoulder pain tells you that she has pain at night that awakens her. After asking a series of follow-up questions, you are able to determine that she had trouble falling asleep because her pain increases when she goes to bed and that once she falls asleep she wakes up as soon as she rolls onto the affected side. What is the most likely explanation for this pain behavior? [Choose all that apply.]

   a. Minimal distractions heighten a person's awareness of musculoskeletal discomfort.

   b. This is a systemic pattern that is associated with a neoplasm.

   c. This represents an acute or subacute clinical presentation of a musculoskeletal problem.

   d. It is impossible to tell.

8. Is this statement true or false? Any spontaneous uterine bleeding after 12 consecutive months without menstrual bleeding requires medical referral.

9. You have just evaluated a 44-year-old man who sprained his ankle in a weekend sporting event. His blood pressure is 154/98 mm Hg, temperature is normal, and pulse rate is 58 bpm. Your ankle rehabilitation protocol includes an aerobic component, and you are concerned about the blood pressure measurement. How should you handle this?

10. A 52-year-old man with low back pain and sciatica on the left side has been referred to you by his family physician. He has had a discectomy and laminectomy on two separate occasions about 5 to 7 years ago. No medical testing has been performed (e.g., x-ray examination or MRI) since that time. What follow-up questions should you ask to screen for medical disease?

References

Bates B: *Guide to physical examination and history taking,* ed 6, Philadelphia, 1995, JB Lippincott.

Christan T., Turnbull T, Cline D: Cardiopulmonary abnormalities after smoking cocaine, *South Med J* 83(3): 335-338, 1990.

Ciccone CD: Geriatric pharmacology. In Guccione AA, editor: *Geriatric physical therapy,* St Louis, 1993, Mosby.

Ciccone CD: *Pharmacology in rehabilitation,* ed 2, Philadelphia, 1996, FA Davis.

Clark T, McKenna LS, Jewell MJ: Physical therapists' recognition of battered women in clinical settings, *Phys Ther* 76(1): 12-19, 1996.

Coulehan JL, Block MR: *The medical interview: mastering skills for clinical practice,* ed 3, Philadelphia, 1997, FA Davis.

Frohlich ED: New blood pressure guidelines, *Health News* (a publication of the New England Journal of Medicine) 3(16): 5, 1997.

Frymoyer JW, Pope MH, Clements JH et al: Risk factors in low back pain, *J Bone Joint Surg* 65-A: 213-218, 1983.

Goodman CC, Boissonnault WG: *Pathology: implications for the physical therapist,* Philadelphia, 1998, WB Saunders.

Heliövaara M, Knekt P, Aromaa A: Incidence and risk factors of herniated lumbar intervertebral disc or sciatica leading to hospitalization, *J Chronic Dis* 40: 251-258, 1987.

Hertling D, Kessler RM: *Management of common musculoskeletal disorders,* ed 2, Philadelphia, 1990, JB Lippincott.

Hillegass E, Sandowsky HS: *The essentials of cardiopulmonary physical therapy,* ed 2, Philadelphia, 1999, WB Saunders.

Holm S, Nachemson A: Nutrition of the intervertebral disc: acute effects of cigarette smoking. An experimental animal study, *Upsala J Med Sci* 83: 91-98, 1998.

Hughes JR, Oliveto AH, Helzer JE et al: Should caffeine abuse, dependence, or withdrawal be added to DSM-IV and ICD-10? *Am J Psychiatry* 149(1): 33-40, 1992.

Hughes JR, Oliveto AH, Liguori A et al: Endorsement of DSM-IV dependence criteria among caffeine users,

Drug Alcohol Depend 52(2): 99-107, October 1998.

Hulme J: Phoenix physical therapy, Personal communication, Missoula, Montana, 1997.

Israel Y, Hollander O, Sanchez-Craig M et al: Screening for problem drinking and counseling by the primary care physician-nurse team, *Alcohol Clin Exp Res* 20(8): 1443-1450, 1996.

Johnson C: Handling the hurt: Physical therapy and domestic violence, *PT Magazine* 5(1): 52-64, 1997.

Ketter P: Physical therapists need to know how to deal with domestic violence issues, *PT Bulletin* 12(31): 6-7, August 1997.

Lane JM: When to consider malignant tumor in the differential diagnosis after athletic trauma. Editorial comment, *J Musculoskel Med* 7(5): 16, 1990.

Majid PA, Cheirif JB, Rokey R et al: Does cocaine cause coronary vasospasm in chronic cocaine abusers? A study of coronary and systemic hemodynamics, *Clin Cardiol* 15(4): 253-258, 1992.

Medications and the PT's Role, *PT Magazine* 3(6): 54-70, 1995.

Melzack R: The McGill Pain Questionnaire: major properties and scoring methods, *Pain* 1: 277, 1975.

Neufeld B: SAFE questions: overcoming barriers to the detection of domestic violence, *Am Fam Physician* 53: 2575-2580, 1996.

Newman LS: Occupational illness, *N Engl J Med* 333: 1128-1134, 1995.

Pauls J: Physical therapy for women, *PT Magazine* 1(2): 64-67, 1993.

Radetsky P: *Allergic to the twentieth century: the explosion in environmental allergies,* Boston, 1997, Little, Brown.

Shapira D: Alcohol abuse and osteoporosis, *Semin Arthritis Rheum* 19(6): 371-376, 1990.

Travell JG, Simons DG: *Myofascial pain and dysfunction: the Trigger Point Manual,* vol 1, Baltimore, 1983, Williams & Wilkins.

VA may see more ailments caused by toxins, *PT Bulletin* 8(3): 3, January 20, 1993.

Wolf GA Jr: *Collecting data from patients,* Baltimore, 1977, University Park Press.

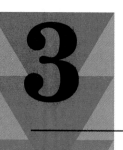

Overview of Cardiovascular Signs and Symptoms

The cardiovascular system consists of the heart, capillaries, veins, and lymphatics and functions in coordination with the pulmonary system to circulate oxygenated blood through the arterial system to all cells. This system then collects deoxygenated blood from the venous system and delivers it to the lungs for reoxygenation (Fig. 3-1).

Heart disease remains the leading cause of death in industrialized nations. In the United States alone, cardiovascular disease (CVD) is responsible for approximately one million deaths each year. More than one in four Americans has some form of cardiovascular disease. The American Heart Association reports that about half of all deaths from heart disease are sudden and unexpected.

Fortunately, during the last two decades cardiovascular research has greatly increased our understanding of the structure and function of the cardiovascular system in health and disease. Despite the formidable statistics regarding the prevalence of CVD, during the last 15 years a steady decline in mortality from cardiovascular disorders has been witnessed. Effective application of the increased knowledge regarding CVD and its risk factors will assist health care professionals to educate clients in achieving and maintaining cardiovascular health.

▼ SIGNS AND SYMPTOMS OF CARDIOVASCULAR DISEASE

Cardinal symptoms of cardiac disease usually include chest, neck and/or arm pain or discomfort, palpitation, dyspnea, syncope (fainting), fatigue, cough, and cyanosis. Edema and leg pain (claudication) are the most common symptoms of the vascular component of a cardiovascular pathologic condition. Symptoms of cardiovascular involvement should also be reviewed by system (Table 3-1).

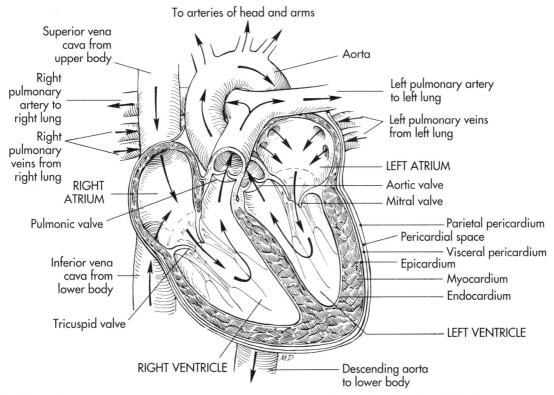

FIGURE 3-1 • Structure and circulation of the heart. Blood entering the left atrium from the right and left pulmonary veins flows into the left ventricle. The left ventricle pumps blood into the systemic circulation through the aorta. From the systemic circulation, blood returns to the heart through the superior and inferior venae cavae. From there the right ventricle pumps blood into the lungs through the right and left pulmonary arteries. (From Black JM, Matassarin-Jacobs E, editors: *Luckmann and Sorenson's medical-surgical nursing,* ed 4, Philadelphia, 1993, WB Saunders, p. 1093.)

TABLE 3-1 ▼ Cardiovascular Signs and Symptoms by System

System	Symptoms	System	Symptoms
General	Weakness Fatigue Weight change Poor exercise tolerance	Genitourinary	Urinary frequency Nocturia Concentrated urine Decreased urinary output
Integumentary	Pressure ulcers Loss of body hair Cyanosis (lips and nail beds)	Musculoskeletal	Chest, shoulder, neck, jaw, or arm pain Myalgias Muscular fatigue Muscle atrophy Edema Claudication
Central nervous system	Headaches Impaired vision Dizziness or syncope		
Respiratory	Labored breathing Productive cough	Gastrointestinal	Nausea and vomiting Ascites (abdominal distension)

Modified from Goodman CC, Boissonnault WG: *Pathology: implications for the physical therapist,* Philadelphia, 1998, WB Saunders.

Chest Pain or Discomfort

Chest pain or discomfort is a common presenting symptom of cardiovascular disease and must be evaluated carefully. Chest pain may be cardiac or noncardiac in origin and may radiate to the neck, jaw, upper trapezius muscle, upper back, shoulder, or arms (most commonly the left arm). Radiating pain down the arm follows the pattern of ulnar nerve distribution. Pain of cardiac origin can be experienced in the somatic areas because the heart is supplied by the C3-T4 spinal segments, referring visceral pain to the corresponding somatic area (Fig. 1-2). For example, the heart and the diaphragm, supplied by the C5-C6 spinal segment, can refer pain to the shoulder (see Figs. 12-5 and 12-6).

Cardiac-related chest pain may arise secondary to angina, myocardial infarction, pericarditis, endocarditis, mitral valve prolapse, or dissecting aortic aneurysm. Location and description (frequency, intensity, and duration) vary according to the underlying pathologic condition (see each individual condition).

Cardiac chest pain is often accompanied by associated signs and symptoms, such as nausea, vomiting, diaphoresis, dyspnea, fatigue, pallor, or syncope. These associated signs and symptoms provide the therapist with red flags to identify musculoskeletal symptoms of a systemic origin. Cardiac chest pain or discomfort can also occur when the coronary circulation is normal, as in the case of clients with anemia, causing lack of oxygenation of the myocardium (heart muscle) during physical exertion.

Noncardiac chest pain can be caused by an extensive list of disorders requiring screening for medical disease. For example, cervical disk disease and arthritic changes can mimic atypical chest pain. Chest pain that is attributed to anxiety, trigger points, cocaine use, and other noncardiac causes is discussed in Chapter 12.

Palpitation

Palpitation, the presence of an irregular heartbeat, may also be referred to as arrhythmia or dysrhythmia, which may be caused by a relatively benign condition (e.g., mitral valve prolapse, "athlete's heart," caffeine, anxiety, exercise) or a severe condition (e.g., coronary artery disease, cardiomyopathy, complete heart block, ventricular aneurysm, atrioventricular valve disease, mitral or aortic stenosis).

The sensation of palpitations has been described as a bump, pound, jump, flop, flutter, or racing sensation of the heart. Associated symptoms may include lightheadedness or syncope. Palpated pulse may feel rapid or irregular, as if the heart "skipped" a beat. Occasionally, a client will report "fluttering" sensations in the neck. Generally, unless accompanied by other symptoms, these sensations in the neck are caused by anxiety, random muscle fasciculation, or minor muscle strain or overuse.

Palpitations can be considered physiologic (i.e., when less than six occur per minute, this may be considered within normal function of the heart). However, palpitation lasting for hours or occurring in association with pain, shortness of breath, fainting, or severe lightheadedness requires medical evaluation. Palpitation in any person with a history of unexplained sudden death in the family requires medical referral.

Clients describing "palpitations" or similar phenomena may not be experiencing symptoms of heart disease. Palpitations may occur as a result of an overactive thyroid, secondary to caffeine sensitivity, as a side effect of some medications, and with the use of drugs such as cocaine. Encourage the client to report any such symptoms to the physician if this information has not already been brought to the physician's attention.

Dyspnea

Dyspnea, also referred to as breathlessness or shortness of breath, can be cardiovascular in origin, but it may also occur secondary to a pulmonary pathologic condition (see also Chapter 4), fever, certain medications, allergies, poor physical conditioning, or obesity. Early onset of dyspnea may be described as having to breathe too much or as an uncomfortable feeling during breathing after exercise or exertion.

Shortness of breath with mild exertion (dyspnea on exertion [DOE]), when caused by an impaired left ventricle that is unable to contract completely, results in the lung's inability to empty itself of blood. Pulmonary congestion and shortness of breath then occur. With severe compromise of the cardiovascular or pulmonary systems, dyspnea may occur at rest.

The severity of dyspnea is determined by the extent of disease. Thus the more severe the heart disease is, the easier it is to bring on dyspnea. Extreme dyspnea includes paroxysmal nocturnal dyspnea (PND) and orthopnea (breathlessness that is relieved by sitting upright with pillows used to prop the trunk and head).

PND and sudden, unexplained episodes of shortness of breath frequently accompany congestive heart failure (CHF). During the day the effects of gravity in the upright position and the shunting of excessive fluid to the lower extremities permit more effective ventilation and perfusion of the lungs, keeping the lungs relatively fluid free, depending on the degree of CHF. PND awakens the person sleeping in the recumbent position because the amount of blood returning to the heart and lungs from the lower extremities increases in this position.

Anyone who cannot climb a single flight of stairs without feeling moderately to severely winded or who awakens at night or experiences shortness of breath when lying down should be evaluated by a physician. Anyone with known cardiac involvement who develops progressively worse dyspnea must also notify the physician of these changes.

Dyspnea relieved by specific breathing patterns (e.g., pursed-lip breathing) or by specific body position (e.g., leaning forward on the arms to lock the shoulder girdle) is more likely to be pulmonary than cardiac in origin. Because breathlessness can be a terrifying experience for many persons, any activity that provokes the sensation is avoided, thus quickly reducing functional activities.

Cardiac Syncope

Cardiac syncope (fainting) or more mild lightheadedness can be caused by reduced oxygen delivery to the brain. Cardiac conditions resulting in syncope include arrhythmias, orthostatic hypotension, poor ventricular function, coronary artery disease, and vertebral artery insufficiency.

Lightheadedness that results from orthostatic hypotension (sudden drop in blood pressure) may occur with any quick change in a prolonged position (e.g., going from a supine position to an upright posture or standing up from a sitting position) or physical exertion involving increased abdominal pressure (e.g., straining with a bowel movement, lifting). Any client with aortic stenosis is likely to experience lightheadedness as a result of these activities.

Noncardiac conditions such as anxiety and emotional stress can cause hyperventilation and subsequent lightheadedness (vasovagal syncope). Side effects such as orthostatic hypotension may also occur during the period of initiation and regulation of cardiac medications (e.g., vasodilators).

Syncope that occurs without any warning period of lightheadedness, dizziness, or nausea may be a sign of heart valve or arrhythmia problems. Since sudden death can thus occur, medical referral is recommended for any unexplained syncope, especially in the presence of heart or circulatory problems or if the client has any risk factors for heart attack or stroke.

Examination of the cervical spine may include vertebral artery tests for compression of the vertebral arteries (see Aspinall, 1989; Magee, 1997; and Rivett, 1995 for specific test procedures).* If signs of eye nystagmus, changes in pupil size, or visual disturbances

---

*The effect of these tests, known as the vertebral basal artery test, the vertebral artery compression test, the Wallenberg test, or the de Kleyn hanging head test on blood flow velocity has been reviewed. It has been suggested that other factors, such as individual sensitivity to extreme head positions, age, and vestibular responsiveness, could affect the results of these tests (Thiel et al, 1994).

and symptoms of dizziness or lightheadedness occur, care must be taken concerning any treatment that follows.

Fatigue

Fatigue provoked by minimal exertion indicates a lack of energy, which may be cardiac in origin (e.g., coronary artery disease, aortic valve dysfunction, cardiomyopathy, or myocarditis) or may occur secondary to a neurologic, muscular, metabolic, or pulmonary pathologic condition. Often fatigue of a cardiac nature is accompanied by associated symptoms, such as dyspnea, chest pain, palpitations, or headache.

Fatigue that goes beyond expectations during or after exercise, especially in a client with a known cardiac condition, must be closely monitored. It should be remembered that beta-blockers prescribed for cardiac problems can also cause unusual fatigue symptoms.

For the client experiencing fatigue without a prior diagnosis of heart disease, monitoring vital signs may indicate a failure of the blood pressure to rise with increasing workloads. Such a situation may indicate cardiac output that is inadequate in meeting the demands of exercise. However, poor exercise tolerance is often the result of deconditioning, especially in the older adult population. Further testing (e.g., exercise treadmill test) may be helpful in determining whether fatigue is cardiac-induced.

Cough

Cough (see also Chapter 4) is usually associated with pulmonary conditions, but it may occur as a pulmonary complication of a cardiovascular pathologic complex. Left ventricular dysfunction, including mitral valve dysfunction resulting from pulmonary edema or left ventricular CHF, may result in a cough when aggravated by exercise, metabolic stress, supine position, or PND. The cough is often hacking and may produce large amounts of frothy, blood-tinged sputum. In the case of CHF, cough develops because a large amount of fluid is trapped in the pulmonary tree, irritating the lung mucosa.

Cyanosis

Cyanosis is a bluish discoloration of the lips and nail beds of the fingers and toes that accompanies inadequate blood oxygen levels (reduced amounts of hemoglobin). Although cyanosis can accompany hematologic or central nervous system disorders, most often visible cyanosis accompanies cardiac and pulmonary problems.

Edema

Edema in the form of a 3-pound or greater weight gain or a gradual, continuous gain over several days that results in swelling of the ankles, abdomen, and hands combined with shortness of breath, fatigue, and dizziness may be red-flag symptoms of CHF.

Other accompanying symptoms may include jugular vein distention (JVD) and cyanosis (of lips and appendages). Right upper quadrant pain described as a constant aching or sharp pain may occur secondary to an enlarged liver in this condition. Right heart failure and subsequent edema can also occur secondary to cardiac surgery, venous valve incompetence or obstruction, cardiac valve stenosis, coronary artery disease, or mitral valve dysfunction.

Noncardiac causes of edema may include pulmonary hypertension, kidney dysfunction, cirrhosis, burns, infection, lymphatic obstruction, use of nonsteroidal antiinflammatory drugs (NSAIDs), or allergic reaction.

When edema and other accompanying symptoms persist despite rest, medical referral is required. Edema of a cardiac origin may require electrocardiogram (ECG) monitoring during exercise or activity (the physician may not want the client stressed when extensive ECG changes are present), whereas edema of peripheral origin requires treatment of the underlying etiologic complex.

Claudication

Claudication or leg pain occurs with peripheral vascular disease (PVD) (arterial or venous), often occurring simultaneously with coronary artery disease. Claudication can be more functionally debilitating than other associated symptoms, such as angina or dyspnea, and may occur in addition to these other symptoms. The presence of pitting edema along with leg pain is usually associated with vascular disease.

Other noncardiac causes of leg pain (e.g., sciatica, pseudoclaudication,* anterior compartment syndrome, gout, peripheral neuropathy) must be differentiated from pain associated with peripheral vascular disease. Vascular claudication may occur in the absence of physical findings but is usually accompanied by skin discoloration and trophic changes (e.g., thin, dry, hairless skin) in the presence of vascular disease. Core temperature, peripheral pulses, and skin temperature should be assessed. Cool skin is more indicative of vascular obstruction; warm to hot skin may indicate inflammation or infection. Abrupt onset of ischemic rest pain or sudden worsening of intermittent claudication may be due to thromboembolism and must be reported to the physician immediately.

If people with intermittent claudication have normal-appearing skin at rest, exercising the extremity to the point of claudication usually produces marked pallor in the skin over the distal third of the extremity. This postexercise cutaneous ischemia occurs in both upper and lower extremities and is due to selective shunting of the available blood to the exercised muscle and away from the more distal parts of the extremity.

---

*Low back pain associated with pseudoclaudication often indicates spinal stenosis. The typical person affected is approximately 60 years old and bothered less by back pain than by a discomfort occurring in the buttock, thigh, or leg that (like true claudication) is brought on by walking but (unlike claudication) can also be elicited by prolonged standing. The discomfort associated with pseudoclaudication is frequently bilateral and improves with rest or flexion of the lumbar spine.

Vital Signs

The physical therapist may see signs of cardiac dysfunction as abnormal responses of heart rate and blood pressure during exercise. The therapist must remain alert to a heart rate that is either too high or too low during exercise, an irregular pulse rate, a systolic blood pressure that does not rise progressively as the work level increases, a systolic blood pressure that falls during exercise, or a change in diastolic pressure greater than 15 to 20 mm Hg.

▼ CARDIAC PATHOPHYSIOLOGY

Three components of cardiac disease are discussed, including diseases affecting the heart muscle, diseases affecting heart valves, and defects of the cardiac nervous system (Table 3-2).

Diseases Affecting the Heart Muscle

In most cases a cardiopulmonary pathologic condition can be traced to at least one of three processes: (1) obstruction or restriction, (2) inflammation, or (3) dilation or distension. Any combination of these can cause chest, neck, back, and/or shoulder pain. Frequently, these conditions occur sequentially.

TABLE 3-2 ▼ Cardiac Diseases

Heart Muscle	Heart Valves	Cardiac Nervous System
Coronary artery disease	Rheumatic fever	Arrhythmias
Myocardial infarct	Endocarditis	Tachycardia
Pericarditis	Mitral valve prolapse	Bradycardia
Congestive heart failure	Congenital deformities	
Aneurysms		

For example, an underlying *obstruction,* such as pulmonary embolus, leads to *congestion,* and subsequent *dilation* of the vessels blocked by the embolus.

The most common cardiovascular conditions to mimic musculoskeletal dysfunction are angina, myocardial infarction, pericarditis, and dissecting aortic aneurysm. Other cardiovascular diseases are not included in this text because they are rare or because they do not mimic musculoskeletal symptoms.

Degenerative heart disease refers to the changes in the heart and blood supply to the heart and major blood vessels that occur with aging. As the population ages, degenerative heart disease becomes the most prevalent form of cardiovascular disease. Degenerative heart disease is also called *atherosclerotic cardiovascular disease, arteriosclerotic cardiovascular disease, coronary heart disease* (CHD), and *coronary artery disease* (CAD).

Coronary Artery Disease

The heart muscle must have an adequate blood supply to contract properly. As mentioned, the coronary arteries carry oxygen and blood to the myocardium. When a coronary artery becomes narrowed or blocked, the area of the heart muscle supplied by that artery becomes ischemic and injured, and infarction may result.

The major disorders caused by insufficient blood supply to the myocardium are angina pectoris, CHF, and myocardial infarction. These disorders are collectively known as coronary artery disease (CAD), also called coronary heart disease or ischemic heart disease.

CAD includes atherosclerosis (fatty buildup), thrombus (blood clot), and spasm (intermittent constriction).

CAD results from a person's complex genetic makeup and interactions with the environment, including nutrition, activity levels, and history of smoking. Susceptibility to CVD may be explained by genetic factors, and it is likely that one or more "heart-attack" genes will be identified. The thera-

peutic use of drugs that act by modifying gene transcription is a well-established practice in the treatment of CAD and essential hypertension (Kurtz and Gardner, 1998).

ATHEROSCLEROSIS

Atherosclerosis is the disease process often called *arteriosclerosis* or *hardening of the arteries.* It is a progressive process that begins in childhood. It can occur in any artery in the body, but it is most common in medium-sized arteries, such as those of the heart, brain, kidneys, and legs. Starting in childhood, the arteries begin to fill with a fatty substance, or lipids such as triglycerides and cholesterol, which then calcify or harden.

This filler, called *plaque,* is made up of fats, calcium, and fibrous scar tissue and lines the usually supple arterial walls (Fig. 3-2), progressively narrowing the arteries. These arteries carry blood rich in oxygen to the myocardium (middle layer of the heart consisting of the heart muscle), but the atherosclerotic process leads to ischemia and to necrosis of the heart muscle. Necrotic tissue gradually forms a scar, but before scar formation, the weakened area is susceptible to aneurysm development.

When fully developed, plaque can cause bleeding, clot formation, and distortion or rupture of a blood vessel. Heart attacks and strokes are the most sudden and often fatal signs of the disease.

THROMBUS

When plaque builds up on the artery walls, the blood flow is slowed and a clot (thrombus) may form on the plaque. When a vessel becomes blocked with a clot, it is called *thrombosis. Coronary thrombosis* refers to the formation of a clot in one of the coronary arteries, usually causing a heart attack.

SPASM

Sudden constriction of a coronary artery is called a spasm; blood flow to that part of the heart is cut off or decreased. A brief spasm may cause mild symptoms that never

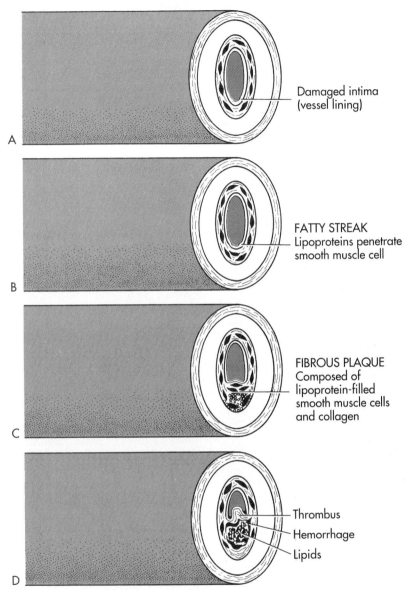

Damaged intima
(vessel lining)

FATTY STREAK
Lipoproteins penetrate
smooth muscle cell

FIBROUS PLAQUE
Composed of
lipoprotein-filled
smooth muscle cells
and collagen

Thrombus
Hemorrhage
Lipids

FIGURE 3-2 • Hardening of the arteries. **A,** Atherosclerosis begins with an injury to the endothelial lining of the artery (intimal layer) that makes the vessel permeable to circulating lipoproteins. **B,** Penetration of lipoproteins into the smooth muscle cells of the intima produces "fatty streaks." **C,** A fibrous plaque large enough to decrease blood flow through the artery develops. **D,** Calcification with rupture or hemorrhage of the fibrous plaque is the final advanced stage. Thrombosis may occur, further occluding the lumen of the blood vessel.

return. A prolonged spasm may cause heart damage, such as an infarct. This process can occur in healthy persons who have no cardiac history, as well as in those who have known atherosclerosis. Chemicals like nicotine and cocaine may lead to coronary artery spasm; other possible factors include anxiety and cold air.

RISK/CONTRIBUTING FACTORS

In 1948 the United States government decided to investigate the etiology, incidence, and pathology of CAD by studying residents of a typical small town in the United States called Framingham, Massachusetts. Over the next multiple decades various aspects of lifestyle, health, and disease were studied.

The research revealed important modifiable and nonmodifiable risk factors associated with death caused by CHD. Since that time, an additional category, contributing factors, has been added (Table 3-3).*

More recent research has identified other possible risk factors for and predictors of cardiac events, especially for those persons who have already had a heart attack. These additional risk factors include (1) exposure to bacteria such as *Chlamydia pneumoniae, Porphyromonas gingivalis,* and *Cytomegalovirus* organisms (Davidson, 1998; Muhlestein, 1998); (2) excess levels of homocysteine, an amino acid by-product of food rich in proteins; (3) high levels of α-lipoprotein, a close cousin of low-density lipoprotein that transports fat throughout the body; (4) high levels of fibrinogen, a protein that

---

*The American Heart Association has also developed a validated health-risk appraisal instrument called the RISKO scale. Anyone can use this tool to assess individual risk (www.americanheart.org/risk/quiz.html).

TABLE 3-3 ▼ Risk Factors and Coronary Artery Disease

Modifiable Risk Factors	Nonmodifiable Risk Factors	Contributing Factors
Physical inactivity	Age	Obesity
Cigarette smoking	Male gender	Response to stress
Elevated serum cholesterol	Family history	Personality
High blood pressure	Race	Peripheral vascular disease
		Diabetes
		Hormonal status
		Alcohol consumption

Modified from Reigle J, Ringel KA: Nursing care of clients with disorders of cardiac function. In Black JM, Matassarin-Jacobs E, editors: *Luckmann and Sorenson's medical-surgical nursing,* ed 4, Philadelphia, 1993, WB Saunders, p 1140.

binds together platelet cells in blood clots (Toss et al, 1998); (5) large amounts of C-reactive protein, a specialized protein necessary for repair of tissue injury (Anderson et al, 1998); (6) the presence of troponin T, a regulatory protein that helps heart muscle contract (Morrow et al, 1998); and (7) the presence of diagonal earlobe creases (Elliot and Powel, 1996).

CLINICAL SIGNS AND SYMPTOMS

Atherosclerosis, by itself, does not necessarily produce symptoms. For manifestations to develop, there must be a critical deficit in blood supply to the heart in proportion to the demands of the myocardium for oxygen and nutrients (supply and demand imbalance). When atherosclerosis develops slowly, collateral circulation develops to meet the heart's demands. Often, symptoms of CAD do not appear until the lumen of the coronary artery narrows by 75% (see also Hypertension).

Although the arteries are rarely completely blocked, the deposits of plaque are often extensive enough to restrict blood flow to the heart, especially during exercise in a physical therapist practice when there is a need to deliver more oxygen-carrying blood to the heart. Like other muscles, the heart, when deprived of oxygen, may ache, causing chest pain or discomfort referred to as *angina.*

CAD is a progressive disorder, especially if left untreated. If the blood flow is entirely disrupted, usually by a clot that has formed in the obstructed region, some of the tissue that is supplied by the vessel can die, and a heart attack or even sudden cardiac death results. When tissue loss is extensive enough to disrupt the electrical impulses that stimulate the heart's contractions, heart failure, chronic arrhythmias, and conduction disturbances may develop.

Angina Pectoris

Acute pain in the chest, called *angina pectoris,* results from the imbalance between cardiac workload and oxygen supply to myocardial tissue. Although the primary cause of angina is CAD, angina can occur in individuals with normal coronary arteries and with other conditions affecting the supply/demand balance (see Causes of Myocardial Ischemia).

As vessels become lined with atherosclerotic plaque, symptoms of inadequate blood supply develop in the tissues supplied by these vessels. A growing mass of plaque in the vessel collects platelets, fibrin, and cellular debris. Platelet aggregations are known

▼
Clinical Symptoms of
Myocardial Ischemia

- May be silent (smokers, diabetics: reduced sensitivity to pain)
- Angina pectoris (chest pain)
- Conduction disturbances
- Arrhythmias
- Eventual myocardial infarct (i.e., necrosis or death of the heart muscle)
- Sudden cardiac death

to release prostaglandin capable of causing vessel spasm. This in turn promotes platelet aggregation, and a vicious spasm/pain cycle begins.

The present theory of heart pain suggests that pain occurs as a result of an accumulation of metabolites within an ischemic segment of the myocardium. The transient ischemia of angina or the prolonged, necrotic ischemia of a myocardial infarction sets off pain impulses secondary to rapid accumulation of these metabolites in the heart muscle.

The imbalance between cardiac workload and oxygen supply can develop as a result of disorders of the coronary vessels, disorders of circulation, increased demands on output of the heart, or damaged myocardium unable to utilize oxygen properly.

TYPES OF ANGINAL PAIN

There are a number of types of anginal pain, including chronic stable angina (also referred to as walk-through angina), resting angina (angina decubitus), unstable angina, nocturnal angina, atypical angina,

CAUSES OF MYOCARDIAL ISCHEMIA

DECREASED BLOOD SUPPLY

Vessels

Atherosclerotic narrowing
Inadequate collateral circulation
Spasm caused by smoking, emotion, or cold
Coronary arteritis
Hypertension
Hypertrophic cardiomyopathy

Circulatory Factors

Arrhythmias ($\downarrow$ blood pressure)
Aortic stenosis
Hypotension
Bleeding

Blood Factors ($\uparrow$ Viscosity)

Anemia
Hypoxemia
Polycythemia

INCREASED BLOOD DEMAND

Hyperthyroidism
Arteriovenous fistula
Thyrotoxicosis
Exercise/exertion
Emotion/excitement
Digestion of a large meal

▼ *Clinical Signs and Symptoms of*
Angina Pectoris

- Gripping, viselike feeling of pain or pressure behind the breast bone
- Pain that may radiate to the neck, jaw, back, shoulder, or arms (most often the left arm)
- Toothache
- Burning indigestion
- Dyspnea (shortness of breath); exercise intolerance
- Nausea
- Belching

Symptoms in women

- Prolonged and repeated palpitations without chest pain
- Left chest pain in the absence of substernal chest pain
- Sensation similar to inhaling cold air
- Extreme fatigue, lethargy, and weakness
- Isolated midthoracic back pain
- Aching in the right biceps muscle
- Chest pain unrelieved by nitroglycerin but relieved by antacids
- Heartburn unrelieved by antacids
- Shortness of breath occurring at night

new-onset angina, and Prinzmetal's or "variant" angina.

Chronic stable angina occurs at a predictable level of physical or emotional stress and responds promptly to rest or to nitroglycerin. No pain occurs at rest, and the location, duration, intensity, and frequency of chest pain are consistent over time.

Resting angina, or *angina decubitus,* is chest pain that occurs at rest in the supine position and frequently at the same time every day. The pain is neither brought on by exercise nor relieved by rest.

Unstable angina, also known as *crescendo angina, preinfarction angina,* or *progressive angina,* is an abrupt change in the intensity and frequency of symptoms or decreased

threshold of stimulus, such as the onset of chest pain while at rest. The duration of these attacks is longer than the usual 1 to 5 minutes; they may last for up to 20 to 30 minutes. Such changes in the pattern of angina require immediate medical follow-up by the client's physician.

Nocturnal angina may awaken a person from sleep with the same sensation experienced during exertion. During sleep this exertion is usually caused by dreams. This type of angina may be associated with underlying CHF.

Atypical angina refers to unusual symptoms (e.g., toothache or earache) related to physical or emotional exertion. These symptoms subside with rest or nitroglycerin. *New-onset angina* describes angina that has developed for the first time within the last 60 days.

Prinzmetal's angina produces symptoms similar to those of typical angina but is caused by coronary artery spasm. These spasms periodically squeeze arteries shut and keep the blood from reaching the heart. Coronary arteries are usually clear of plaque or physiologic changes causing obstruction of the blood vessels. This form of angina occurs at rest, especially in the early hours of the morning, and can be difficult to induce by exercise. It is cyclic and frequently occurs at the same time each day. In postmenopausal women who are not undergoing hormone replacement therapy, the reduction in estrogen may cause coronary arteries to spasm, resulting in vasospastic (Prinzmetal's) angina.

CLINICAL SIGNS AND SYMPTOMS

The client may indicate the location of the symptoms by placing a clenched fist against the sternum. Angina radiates most commonly to the left shoulder and down the inside of the arm to the fingers; but it can also refer pain to the neck, jaw, teeth, upper back, possibly down the right arm, and occasionally to the abdomen (see Fig. 3-7).

Recognizing heart pain in women is more difficult because the symptoms are less reliable and often do not follow the classic pattern described earlier. Many women describe the pain in ways consistent with unstable angina, suggesting that they first become aware of their chest discomfort or have it diagnosed only after it reaches more advanced stages. Some experience a sensation similar to inhaling cold air, rather than the more typical shortness of breath. Other women complain only of weakness and lethargy, and some have noted isolated pain in the midthoracic spine or throbbing and aching in the right biceps muscle.

Pain associated with the angina and myocardial infarction occurring along the inner aspect of the arm and corresponding to the ulnar nerve distribution results from common connections between the cardiac and brachial plexuses.

Cardiac pain referred to the jaw occurs through internuncial (neurons connecting other neurons) fibers from cervical spinal cord posterior horns to the spinal nucleus of the trigeminal nerve. Abdominal pain produced by referred cardiac pain is more difficult to explain and may be due to the overflow of segmental levels to which visceral afferent nerve pathways flow (see Fig. 1-2). This overflow increases the chances that final common pain pathways between the chest and the abdomen may occur.

The *sensation* of angina is described as squeezing, burning, pressing, choking, aching, or bursting. Chest pain can be brought on by a wide variety of noncardiac causes (see discussion of Chest Pain, Chapter 12). In particular, angina is often confused with heartburn or indigestion, hiatal hernia, esophageal spasm, or gallbladder disease, but the pain of these other conditions is not described as sharp or knifelike. The client often says the pain feels like "gas" or "heartburn" or "indigestion." Referred pain from the external oblique abdominal muscle can cause heartburn in the anterior chest wall.

A physician must make the differentiation between angina and heartburn, hiatal hernia, and gallbladder disease.

Severity is usually mild or moderate. Rarely is the pain described as severe. As to *location,* 80% to 90% of clients experience the pain as retrosternal or slightly to the left of the sternum. The *duration* of angina as a direct result of myocardial ischemia is typically 1 to 3 min-

---

▼ **Clinical Signs and Symptoms of**
Heartburn

- Frequent "heartburn" attacks
- Frequent use of antacids to relieve symptoms
- Heartburn wakes client up at night
- Acid or bitter taste in the mouth
- Burning sensation in the chest
- Discomfort after eating spicy foods
- Abdominal bloating and gas
- Difficulty in swallowing

---

utes and no longer than 3 to 5 minutes. However, attacks precipitated by a heavy meal or extreme anger may last 15 to 20 minutes. Angina is relieved by rest or nitroglycerin (a coronary artery vasodilator).

Severity of pain is not a good prognostic indicator; some persons with severe discomfort live for many years, whereas others with mild symptoms may die suddenly. If the pain is not relieved by rest or up to 3 nitroglycerin tablets (taken one at a time at 5-minute intervals) in 10 to 15 minutes, the physician should be notified and the client taken to a cardiac care unit. (Nitroglycerin dilates the coronary arteries and improves collateral cardiac circulation, thus providing an increase in oxygen to the heart muscle and a decrease in symptoms of angina.)

Myocardial Infarct

Myocardial infarct (MI), also known as a heart attack, coronary occlusion, or "a coronary," is the development of ischemia and necrosis of myocardial tissue. It results from a sudden decrease in coronary perfusion or an increase in myocardial oxygen demand without adequate blood supply. If the requirements for blood are not eased (e.g., by decreased activity), the heart attempts to continue meeting the increased demands for oxygen with an inadequate blood supply, which leads to an MI. Myocardial tissue death is usually preceded by a sudden occlusion of one of the major coronary arteries.

The myocardium receives its blood supply from the two large coronary arteries and their branches. Occlusion of one or more of these blood vessels (coronary occlusion) is one of the major causes of MI. The occlusion may result from the formation of a clot that develops suddenly when an atheromatous plaque ruptures through the sublayers of a blood vessel, or when the narrow, roughened inner lining of a sclerosed artery leads to complete thrombosis.

Although coronary thrombosis is the most common cause of infarction, many inter-related factors may be responsible, including coronary artery spasm, platelet aggregation and embolism, thrombus secondary to rheumatic heart disease, endocarditis, aortic stenosis, a thrombus on a prosthetic mitral or aortic valve, or a dislodged calcium plaque from a calcified aortic or mitral valve.

Coronary blood flow is affected by the tonus (tone) of the coronary arteries. Arteries "clogged" by plaque formation become rigid, and resultant spasm may be provoked by cold and by exercise, which explains the adverse effect of both factors on clients with angina.

CLINICAL SIGNS AND SYMPTOMS

The onset of an infarct may be characterized by severe fatigue for several days before the infarct.

The likelihood of having a heart attack in the morning hours is 40% higher than during the rest of the day (Cohen et al, 1997). The morning is when the body's clotting system is more active, blood pressure surges, heart rate increases, and there may be reduced blood flow to the heart. Additionally, the levels and activity of stress hormones (e.g., catecholamines), which can induce vasoconstriction, increase in the morning.* Combined with these factors are the increased mental and physical stresses that typically occur after waking.

Persons who have MIs may not experience any pain and may be unaware that damage is occurring to the heart muscle as a result of prolonged ischemia. The presence of silent

infarction (SI) increases with advancing age, especially SI without a history of CAD.

Those who do have warning signs of MI may have severe unrelenting chest pain described as "crushing pain" lasting 30 or more minutes that is not alleviated by rest or by nitroglycerin. This chest pain may radiate to the arms, throat, and back, persisting for hours (see Fig. 3-8). Other symptoms include pallor, profuse perspiration, and possibly nausea and vomiting. The pain of an MI may be misinterpreted as indigestion because of the nausea and vomiting. A medical evaluation may be difficult because many clients have coexisting hiatal hernia, peptic ulcer, or gallbladder disease.

The shoulder-hand syndrome (more accurately termed reflex sympathetic dystrophy, or RSD) was a common complication of MI when clients were treated with strict, prolonged bed rest and immobilization. The change from prolonged bed rest to early ambulation has almost eliminated this problem. Rarely, clients with preexisting disease of the shoulder and medical complications requiring prolonged bed rest develop RSD.

▼ *Clinical Signs and Symptoms of*
Myocardial Infarction

- Severe substernal chest pain or squeezing pressure
- Pain possibly radiating down both arms
- Feeling of indigestion
- Angina lasting for 30 minutes or more
- Angina unrelieved by rest or nitroglycerin
- Pain of infarct unrelieved by a change in position
- Nausea
- Sudden dimness or loss of vision or loss of speech
- Pallor
- Diaphoresis (heavy perspiration)
- Shortness of breath
- Weakness, numbness, and feelings of faintness
- Painful shoulder-hand syndrome (RSD)

*The shift worker would experience this same phenomenon in the evening or on arising.

It begins 1 to 3 months after infarction with shoulder pain, stiffness, and marked limitation of motion of the shoulder joint, shoulder girdle, and arm. The hand may become swollen, shiny, stiff, and discolored.

An MI may occur during exertion, exercise, or exposure to extremes of temperature, or it may occur while the person is at rest. A subtle variation on ischemia during exertion is an important one for the physical therapist. The onset of an MI is known to be precipitated when one is working with the arms extended over the head. If the person becomes weak or short of breath while in this position, ischemia or infarction may be the cause of the pain and associated symptoms.

Because the infarction process may take up to 6 hours to complete, restoration of adequate myocardial perfusion is important if significant necrosis is to be limited. Deaths generally result from severe arrhythmias, cardiogenic shock, CHF, rupture of the heart, and recurrent MI.

Pericarditis

Pericarditis is an inflammation of the parietal pericardium (fluidlike membrane between the [fibrous] pericardium and the epicardium) and the visceral (epicardium) pericardium (Fig. 3-3). This inflammatory process may develop either as a primary

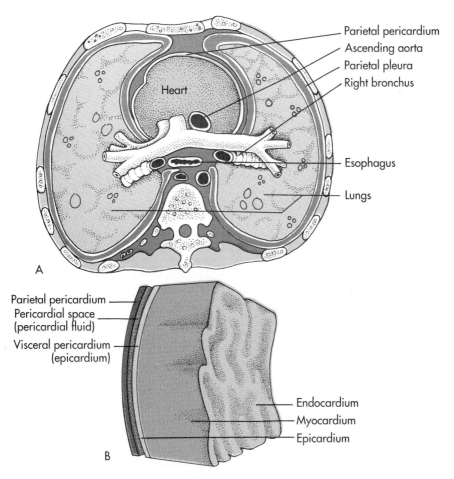

FIGURE 3-3 • The heart and associated layers of membranes. **A,** Cross section through the thorax just above the heart, emphasizing the lining of the cavity that contains the lungs (parietal pleura) and the lining of the cavity that contains the heart (parietal pericardium). **B,** Sagittal view of the layers of the heart.

CAUSES OF PERICARDITIS

INFECTIONS

Viral: Coxsackie, influenza
Bacterial: Tuberculosis, staph, strep, meningococcus, pneumonia
Parasitic
Fungal

MYOCARDIAL INJURY

Myocardial infarction
Cardiac trauma: Blunt or penetrating pericardium; rib fracture
Postcardiac surgery
Irradiation

HYPERSENSITIVITY

Collagen diseases: Rheumatic fever, scleroderma, systemic lupus erythematosus, rheumatoid arthritis
Drug reaction
Radiation/cobalt therapy

METABOLIC DISORDERS

Uremia
Myxedema
Chronic anemia

NEOPLASM

Lymphoma, lung or breast cancer

AORTIC DISSECTION

Modified from Ott B: Nursing care of clients with cardiac structure disorders. In Black JM, Matassarin-Jacobs E, editors: *Luckmann and Sorensen's medical-surgical nursing,* ed 4, Philadelphia, 1993, WB Saunders, p 1221.

condition or secondary to a number of diseases and circumstances.

Pericarditis may be acute or chronic (recurring); it is not known why pericarditis may be a single illness in some persons and recurrent in others.

Previous infection may be mild or asymptomatic with postinfectious onset of pain occurring 1 to 3 weeks later. Since this condition can occur in any age group, a history of recent pericarditis in the presence of new onset of chest, neck, or left shoulder pain is important.

CLINICAL SIGNS AND SYMPTOMS

At first, pericarditis may have no external signs or symptoms. The symptoms of acute pericarditis vary with the cause but usually include chest pain and dyspnea, an increase in the pulse rate, and a rise in temperature. Malaise and myalgia may occur.

Over time, the inflammatory process may result in an accumulation of fluid in the pericardial sac, preventing the heart from expanding fully. The subsequent chest pain of pericarditis (see Fig. 3-9) closely mimics that of an MI since it is substernal, is associated with cough, and may radiate to the left shoulder or supraclavicular area. It can be differentiated from MI by the pattern of relieving and aggravating factors (Table 3-4).

For example, the pain of an MI is unaffected by position, breathing, or movement, whereas the pain associated with pericardi-

TABLE 3-4 ▼ Characteristics of Cardiac Chest Pain

Angina	Myocardial Infarct	Mitral Valve Prolapse	Pericarditis
1–5 minutes	30 minutes–hours	Minutes to hours	Hours to days
Moderate intensity	Severe (can be painless)	Rarely severe	Varies; mild to severe
Tightness; chest discomfort	Crushing pain; intolerable (can be painless)	May be asymptomatic; "sticking" sensation, not substernal	Asymptomatic; sharp or cutting; can mimic MI
Can occur at rest or during sleep	Exertion	Often occurs at rest	Worse with breathing, swallowing, belching, neck or trunk movement
Usually occurs with exertion, emotion, cold, or large meal			
Subsides with rest or nitroglycerin; worse when lying down	Unrelieved by rest or nitroglycerin	Unrelieved by rest or nitroglycerin; may be relieved by lying down	Relieved by kneeling on all fours, leaning forward, sitting upright, or breathholding
Pain related to tone of arteries (spasm)	Pain related to heart ischemia	Mechanism of pain unknown	Pain related to inflammatory process

▼ **Clinical Signs and Symptoms of**
Pericarditis

- Substernal pain that may radiate to the neck, upper back, upper trapezius muscle, left supraclavicular area, down the left arm to the costal margins
- Difficulty in swallowing
- Pain relieved by leaning forward or sitting upright
- Pain aggravated by movement associated with deep breathing (laughing, coughing, deep inspiration)
- Pain relieved or reduced by holding the breath
- Pain aggravated by trunk movements (side bending or rotation)
- History of fever, chills, weakness, or heart disease (a recent myocardial infarction accompanying the pattern of symptoms may alert the physical therapist to the need for medical referral to rule out cardiac involvement)

tis may be relieved by kneeling on all fours, leaning forward, or sitting upright. Pericardial chest pain is often worse with breathing, swallowing, belching, or neck or trunk movements, especially side bending or rotation. The pain tends to be sharp or cutting and may recur in intermittent bursts that are usually precipitated by a change in body position. Pericarditis pain may diminish if the breath is held.

Congestive Heart Failure or Heart Failure

Heart failure, also called *cardiac decompensation* and *cardiac insufficiency,* can be defined as a physiologic state in which the heart is unable to pump enough blood to meet the metabolic needs of the body (determined as oxygen consumption) at rest or during exercise, even though filling pressures are adequate.

The heart fails when, because of intrinsic disease or structural defects, it cannot handle a normal blood volume, or in the absence of disease cannot tolerate a sudden expansion in blood volume (e.g., exercise). Heart failure is not a disease itself; instead, the term denotes a group of manifestations related to inadequate pump performance from either the cardiac valves or the myocardium.

Whatever the cause, when the heart fails to propel blood forward normally, congestion occurs in the pulmonary circulation as blood accumulates in the lungs. The right ventricle, which is not yet affected by congestive heart disease, continues to pump more blood into the lungs. The immediate result is shortness of breath and, if the process continues, actual flooding of the air spaces of the lungs with fluid seeping from the distended blood vessels. This last phenomenon is called pulmonary congestion or pulmonary edema.

Because a properly functioning heart depends on both ventricles, failure of one ventricle almost always leads to failure of the other ventricle. This is called ventricular interdependence. Right-sided ventricular failure (right-sided heart failure) causes congestion of the peripheral tissues and viscera. The liver may enlarge, the ankles may swell, and the client develops ascites (fluid accumulates in the abdomen).

Some clients have preexisting mild-to-moderate heart disease with no evidence of CHF. However, when the heart undergoes undue stress or deterioration from risk factors, compensatory mechanisms may be inadequate, and the heart fails.

Conditions that precipitate or exacerbate heart failure include hypertension, CAD, cardiomyopathy, heart valve abnormalities, arrhythmia, fever, infection, anemia, thyroid disorders, pregnancy, Paget's disease, nutritional deficiency (e.g., thiamine deficiency secondary to alcoholism), pulmonary disease, spinal cord injury, and hypervolemia from poor renal function.

Medications are frequently implicated in the development of CHF. Examples include cardiovascular drugs, antibiotics, central nervous system drugs (e.g., sedatives, hypnotics, antidepressants, narcotic analgesics), and antiinflammatory drugs (both nonsteroidal and steroidal).

CLINICAL SIGNS AND SYMPTOMS

The incidence of CHF increases with advancing age. Because of the increasing age of the U.S. population and newer medications and technologies that have increased survival at the expense of increased cardiovascular morbidity, the population affected by CHF is markedly increasing. In view of this increase, many individuals with a wide variety of heart and lung diseases will very likely develop CHF at some during their lives, manifesting itself as pulmonary congestion or edema (Cahalin, 1996).

Left Ventricular Failure. Failure of the left ventricle causes either pulmonary congestion or a disturbance in the respiratory control mechanisms. These problems in turn precipitate respiratory distress. The degree of distress varies with the client's position, activity, and level of stress.

However, many persons with severely impaired ventricular performance may have few or no symptoms, particularly if heart failure has developed gradually. Breathlessness, exhaustion, and lower extremity edema are the most common signs and symptoms of CHF.

Dyspnea is subjective and does not always correlate with the extent of heart failure. To some degree, exertional dyspnea occurs in all clients. The increased fluid in the tissue spaces causes dyspnea, at first on effort and then at rest, by stimulation of stretch receptors in the lung and chest wall and by the increased work of breathing with stiff lungs.

Paroxysmal nocturnal dyspnea (PND) resembles the frightening sensation of suffocation. The client suddenly awakens with the feeling of severe suffocation. Once the client is in the upright position, relief from the attack may not occur for 30 minutes or longer.

Orthopnea is a more advanced stage of dyspnea. The client often assumes a "three-point position," sitting up with both hands on the knees and leaning forward. Orthopnea develops because the supine position increases the amount of blood returning from the lower extremities to the heart and lungs. This gravitational redistribution of blood increases pulmonary congestion and dyspnea. The client learns to avoid respiratory distress at night by supporting the head and thorax on pillows. In severe heart failure the client may resort to sleeping upright in a chair.

Cough is a common symptom of left ventricular failure and is often hacking, producing large amounts of frothy, blood-tinged sputum. The client coughs because a large amount of fluid is trapped in the pulmonary tree, irritating the lung mucosa.

Pulmonary edema may develop when rapidly rising pulmonary capillary pressure causes fluid to move into the alveoli, resulting in extreme breathlessness, anxiety, frothy sputum, nasal flaring, use of accessory breathing muscles, tachypnea, noisy and wet breathing, and diaphoresis.

Cerebral hypoxia may occur as a result of a decrease in cardiac output, causing inadequate brain perfusion. Depressed cerebral function can cause anxiety, irritability, restlessness, confusion, impaired memory, bad dreams, and insomnia.

Fatigue and muscular weakness are often associated with left ventricular failure. Inadequate cardiac output leads to hypoxic tissue and slowed removal of metabolic wastes, which in turn causes the client to tire easily. A common report is feeling tired after an activity or type of exertion that was easily accomplished previously. Disturbances in sleep and rest patterns may aggravate fatigue.

Nocturia (urination at night) develops as a result of renal changes that can occur in both right- and left-sided heart failure (but more evident in left-sided failure). During the day the affected individual is upright and blood flow is away from the kidneys with reduced formation of urine. At night urine formation increases as blood flow to the kidneys improves.

Nocturia may interfere with effective sleep patterns, contributing to the fatigue associated with CHF. As cardiac output falls, decreased renal blood flow may result in oliguria (reduced urine output), a late sign of heart failure.

Right Ventricular Failure. Failure of the right ventricle may occur in response to left-sided CHF or as a result of pulmonary embolism (see Cor Pulmonale, Chapter 4). Right ventricular failure results in peripheral edema and venous congestion of the organs. For example, as the liver becomes congested with venous blood, it becomes enlarged and abdominal pain occurs. If this occurs rapidly, stretching of the capsule surrounding the liver causes severe discomfort. The client may notice either a constant

▼ *Clinical Signs and Symptoms of*
Left-Sided Heart Failure

- Fatigue and dyspnea after mild physical exertion or exercise
- Persistent spasmodic cough, especially when lying down, while fluid moves from the extremities to the lungs
- Paroxysmal nocturnal dyspnea (occurring suddenly at night)
- Orthopnea (person must be in the upright position to breathe)
- Tachycardia
- Fatigue and muscle weakness
- Edema (especially of the legs and ankles) and weight gain
- Irritability/restlessness
- Decreased renal function or frequent urination at night

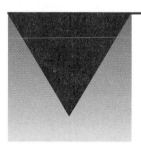

Case Example. A 74-year-old retired homemaker had a total hip replacement (THR) 2 days ago and remains as an inpatient with complications related to congestive heart failure. She has a previous medical history of gallbladder removal 20 years ago, total hysterectomy 30 years ago, and surgically induced menopause with subsequent onset of hypertension. Her medications include intravenous furosemide (Lasix), digoxin, and potassium replacement.

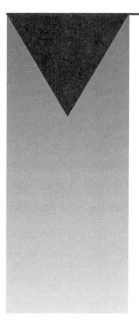

During the initial physical therapy treatment session, the client complained of muscle cramping and headache but was able to complete the entire exercise protocol. Blood pressure was 100/76 mm Hg. Systolic measurement dropped to 90 mm Hg when the client moved from supine to standing. Pulse rate was 56 bpm with a pattern of irregular beats. Pulse rate did not change with postural change. Platelet count was 98,000 cells/mm^3.

Result. With congestive heart failure, the heart will try to compensate by increasing the heart rate. However, the digoxin is designed to increase cardiac output and lower heart rate. In normal circumstances postural changes result in an increase in heart rate, but when digoxin is used, this increase cannot occur so the person becomes symptomatic. Most of the clients like this one are also taking beta-blockers, which also prevent the heart rate from increasing when the blood pressure drops.

In a clinical situation such as this one, the response of vital signs to exercise must be monitored carefully and charted. Any unusual symptoms, such as the muscle cramping and headaches, and any irregular pulse patterns must also be reported and documented.

Clinical Signs and Symptoms of
Right-Sided Heart Failure

- Increased fatigue
- Dependent edema (usually beginning in the ankles)
- Pitting edema (after 5 to 10 pounds of edema accumulate)
- Edema in the sacral area or the back of the thighs
- Right upper quadrant pain
- Cyanosis of nail beds

aching or a sharp pain in the right upper quadrant.

Dependent edema is one of the early signs of right ventricular failure. Edema is usually symmetric and occurs in the dependent parts of the body, where venous pressure is the highest. In ambulatory individuals, edema begins in the feet and ankles and ascends the lower legs. It is most noticeable at the end of a day and often decreases after a night's rest. Many people experiencing this type of edema assume that it is a normal sign of aging and fail to report it to their physician. In the recumbent person, pitting edema may develop in the presacral area and, as it worsens, progress to the genital area and medial thighs.

Cyanosis of the nail beds appears as venous congestion reduces peripheral blood flow. Clients with CHF often feel anxious, frightened, and depressed. Fears may be expressed as frightening nightmares, insomnia, acute anxiety states, depression, or withdrawal from reality.

Aneurysm

An aneurysm is an abnormal dilatation (commonly a saclike formation) in the wall of an artery, a vein, or the heart. Aneurysms occur when the vessel or heart wall becomes weakened from trauma, congenital vascular disease, infection, or atherosclerosis. This section could also be discussed under Peripheral Vascular Diseases because aneurysms of arterial blood vessels can result in some form of PVD.

Case Example. A 65-year-old man came to the clinic with a referral from his family doctor for "Hip pain—evaluate and treat." Past medical history included three total hip replacements of the right hip, open heart surgery 6 years ago, and persistent hypertension currently being treated with beta-blockers. During the interview it was discovered that the client had experienced many bouts of hip pain, leg weakness, and loss of hip motion. He was not actually examined by his doctor but had contacted the physician's office by phone, requesting a new P.T. referral.

On examination, large adhesed scars were noted along the anterior, lateral, and posterior aspects of the right hip, with significant bilateral hip flexion contractures. Pitting edema was noted in the right ankle, with mild swelling also observed around the left ankle. The client was unaware of this swelling. Further questions were negative for shortness of breath, difficulty in sleeping, cough, or other symptoms of cardiopulmonary involvement.

The bilateral edema could have been from compromise of the lymphatic drainage system following the multiple surgeries and adhesive scarring. However, with the positive history for cardiovascular involvement, bilateral edema, and telephone-derived referral, the physician was contacted by phone to notify him of the edema, and the client was directed by the physician to make an appointment. The client was diagnosed in the early stages of congestive heart failure. Physical therapy to address the appropriate hip musculoskeletal problems was continued.

Aneurysms are designated either venous or arterial and are also described according to the specific vessel in which they develop. *Thoracic aneurysms* usually involve the ascending, transverse, or descending portion of the aorta; *abdominal aneurysms* generally involve the aorta between the renal arteries and the iliac branches; *peripheral arterial aneurysms* affect the femoral and popliteal arteries.

THORACIC AND PERIPHERAL ARTERIAL ANEURYSMS

A dissecting aneurysm (most often a thoracic aneurysm) splits and penetrates the arterial wall, creating a false vessel. Thoracic aneurysms occur most frequently in hypertensive men between the ages of 40 and 70 years. Marked elevation of blood pressure may facilitate rapid disruption and final rupture of the aortic wall when a small tear in the intima has occurred.

The most common site for peripheral arterial aneurysms is the popliteal space in the lower extremities. Popliteal aneurysms cause ischemic symptoms in the lower limbs and an easily palpable pulse of larger amplitude. An enlarged area behind the knee may be present, seldom with discomfort.

ABDOMINAL AORTIC ANEURYSMS

Abdominal aortic aneurysms (AAAs) occur about four times more often than thoracic aneurysms. The natural course of an untreated AAA is expansion and rupture in one of several places, including the peritoneal cavity, the mesentery, behind the peritoneum, into the inferior vena cava, or into the duodenum or rectum. The most common site for an AAA is just below the kidney (immediately below the takeoff of the renal arteries), with referred pain to the thoraco-lumbar junction (see Fig. 3-10).

CLINICAL SIGNS AND SYMPTOMS

Most AAAs are asymptomatic; discovery occurs on physical or x-ray examination of

▼ *Clinical Signs and Symptoms of*
Aneurysm

- Chest pain with any of the following:
  - Palpable, pulsating mass (abdomen, popliteal space)
  - Abdominal "heartbeat" felt by the client when lying down
  - Dull ache in the midabdominal left flank or low back
  - Groin and/or leg pain
  - Weakness or transient paralysis of legs

▼ *Clinical Signs and Symptoms of*
Ruptured Aneurysm

- Sudden, severe chest pain with a tearing sensation (see Fig. 3-10)
- Pain may extend to the neck, shoulders, lower back, or abdomen but rarely to the joints and arms, which distinguishes it from myocardial infarction
- Pulsating abdominal mass
- Systolic blood pressure <100 mm Hg
- Pulse rate >100 beats/min
- Ecchymoses in the flank and perianal area
- Lightheadedness and nausea

the abdomen or lower spine for some other reason.

The most common symptom is awareness of a pulsating mass in the abdomen, with or without pain, followed by abdominal pain and back pain. Back pain may be the only presenting feature. Groin pain and flank pain may be experienced because of increasing pressure on other structures.

Extreme pain may be felt at the base of the neck along the back, particularly in the interscapular area, while dissection proceeds over the aortic arch and into the descending aorta.

The physical therapist can palpate the width of the arterial pulses; these pulses (e.g., aortic, femoral) should be uniform in width from the midline outward on either side. In adults older than 50, a normal aorta is not more than 3 cm (average 2.5 cm) wide.

The ease with which the aortic pulsations can be felt varies greatly with the thickness of the abdominal wall and the anteroposterior diameter of the abdomen. To palpate the aortic pulse, the therapist should press firmly deep in the upper abdomen (slightly to the left of the midline) to find the aortic pulsations.

By using both hands (one on each side of the aorta) and pressing deeply, one can assess the width of the aorta. Where the aorta

bifurcates (usually near the umbilicus), the width of the pulse should expand. Throbbing pain that increases with exertion and is accompanied by a sensation of a heartbeat when lying down and of a palpable pulsating abdominal mass requires immediate medical attention.

Systolic blood pressure below 100 mm Hg and pulse rate over 100 beats per minute may indicate signs of shock. Other symptoms may include ecchymoses in the flank and perianal area; severe and sudden pain in the abdomen, paravertebral area, or flank; and lightheadedness and nausea with sudden hypotension.

Diseases Affecting the Heart Valves

The second category of heart problems includes those that occur secondary to impairment of the valves caused by disease (e.g., rheumatic fever or coronary thrombosis), congenital deformity, or infection such as endocarditis. Three types of valve deformities may affect aortic, mitral, tricuspid, or pulmonic valves: *stenosis, insufficiency,* or *prolapse.*

Stenosis is a narrowing or constriction that prevents the valve from opening fully and may be caused by growths, scars, or

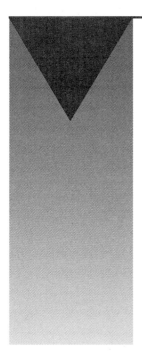

Case Example. A 72-year-old retired farmer has come to the physical therapist for recommendations about weight lifting. He had been following a regular program of weight lifting for almost 30 years, using a set of dead weights purchased at a garage sale. One year ago he experienced an abdominal aortic aneurysm that ruptured and required surgery (Date of surgery [DOS]: 7/7/97). Symptoms at the time of the diagnosis were back pain at the thoracolumbar junction radiating outward toward the flanks bilaterally. The client is symptom-free and in apparent good health, taking no medications, and receiving no medical treatment at this time.

Result. The hemodynamic stresses of weight lifting involve a rapid increase in systemic arterial blood pressure without a decrease in total peripheral vascular resistance. This principle combined with aortic degeneration may have contributed to the aortic dissection (de Virgilio, 1990).

Weight lifting in anyone with a history of aortic aneurysm is considered a contraindication. The therapist suggested a conditioning program combining a walking/biking program with resistive exercises using a lightweight elastic band alternating with an aquatic program for cardiac clients. Given this client's history, a medical evaluation before initiating an exercise program is necessary.

abnormal deposits on the leaflets. *Insufficiency* (also referred to as regurgitation) occurs when the valve does not close properly and causes blood to flow back into the heart chamber. *Prolapse* affects only the mitral valve and occurs when enlarged valve leaflets bulge backward into the left atrium.

These valve conditions increase the workload of the heart and require the heart to pump harder to force blood through a stenosed valve or to maintain adequate flow if blood is seeping back. Further complications for individuals with a malfunctioning valve may occur secondary to a bacterial infection of the valves (endocarditis).

Persons affected by diseases of the heart valves may be asymptomatic, and extensive auscultation with a stethoscope and diagnostic study may be required to differentiate one condition from another. In its early symptomatic stages cardiac valvular disease causes the person to become fatigued easily. As stenosis or insufficiency progresses, the main symptom of heart failure (breathlessness or dyspnea) appears.

▼ *Clinical Signs and Symptoms of*
Cardiac Valvular Disease

- Easy fatigue
- Dyspnea
- Palpitation (subjective sensation of throbbing, skipping, rapid or forcible pulsation of the heart)
- Chest pain
- Pitting edema
- Orthopnea or paroxysmal dyspnea
- Dizziness and syncope (episodes of fainting or loss of consciousness)

Rheumatic Fever

Rheumatic fever is an infection caused by streptococcal bacteria that can be fatal or may lead to rheumatic heart disease, a chronic condition caused by scarring and deformity of the heart valves (Fig. 3-4). It is called rheumatic fever because two of the

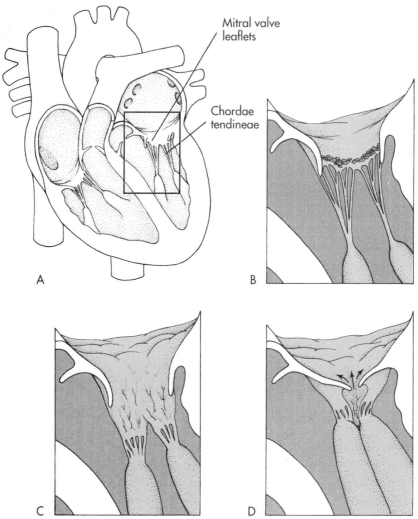

Mitral valve
leaflets

Chordae
tendineae

A

B

C

D

FIGURE 3-4 • Cardiac valvular disease caused by rheumatic fever. **A,** Inflammation of the membrane over the mitral (and aortic) valves may cause edema and accumulation of fibrin and platelets on the chordae tendineae. **B,** This accumulation of inflammatory materials produces rheumatic vegetations that affect the support provided by the chordae tendineae to the atrioventricular valves. **C,** In this view the mitral valve leaflets have become thickened with scar tissue so that the valves fail to close properly (mitral stenosis). **D,** Regurgitation or backflow of blood into the atrium develops when the scarred valve fails to close tightly. Prolonged severe stenosis with mitral regurgitation leads to symptoms of CHF.

most common symptoms are fever and joint pain.

The infection generally starts with strep throat in children between the ages of 5 and 15 years and damages the heart in approximately 50% of cases. Rheumatic fever produces a diffuse, proliferative, and exudative inflammatory process.

The aggressive use of specific antibiotics in the United States had effectively removed rheumatic fever as the primary cause of valvular damage. However, in 1985 a series of epidemics of rheumatic fever occurred in several widely diverse geographic regions of the continental United States. Currently, the prevalence and incidence of cases have not approximated the 1985 record, but they have remained above baseline levels.

CLINICAL SIGNS AND SYMPTOMS

The most typical clinical profile of a child or young adult with acute rheumatic fever is an initial cold or sore throat followed 2 or 3 weeks later by sudden or gradual onset of painful migratory joint symptoms in the knees, shoulders, feet, ankles, elbows, fingers, or neck. Fever of 37.2°C to 39.4°C (99°F to 103°F) and palpitations and fatigue are also present. Malaise, weakness, weight loss, and anorexia may accompany the fever.

The migratory arthralgias may last only 24 hours, or they may persist for several weeks. Joints that are sore and hot and contain fluid completely resolve, followed by acute synovitis, heat, synovial space tenderness, swelling, and effusion present in a different area the next day. The persistence of swelling, heat, and synovitis in a single joint or joints for more than 2 to 3 weeks is extremely unusual in acute rheumatic fever.

In the acute full-blown sequelae, shortness of breath and increasing nocturnal cough will also occur. A rash on the skin of the limbs or trunk is present in fewer than 2% of clients with acute rheumatic fever. Subcutaneous nodules over the extensor surfaces of the arms, heels, knees, or back of the head may occur.

All layers of the heart (epicardium, endocardium, myocardium, and pericardium) may be involved, and the heart valves are affected by this inflammatory reaction. The most characteristic and potentially dangerous anatomic lesion of rheumatic inflammation is the gross effect on cardiac valves, most commonly the mitral and aortic valves. If untreated, as many as 25% of clients will have mitral valvular disease 25 to 30 years later.

Rheumatic chorea (also called chorea or St. Vitus' dance) may occur 1 to 3 months after the strep infection and always is noted after polyarthritis. Chorea in a child, teenager, or young adult is almost always a manifestation of acute rheumatic fever. Other uncommon causes of chorea are systemic lupus erythematosus, thyrotoxicosis,

▼ **Clinical Signs and Symptoms of**
Rheumatic Fever

- Migratory arthralgias
- Subcutaneous nodules on extensor surfaces
- Fever and sore throat
- Flat, painless skin rash (short duration)
- Carditis
- Chorea
- Weakness, malaise, weight loss, and anorexia

and cerebrovascular accident, but these are unlikely in a child.

The client develops rapid, purposeless, nonrepetitive movements that may involve all muscles except the eyes. This chorea may last for 1 week or several months or may persist for several years without permanent impairment of the central nervous system.

Initial episodes of rheumatic fever last months in children and weeks in adults. Twenty percent of children have recurrences within 5 years. Recurrences are uncommon after 5 years of good health and are rare after age 21 years.

Endocarditis

Bacterial endocarditis, another common heart infection, causes inflammation of the cardiac endothelium (layer of cells lining the cavities of the heart) and damages the tricuspid, aortic, or mitral valve.

This infection may be caused by bacteria, or it may occur as a result of abnormal growths on the closure lines of previously damaged valves. These growths consist of collagen fibers and may separate from the valve, embolize, and cause infarction in the myocardium, kidney, brain, spleen, abdomen, or extremities.

In addition to clients with previous valvular damage, injection drug users and postcardiac surgical clients are at high risk for developing endocarditis. Congenital heart disease and degenerative heart disease, such as calcific aortic stenosis, may also cause bacterial endocarditis. The prosthetic cardiac valve has become more important as a predisposing factor for endocarditis because cardiac surgery is performed on a much larger scale than in the past.

This infection is often the consequence of invasive diagnostic procedures, such as renal shunts and urinary catheters, long-term indwelling catheters, or dental treatment (because of the increased opportunities for normal oral microorganisms to gain entrance to the circulatory system by way of highly vascularized oral structures). Individuals who are susceptible may take antibiotics as a precaution before undergoing any of these procedures.

A significant number of clients (up to 45%) with bacterial endocarditis initially have musculoskeletal symptoms, including arthralgia, arthritis, low back pain, and myalgias. Half these clients will have only musculoskeletal symptoms without other signs of endocarditis.

The early onset of joint pain and myalgia is more likely if the client is older and has had a previously diagnosed heart murmur. Musculoskeletal problems make up a significant part of the clinical picture of infective endocarditis diagnosed in an injection drug user.

The most common musculoskeletal symptom in clients with bacterial endocarditis is *arthralgia,* generally in the proximal joints. The shoulder is the most commonly affected site, followed (in declining incidence) by the knee, hip, wrist, ankle, metatarsophalangeal and metacarpophalangeal joints, and acromioclavicular joints.

Most endocarditis clients with arthralgias have only one or two painful joints, although some may have pain in several joints. Painful symptoms begin suddenly in one or two joints, accompanied by warmth, tenderness, and redness. Symmetric arthralgia in the knees or ankles may lead to a diagnosis of rheumatoid arthritis. One helpful clue: as a rule, morning stiffness is not as prevalent in clients with endocarditis as in those with rheumatoid arthritis or polymyalgia rheumatica.

Osteoarticular infections are the most common initial presentation when associated with endocarditis caused by injection drug use. Most commonly affected sites include the vertebrae, the wrist, the sternoclavicular joints, and the sacroiliac joints. Often multiple joint involvement occurs (Sapico et al, 1996).

Endocarditis may produce destructive changes in the *sacroiliac joint,* probably as a result of seeding the joint by septic emboli. The pain will be localized over the SI joint, and the physician will use roentgenograms and bone scans to verify this diagnosis.

Almost one third of clients with bacterial endocarditis have *low back pain;* in many clients it is the principal musculoskeletal symptom reported. Back pain is accompanied by decreased range of motion and spinal tenderness. Pain may affect only one side, and it may be limited to the paraspinal muscles. Endocarditis-induced low back pain may be very similar to that associated with a herniated lumbar disk: it radiates to the leg and may be accentuated by raising the leg or by sneezing. The key difference is that neurologic deficits are usually absent in clients with bacterial endocarditis.

Widespread diffuse *myalgias* may occur during periods of fever, but these are not appreciably different from the general myalgia seen in clients with other febrile illnesses. More commonly, myalgia will be restricted to the calf or thigh. Bilateral or unilateral leg

▼ **Clinical Signs and Symptoms of**
Endocarditis

- Constitutional symptoms
- Dyspnea, chest pain
- Cold and painful extremities
- Petechiae/splinter hemorrhages
- Musculoskeletal symptoms
- Myalgias
- Arthralgias
- Low back/sacroiliac pain
- Arthritis

myalgias occur in approximately 10% to 15% of all clients with bacterial endocarditis.

The cause of back pain and leg myalgia associated with bacterial endocarditis has not been determined. Some suggest that concurrent aseptic meningitis may contribute to both leg and back pain. Others suggest that leg pain is related to emboli that break off from the infected cardiac valves. The latter theory is supported by biopsy evidence of muscle necrosis or vasculitis in clients with bacterial endocarditis.

Rarely, other musculoskeletal symptoms, such as osteomyelitis, nail clubbing, tendinitis, hypertrophic osteoarthropathy, bone infarcts, and ischemic bone necrosis, may occur.

Lupus Carditis

Systemic lupus erythematosus (SLE) is a multisystem clinical illness associated with the release of a broad spectrum of autoantibodies into the circulation (see Chapter 11). The inflammatory process mediated by the immune response can target the heart and vasculature of the client with SLE.

Except for pericarditis, clinically significant cardiac disease directly associated with systemic lupus erythematosus (SLE) is relatively infrequent, but because of the musculoskeletal involvement, it may be of major importance for the physical therapist. Primary lupus cardiac involvement may include pericarditis, myocarditis, endocarditis, or a combination of the three.

Pericarditis is the most common cardiac lesion associated with SLE, appearing with the characteristic substernal chest pain that varies with posture, becoming worse in recumbency and improving with sitting or bending forward. *Myocarditis* may occur and is strongly associated with skeletal myositis in SLE.

Congenital Valvular Defects

Congenital malformations of the heart occur in approximately 1 of every 100 infants born in the United States. The most common defects include ventricular or atrial septal defect (hole between the ventricles or atria), tetralogy of Fallot (combination of four defects), patent ductus arteriosus (shunt caused by an opening between the aorta and the pulmonary artery), and congenital stenosis of the pulmonary, aortic, and tricuspid valves (Fig. 3-5). These congenital defects require surgical correction and may be part of the client's *past medical history*. They are not conditions that are likely to mimic musculoskeletal lesions and are therefore not covered in detail in this text.

Congenital cardiovascular abnormalities, which are usually asymptomatic and often undiagnosed during life, are the main cause of sudden death in athletes. Aortic stenosis, hypertrophic cardiomyopathy, Marfan's syndrome, congenital coronary artery anomalies, and ruptured aorta are the most commonly reported causes of sudden death during the practice of a sports activity. Family history of any of these conditions or premature sudden unexpected syncope or death is an indication for a thorough cardiovascular evaluation before participation in sports (Costa et al, 1998).

Mitral valve prolapse (MVP) is included in this section because of its increasing prevalence in the physical therapy client population. At presentation, usually the client with MVP has some other unrelated primary (musculoskeletal) diagnosis. During physical therapy treatment, the symptomatic MVP client may experience symptoms associated with MVP and require assurance or education regarding exercise and MVP.

MITRAL VALVE PROLAPSE

In a little more than 10% of the population, there is a slight variation in the shape or structure of the mitral valve of the heart that could cause mitral valve prolapse. This structural variation has many other names, including floppy valve syndrome, Barlow's syndrome, and click-murmur syndrome.

The incidence of MVP appears to be increasing dramatically in recent years. This increase may be attributed to nutritional changes and ever-increasing continual stress

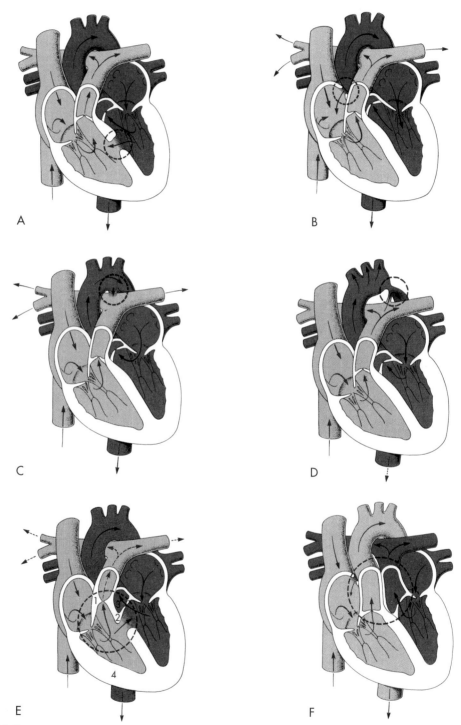

FIGURE 3-5 • Congenital malformations of the heart. **A,** Ventricular septal defect. **B,** Atrial septal defect. **C,** Patent ductus arteriosus. **D,** Coarctation of the aorta. **E,** Tetralogy of Fallot: *1,* Stenosis of the pulmonary valve: *2,* ventricular septal defect; *3,* aorta communicates with both ventricles; *4,* enlargement of the right ventricle wall. **F,** Transposition of the great arteries.

levels in our society or possibly to better diagnostic testing, which permits documenting the true incidence for the first time.

Occurring most often in young women, MVP is a benign condition in isolation; however, it can be associated with a number of other conditions, including endocarditis, myocarditis, atherosclerosis, systemic lupus erythematosus, muscular dystrophy, acromegaly, and cardiac sarcoidosis.

MVP appears to be due to connective tissue abnormalities in the valve leaflets. Normally, when the lower part of the heart contracts, the mitral valve remains firm and allows no blood to leak back into the upper chambers. In MVP the slight variation in shape of the mitral valve allows one part of the valve, the leaflet, to billow back into the upper chamber during contraction of the ventricle. One or both of the valve leaflets may bulge into the left atrium during ventricular systole. This protrusion can often be heard through a stethoscope as a sound known as a "click." Leaking of blood backward through the mitral valve can also be heard and is referred to as a heart murmur.

Approximately 60% of all clients with MVP experience no symptoms. Another 39% experience occasional symptoms that are mildly to moderately uncomfortable enough to interfere with the person's ability to enjoy an unrestricted life; approximately 1% suffer severe symptoms and lifestyle restrictions.

Clinical Signs and Symptoms. Almost all the symptoms of MVP syndrome are due to an imbalance in the autonomic nervous system, called *dysautonomia*. Frequently, when there is a slight variation in structure of the heart valve, there is also a slight variation in the function or balance of the autonomic nervous system (ANS). This description in the autonomic innervation of the heart may account for the high incidence of MVP in fibromyalgia, a condition known to be associated with dysregulation or dysautonomia of the ANS.

Symptoms include profound fatigue that cannot be correlated with exercise or stress, cold hands and feet, shortness of breath, chest pain, and heart palpitations. The most

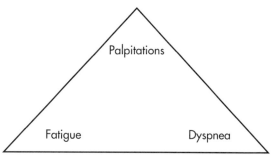

FIGURE 3-6 • The triad of symptoms associated with mitral valve prolapse.

common triad of symptoms associated with MVP is fatigue, palpitations, and dyspnea (Fig. 3-6).

Although the fatigue that accompanies MVP is not related to exertion, deconditioning from prolonged inactivity may develop, further complicating the picture. Minor symptoms associated with MVP may include tremors, swelling of extremities, sleep disturbances, low back pain, irritable bowel syndrome, numbness in any part of the body, excessive perspiration or inability to perspire, skin rashes, muscular fasciculations, visual changes or disturbances, difficulty in concentrating, memory lapses, and dizziness.

Although the chest pain associated with MVP can be severe, it differs from pain associated with MI (see Table 3-4). When there is an imbalance in the ANS, which controls contraction and relaxation of the chest wall muscles (the muscles of breathing), there may be inadequate relaxation between respirations. Over time these chest wall muscles go into spasm, resulting in chest pain.

It is important that the physical therapist evaluate the client with chest pain for trigger points. If palpation of the chest reproduces symptoms, especially radiating pain, deactivation of trigger points must be carried out followed by a reevaluation as part of the screening process for pain of a cardiac origin.

Frequently occurring musculoskeletal findings in clients with MVP include joint hypermobility, temporomandibular joint (TMJ) syndrome, and myalgias.

▼ *Clinical Signs and Symptoms of*
Mitral Valve Prolapse

- Profound fatigue
- Chest pain
- Palpitations or irregular heartbeat
- Tachycardia
- Migraine headache
- Anxiety, depression, panic attacks
- Dyspnea

MVP is not life-threatening but may be lifestyle-threatening for the small number of persons (rare) who have more severe structural problems that may progress to the point at which surgical replacement of the valve is required. To prevent infective endocarditis, the client may be given antibiotics prophylactically before any invasive procedures.

Clients with MVP are often referred to an exercise physiologist for a treatment program, but more and more are also going to physical therapy clinics for conditioning and exercise programs. Caution is advised in the use of weight training for the MVP client. Gradual buildup using light weights and increased repetitions is recommended.

Defects of the Cardiac Nervous System

The third component of cardiac disease is caused by failure of the heart's nervous system to conduct normal electrical impulses. The heart has its own intrinsic conduction system that allows the orderly depolarization of cardiac muscle tissue. Arrhythmias, also called *dysrhythmias,* are disorders of the heart rate and rhythm caused by disturbances in the conduction system.

Arrhythmias may cause the heart to beat too quickly (tachycardia), too slowly (bradycardia), or with extra beats and fibrillations. Arrhythmias can lead to dramatic changes in circulatory dynamics, such as hypotension, heart failure, and shock.

Clients who are neurologically unstable owing to recent cerebrovascular accident, head trauma, spinal cord injury, or other central nervous system insult often exhibit new arrhythmias during the period of instability. These may be due to elevation of intracranial pressure, and once this has been controlled and returned to normal range, arrhythmias usually disappear.

However, in clients who have preexisting arrhythmias, preexisting CAD, or CHF, these "transient arrhythmias" may not disappear and may lead to serious complications. Dizziness and loss of consciousness may occur, owing to loss of brain perfusion (not caused by transient ischemic attacks, as is often suspected) when the arrhythmia results in a serious reduction in cardiac output.

The physical therapist working with a client who has had a stroke may be the first health care professional to identify an arrhythmia that appears during exercise. In the early recovery period the therapist should monitor for these arrhythmias by taking the client's pulse. New arrhythmias should be reported to the physician.

Fibrillation

The sinoatrial (SA) node (or cardiac pacemaker) initiates and paces the heartbeat. During an MI, damaged heart muscle cells, deprived of oxygen, release small electrical impulses that may disrupt the heart's normal conduction pathway between the ventricles. The heart attack may develop suddenly into ventricular fibrillation that can result in sudden death. Similarly, a heart damaged by CAD (with or without previous infarcts) can go into ventricular fibrillation.

Atrial fibrillation is characterized by a total disorganization of atrial activity without effective atrial contraction. The upper chambers of the heart contract in an unsynchronized pattern, causing the atrium to quiver rather than to contract and often causing blood to pool, which allows for clots to form. These clots can break loose and travel to the brain, causing a stroke.

The physical therapist can easily and quickly screen individuals at risk and teach them to screen themselves by checking the pulse for the telltale signs of an irregular heartbeat. A regular heartbeat is characterized by a series of even and continuous pulsations, whereas an irregular heartbeat often feels like an extra or missed beat. To help determine the steadiness of the heartbeat, the therapist or individual keeps time by tapping the foot.

Persons at risk who require screening include those who have had a previous heart attack or a history that includes high blood pressure, CHF, digitalis toxicity, pericarditis, or rheumatic mitral stenosis.

Other factors that can overstimulate the sinus node include excessive production of thyroid hormone (hyperthyroidism), alcohol and caffeine consumption, and high fevers. In many instances, particularly in younger persons, there is no apparent cause.

CLINICAL SIGNS AND SYMPTOMS

Symptoms of fibrillation vary depending on the functional state of the heart, and fibrillation may exist without symptoms. The affected individual is usually aware of the irregular heart action and reports feeling "palpitations." Careful questioning may be required to pinpoint the exact description of sensations reported by the client.

Some individuals experience the symptoms of inadequate blood flow and low oxygen levels, such as dizziness, chest pain, and fainting. Chronic atrial fibrillation may cause CHF, which is often experienced as shortness of breath during exercise and fluid accumulation in the feet and legs.

More than six palpitations occurring in a minute or prolonged, repeated palpitations—especially if accompanied by chest pain, dyspnea, fainting, or other associated signs and symptoms—should be reported to the physician.

Sinus Tachycardia

Sinus tachycardia, defined as an abnormally rapid heart rate, usually taken to be more than 100 beats per minute, is the normal physiologic response to such stressors as fever, hypotension, thyrotoxicosis, anemia, anxiety, exertion, hypovolemia, pulmonary emboli, myocardial ischemia, CHF, and shock.

Sinus tachycardia is usually of no physiologic significance; however, in clients with organic myocardial disease, the result may be reduced cardiac output, CFH, or arrhythmias. Because heart rate is a major determinant of oxygen requirements, angina or perhaps an increase in the size of an infarction may accompany persistent tachycardia in clients with CAD.

CLINICAL SIGNS AND SYMPTOMS

The symptoms of tachycardia vary from one person to another and may range from an increased pulse to a group of symptoms that would restrict normal activity of the client. Anxiety and apprehension may occur, depending on the pain threshold and emotional reaction of the client.

▼ **Clinical Signs and Symptoms of**
Fibrillation

- Subjective report of palpitations
- Sensations of fluttering, skipping, irregular beating or pounding, heaving action
- Dyspnea
- Chest pain
- Anxiety
- Pallor
- Nervousness
- Cyanosis

▼ **Clinical Signs and Symptoms of**
Sinus Tachycardia

- Palpitation (most common symptom)
- Restlessness
- Chest discomfort or pain
- Agitation
- Anxiety and apprehension

▼ *Clinical Signs and Symptoms of*

Sinus Bradycardia

- Reduced pulse rate
- Syncope

Sinus Bradycardia

In sinus bradycardia, impulses travel down the same pathway as in sinus rhythm, but the sinus node discharges at a rate less than 60 beats per minute. Bradycardia may be normal in athletes or young adults and is therefore asymptomatic.

In most cases sinus bradycardia is a benign arrhythmia and may actually be beneficial by producing a longer period of diastole and increased ventricular filling. In some clients who have acute MI, it reduces oxygen demands and may help minimize the size of the infarction.

Eye surgery, meningitis, intracranial tumors, cervical and mediastinal tumors, and certain disease states (e.g., MI, myxedema, obstructive jaundice, and cardiac fibrosis) may produce sinus bradycardia.

CLINICAL SIGNS AND SYMPTOMS

Syncope may be preceded by sudden onset of weakness, sweating, nausea, pallor, vomiting, and distortion or dimming of vision. Signs and symptoms remit promptly when the client is placed in the horizontal position.

Physician referral for sinus bradycardia is needed only when symptoms such as chest pain, dyspnea, lightheadedness, or hypotension occur.

▼ CARDIOVASCULAR DISORDERS

Peripheral Vascular Disorders

Impaired circulation may be caused by a number of acute or chronic medical conditions known as *peripheral vascular diseases* (PVDs). PVDs can affect the arterial, venous, or lymphatic circulatory system.

Vascular disorders secondary to occlusive arterial disease usually have an underlying atherosclerotic process that causes disturbances of circulation to the extremities and can result in significant loss of function of either the upper or lower extremities.

Peripheral arterial occlusive diseases also can be caused by embolism, thrombosis, trauma, vasospasm, inflammation, or autoimmunity. The cause of some disorders is unknown.

Arterial (Occlusive) Disease

Arterial diseases include acute and chronic arterial occlusion (Table 3-5). Acute arterial occlusion may be caused by (1) thrombus, embolism, or trauma to an artery, (2) arteriosclerosis obliterans, (3) thromboangiitis obliterans or Buerger's disease, or (4) Raynaud's disease.

Clinical manifestations of chronic arterial occlusion caused by peripheral vascular disease may not appear for 20 to 40 years. The lower limbs are far more susceptible to arterial occlusive disorders and atherosclerosis than are the upper limbs.

Diabetes mellitus increases the susceptibility to coronary heart disease. People with diabetes have abnormalities that affect a number of steps in the development of atherosclerosis. Only the combination of factors, such as hypertension, abnormal platelet activation, and metabolic disturbances affecting fat and serum cholesterol, account for the increased risk.

Other risk factors include smoking, hypertension, hyperlipidemia (elevated levels of fats in the blood), and older age. Peripheral artery disease most often afflicts men older than 50, although women are at significant risk because of their increased smoking habits.

CLINICAL SIGNS AND SYMPTOMS

The first sign of vascular occlusive disease is the loss of hair on the toes. The most important symptoms of chronic arterial occlusive disease are intermittent claudication (limping resulting from pain, ache, or cramp

TABLE 3-5 ▼ Comparison of Acute and Chronic Arterial Symptoms

Symptom Analysis	Acute Arterial Symptoms	Chronic Arterial Symptoms
Location	Varies; distal to occlusion; may involve entire leg	Deep muscle pain, usually in calf; may be in lower leg or dorsum of foot
Character	Throbbing	Intermittent claudication; feels like cramp, numbness, and tingling; feeling of cold
Onset and duration	Sudden onset (within 1 hour)	Chronic pain; onset gradual following exertion
Aggravating factors		Activity such as walking or stairs; elevation
Relieving factors		Rest (usually within 2 minutes); dangling (severe involvement)
Associated symptoms	6 P's: Pain, pallor, pulselessness, paresthesia, poikilothermia (coldness), paralysis (severe)	Cool, pale skin
At risk	History of vascular surgery, arterial invasive procedure, abdominal aneurysm, trauma (including injured arteries), chronic atrial fibrillation	Older adults; more males than females; inherited predisposition; history of hypertension, smoking, diabetes, hypercholesterolemia, obesity, vascular disease

Modified from Jarvis C: *Physical examination and health assessment,* Philadelphia, 1992, WB Saunders, p. 658.

in the muscles of the lower extremities caused by ischemia or insufficient blood flow) and ischemic rest pain.

The pain associated with arterial disease is generally felt as a dull, aching tightness deep in the muscle, but it may be described as a boring, stabbing, squeezing, pulling, or even burning sensation. Although the pain is sometimes referred to as a cramp, there is no actual spasm in the painful muscles.

The location of the pain is determined by the site of the major arterial occlusion (Table 3-6). Aortoiliac occlusive disease induces pain in the gluteal and quadriceps muscles.

The most frequent lesion, which is present in about two thirds of clients, is occlusion of the superficial femoral artery between the groin and the knee, producing pain in the calf that sometimes radiates upward to the popliteal region and to the lower thigh. Occlusion of the popliteal or more distal arteries causes pain in the foot.

In the typical case of superficial femoral artery occlusion, there is a good femoral pulse at the groin but arterial pulses are absent at the knee and foot, although resting circulation appears to be good in the foot.

After exercise the client may have numbness in the foot as well as pain in the calf. The foot may be cold, pale, and chalky white, which is an indication that the circulation has been diverted to the arteriolar bed of the leg muscles. Blood in regions of sluggish flow becomes deoxygenated, inducing a red-purple mottling of the skin.

Painful, cramping symptoms occur during walking and disappear quickly with rest. Ischemic rest pain is relieved by placing the limb in a dependent position, using gravity to enhance blood flow. In most clients the symptoms are constant and reproducible, that is, the client who cannot walk the length of the house because of leg pain one day but is able to walk indefinitely the next does not have intermittent claudication.

Intermittent claudication is influenced by the speed, incline, and surface of the walk. Exercise tolerance decreases over time, so that episodes of claudication occur more frequently with less exertion. The differentiation between vascular claudication and neurogenic claudication is presented in Chapter 12 (see Table 12-2).

TABLE 3-6 ▼ Arterial Occlusive Disease

Site of Occlusion	Signs and Symptoms

Aortic bifurcation	Sensory and motor deficits
	  Muscle weakness
	  Numbness (loss of sensation)
	  Paresthesias (burning, pricking)
	  Paralysis
	Intermittent claudication (lower back, gluteal muscles, quadriceps, calves; relieved by rest)
	Cold, pale legs with decreased or absent peripheral pulses

Iliac artery	Intermittent claudication (buttock, hip, thigh; relieved by rest) Diminished or absent femoral or distal pulses Impotence in males
Femoral and popliteal artery	Intermittent claudication (calf and foot; may radiate) Leg pallor and coolness Dependent rubor Blanching of feet on elevation No palpable pulses in ankles and feet Gangrene
Tibial and common peroneal artery	Intermittent claudication (calf; feet occasionally) Pain at rest (severe disease); possibly relieved by dangling leg Same skin and temperature changes in lower leg and foot as described above Pedal pulses absent; popliteal pulses may be present

From Goodman CC, Boissonnault WG: *Pathology: implications for the physical therapist,* Philadelphia, 1998, WB Saunders, p 321.

▼ **Clinical Signs and Symptoms of Arterial Disease**

- Intermittent claudication
- Burning, ischemic pain at rest
- Rest pain aggravated by elevating the extremity; relieved by hanging the foot over the side of the bed or chair
- Color, temperature, skin, nail bed changes
  Decreased skin temperature
  Dry, scaly, or shiny skin
  Poor nail and hair growth
- Possible ulcerations and gangrene on weight bearing surfaces (e.g., toes, heel)
- Vision changes (diabetic atherosclerosis)
- Fatigue on exertion (diabetic atherosclerosis)

Ulceration and gangrene are common complications and may occur early in the course of some arterial diseases (e.g., Buerger's disease). Gangrene usually occurs in one extremity at a time. In advanced cases the extremities may be abnormally red or cyanotic, particularly when dependent. Edema of the legs is fairly common. Color or temperature changes and changes in nail bed and skin may also appear.

Raynaud's Phenomenon and Disease

The term *Raynaud's phenomenon* refers to intermittent episodes during which small arteries or arterioles in extremities constrict, causing temporary pallor and cyanosis of the digits and changes in skin temperature. These episodes occur in response to cold temperature or strong emotion (anxiety, excitement). As the episode passes, the changes in color are replaced by redness. If the disorder is secondary to another disease or underlying cause, the term *Raynaud's phenomenon* is used.

Secondary Raynaud's phenomenon is often associated with connective tissue or collagen vascular disease, such as scleroderma, polymyositis/dermatomyositis, systemic lupus erythematosus, or rheumatoid arthritis. Raynaud's phenomenon may occur after trauma or use of vibrating equipment such as jackhammers, or it may be related to various neurogenic lesions (e.g., thoracic outlet syndrome) and occlusive arterial diseases.

Raynaud's disease is a primary vasospastic or vasomotor disorder, although it is included in this section under occlusive arterial because of the arterial involvement. It appears to be caused by (1) hypersensitivity of digital arteries to cold, (2) release of serotonin, and (3) congenital predisposition to vasospasm. Eighty percent of clients with Raynaud's disease are women between the ages of 20 and 49 years. Primary Raynaud's disease rarely leads to tissue necrosis.

▼ *Clinical Signs and Symptoms of*
Raynaud's Phenomenon and Disease

- Pallor in the digits
- Cyanotic, blue digits
- Cold, numbness, pain of digits
- Intense redness of digits

Idiopathic Raynaud's disease is differentiated from secondary Raynaud's phenomenon by a history of symptoms for at least 2 years with no progression of the symptoms and no evidence of underlying cause.

CLINICAL SIGNS AND SYMPTOMS

The typical progression of Raynaud's phenomenon is pallor in the digits, followed by cyanosis accompanied by feelings of cold, numbness, and occasionally pain, and, finally, intense redness with tingling or throbbing.

The pallor is caused by vasoconstriction of the arterioles in the extremity, which leads to decreased capillary blood flow. Blood flow becomes sluggish and cyanosis appears; the digits turn blue. The intense redness (rubor) results from the end of vasospasm and a period of hyperemia as oxygenated blood rushes through the capillaries.

Venous Disorders

Venous disorders can be separated into acute and chronic conditions. Acute venous disorders include thromboembolism. Chronic venous disorders can be separated further into varicose vein formation and chronic venous insufficiency.

Acute venous disorders are due to formation of thrombi (clots), which obstruct venous flow. Blockage may occur in both superficial and deep veins. Superficial thrombophlebitis is often iatrogenic, resulting from insertion of intravenous catheters or as a complication of intravenous sites.

Deep venous thrombosis is a common disorder affecting women more than men and adults more than children. Approximately one third of clients older than 40 who have had either major surgery or an acute MI develop deep venous thrombosis.

Chronic venous insufficiency, also known as postphlebitic syndrome, is identified by chronic swollen limbs; thick, coarse, brownish skin around the ankles; and venous stasis ulceration. Chronic venous insufficiency is the result of dysfunctional valves that reduce venous return, which thus increases venous pressure and causes venous stasis and skin ulcerations.

Chronic venous insufficiency follows most severe cases of deep venous thrombosis but may take as long as 5 to 10 years to develop. Education and prevention are essential, and clients with a history of deep venous thrombosis must be monitored periodically for life.

Thrombus formation is usually attributed to venous stasis, hypercoagulability, or injury to the venous wall. *Venous stasis* is caused by immobilization or absence of the calf muscle pump (e.g., because of illness, paralysis, or inactivity), surgery,* obesity, pregnancy, and CHF.

Hypercoagulability often accompanies malignant neoplasms, especially visceral and ovarian tumors. Oral contraceptives, selective estrogen-receptor modulators (SERMs) (e.g., raloxifene) used for estrogen replacement therapy, and hematologic disorders also may increase the coagulability of the blood. In addition, previous spontaneous thromboembolism and increased levels of homocysteine are newly discovered risk factors (Goodnight and Feinstein, 1998).

Currently, the observed relationship of higher venous thrombosis risk with the use of third-generation oral contraceptives† is under investigation (Farmer and Lawrenson, 1998; Thorogood, 1998). The venous clots associated with the newest oral contraceptives typically develop in superficial leg veins and rarely result in pulmonary emboli.

Vein wall trauma may occur as a result of intravenous injections, Buerger's disease,

---

*Especially orthopedic surgery, gynecologic cancer surgery, major abdominal surgery, coronary artery bypass grafting, renal transplantation, and splenectomy.
†The term *third-generation* refers to the newest formulation of oral contraceptives with much lower levels of estrogen than first administered.

fractures and dislocations, sclerosing agents, and opaque mediator radiography.

CLINICAL SIGNS AND SYMPTOMS

Superficial thrombophlebitis appears as a local, raised, red, slightly indurated (hard), warm, tender cord along the course of the involved vein.

In contrast, symptoms of deep venous thrombosis are less distinctive; about one half of clients are asymptomatic. The most common symptoms are pain in the region of the thrombus and unilateral swelling distal to the site.

Other symptoms include redness or warmth of the leg, dilated veins, or low-grade fever possibly accompanied by chills and malaise. Unfortunately, the first clinical manifestation may be pulmonary embolism. Frequently, clients have thrombi in both legs even though the symptoms are unilateral.

Homans' sign (discomfort in the upper calf during gentle, forced dorsiflexion of the foot)

is commonly assessed during physical examination. Unfortunately, it is insensitive and nonspecific. It is present in less than one third of clients with documented deep venous thrombosis. In addition, more than 50% of clients with a positive finding of Homans' sign do not have evidence of venous thrombosis.

Pulmonary emboli (see Chapter 4), most of which start as thrombi in the large deep veins of the legs, are an acute and potentially lethal complication of deep venous thrombosis.

Symptoms of superficial thrombophlebitis are relieved by bed rest with elevation of the legs and the application of heat for 7 to 15 days. When local signs of inflammation subside, the client is usually allowed to ambulate wearing elastic stockings.

Sometimes antiinflammatory medications are required. Anticoagulants such as heparin and warfarin are used to prevent clot extension.

Lymphedema

The third type of peripheral vascular disorder, lymphedema, is defined as an excessive accumulation of fluid in tissue spaces. Lymphedema typically occurs secondary to an obstruction of the lymphatic system from trauma, infection, radiation, or surgery.

Postsurgical lymphedema is usually seen after surgical excision of axillary, inguinal, or iliac nodes, usually performed as a prophylactic or therapeutic measure for metastatic tumor. Lymphedema secondary to primary or metastatic neoplasms in the lymph nodes is common.

▼ *Clinical Signs and Symptoms of*
Superficial Venous Thrombosis

- Subcutaneous venous distention
- Palpable cord
- Warmth, redness
- Indurated (hard)

▼ *Clinical Signs and Symptoms of*
Deep Venous Thrombosis

- Unilateral tenderness or leg pain
- Unilateral swelling (difference in leg circumference)
- Warmth
- Positive Homans' sign
- Discoloration
- Pain with placement of blood pressure cuff around calf inflated to 160 to 180 mm Hg

▼ *Clinical Signs and Symptoms of*
Lymphedema

- Edema of the dorsum of the foot or hand
- Decreased range of motion and function
- Usually unilateral
- Worse after prolonged dependency
- No discomfort or a dull, heavy sensation

Hypertension*

Blood pressure is the force against the walls of the arteries and arterioles as these vessels carry blood away from the heart. When these muscular walls constrict, reducing the diameter of the vessel, blood pressure rises; when they relax, increasing the vessel diameter, blood pressure falls.

A high blood pressure reading is usually a sign that the vessels cannot relax fully and remain somewhat constricted, requiring the heart to work harder to pump blood through the vessels. Over time the extra effort can cause the heart muscle to become enlarged and eventually weakened. The force of blood pumped at high pressure can also produce small tears in the lining of the arteries, weakening the arterial vessels. The evidence of this effect is most pronounced in the vessels of the brain, the kidneys, and the small vessels of the eye.

Hypertension is a major cardiovascular risk factor, associated with elevated risks of cardiovascular diseases, especially MI, stroke, and cardiovascular death. Although diastolic changes were always evaluated closely, research now shows that the risks increase progressively as systolic pressure goes up and increased cardiovascular risk is consistent for men whose systolic blood pressure levels are near or slightly above normal (O'Donnell et al, 1997).

Hypertension is defined by an elevation of diastolic pressure, systolic pressure, or both measured on at least two separate occasions at least 2 weeks apart—in other words, sustained elevation of blood pressure. Medical researchers have developed classifications for blood pressure based on risk (Table 3-7). These new guidelines were issued in 1997 by the Joint National Committee on Prevention, Detection, Evaluation, and Treatment of Hypertension (Sixth Report of the Joint National Committee, 1997).

---

*Hypertension is often considered in conjunction with peripheral vascular disorders for several reasons: both are disorders of the circulatory system; the course of both diseases are affected by similar factors; and hypertension is a major risk factor in atherosclerosis, the largest single cause of peripheral vascular disease.

TABLE 3-7 ▼ Classification of Blood Pressure†

Stages	Blood Pressure (mm Hg)
Optimal	<120/<80
Normal	<130/<85
High normal	130-139/85-89
Hypertension	
Stage 1 (mild)	140-159/90-99
Stage 2 (moderate)	160-179/100-109
Stage 3 (severe)	≥180/≥110

†For adults aged 18 and older who are not taking antihypertensive drugs and are not acutely ill.

From Sixth Report of the Joint National Committee on Prevention, Detection, Evaluation and Treatment of High Blood Pressure, *Arch Intern Med* 157(21):2413-2446, 1997.

Hypertension can also be classified according to type (systolic or diastolic), cause, and degree of severity. *Primary* (or *essential) hypertension* is also known as *idiopathic hypertension* and accounts for 90% to 95% of all hypertensive clients.

Secondary hypertension results from an identifiable cause, including a variety of specific diseases or problems such as renal artery stenosis, oral contraceptive use,‡ hyperthyroidism, adrenal tumors, and medication use.

Drugs that constrict blood vessels can contribute to hypertension. Among the most common are phenylpropanolamine in over-the-counter appetite suppressants, including herbal ephedra, pseudoephedrine in cold and allergy remedies, and prescription drugs such as monoamine oxidase (MAO) inhibitors (a class of antidepressant) and corticosteroids when used over a long period.

Intermittent elevation of blood pressure interspersed with normal readings is called *labile hypertension* or *borderline hypertension*.

---

‡Originally, birth-control pills contained higher levels of estrogen, but today the estrogen and progestin (synthetic progesterone) contents of the pill are greatly reduced. The risk of high blood pressure with oral contraceptive use is considered quite low (Heinemann et al, 1998; WHO, 1998). The risk may be increased for older women who smoke, but the risk for all women returns to normal after they discontinue the pill. The risk of venous thromboembolism associated with newer oral contraceptives remains under investigation (see previous discussion).

▼ *Clinical Signs and Symptoms of*
Hypertension

- Occipital headache
- Vertigo (dizziness)
- Flushed face
- Spontaneous epistaxis
- Vision changes
- Nocturnal urinary frequency

▼ *Clinical Signs and Symptoms of*
Transient Ischemic Attack

- Slurred speech or sudden difficulty with speech
- Temporary blindness or other dramatic visual changes
- Paralysis or extreme weakness, usually affecting one side of the body

RISK FACTORS

Modifiable risk factors include stress, obesity, and insufficient intake of nutrients. Stress has shown to cause increased peripheral vascular resistance and cardiac output and to stimulate sympathetic nervous system activity. Potassium deficiency can also contribute to hypertension.

Nonmodifiable risk factors include family history, age, gender, and race. The risk of hypertension increases with age as arteries lose elasticity and become less able to relax. There is a poorer prognosis associated with early onset of hypertension.

A sex-specific gene for hypertension may exist (O'Donnell et al, 1998) because men experience hypertension at higher rates and at an earlier age than women do until after menopause. Hypertension is the most serious health problem for African-Americans (both men and women and at earlier ages than for whites) in the United States.

CLINICAL SIGNS AND SYMPTOMS

Clients with hypertension are usually asymptomatic in the early stages, but when symptoms do occur, they include occipital headache (usually present in the early morning), vertigo, flushed face, nocturnal urinary frequency, spontaneous nosebleeds, and blurred vision.

Transient Ischemic Attack

Hypertension is a major cause of heart failure, stroke, and kidney failure. Aneurysm

formation and CHF are also associated with hypertension. Persistent elevated diastolic pressure damages the intimal layer of the small vessels, which causes an accumulation of fibrin, local edema, and, possibly, intravascular clotting.

Eventually, these damaging changes diminish blood flow to vital organs, such as the heart, kidneys, and brain, resulting in complications such as heart failure, renal failure, and cerebrovascular accidents or stroke.

Many persons have brief episodes of transient ischemic attacks (TIAs) before they have an actual stroke. The attacks occur when the blood supply to part of the brain has been temporarily disrupted. These ischemic episodes last from 5 to 20 minutes, although they may last for as long as 24 hours. TIAs are important warning signals that an obstruction exists in an artery leading to the brain.

Orthostatic Hypotension

Orthostatic hypotension is an excessive fall in blood pressure of 20 mm Hg or more in systolic blood pressure or a drop of 10 mm Hg or more of both systolic and diastolic arterial blood pressure on assumption of the erect position with a concomitant rise in pulse rate of 15 beats per minute. It is not a disease but a manifestation of abnormalities in normal blood pressure regulation.

This condition may occur as a normal part of aging or secondary to the effects of drugs such as hypertensives, diuretics, and antidepressants; as a result of venous pooling (e.g., pregnancy, prolonged bed rest, or standing); or in association with neurogenic origins. The last category includes diseases affecting the autonomic nervous system, such as Guillain-Barré syndrome, diabetes mellitus, or multiple sclerosis.

Orthostatic intolerance is the most common cause of lightheadedness in clients, especially those who have been on prolonged bed rest or those who have had prolonged anesthesia for surgery. When such a client is getting up out of bed for the first time, blood pressure and heart rate should be monitored with the person in the supine position and repeated after the person is upright. If the legs are dangled off the bed, a significant drop in blood pressure may occur with or without compensatory tachycardia. This drop may provoke lightheadedness, and standing may even produce loss of consciousness.

These postural symptoms are often accentuated in the morning and are aggravated by heat, humidity, heavy meals, and exercise.

Text continued on p. 130

▼ ***Clinical Signs and Symptoms of***
Orthostatic Hypotension

- Lightheadedness, dizziness
- Syncope or fainting
- Mental or visual blurring
- Sense of weakness or "rubbery" legs

OVERVIEW | CARDIAC CHEST PAIN PATTERNS

▼ ANGINA (Fig. 3-7)

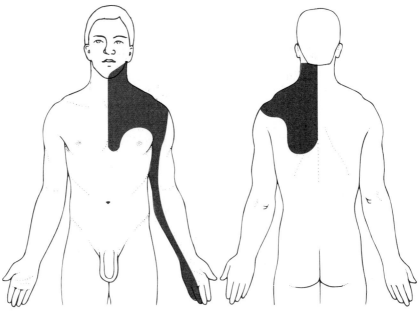

FIGURE 3-7 • Pain patterns associated with angina. *Left,* Area of substernal discomfort projected to the left shoulder and arm over the distribution of the ulnar nerve. Referred pain may be present only in the left shoulder or in the shoulder and along the arm only to the elbow. *Right,* Occasionally, anginal pain may be referred to the back in the area of the left scapula or the interscapular region.

continued

Location:	Substernal/retrosternal (beneath the sternum)
	Left chest pain in the absence of substernal chest pain (women)
	Isolated midthoracic back pain (women)
	Aching in the right biceps muscle (women)
Referral:	Neck, jaw, back, shoulder, or arms (most commonly the left arm)
	May have only a toothache
	Occasionally to the abdomen
Description:	Viselike pressure, squeezing, heaviness, burning indigestion
Intensity:*	Mild to moderate
	Builds up gradually or may be sudden
Duration:	Usually less than 10 minutes
	Never more than 30 minutes
	Average: 3-5 minutes
Associated signs and symptoms:	Extreme fatigue, lethargy, weakness (women)
	Shortness of breath (dyspnea)
	Nausea
	Diaphoresis (heavy perspiration)
	Anxiety or apprehension
	Belching (eructation)
	"Heartburn" (unrelieved by antacids) (women)
	Sensation similar to inhaling cold air (women)
	Prolonged and repeated palpitations without chest pain (women)
Relieving factors:	Rest or nitroglycerin
	Antacids (women)
Aggravating factors:	Exercise or physical exertion
	Cold weather or wind
	Heavy meals
	Emotional stress

---

*For each pattern reviewed throughout this text, intensity is related directly to the degree of noxious stimuli.

▼ MYOCARDIAL INFARCTION (Fig. 3-8)

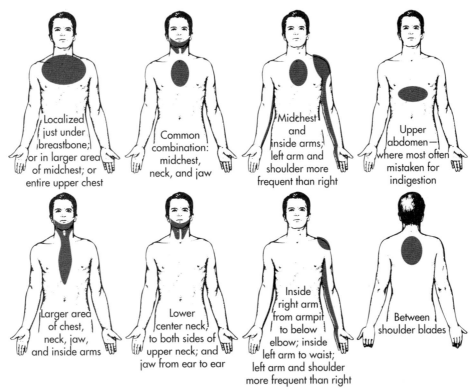

FIGURE 3-8 • Early warning signs of a heart attack.

Location:	Substernal, anterior chest
Referral:	May radiate like angina, frequently down both arms
Description:	Burning, stabbing, viselike pressure, squeezing, heaviness
Intensity:	Severe
Duration:	Usually at least 30 minutes; may last 1 to 2 hours
	Residual soreness 1 to 3 days
Associated signs and symptoms:	None with a silent myocardial infarction
	Dizziness, feeling faint
	Nausea, vomiting
	Pallor
	Diaphoresis (heavy perspiration)
	Apprehension, severe anxiety
	Fatigue, sudden weakness
	Dyspnea
	May be followed by painful shoulder-hand syndrome (see text)

| Relieving factors: | None; unrelieved by rest or nitroglycerin taken every 5 minutes for 20 minutes |
| Aggravating factors: | Not necessarily anything; may occur at rest or may follow emotional stress or physical exertion |

▼ PERICARDITIS (Fig. 3-9)

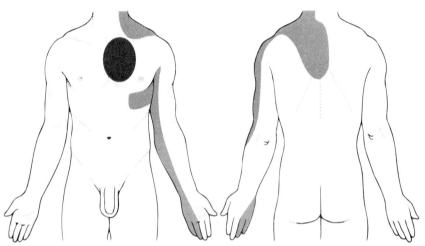

FIGURE 3-9 • Substernal pain associated with pericarditis *(dark red)* may radiate anteriorly *(light red)* to the costal margins, neck, upper back, upper trapezius muscle, and left supraclavicular area or down the left arm.

Location:	Substernal or over the sternum, sometimes to the left of midline toward the cardiac apex
Referral:	Neck, upper back, upper trapezious muscle, left supraclavicular area, down the left arm, costal margins
Description:	More localized than pain of myocardial infarction Sharp, stabbing, knifelike
Intensity:	Moderate to severe
Duration:	Continuous; may last hours or days with residual soreness following
Associated signs and symptoms:	Usually medically determined associated symptoms (e.g., by chest auscultation using a stethoscope)
Relieving factors:	Sitting upright or leaning forward
Aggravating factors:	Muscle movement associated with deep breathing (e.g., laughter, inspiration, coughing) Left lateral (side) bending of the upper trunk Trunk rotation (either to the right or to the left) Supine position

▼ DISSECTING AORTIC ANEURYSM (Fig. 3-10)

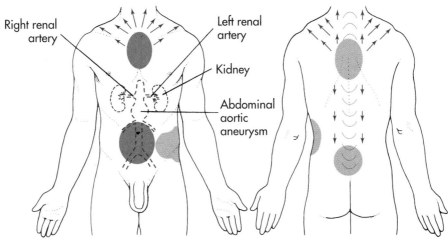

FIGURE 3-10 • Most aortic aneurysms (more than 95%) are located just below the renal arteries and extend to the umbilicus, causing low back pain. Chest pain *(dark red)* associated with thoracic aneurysms may radiate *(light red)* to the neck, interscapular area, shoulders, lower back, or abdomen. Early warning signs of an impending rupture may include an abdominal heartbeat when lying down (not shown) or a dull ache in the midabdominal left flank or lower back *(light red)*.

Location:	Anterior chest (thoracic aneurysm)
	Abdomen (abdominal aneurysm)
	Thoracic area of back
Referral:	Pain may move in the chest as dissection progresses
	Pain may extend to the neck, shoulders, interscapular area, or lower back
Description:	Knifelike, tearing (thoracic aneurysm)
	Dull ache in the lower back or midabdominal left flank (abdominal aneurysm)
Intensity:	Severe, excruciating
Duration:	Hours
Associated signs and symptoms:	Pulses absent
	Person senses "heartbeat" when lying down
	Palpable, pulsating abdominal mass
	Lower blood pressure in one arm
	Other medically determined symptoms
Relieving factors:	None
Aggravating factors:	Supine position accentuates symptoms

OVERVIEW	NONCARDIAC CHEST PAIN PATTERNS

▼ MUSCULOSKELETAL DISORDERS See Chapter 12.

▼ NEUROLOGIC DISORDERS See Chapter 12.

▼ PLEUROPULMONARY DISORDERS See Chapter 12.

▼ GASTROINTESTINAL DISORDERS See Chapter 12.

▼ BREAST DISEASES See Chapter 12.

▼ ANXIETY STATES See Chapter 12.

▼ LABORATORY VALUES

The results of diagnostic tests can provide the therapist with information to assist in client education. The client often reports test results to the therapist and asks for information regarding the significance of those results. The information presented in this text discusses potential reasons for abnormal laboratory values relevant to clients with cardiovascular problems.

A basic understanding of laboratory tests used specifically in the diagnosis and monitoring of cardiovascular problems can provide the therapist with additional information regarding the client's status.

Some of the tests commonly used in the management and diagnosis of cardiovascular problems include lipid screening (cholesterol levels, low-density lipoprotein/LDL levels, high-density lipoprotein/HDL levels, and triglyceride levels), serum electrolytes, and arterial blood gases (see Chapter 4).

Other laboratory measurements of importance in the overall evaluation of the client with cardiovascular disease include red blood cell values (e.g., red blood cell count, hemoglobin, and hematocrit). Those values (see Chapter 5) provide valuable information regarding the oxygen-carrying capability of the blood and the subsequent oxygenation of body tissues, such as the heart muscle.

Serum Electrolytes

Measurement of serum electrolyte values is particularly important in diagnosis, management, and monitoring of the client with cardiovascular disease, since electrolyte levels have a direct influence on the function of cardiac muscle (in a manner similar to that of skeletal muscle). Abnormalities in serum electrolytes, even in noncardiac clients, can result in significant cardiac arrhythmias and even cardiac arrest.

In addition, certain medications prescribed for cardiac clients can alter serum electrolytes in such a way that rhythm problems can occur as a result of the medication. The electrolyte levels most important to monitor include potassium, sodium, calcium, and magnesium (see inside back cover).

Potassium

Serum potassium levels can be lowered significantly as a result of diuretic therapy (particularly with loop diuretics such as Lasix [furosemide]), vomiting, diarrhea, sweating, and alkalosis.

Low potassium levels cause increased electrical instability of the myocardium, life-threatening ventricular arrhythmias, and increased risk of digitalis toxicity.

Serum potassium levels must be measured frequently by the physician in any client taking a digitalis preparation (e.g., Digoxin), since most of these clients are also undergoing diuretic therapy. Low potassium levels in clients taking digitalis can cause digitalis toxicity and precipitate life-threatening arrhythmias.

Increased potassium levels most commonly occur because of renal and endocrine problems or as a result of potassium replacement overdose. Cardiac effects of increased potassium levels include ventricular arrhythmias and asystole/flat line (complete cessation of electrical activity of the heart).

Sodium

Serum sodium levels indicate the client's state of water/fluid balance, which is particularly important in CHF and other pathologic states related to fluid imbalances. A low serum sodium level can indicate water overload or extensive loss of sodium through diuretic use, vomiting, diarrhea, or diaphoresis.

A high serum sodium level can indicate a water deficit state such as dehydration or water loss (e.g., lack of antidiuretic hormone [ADH]).

Calcium

Serum calcium levels can be decreased as a result of multiple transfusions of citrated blood, renal failure, alkalosis, laxative or antacid abuse, and parathyroid damage or removal. A decreased calcium level provokes serious and often life-threatening ventricular arrhythmias and cardiac arrest.

Increased calcium levels are less common but can be caused by a variety of situations, including thiazide diuretic use (e.g., Diuril [chlorothiazide]), acidosis, adrenal insufficiency, immobility, and vitamin D excess.

Calcium excess causes atrioventricular conduction blocks or tachycardia and ultimately can result in cardiac arrest.

Magnesium

Serum magnesium levels are rarely changed in healthy individuals because magnesium is abundant in foods and water. However, magnesium deficits are often seen in alcoholic clients or clients with critical illnesses that involve shifting of a variety of electrolytes. Magnesium deficits often accompany potassium and calcium deficits. A decrease in serum magnesium results in myocardial irritability and cardiac arrhythmias, such as atrial or ventricular fibrillation or premature ventricular beats (PVCs).

▼
EFFECTS OF CARDIOVASCULAR MEDICATIONS

When a client is physically challenged, as often occurs in physical therapy, signs and symptoms develop from side effects of various classes of cardiovascular medications (Table 3-8; box on following page).* For example, medications that cause peripheral vasodilation can produce hypotension, dizziness, and syncope when combined with physical therapy interventions that also produce peripheral vasodilation (e.g., hydrotherapy, aquatics, aerobic exercise).

On the other hand, cardiovascular responses to exercise can be limited in clients who are taking beta-blockers because these drugs limit the increase in heart rate that can occur as exercise increases the workload of the heart.

---

*The available pharmaceuticals used in the treatment of the conditions listed in Table 3-8 are extensive. Only a basic overview is provided in this text as a screening tool for possible medication side effects. The physical therapist is advised to rely on more specific texts for a complete understanding of drug interactions and the implications of drug treatment in clinical practice.

POTENTIAL SIDE EFFECTS OF CARDIOVASCULAR MEDICATIONS

Abdominal pain*
Asthmatic attacks*
Bradycardia*
Cough
Dehydration
Difficulty breathing or swallowing*
Dizziness or fainting*
Drowsiness
Easy bruising
Fatigue
Headache
Insomnia†
Joint pain*
Loss of taste
Muscle cramps†
Nausea
Nightmares†

Orthostatic hypotension†
Palpitations†
Paralysis*
Sexual dysfunction†
Skin rash†
Stomach irritation†
Swelling of feet or abdomen†
Symptoms of congestive heart failure*
   Shortness of breath
   Swollen ankles
   Coughing up blood
Tachycardia†
Unexplained swelling, unusual or uncontrolled bleeding
Vomiting
Weakness

*Immediate physician referral.
†Notify physician.

TABLE 3-8 ▼ Cardiovascular Medications

Condition	Drug Class
Angina pectoris	Organic nitrates
	Beta-blockers
	Calcium channel (Ca^{2+}) blockers
Arrhythmias	Sodium channel blockers
	Beta-blockers
	Calcium channel (Ca^{2+}) blockers
	Agents prolonging depolarization
Congestive heart failure	Cardiac glycosides (digitalis)
	Diuretics
	ACE inhibitors
	Vasodilators
Hypertension	Diuretics
	Beta-blockers
	ACE inhibitors
	Vasodilators
	Calcium (Ca^{2+}) channel blockers
	Alpha (α_1)-blockers

Courtesy Susan Queen, Ph.D., P.T., School of Pharmacy and Allied Health Sciences, Physical Therapy Department, University of Montana, Missoula, Montana, 1998.

The physical therapist must especially keep in mind that nonsteroidal antiinflammatory drugs (NSAIDs), often used in the treatment of inflammatory conditions, have the ability to negate the antihypertensive effects of angiotensin-converting enzyme (ACE) inhibitors. Anyone being treated with both NSAIDs and ACE inhibitors must be monitored closely during exercise for elevated blood pressure.

Likewise, NSAIDs have the ability to decrease the excretion of digitalis glycosides (e.g., digoxin[Lanoxin] and digitoxin [Crystodigin]). Therefore levels of these glycosides can increase, thus producing digitalis toxicity (e.g., fatigue, confusion, gastrointestinal problems, arrhythmias). Digitalis and diuretics in combination with NSAIDs exacerbate the side effects of NSAIDs. Anyone receiving any of these combinations must be monitored for lower-extremity (especially ankle) and abdominal swelling.

Diuretics, usually referred to by clients as "water pills," lower blood pressure by eliminating sodium and water and thus reducing the blood volume. Thiazide diuretics may also be used to prevent osteoporosis by increasing calcium reabsorption by the kidneys. Some diuretics remove potassium from the body, causing potentially life-threatening arrhythmias. The primary adverse effects associated with diuretics are fluid and electrolyte imbalances, such as muscle weakness and spasms, dizziness, headache, incoordination, and nausea.

Beta-blockers relax the blood vessels and the heart muscle by blocking the beta-receptors on the sinoatrial node and myocardial cells, producing a decline in the force of contraction and a reduction in heart rate. This effect eases the strain on the heart by reducing its workload and reducing oxygen consumption.

The therapist must monitor the client's perceived exertion and watch for excessive slowing of the heart rate (bradycardia) and contractility, resulting in depressed cardiac function. Other potential side effects include depression, worsening of asthma symptoms, sexual dysfunction, and fatigue. The generic names of beta-blockers end in "olol" (e.g., propranolol, metoprolol, atenolol, labetalol). Trade names include Inderal, Lopressor, and Tenormin.

Alpha-1 blockers lower the blood pressure by dilating blood vessels. The therapist must be observant for signs of hypotension and reflex tachycardia (i.e., the heart rate increases to compensate for the hypotension). Alpha-1 blockers all have the last name "zocin" (e.g., prazocin, terazocin, doxazocin; trade names include Minipress, Hytrin, Cardura).

Angiotensin-converting enzyme (ACE) inhibitors are highly selective drugs that interrupt a chain of molecular messengers that constrict blood vessels. They can improve cardiac function in individuals with heart failure and are used for persons with diabetes or early kidney damage. Rash and a persistent dry cough are common side effects. The generic names of ACE inhibitors end in "pril" (e.g., benazepril, captopril, enalapril, lisinopril). Trade names include Lotensin, Capoten, Vasotec, Prinivil, and Zestril. Newest on the market are ACE II inhibitors, such a Cozaar (losartan potassium) and Hyzaar (losartan potassium-hydrochlorothiazide).

Calcium channel blockers inhibit calcium from entering the blood vessel walls, where calcium works to constrict blood vessels. Side effects may include swelling in the feet and ankles, orthostatic hypotension, headache, and nausea.

There are several groups of calcium channel blockers. Those in the group that primarily interact with calcium channels on the smooth muscle of the peripheral arterioles all end with "pine" (e.g., amlodipine, felodipine, nisoldipine, nifedipine). Trade names include Norvasc, Plendil, Sular, and Adalat or Procardia.

A second group of calcium channel blockers work to dilate coronary arteries to lower blood pressure and suppress some arrhythmias. This group includes verapamil (Verelan, Calan, Isoptin) and diltiazem (Cardizem, Dilacor).

Nitrates such as nitroglycerin (e.g., nitroglycerin [Nitrostat, Nitro-Bid], isosorbide dinitrate [Iso-Bid, Isordil] dilate the coronary arteries and are used to prevent or relieve the symptoms of angina. Headache, dizziness, tachycardia, and orthostatic hypotension may occur as a result of the vasodilating properties of these drugs.

There are other classes of drugs to treat various aspects of cardiovascular diseases separate from those listed in Table 3-8. Hyperlipidemia is often treated with medications to inhibit cholesterol synthesis. Platelet aggregation and clot formation are prevented with anticoagulant drugs such as heparin, warfarin (Coumadin), and aspirin, whereas thrombolytic drugs such as streptokinase, urokinase, and tissue-type plasminogen activator (t-PA) are used to break down and dissolve clots already formed in the coronary arteries.

Anyone receiving cardiovascular medications, especially in combination with other medications or over-the-counter drugs, must be monitored during physical therapy for unusual vital signs. Any of the signs or

CLUES TO CARDIOVASCULAR SIGNS AND SYMPTOMS*

- Watch for the three P's†:

  (1) Pleuritic pain (exacerbated by respiratory movement involving the diaphragm, such as sighing, deep breathing, coughing, sneezing, laughing, or the hiccups; this may be cardiac if pericarditis or it may be pulmonary); have the client hold his or her breath and reassess symptoms—any reduction or elimination of symptoms with breath holding or the Valsalva maneuver suggests pulmonary or cardiac source of symptoms.

  (2) Pain on palpation (musculoskeletal origin).

  (3) Pain with changes in position (musculoskeletal or pulmonary origin; pain that is worse when lying down and improves when sitting up or leaning forward is often pleuritic in origin).

- Chest pain may occur from intercostal muscle or periosteal trauma with protracted or vigorous coughing. Palpation of local chest wall will reproduce tenderness. However, a client can have both a pulmonary/cardiac condition with subsequent musculoskeletal trauma from coughing. Look for associated signs and symptoms (e.g., fever, sweats, blood in sputum).

- Angina is activated by physical exertion, emotional reactions, a large meal, or exposure to cold and has a lag time of 5 to 10 minutes. Angina does not occur immediately after physical activity. Immediate pain with activity is more likely musculoskeletal or psychologic (e.g., "I do not want to shovel today").

- Chest pain, shoulder pain, neck pain, or temporomandibular pain occurring in the presence of coronary artery disease or previous history of myocardial infarction, especially if accompanied by associated signs and symptoms, may be cardiac.

- Upper quadrant pain that can be induced or reproduced by lower quadrant activity, such as biking, stair climbing, or walking without using the arms, is usually cardiac in origin.

- If an individual with known risk factors for congestive heart disease, especially a history of angina, becomes weak or short of breath while working with the arms extended over the head, ischemia or infarction is a likely cause of the pain and associated symptoms.

- Insidious onset of joint or muscle pain in the older client who has had a previously diagnosed heart murmur may be caused by bacterial endocarditis. Usually there is no morning stiffness to differentiate it from rheumatoid arthritis.

- Back pain similar to that associated with a herniated lumbar disk but without neurologic deficits, especially in the presence of a diagnosed heart murmur, may be caused by bacterial endocarditis.

- Anyone with chest pain must be evaluated for trigger points. If palpation of the chest reproduces symptoms, especially symptoms of radiating pain, deactivation of the trigger points must be carried out and followed by a reevaluation as part of the screening process for pain of a cardiac origin (see Fig. 12-4 and Table 12-10).

- Symptoms of vascular occlusive disease include exertional calf pain that is relieved by rest (intermittent claudication), nocturnal aching of the foot and forefoot (rest pain), and classic skin changes, especially hair loss of the ankle and foot. Ischemic rest pain is relieved by placing the limb in a dependent position.

- Throbbing pain at the base of the neck and/or along the back into the interscapular areas that increases with exertion requires monitoring of vital signs and palpation of peripheral pulses to screen for aneurysm. Check for a palpable abdominal heartbeat that increases in the supine position.

---

*See also "Clues to Differentiating Chest Pain," Chapter 12.

†If two of the three P's are present, a myocardial infarction is very unlikely. A myocardial infarction or anginal pain occurs in approximately 5 to 7% of clients whose pain is reproducible by palpation. If the symptoms are altered by a change in positioning, this percentage drops to 2%, and if the chest pain is reproducible by respiratory movements, the likelihood of a coronary event is only 1% (Bancroft, 1996).

symptoms listed in the box on p. 132 must be monitored. The therapist should be familiar with the signs or symptoms that require immediate physician referral and those that must be reported to the physician.

▼ PHYSICIAN REFERRAL

The description and location of chest pain associated with pericarditis, MI, angina, breast pain, gastrointestinal disorders, and anxiety are often similar. The physician is able to distinguish among these conditions through a careful history, medical examination, and medical testing.

For example, the severe substernal pain of pericarditis closely mimics the pain of acute MI, but the two disorders differ in aggravating and relieving factors.

Pain associated with gastrointestinal disorders involving the esophagus may create pain like that of angina pectoris, with discomfort precipitated by recumbency or by meals. However, the esophageal pain is not aggravated by exercise, whereas true angina is caused by exercise or by physical exertion and is relieved by rest. In both these examples, chest auscultation and an ECG provide the physician with valuable diagnostic information.

It is not the physical therapist's responsibility to differentiate diagnostically among the various causes of chest pain, but rather to recognize the systemic origin of signs and symptoms that may mimic musculoskeletal disorders.

For example, compared with angina, the pain of true musculoskeletal disorders may last for seconds or for hours, is not relieved by nitroglycerin, and may be aggravated by local palpation or by exertion of just the upper body.

The physical therapy interview presented in Chapter 2 is the primary mechanism used to begin exploring a client's reported symptoms and is accomplished by carefully questioning the client to determine the location, duration, intensity, frequency, associated symptoms, and relieving or aggravating factors related to pain or symptoms.

When to Refer a Client to the Physician

When a client mentions signs and symptoms, these may be clues to systemic disease processes that mimic musculoskeletal pain and dysfunction. Clients often confide in physical therapists and describe symptoms of a more serious nature. Cardiac symptoms unknown to the physician may be mentioned to the therapist during the opening interview or in subsequent visits.

The materials presented in this chapter help prepare the therapist for making referral decisions. An understanding of the nature of thoracic pain provides a knowledge base for recognizing cardiac and noncardiac chest pain patterns and the systemic signs and symptoms associated with these patterns.

Immediate Medical Attention

In the clinic setting the onset of an anginal attack requires immediate cessation of exercise. If the client is currently taking nitroglycerin, self-administration of medication is recommended. Relief from pain should occur within 1 to 2 minutes. The dose may be repeated according to the prescribed direction. If anginal pain is not relieved in 20 minutes or if the client has nausea, vomiting, or profuse sweating, immediate medical intervention may be indicated.

Changes in the pattern of angina, such as increased intensity, decreased threshold of stimulus, or longer duration of pain, require immediate intervention by the physician.

Clients in treatment under these circumstances should either be returned to the care of the nursing staff or, in the case of an outpatient, should be encouraged to contact their physicians by telephone for further instructions before leaving the physical therapy department. The client should be advised not to leave unaccompanied.

Systemic Signs and Symptoms Requiring Physician Referral

Referral by the therapist to the physician is recommended when the client has any combination of systemic signs or symptoms discussed throughout this chapter at presentation. These signs and symptoms should always be correlated with the client's history to rule out systemic involvement or to identify musculoskeletal or neurologic disorders

---

GUIDELINES FOR PHYSICIAN REFERRAL

- When a client has any combination of systemic signs or symptoms at presentation, refer him or her to a physician.
- Women with chest or breast pain who have a positive family history of breast cancer should always be referred to a physician for a follow-up examination.
- Palpitation in any person with a history of unexplained sudden death in the family requires medical evaluation. More than six episodes of palpitations in 1 minute or palpitations lasting for hours or occurring in association with pain, shortness of breath, fainting, or severe lightheadedness require medical evaluation.
- Anyone who cannot climb a single flight of stairs without feeling moderately to severely winded or who awakens at night or experiences shortness of breath when lying down should be evaluated by a physician.
- Fainting (syncope) without any warning period of lightheadedness, dizziness, or nausea may be a sign of heart valve or arrhythmia problems. Unexplained syncope in the presence of heart or circulatory problems (or risk factors for heart attack or stroke) should be evaluated by a physician.
- Clients who are neurologically unstable as a result of a recent cerebrovascular accident, head trauma, spinal cord injury, or other central nervous system insult often exhibit new arrhythmias during the period of instability. When the client's pulse is monitored, any new arrhythmias noted should be reported to the nursing staff or the physician.
- Cardiac clients should be sent back to their physician under the following conditions:
  - Nitroglycerin tablets do not relieve anginal pain.
  - Pattern of angina changes is noted.
  - Client has abnormally severe chest pain with nausea and vomiting.
  - Anginal pain radiates to the jaw or to the left arm.
  - Anginal pain is not relieved by rest.
  - Upper back feels abnormally cool, sweaty, or moist to touch.
  - Client develops progressively worse dyspnea.
  - Client has any doubt about his or her present condition.

GUIDELINES FOR IMMEDIATE MEDICAL ATTENTION

- If anginal pain is not relieved in 20 minutes, seek medical help.
- If the client has nausea, vomiting, or profuse sweating, medical attention is necessary.
- Throbbing chest, back, or abdominal pain that increases with exertion, accompanied by a sensation of a heartbeat when lying down, and palpable pulsating abdominal mass, may be an aneurysm.
- Sudden worsening of intermittent claudication may be due to thromboembolism and must be reported to the physician immediately.

that would be appropriate for physical therapy treatment.

Absent pulses
Anxiety or apprehension
Bradycardia
Breast lumps or nodules
Chest pain caused by exertion
Chest pressure
Claudication
Cold sweat
Diaphoresis
Difficulty in swallowing
Distortion of vision or speech
Dyspnea
Edema and weight gain
Eructation
Fatigue, severe
Fever
"Heartbeat" in the back or abdomen
Heart fibrillation

Heart palpitations
Hemoptysis
Homans' sign positive
Irritability
Migratory joint pain
Nausea/vomiting
Night sweats
Nocturnal dyspnea
Orthopnea
Painful shoulder-hand syndrome (RSD)
Pallor
Persistent cough
Restlessness
Skin rashes or petechiae
Skipped heartbeats
Sudden incoordination
Sudden weakness
Syncope
Tachycardia
Transient paralysis

 KEY POINTS TO REMEMBER

▶ Fatigue beyond expectations during or after exercise is a red-flag symptom.

▶ Be on the alert for cardiac risk factors in older adults, especially women, and begin a conditioning program before an exercise program.

▶ The client with stable angina typically has a normal blood pressure; it may be low, depending on medications. Blood pressure may be elevated when anxiety accompanies chest pain or during acute coronary insufficiency; systolic blood pressure may be low if there is heart failure.

▶ Cervical disk disease and arthritic changes can mimic atypical chest pain of angina pectoris, requiring screening through questions and musculoskeletal evaluation.

▶ If a client uses nitroglycerin, make sure that he or she has a fresh supply, and check that the physical therapy department has a fresh supply in a readily accessible location.

▶ Make sure that a client with cardiac compromise has not smoked a cigarette or eaten a large meal just before exercise.

▶ A person taking medications, such as beta-blockers or calcium channel blockers, may not be able to achieve a target heart rate (THR) above 90 beats per minute. To determine a safe rate of exercise, the heart rate should return to the resting level 2 minutes after stopping exercise.

▶ A 3-pound or greater weight gain or gradual, continuous gain over several days, resulting in swelling of the ankles, abdomen, and hands, combined with shortness of breath, fatigue, and dizziness that persist despite rest, may be red-flag symptoms of CHF.

▶ The pericardium (sac around the entire heart) is adjacent to the diaphragm. Pain of cardiac and diaphragmatic origin is often experienced in the shoulder because the heart and the diaphragm are supplied by the C5-C6 spinal segment. The visceral pain is referred to the corresponding somatic area.

SUBJECTIVE EXAMINATION

• SPECIAL QUESTIONS TO ASK

Past Medical History

- Has a doctor ever said that you have heart trouble?
- Have you ever had a heart attack?
  - If yes, when? Please describe.
- Do you associate your current symptoms with your heart problems?
- Have you ever had rheumatic fever, twitching of the limbs called St. Vitus' dance, or rheumatic heart disease?
- Have you ever had an abnormal electrocardiogram (ECG)?
- Have you ever had an ECG taken while you were exercising (e.g., climbing up and down steps or walking on a treadmill) that was not normal?
- Do you have a pacemaker, artificial heart, or any other device to assist your heart?
- For the therapist: Remember to review smoking, diet, lifestyle, exercise, and stress history (see Family/Personal History, Chapter 2).

Angina/Myocardial Infarct

- Do you have angina (pectoris) or chest pain or tightness?
  - If yes, please describe the symptoms and tell me when it occurs.
- Can you point to the area of pain with one finger? **(Anginal pain is characteristically demonstrated with the hand or fist on the chest.)**
- Is the pain close to the surface or deep inside? **(Pleuritic pain is close to the surface; anginal pain can be close to the surface but always also has a "deep inside" sensation.)**
  - If yes, what makes it better?
  - If no, pursue further with the following questions:
    - Do you ever have discomfort or tightness in your chest?
    - Have you ever had a crushing sensation in your chest with or without pain down your left arm?
    - Do you have pain in your jaw either alone or in combination with chest pain?

- If you climb a few flights of stairs fairly rapidly, do you have tightness or pressing pain in your chest?
- Do you get pressure or pain or tightness in the chest as if you were walking in the cold wind or facing a cold blast of air?
- Have you ever had pain or pressure or a squeezing feeling in the chest that occurred during exercise, walking, or any other physical or sexual activity?

Associated Symptoms

- Do you ever have bouts of rapid heart action, irregular heartbeats, or palpitations of your heart?
- Have you ever felt a "heartbeat" in your abdomen when you lie down?
  - If yes, is this associated with low back pain or left flank pain? **(Abdominal aneurysm)**
- Do you ever notice sweating, nausea, or chest pain when your current symptoms (e.g., back pain, shoulder pain) occur?
- Do you have frequent attacks of heartburn, or do you take antacids to relieve heartburn or acid indigestion? **(Noncardiac cause of chest pain [men], abdominal muscle trigger point, gastrointestinal disorder)**
- Do you get very short of breath during activities that do not make other people short of breath? **(Dyspnea)**
- Do you ever wake up at night gasping for air or have short breaths? **(paroxysmal nocturnal dyspnea)**
- Do you ever need to sleep on more than one pillow to breathe comfortably? **(Orthopnea)**
- Do you ever get cramps in your legs if you walk for several blocks? **(Intermittent claudication)**
- Do you ever have swollen feet or ankles?
  - If yes, are they swollen when you get up in the morning? **(Edema/congestive heart failure; NSAIDs)**
- Have you gained unexpected weight during a fairly short period of time (i.e., less than 1 week)? **(Edema, congestive heart failure)**
- Do you ever feel dizzy or have fainting spells? **(Valvular insufficiency, bradycardia, pulmonary hypertension, orthostatic hypotension)**
- Have you had any significant changes in your urine (e.g., increased amount, concentrated urine, frequency at night, or decreased amount)? **(Congestive heart failure, diabetes, hypertension)**
- Do you ever have sudden difficulty with speech, temporary blindness, or other changes in your vision? **(Transient ischemic attacks)**
- Have you ever had sudden weakness or paralysis down one side of your body or just in an arm or a leg? **(Transient ischemic attacks)**

continued

Medications

- Have you ever taken digitalis, nitroglycerin, or any other drug for your heart?
- Have you been on a diet or taken medications to lower your blood cholesterol?
- For the therapist: Any clients taking anticlotting drugs should be examined for hematoma, nosebleed, or other sites of bleeding. Protect client from trauma.
- Anyone taking cardiovascular medications (especially ACE inhibitors or digitalis glycosides) in combination with NSAIDs must be monitored closely (see text explanation).
- Any woman older than 35 and taking oral contraceptives who has a history of smoking should be monitored for increases in blood pressure.
- Any woman taking third-generation oral contraceptives should be monitored for venous thrombosis.

For clients taking nitroglycerin:

- Do you ever have headaches, dizziness, or a flushed sensation after taking nitroglycerin? (Most common side effects)
- How quickly does your nitroglycerin reduce or eliminate your chest pain? (Use as a guideline in the clinic when the client has angina during exercise; refer to a physician if angina is consistently unrelieved with nitroglycerin or rest after the usual period of time.)

For Clients With Breast Pain (see Questions, Chapter 12)

For Clients With Joint Pain

- Have you had any recent skin rashes or dotlike hemorrhages under the skin? **(Rheumatic fever, endocarditis)**
    - If yes, did this occur after a visit to the dentist? **(Endocarditis)**
- Do you notice any increase in your joint pain or symptoms 1 to 2 hours after you take your medication? **(Allergic response)**
- For new onset of left upper trapezius muscle/left shoulder pain: Have you been treated for any infection in the last 3 weeks?

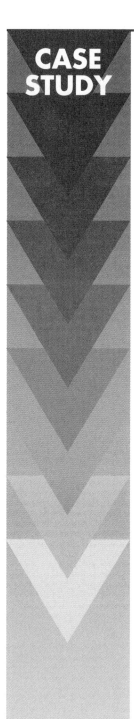

CASE STUDY

REFERRAL

A 30-year-old woman with five children comes to you for an evaluation on the recommendation of her friend, who received physical therapy from you last year. She has not been to a physician since her last child was delivered by her obstetrician 4 years ago. Her chief complaint is pain in the left shoulder and left upper trapezius muscle with pain radiating into the chest and referred pain down the medial aspect of the arm to the thumb and first two fingers. When the medical history is being taken, the client mentions that she was told 5 years ago that she had a mitral valve prolapse secondary to rheumatic fever, which she had when she was 12 years old.

There is no reported injury or trauma to the neck or shoulder, and the symptoms subside with rest. Physical exertion, such as carrying groceries up the stairs or laundry outside, aggravates the symptoms, but she is uncertain whether just using her upper body has the same effect. She is not taking any medication, denies any palpitations, but complains of fatigue and has dyspnea after playing ball with her son for 10 or 15 minutes.

Despite the client's denial of injury or trauma, the neck and shoulder should be screened for any possible musculoskeletal or neurologic origin of symptoms. Your observation of the woman indicates that she is 30 to 40 pounds overweight. She confides that she is under physical and emotional stress by the daily demands made by seven people in her house. She is not involved in any kind of exercise program outside of her play activities with the children. These two factors (obesity and stress) could account for her chronic fatigue and dyspnea, but that determination must be made by a physician. Even if you can identify a musculoskeletal basis for this woman's symptoms, the past medical history of rheumatic heart disease and absence of medical follow-up would support your recommendation that the client should go to the physician for a medical checkup.

How do you rule the possibility that this pain is not associated with a mitral valve prolapse and is caused instead by true cervical spine or shoulder pain?

It should be pointed out here that the physical therapist is not equipped with the skills, knowledge, or expertise to determine that the mitral valve prolapse is the cause of the client's symptoms. However, a thorough subjective and objective evaluation can assist the therapist both in making a determination regarding the client's musculoskeletal condition and in providing clear and thorough feedback for the physician on referral.

SCREENING FOR MITRAL VALVE PROLAPSE

- Pain of a mitral valve must be diagnosed by a physician
- Mitral valve may be asymptomatic
- Positive history for rheumatic fever
- Carefully ask the client about a history of possible neck or shoulder pain, which the person may not mention otherwise
- Musculoskeletal pain associated with the neck or shoulder is more superficial than cardiac pain
- Total body exertion causing shoulder pain may be secondary to angina or myocardial ischemia and subsequent infarction, whereas movements of just the upper extremity causing shoulder pain are more indicative of a primary musculoskeletal lesion

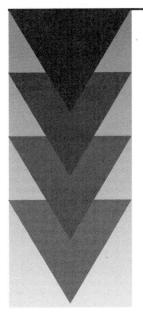

Does your shoulder pain occur during exercise, such as walking, climbing stairs, mowing the lawn, or during any other physical or sexual activity that does not require the use of your arm or shoulder?

- Presence of associated signs and symptoms, such as dyspnea, fatigue, or heart palpitations
- X-ray findings, if available, may confirm osteophyte formation with decreased intraforaminal spaces, which may contribute to cervical spine pain
- History of neck injury or overuse
- History of shoulder injury or overuse
- Results of objective tests to clear or rule out the cervical spine and shoulder as the cause of symptoms
- Presence of other neurologic signs to implicate the cervical spine or thoracic outlet type of symptoms (e.g., abnormal deep tendon reflexes, subjective report of numbness and tingling, objective sensory changes, muscle wasting or atrophy)
- Pattern of symptoms: A change in position may relieve symptoms associated with a cervical disorder

PRACTICE QUESTIONS

1. Pursed-lip breathing in the sitting position while leaning forward on the arms relieves symptoms of dyspnea for the client with

   a. Orthopnea

   b. Emphysema

   c. Congestive heart failure

   d. (a) and (c)

2. Briefly describe the difference between myocardial ischemia, angina pectoris, and myocardial infarction.

3. What should you do if a client complains of throbbing pain at the base of the neck that radiates into the interscapular areas and increases with exertion?

4. What are the 3 Ps? What is the significance of each one?

5. When are palpitations clinically significant?

6. A 48-year-old woman with temporomandibular joint syndrome has been referred to you by her dentist. How do you screen for the possibility of medical (specifically cardiac) disease?

7. A 55-year-old male grocery store manager reports that he becomes extremely weak and breathless when he is stocking groceries on overhead shelves. What is the possible significance of this complaint?

8. You are seeing an 83-year-old woman for a home health evaluation after a motor vehicle accident (MVA) that required a long hospitalization followed by transition care in an intermediate care nursing facility and now home health care.

She is ambulating short distances with a wheeled walker, but she becomes short of breath quickly and requires lengthy rest periods. At each visit the client is wearing her slippers and housecoat, so you suggest that she start dressing each day as if she intended to go out. She replies that she can no longer fit into her loosest slacks and she cannot tie her shoes. Is there any significance to this client's comments, or is this consistent with her age and obvious deconditioning? Briefly explain your answer.

9. Peripheral vascular diseases include

   a. Arterial and occlusive diseases

   b. Arterial and venous disorders

   c. Acute and chronic arterial diseases

   d. All of the above

   e. None of the above

10 Which statement is the *most* accurate?

   a. Arterial disease is characterized by intermittent claudication, pain relieved by elevating the extremity, and history of smoking.

   b. Arterial disease is characterized by loss of hair on the lower extremities and throbbing pain in the calf muscles that goes away by using heat and elevation.

   c. Arterial disease is characterized by painful throbbing of the feet at night that goes away by dangling the feet over the bed.

   d. Arterial disease is characterized by loss of hair on the toes, intermittent claudication, and redness or warmth of the legs that is accompanied by a burning sensation.

References

Anderson JL, Carlquist JF, Muhlestein JB et al: Evaluation of C-reactive protein, an inflammatory marker, and infectious serology as risk factors of coronary artery disease and myocardial infarction, *J Am Coll Cardiol* 32(1):35-41, 1998.

Aspinall W: Clinical testing for the craniovertebral hypermobility syndrome, *J Orthop Sports Phys Ther* 12:180-131, 1989.

Bancroft B: Chest pain and the 3 P's, *Pathophysiol Perspect,* March/April 1996.

Cahalin LP: Heart failure, *Phys Ther* 76(5):517-533, 1996.

Cohen MC, Rohtla KM, Mittleman MA et al: Meta-analysis of the morning excess of acute myocardial infarction and sudden cardiac death, *Am J Cardiol* 79(11):1512-1516, 1997.

Costa O, Freitas J, Sa I et al: Current perspectives in screening for cardiac diseases which most frequently cause sudden death during the practice of a sports activity, *Rev Port Cardiol* 17(3):273-283, 1998.

Davidson M: Confirmed previous infection with *Chlamydia pneumoniae* (TWAR) and its presence in early coronary atherosclerosis, *Circulation* 98(7):628-633, 1998.

de Virgilio C: Ascending aortic dissection in weight lifters with cystic medial degeneration, *Ann Thorac Surg* 49(4):638-642, 1990.

Elliot WJ, Powel LH: Diagonal earlobe creases and prognosis in patients with suspected coronary artery disease, *Am J Med* 100(2):205-211, 1996.

Farmer RD, Lawrenson RA: Oral contraceptives and venous thromboembolic disease, *Am J Obstet Gynecol* 179(3 Pt 2):S78-S86, 1998.

Goodnight SH, Feinstein DI: Update in hematology, *Ann Intern Med* 128(7):545-551, 1998.

Heinemann LA, Lewis MA, Spitzer WO et al: Thromboembolic stroke in young women, *Contraception* 57(1):29-37, 1998.

Kurtz TW, Gardner DG: Transcription-modulating drugs: a new frontier in the treatment of essential hypertension, *Hypertension* 32(3):380-386, 1998.

Magee DJ: *Orthopedic physical assessment,* ed 3, Philadelphia, 1997, WB Saunders.

Morrow DA, Rifai N, Antman EM et al: C-reactive protein is a potent predictor of mortality independently of and in combination with troponin T in acute coronary syndromes: a TIMI 11A substudy—thrombolysis in myocardial infarction, *J Am Coll Cardiol* 31(7):1460-1465, 1998.

Muhlestein JB: Bacterial infections and atherosclerosis, *J Invest Med* 46(8):396-402, 1998.

O'Donnell CJ, Lindpaintner K, Larson MG et al: Evidence for association and genetic linkage with hypertension and blood pressure in men but not women in the Framingham heart study, *Circulation* 97(18):1766-1772, 1998.

O'Donnell CJ, Ridker PM, Glynn RJ: Hypertension and borderline isolated systolic hypertension increase risks of cardiovascular disease and mortality in male physicians, *Circulation* 95(5):1132-1137, 1997.

Rivett DA: The premanipulative vertebral artery testing protocol: a brief review, *Physiotherapy* 23:9-12, 1995.

Sapico FL, Liquette JA, Sarma RJ: Bone and joint infections in patients with infective endocarditis: review of a 4-year experience, *Clin Infect Dis* 22: 783- 787, 1996.

Sixth Report of the Joint National Committee on Prevention, Detection, Evaluation and Treatment of High Blood Pressure, *Arch Intern Med* 157(21): 2413- 2446, 1997.

Thiel H, Wallace K, Donut J et al: Effect of various head and neck positions on vertebral artery blood flow, *Clin Biomech* 9:105-110, 1994.

Thorogood M: Oral contraceptives and thrombosis, *Curr Opin Hematol* 5(5):350-354, 1998.

Toss H, Gnarpe J, Gnarpe H: Increased fibrinogen levels are associated with persistent *Chlamydia pneumoniae* infection in unstable coronary artery disease, *Eur Heart J* 19(4):570-577, 1998.

World Health Organization (WHO) Collaborative Study of Cardiovascular Disease and Steroid Hormone Contraception: Cardiovascular disease and use of oral and injectable progestogen-only contraceptives and combined injectable contraceptives, *Contraception* 57(5):315-324, 1998.

Overview of Pulmonary Signs and Symptoms

4

Pulmonary pain patterns are usually localized in the substernal or chest region over involved lung fields that may include the anterior chest, side, or back. However, pulmonary pain can radiate to the neck, upper trapezius muscle, costal margins, thoracic back, scapulae, or shoulder. Shoulder pain may radiate along the medial aspect of the arm, mimicking other neuromuscular causes of neck or shoulder pain. Pulmonary pain usually increases with inspiratory movements, such as laughing, coughing, sneezing, or deep breathing, and the client notes the presence of associated symptoms, such as dyspnea (exertional or at rest), persistent cough, fever, and chills.

For the client with neck, shoulder, or back pain at presentation, it may be necessary to consider the possibility of a pulmonary cause requiring medical referral.

The most common pulmonary conditions to mimic those of the musculoskeletal system include pulmonary artery hypertension, pulmonary embolism, pleurisy, pneumothorax, and pneumonia.

The material in this chapter will assist the physical therapist in treating both the client with a known pulmonary problem and the client having musculoskeletal signs and symptoms that may have an underlying systemic basis (see Case Example on p. 146).

In the case of pleuropulmonary disorders, the client's recent personal medical history may include a previous or recurrent upper respiratory infection or pneumonia.

Central nervous system (CNS) symptoms, such as muscle weakness, muscle atrophy, headache, loss of lower extremity sensation, and localized or radicular back pain may be associated with lung cancer and must be investigated by a physician for diagnosis.

▼ PULMONARY PAIN PATTERNS

As discussed earlier in the section on chest pain in Chapter 3, the parietal pleura* is sensitive to painful stimulation, but the visceral

---

*The thoracic cavity is lined with pleura, or serous membrane. One surface of the pleura lines the inside of the rib cage (parietal pleura), and the other surface, the visceral pleura, covers the lungs.

pleura is insensitive. Within the pulmonary system, the trachea and large bronchi are innervated by the vagus trunks, whereas the finer bronchi and lung parenchyma appear to be free of pain innervation.

Tracheobronchial pain is referred to sites in the neck or anterior chest at the same levels as the points of irritation in the air passages (Fig. 4-1). This irritation may be caused by inflammatory lesions, irritating foreign materials, or cancerous tumors.

Extensive disease may occur in the periphery of the lung without occurrence of pain until the process extends to the parietal pleura. Pleural irritation then results in sharp, localized pain that is aggravated by any respiratory movement. Clients usually note that the pain is alleviated by lying on the affected side, which diminishes the movement of that side of the chest ("autosplinting").

Debate continues concerning the mechanism by which pain occurs in the parietal

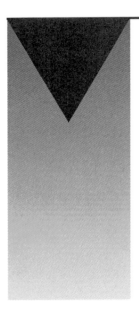

Case Example. A 67-year-old woman with a known diagnosis of rheumatoid arthritis has been treated as needed in a physical therapy clinic for the last 8 years. She has reported occasional chest pain described as "coming on suddenly, like a knife pushing from the inside out—it takes my breath away." She missed 2 days of treatment because of illness, and when she returned to the clinic, the physical therapist noticed that she had a newly developed cough and that her rheumatoid arthritis was much worse. She says that she missed her appointments because she had the "flu."

Further questioning to elicit the potential development of chest pain on inspiration, the presence of ongoing fever and chills, and the changes in breathing pattern is recommended. Positive findings beyond the reasonable duration of influenza (7 to 10 days) or an increase in pulmonary symptoms (shortness of breath, hacking cough, hemoptysis, wheezing or other changes in breathing pattern) raises a red flag indicating the need for medical referral. This clinical case points out that clients currently undergoing physical therapy for a known musculoskeletal problem may be describing signs and symptoms of systemic disease.

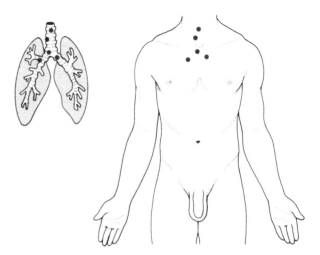

FIGURE 4-1 • Tracheobronchial pain is referred to sites in the neck or anterior chest at the same levels as the points of irritation in the air passages. The points of pain are on the same side as the areas of irritation.

membrane. It has been long thought that friction between the two pleural surfaces (when the membranes are irritated and covered with fibrinous exudate) causes sharp pain. Other theories suggest that intercostal muscle spasm resulting from pleurisy or stretching of the parietal pleura causes this pain.

Pleural pain is present in pulmonary disease processes including pleurisy, pneumonia, pulmonary infarct (when it extends to the pleural surface, thus causing pleurisy), tumor (when it invades the parietal pleura), and pneumothorax. Tumor, especially bronchogenic carcinoma, may be accompanied by severe, continuous pain when the tumor tissue, extending to the parietal pleura through the lung, constantly irritates the pain nerve endings in the pleura.

The *diaphragmatic pleura* receives dual pain innervation through the phrenic and intercostal nerves. Damage to the phrenic nerve produces paralysis of the corresponding half of the diaphragm. The phrenic nerves are sensory and motor from both surfaces of the diaphragm.

Stimulation of the peripheral portions of the diaphragmatic pleura results in sharp pain felt along the costal margins, which can be referred to the lumbar region by the lower thoracic somatic nerves. Stimulation of the central portion of the diaphragmatic pleura results in sharp pain referred to the upper trapezius muscle and shoulder on the ipsilateral side of the stimulation (see Fig. 12-6).

Pain of cardiac and diaphragmatic origin is often experienced in the shoulder because the heart and diaphragm are supplied by the C5-C6 spinal segment, and the visceral pain is referred to the corresponding somatic area.

Diaphragmatic pleurisy secondary to pneumonia is common and refers sharp pain along the costal margins or upper trapezius, which is aggravated by any diaphragmatic motion, such as coughing, laughing, or deep breathing.

There may be tenderness to palpation along the costal margins, and sharp pain occurs when the client is asked to take a deep breath. A change in position (side bending or rotation of the trunk) does not reproduce the symptoms, which would be the case with a true intercostal lesion or tear. Forceful, repeated coughing can result in an intercostal lesion in the presence of referred intercostal pain from diaphragmatic pleurisy, which can make differentiation between these two entities impossible without a medical referral and further diagnostic testing.

▼ PULMONARY PHYSIOLOGY

The primary function of the respiratory system is to provide oxygen to and to remove carbon dioxide from cells in the body. The act of breathing, in which the oxygen and carbon dioxide exchange occurs, involves the two interrelated processes of ventilation and respiration. Ventilation is the movement of air from outside the body to the alveoli of the lungs. Respiration is the process of oxygen uptake and carbon dioxide elimination between the body and the outside environment.

Breathing is an automatic process by which sensors detect changes in the levels of carbon dioxide and continuously direct data to the medulla. The medulla then directs respiratory muscles that adjust ventilation. Breathing patterns can be altered voluntarily when this automatic response is overridden by conscious thought.

The major sensors mentioned here are the central chemoreceptors (located near the medulla) and the peripheral sensors (located in the carotid body and aortic arch). The central chemoreceptors respond to increases in carbon dioxide and decreases in pH in cerebrospinal fluid.

As carbon dioxide increases, the medulla signals a response to increase respiration. The peripheral chemoreceptor system responds to low arterial blood oxygen and is believed to function only in pathologic situations, such as when there are chronically

CLUES TO SCREENING FOR PULMONARY DISEASE

- Age over 40 years
- History of cigarette smoking for many years
- Past medical history of breast, prostate, kidney, pancreas, colon, or uterine cancer
- Recent history of upper respiratory infection
- Musculoskeletal pain exacerbated by respiratory movements (e.g., deep breathing, coughing, laughing)
- Respiratory movements are diminished or absent on one side (pneumothorax)
- Unable to localize pain by palpation
- Pain does not change with alterations in position
- Symptoms are increased with recumbency (lying supine shifts the contents of the abdominal cavity in an upward direction, thereby placing pressure on the diaphragm and, in turn, the lungs, referring pain from a lower lung pathologic condition)
- Presence of associated signs and symptoms, especially persistent cough, hemoptysis, dyspnea, and consitutional symptoms, most commonly sore throat, fever, and chills
- Autosplinting decreases pain
- Elimination of trigger points resolves symptoms
- Range of motion does not reproduce symptoms* (e.g., trunk rotation, trunk side bending, shoulder motions)
- See also Key Points to Remember and Overview: Pulmonary Pain Patterns

*There are two possible exceptions to this guideline. Painful symptoms from an intercostal tear (secondary to forceful coughing caused by diaphragmatic pleurisy) will be reproduced by trunk side bending to the opposite side and trunk rotation to one or both sides. In such a case there is an underlying pulmonary pathologic condition, and a musculoskeletal component. Pleuritic pain can also be reproduced by trunk movements, but the therapist will be unable to localize the pain on palpation.

---

elevated carbon dioxide levels (e.g., chronic obstructive pulmonary disease [COPD]).

Acid-Base Regulation

The proper balance of acids and bases in the body is essential to life. This balance is very complex and must be kept within the narrow parameters of a pH of 7.35 to 7.45 in the extracellular fluid. This number (or pH value) represents the hydrogen ion concentration in body fluid. A reading of less than 7.35 is considered *acidosis* and a reading greater than 7.45 is called *alkalosis*. Life cannot be sustained if the pH values are less than 7 or greater than 7.8.

Living human cells are extremely sensitive to alterations in body fluid pH (hydrogen ion concentration); thus various mechanisms are in operation to keep the pH at a relatively constant level. Acid-base regulatory mechanisms include chemical buffer systems, the respiratory system, and the renal system. These systems interact very closely to maintain a normal acid-base ratio of 20 parts of bicarbonate to 1 part of carbonic acid and thus to maintain normal body fluid pH.

The blood test used most often to measure the effectiveness of ventilation and oxygen transport is the arterial blood gas (ABG) test (Table 4-1). The measurement of arterial blood gases is important in the diagnosis and treatment of ventilation, oxygen transport, and acid-base problems. The arterial blood gas test measures the amount of dissolved oxygen and carbon dioxide in arterial blood and indicates acid-base status by measurement of the arterial blood pH.

TABLE 4-1 ▼ Arterial Blood Gas Values*

pH	7.35-7.45
pCO₂ (partial pressure of carbon dioxide)	35-45 mm Hg
HCO₃ (bicarbonate ion)	22-26 mEq/L
pO₂ (partial pressure of oxygen)	75-100 mm Hg
O₂ saturation (oxygen saturation)	96%-100%

Panic Values

pH	≤ 7.20 or > 7.6
pCO₂	≤ 20 or > 70 mm Hg
HCO₃	≤ 10 or > 40 mEq/L
pO₂	≤ 40 mm Hg
O₂ saturation	≤ 60%

Normal pH level: *The pH is inversely proportional to the hydrogen ion concentration in the blood. As the hydrogen ion concentration increases (acidosis), the pH decreases; as the hydrogen ion concentration decreases (alkalosis), the pH increases.*

Normal pCO₂: *The pCO₂ is a measure of the partial pressure of carbon dioxide in the blood. As the carbon dioxide level increases, the pH decreases (respiratory acidosis); as the carbon dioxide level decreases, the pH increases (respiratory alkalosis).*

Bicarbonate ion: *HCO₃ is a measure of the metabolic portion of the acid-base function. As the bicarbonate value increases, the pH increases (metabolic acidosis); as the bicarbonate value decreases, the pH decreases (metabolic acidosis).*

Partial pressure of oxygen: *The pO₂ is a measure of the partial pressure of oxygen in the blood and represents the status of alveolar gas exchange.*

Oxygen saturation: *O₂ saturation is an indication of the percentage of hemoglobin saturated with oxygen. When 95% to 100% of the hemoglobin binds and carries oxygen, the tissues are adequately perfused with oxygen. As the pO₂ decreases, the percentage of hemoglobin saturation also decreases. At oxygen saturation levels of less than 70%, the tissues are unable to carry out vital functions.*

*Modified from Chernecky C, Berger B: *Laboratory tests and diagnostic procedures,* ed 2, Philadelphia, 1997, WB Saunders, p 252.

▼ PULMONARY PATHOPHYSIOLOGY

Respiratory Acidosis

Any condition that decreases pulmonary ventilation increases the retention and con-

▼ ***Clinical Signs and Symptoms of***
Respiratory Acidosis

- Decreased ventilation
- Confusion
- Sleepiness and unconsciousness
- Diaphoresis
- Shallow, rapid breathing
- Restlessness
- Cyanosis

centration of carbon dioxide (CO_2), hydrogen, and carbonic acid; this results in an increase in the amount of circulating hydrogen and is called respiratory acidosis.

If ventilation is severely compromised, CO_2 levels become extremely high and respiration is depressed even further, causing hypoxia as well.

During respiratory acidosis, potassium moves out of cells into the extracellular fluid to exchange with circulating hydrogen. This results in hyperkalemia (abnormally high potassium concentration in the blood) and cardiac changes that can cause cardiac arrest.

Respiratory acidosis can result from pathologic conditions that decrease the efficiency of the respiratory system. These pathologies can include damage to the medulla, which controls respiration, obstruction of airways (e.g., neoplasm, foreign bodies, pulmonary disease such as COPD, pneumonia), loss of lung surface ventilation (e.g., pneumothorax, pulmonary fibrosis), weakness of respiratory muscles (e.g., poliomyelitis, spinal cord injury, Guillain-Barré syndrome), or overdose of respiratory depressant drugs.

As hypoxia becomes more severe, diaphoresis, shallow rapid breathing, restlessness, and cyanosis may appear. Cardiac arrhythmias may also be present as the potassium level in the blood serum rises.

Treatment is directed at restoration of efficient ventilation. If the respiratory depression and acidosis are severe, injection of intravenous sodium bicarbonate and use of a mechanical ventilator may be necessary.

Any client with symptoms of inadequate ventilation or CO_2 retention needs immediate medical referral.

Respiratory Alkalosis

Increased respiratory rate and depth decrease the amount of available CO_2 and hydrogen and create a condition of increased pH, or alkalosis. When pulmonary ventilation is increased, CO_2 and hydrogen are eliminated from the body too quickly and are not available to buffer the increasingly alkaline environment.

Respiratory alkalosis is usually due to *hyperventilation*. Rapid, deep respirations are often caused by neurogenic or psychogenic problems, including anxiety, pain, and cerebral trauma or lesions. Other causes can be related to conditions that greatly increase metabolism (e.g., hyperthyroidism) or overventilation of clients with a mechanical ventilator.

If the alkalosis becomes more severe, muscular tetany and convulsions can occur. Cardiac arrhythmias caused by serum potassium loss through the kidneys may also occur. The kidneys keep hydrogen in exchange for potassium.

Treatment of respiratory alkalosis includes reassurance, assistance in slowing breathing and facilitating relaxation, sedation, pain control, CO_2 administration, and use of a rebreathing device such as a rebreathing mask or paper bag. A rebreathing device allows the client to inhale and "rebreathe" the exhaled CO_2.

▼ *Clinical Signs and Symptoms of*
Respiratory Alkalosis

- Hyperventilation
- Lightheadedness
- Dizziness
- Numbness and tingling of the face, fingers, and toes
- Syncope (fainting)

Respiratory alkalosis related to hyperventilation is a relatively common condition and might be present more often in the physical therapy setting than is respiratory acidosis. Pain and anxiety are common causes of hyperventilation, and treatment needs to be focused toward reduction of both of these interrelated elements. If hyperventilation continues in the absence of pain or anxiety, serious systemic problems may be the cause, and immediate physician referral is necessary.

If either respiratory acidosis or alkalosis persist for hours to days in a chronic and not life-threatening manner, the kidneys then begin to assist in the restoration of normal body fluid pH by selective excretion or retention of hydrogen ions or bicarbonate. This process is called *renal compensation*. When the kidneys compensate effectively, blood pH values are within normal limits (7.35 to 7.45) even though the underlying problem may still cause the respiratory imbalance.

Chronic Obstructive Pulmonary Disease

COPD, also called chronic obstructive lung disease (COLD), refers to a number of disorders that have in common abnormal airway structure resulting in obstruction of air in and out of the lungs. The most important of these disorders are obstructive bronchitis, emphysema, and asthma. Although bronchitis, emphysema, and asthma may occur in a "pure form," they most commonly coexist. Although the term *COPD* is commonly used, specialists in pulmonary medicine believe that it is not completely accurate, and the term *chronic airflow limitation (CAL)* may be used in its place.

COPD is a leading cause of morbidity and mortality among cigarette smokers. Other factors predisposing to COPD include air pollution, occupational exposure to irritating dusts or gases, hereditary factors, infection, allergies, aging, and potentially harmful drugs and chemicals. COPD rarely occurs in nonsmokers; however, only a minority of cigarette smokers develop symptomatic disease, suggesting that genetic factors may contribute to the development of COPD (Sandford et al, 1997).

TABLE 4-2 ▼ Respiratory Diseases: Summary of Differences

Disease	Primary Area Affected	Result
Bronchitis	Membrane lining bronchial tubes	Inflammation of lining
Bronchiectasis	Bronchial tubes (bronchi or air passages)	Bronchial dilation with inflammation
Pneumonia	Alveoli (air sacs)	Causative agent invades alveoli with resultant outpouring from lung capillaries into air spaces and continued healing process
Emphysema	Air spaces beyond terminal bronchioles (alveoli)	Breakdown of alveolar walls Air spaces enlarged
Asthma	Bronchioles (small airways)	Bronchioles obstructed by muscle spasm, swelling of mucosa, thick secretions
Cystic fibrosis	Bronchioles	Bronchioles become obstructed and obliterated. Later, larger airways become involved. Plugs of mucus cling to airway walls, leading to bronchitis, bronchiectasis, atelectasis, pneumonia, or pulmonary abscess

In all forms of COPD narrowing of the airways obstructs airflow to and from the lungs (Table 4-2). This narrowing impairs ventilation by trapping air in the bronchioles and alveoli. The obstruction increases the resistance to airflow. Trapped air hinders normal gas exchange and causes distention of the alveoli. Other mechanisms of COPD vary with each form of the disease.

Bronchitis

ACUTE

Acute bronchitis is an inflammation of the trachea and bronchi (tracheobronchial tree) that is self-limiting and of short duration with few pulmonary signs. This condition may result from chemical irritation (e.g., smoke, fumes, gas) or may occur with viral infections such as influenza, measles, chickenpox, or whooping cough. These predisposing conditions may become apparent during the subjective examination (i.e., Personal/Family History form or the Physical Therapy Interview). Although bronchitis is usually mild, it can become complicated in older clients and clients with chronic lung or heart disease. Pneumonia is a critical complication.

Treatment is symptomatic, involving cough suppressants, rest, and hydration.

▼ *Clinical Signs and Symptoms of*
Acute Bronchitis

- Mild fever from 1 to 3 days
- Malaise
- Back and muscle pain
- Sore throat
- Cough with sputum production, followed by wheezing
- Possibly laryngitis

CHRONIC

Chronic bronchitis is a condition associated with prolonged exposure to nonspecific bronchial irritants and is accompanied by mucous hypersecretion and structural changes in the bronchi (large air passages leading into the lungs). This irritation of the tissue usually results from exposure to cigarette smoke, long-term inhalation of dust or air pollution, and causes hypertrophy of mucus-producing cells in the bronchi. The swollen mucous membrane and thick sputum obstruct the airways, causing wheezing, and the client develops a cough to clear the airways. The clinical definition of a person with chronic bronchitis is anyone who coughs for at least 3 months per year for 2

Clinical Signs and Symptoms of
Chronic Bronchitis

- Persistent cough with production of sputum (worse in the morning and evening than at midday)
- Reduced chest expansion
- Wheezing
- Fever
- Dyspnea (shortness of breath)
- Cyanosis (blue discoloration of skin and mucous membranes)
- Decreased exercise tolerance

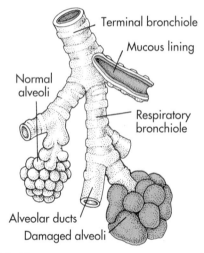

FIGURE 4-2 • Chronic bronchitis may lead to the formation of misshapen or large alveolar sacs with reduced space for oxygen and carbon dioxide exchange. The client may develop cyanosis and pulmonary edema.

consecutive years without having had a precipitating disease.

In bronchitis, partial or complete blockage of the airways from mucous secretions causes insufficient oxygenation in the alveoli (Fig. 4-2).

To confirm that the condition is chronic bronchitis, tests are performed to determine whether the airways are obstructed and to exclude other diseases that may cause similar symptoms, such as silicosis, tuberculosis, or a tumor in the upper airway. Sputum samples will be analyzed, and lung function tests may be performed.

Treatment is aimed at keeping the airways as clear as possible. Smokers are encouraged and helped to stop smoking. A combination of drugs may be prescribed to relieve the symptoms, including bronchodilators to open the obstructed airways and to thin the obstructive mucus so that it can be coughed up more easily.

Chronic bronchitis may develop slowly over a period of years, but it will not go away if untreated. Eventually, the bronchial walls thicken, and the number of mucous glands increases. The client is increasingly susceptible to respiratory infections, during which the bronchial tissue becomes inflamed and the mucus becomes even thicker and more profuse.

Chronic bronchitis can be incapacitating and lead to more serious and potentially fatal lung disease. Influenza and pneumococcal vaccines are recommended for these clients.

Bronchiectasis

Bronchiectasis is a form of obstructive lung disease that is actually a type of bronchitis. It is a progressive and chronic pulmonary condition that occurs after infections such as childhood pneumonia or cystic fibrosis. Although bronchiectasis was once a common disease because of measles, pertussis, tuberculosis, and poorly treated bacterial pneumonias, the prevalence of bronchiectasis has diminished greatly since the introduction of antibiotics. It is characterized by abnormal and permanent dilatation of the large air passages leading into the lungs (bronchi) and by destruction of bronchial walls.

Bronchiectasis is caused by repeated damage to bronchial walls. The resultant destruction and bronchial dilatation reduce bronchial wall movement so that secretions cannot be removed effectively from the lungs, and the person is predisposed to frequent respiratory infections.

Clinical Signs and Symptoms of
Bronchiectasis

Clinical signs and symptoms of bronchiectasis vary widely, depending on the extent of the disease and on the presence of complicating infection, but may include:

- Chronic "wet" cough with copious foul-smelling secretions; generally worse in the morning after the individual has been recumbent for a length of time
- Hemoptysis (bloody sputum)
- Occasional wheezing sounds
- Dyspnea
- Sinusitis (inflammation of one or more paranasal sinuses)
- Weight loss
- Anemia
- Malaise
- Recurrent fever and chills
- Fatigue

This vicious cycle of bacterial infection and inflammation of the bronchial wall leads to loss of ventilation and irreversible lung damage. Advanced bronchiectasis may cause pneumonia, cor pulmonale, or right-sided ventricular failure.

All pulmonary irritants, especially cigarette smoke, should be avoided. Postural drainage, adequate hydration, good nutrition, and bronchodilator therapy in bronchospasm are important components in treatment. Antibiotics are used during disease exacerbations (e.g., increased cough, purulent sputum, hemoptysis, malaise, and weight loss). Future treatment through immunomodulatory therapy to alter the host response directly and thereby reduce tissue damage is under investigation.

Emphysema

Emphysema may develop in a person after a long history of chronic bronchitis in which the alveolar walls are destroyed, leading to permanent overdistension of the air spaces and loss of normal elastic tension in the lung tissue.

Air passages are obstructed as a result of these changes (rather than as a result of mucous production, as in chronic bronchitis). Difficult expiration in emphysema is due to the destruction of the walls (septa) between the alveoli, partial airway collapse, and loss of elastic recoil.

As the alveoli and septa collapse, pockets of air form between the alveolar spaces (called *blebs*) and within the lung parenchyma (called *bullae*). This process leads to increased ventilatory "dead space," or areas that do not participate in gas or blood exchange. The work of breathing is increased because there is less functional lung tissue to exchange oxygen and CO_2. Emphysema also causes destruction of the pulmonary capillaries, further decreasing oxygen perfusion and ventilation.

There are three types of emphysema. *Centrilobular emphysema* (Fig. 4-3), the most common type, destroys the bronchioles, usually in the upper lung regions. Inflammation develops in the bronchioles, but usually the alveolar sac remains intact. *Panlobular emphysema* destroys the more distal alveolar walls, most commonly involving the lower lung. This destruction of alveolar walls may occur secondary to infection or to irritants (most commonly, cigarette smoke). These two forms of emphysema, collectively called centriacinar emphysema, occur most often in smokers. *Paraseptal* (or *panacinar*) *emphysema* destroys the alveoli in the lower lobes of the lungs, resulting in isolated blebs along the lung periphery. Paraseptal emphysema is believed to be the likely cause of spontaneous pneumothorax.

CLINICAL SIGNS AND SYMPTOMS

The irreversible destruction reduces elasticity of the lung and increases the effort to exhale trapped air, causing marked dyspnea on exertion that later progresses to dyspnea at rest. Cough is uncommon. The client is often thin, has tachypnea with prolonged expiration, and uses the accessory muscles for

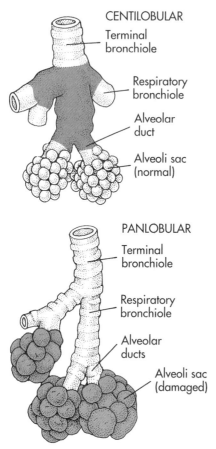

FIGURE 4-3 • Emphysema traps air in the lungs so that expelling air becomes increasingly difficult. Centrilobular emphysema affects the upper airways and produces destructive changes in the bronchioles. Panlobular emphysema affects the lower airways and is more diffusely scattered throughout the alveoli.

▼ *Clinical Signs and Symptoms of*
Emphysema

- Shortness of breath
- Dyspnea on exertion
- Orthopnea (only able to breathe in the upright position) immediately after assuming the supine position
- Chronic cough
- Barrel chest
- Weight loss
- Malaise
- Use of accessory muscles of respiration
- Prolonged expiratory period (with grunting)
- Wheezing
- Pursed-lip breathing
- Increased respiratory rate
- Peripheral cyanosis

The most important factor in the treatment of emphysema is cessation of smoking. The main goals for the client with emphysema are to improve oxygenation and decrease CO_2 retention.

Pursed-lip breathing causes resistance to outflow at the lips, which in turn maintains intrabronchial pressure and improves the mixing of gases in the lungs. This type of breathing should be encouraged to help the client get rid of the stale air trapped in the lungs.

Exercise will not improve pulmonary function but is used to enhance cardiovascular fitness and train skeletal muscles to function more effectively. Routine progressive walking is the most common form of exercise.

respiration. The client often leans forward with the arms braced on the knees to support the shoulders and chest for breathing. The combined effects of trapped air and alveolar distension change the size and shape of the client's chest, causing a barrel chest and increased expiratory effort.

As the disease progresses, there is a loss of surface area available for gas exchange. In the final stages of emphysema, cardiac complications, especially enlargement and dilatation of the right ventricle, may develop. The overloaded heart reaches its limit of muscular compensation and begins to fail (cor pulmonale).

Inflammatory/Infectious Disease

Asthma

Asthma is a reversible obstructive lung disease caused by increased reaction of the airways to various stimuli. It is a chronic inflammatory condition* with acute exacerbations that can be life-threatening if not properly managed.

Fifteen million persons of all ages are affected by asthma in the United States. This represents a 61% increase over the last 15 years with a 45% increase in mortality during the last decade. The exact cause of asthma

*Our understanding of asthma has changed dramatically over the last decade. Previously asthma was viewed as a bronchoconstrictive disorder in which the airways narrowed, causing wheezing and breathing difficulties. Treatment with bronchodilators to open airways was the primary focus. Scientific evidence now supports the idea that asthma is primarily an inflammatory disorder in which the constriction of airways is only a symptom of the underlying inflammation.

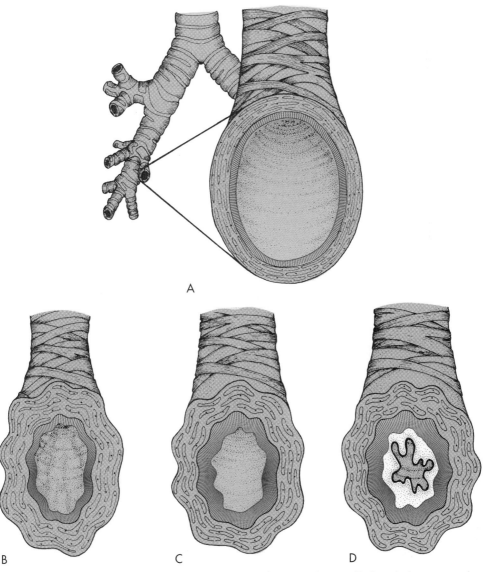

FIGURE 4-4 • **A,** Cross-section of a normal bronchus (mucous membrane in color). Healthy bronchioles accommodate a constant flow of air when open and relaxed. **B,** Asthma: Airway inflammation begins. The smooth muscle surrounding the bronchus contracts and causes narrowing of the airway, called *bronchospasm*. **C,** The airway tissue swells; this edema of the mucous membrane further narrows airways. **D,** Mucous is produced, further compromising airflow.

remains unknown, but current theories suggest genetic and environmental factors.

There are two major components to asthma. When the immune system becomes sensitized to an allergen, usually through heavy exposure in early life, an inflammatory cascade occurs, extending beyond the upper airways into the lungs.

The lungs become hyperreactive, responding to allergens and other irritants in an exaggerated way. This hyperresponsiveness causes the muscles of the airways to constrict, making breathing more difficult (Fig. 4-4). The second component is inflammation, which causes the air passages to swell and the cells lining the passages to produce excess mucus, further impairing breathing.

Asthma may be categorized as conventional asthma, occupational asthma, or exercise-induced asthma (EIA), but the underlying pathophysiologic complex remains the same. Since the triggers or allergens vary, each person reacts differently. Shortness of breath, wheezing, tightness in the chest, and cough are the most commonly reported symptoms, but other symptoms may also occur.

Anytime a client experiences shortness of breath, wheezing, and cough and comments, "I'm more out of shape that I thought," the therapist should ask about a past medical history of asthma and review the list of symptoms with the client. Physical therapists working with known asthmatic clients should encourage them to maintain hydration by drinking fluids to prevent mucous plugs from hardening and to take prescribed medications.

Exercise- or hyperventilation-induced asthma potentially can be prevented by exercising in a moist, humid environment and by grading exercise according to client tolerance using diaphragmatic breathing. Any type of sustained running or cycling

---

▼ Clinical Signs and Symptoms of
Asthma

Listen for
- Wheezing, however light
- Irregular breathing with prolonged expiration
- Noisy, difficult breathing
- Episodes of dyspnea
- Clearing the throat (tickle at the back of the throat or neck)
- Cough with or without sputum production, especially in the absence of a cold and/or occurring 5 to 10 minutes after exercise

Look for
- Skin retraction (clavicles, ribs, sternum)
- Hunched-over body posture; inability to stand, sit straight, or relax
- Pursed-lip breathing
- Nostrils flaring
- Unusual pallor or unexplained sweating

Ask about
- Restlessness during sleep
- Vomiting
- Fatigue unrelated to working or playing

FACTORS THAT MAY TRIGGER ASTHMA

- Respiratory infections, colds
- Cigarette smoke
- Allergic reactions to pollen, mold, animal dander, feather, dust, food, insects
- Indoor and outdoor air pollutants, including ozone
- Physical exertion or vigorous exercise
- Exposure to cold air or sudden temperature change
- Excitement or strong emotion, psychologic or emotional stress

or activity in the cold is more likely to precipitate EIA (see "Factors That May Trigger Asthma" box on p. 156).

COMPLICATIONS

Status asthmaticus is a severe, life-threatening complication of asthma. With severe bronchospasm the workload of breathing increases five to ten times, which can lead to acute cor pulmonale. When air is trapped, a severe paradoxic pulse develops as venous return is obstructed. This condition is seen as a blood pressure drop of more than 10 mm Hg during inspiration.

Pneumothorax can develop. If status asthmaticus continues, hypoxemia worsens and acidosis begins. If the condition is untreated or not reversed, respiratory or cardiac arrest will occur. An acute asthma episode may constitute a medical emergency.

Medical treatment for the underlying inflammation and resulting airway obstruction is with antiinflammatory agents* and bronchodilators to prevent, interrupt, or terminate ongoing inflammatory reactions in the airways. Reducing, eliminating, or avoiding allergens or triggers is an important part of self-care.

Pneumonia

Pneumonia is an inflammation of the lungs and can be caused by (1) aspiration of food, fluids, or vomitus; (2) inhalation of toxic or caustic chemicals, smoke, dust, or gases; or (3) a bacterial, viral, or mycoplasmal infection. It may be primary or secondary (a complication of another disease); it often follows influenza.

The common feature of all types of pneumonia is an inflammatory pulmonary response to the offending organism or agent. This response may involve one or both lungs at the level of the lobe (lobar pneumonia) or more distally beginning in the terminal bronchioles and alveoli (bronchopneumonia). Bronchopneumonia is seen more frequently than lobar pneumonia and is common in clients postoperatively and in clients with chronic bronchitis, particularly when these two situations coexist.

Infectious agents responsible for pneumonia are typically present in the upper respiratory tract and cause no harm unless resistance is lowered severely by some other factor, such as a severe cold, disease, alcoholism, or generally poor health (e.g., poorly controlled diabetes, chronic renal problems). Older or bedridden clients are particularly at risk because of physical inactivity and immobility. Limited mobility causes normal secretions to pool in the airways and facilitates bacterial growth.

Pneumocystis carinii is a protozoan organism that rarely causes pneumonia in healthy individuals. *Pneumocystis carinii* pneumonia (PCP) has been the most common life-threatening opportunistic infection in persons with acquired immune deficiency syndrome (AIDS). PCP also has been shown to be the first indicator of conversion from human immunodeficiency virus (HIV) infection to the designation of AIDS in 60% of individuals with HIV disease.

CLINICAL SIGNS AND SYMPTOMS

The onset of all pneumonias is generally marked by any of the following†: fever, chills, sweats, pleuritic chest pain, cough, sputum production, hemoptysis, dyspnea, headache or fatigue. The older client can have full-blown pneumonia and may appear with altered mental status (especially confusion) rather than fever or respiratory symptoms because of the changes in temperature regulation as we age. Anytime an older person has shoulder pain and confusion at presentation, consider the possibility

---

*A new class of antiinflammatory medications known as leukotriene modifiers has recently come on the market. These drugs work by blocking the activity of chemicals called leukotrienes, which are involved in airway inflammation.

†Pneumocystis pneumonia causes a dry, hacking cough without sputum production.

RISK FACTORS PREDISPOSING A CLIENT TO PNEUMONIA

- Smoking
- Air pollution
- Upper respiratory infection (URI)
- Altered consciousness: alcoholism, head injury, seizure disorder, drug overdose, general anesthesia
- Tracheal intubation
- Prolonged immobility
- Immunosuppressive therapy: corticosteroids, cancer chemotherapy
- Nonfunctional immune system: AIDS
- Severe periodontal disease
- Prolonged exposure to virulent organisms
- Malnutrition
- Dehydration
- Chronic diseases: diabetes mellitus, heart disease, chronic lung disease, renal disease, cancer
- Prolonged debilitating disease
- Inhalation of noxious substances
- Aspiration of oral/gastric material
- Aspiration of foreign materials (e.g., petroleum products)
- Chronically ill, older clients who have poor immune systems, often residing in group-living situations

Clinical Signs and Symptoms of Pneumonia

- Sudden and sharp pleuritic chest pain that is aggravated by chest movement
- Shoulder pain
- Hacking, productive cough (rust-colored or green, purulent sputum)
- Dyspnea
- Tachypnea (rapid respirations associated with fever or pneumonia) accompanied by decreased chest excursion on the affected side
- Cyanosis
- Headache
- Fever and chills
- Generalized aches and myalgia that may extend to the thighs and calves
- Knees may be painful and swollen
- Fatigue

of diaphragmatic impingement by an underlying lung pathologic condition.

The clinical manifestations of PCP are slow to develop; they include fever, tachypnea, tachycardia, dyspnea, nonproductive cough, and hypoxemia. A diffuse, bilateral pattern of alveolar infiltration is apparent on chest radiograph.

Hospitalization may be required for the immunocompromised client. Otherwise, if the client has an intact defense system and good general health, recuperation can take place at home with rest and supportive treatment. In the hospital rigorous handwashing by medical personnel is essential for reducing the transmission of infectious agents.

Tuberculosis

Tuberculosis (TB) is a bacterial infectious disease transmitted by the gram-positive, acid-fast bacillus *Mycobacterium tuberculo-*

Case Example. A 42-year-old man comes to an outpatient physical therapy clinic with complaints of painful swollen knees. Symptoms were first observed 10 days ago, and the left knee was reportedly worse than the right. Stiffness was reported in the morning on rising, with pain increasing as the day progressed. As a nonsmoker, the man reported his general health as "good" and noted that he had sprained his left ankle 2 months before the onset of knee pain.

The knee joints were not tender, warm, or red. Observable and palpable "boggy" fluid could be demonstrated in the popliteal spaces bilaterally. There was no sign of effusion when viewed anteriorly, and the test for a wave of fluid was negative. All special tests for the hip and knee were negative, with full active and passive range of motion present. There was no known history of Baker's cysts (herniation of synovial tissue through a weakening in the posterior capsule wall) reported. There were no palpable myalgias of the lower leg musculature and no trigger points present. The left ankle demonstrated some residual stiffness with a mild loss of plantar flexion. Joint accessory motions were consistent with a grade 1 lateral ankle sprain. Standing posture was unremarkable for possible contributing alignment problems.

The clinical presentation of this client was puzzling to the evaluating physical therapist. A brief screening for possible systemic origin of symptoms elicited no red-flag symptoms or history. Ongoing evaluation continued as treatment for both knees and the left ankle was initiated. After 3 weeks there were no changes in the clinical presentation of the knees. At that time the client developed a noticeable productive cough with greenish/yellow sputum but no other reported symptoms. Vital signs (including temperature) were unremarkable.

Given the unusual clinical presentation, lack of progress with treatment, and development of a productive cough, this client was referred to his family physician for a medical evaluation. A one-page letter outlining the physical therapist's findings and treatment protocol was sent with the client. A medical diagnosis of pneumonia was established. The physician noted that although the clinical presentation was unusual, knee involvement can occur with pneumonia. The pathophysiologic mechanism for this is unknown.

sis. Despite improved methods of detection and treatment, TB remains a worldwide health problem with increasing spread of a highly drug-resistant strain of TB present in almost every state in the United States.

Before the development of anti-TB drugs in the late 1940s, TB was the leading cause of death in the United States. Drug therapy, along with improvements in public health and general living standards, resulted in a marked decline in incidence. However, recent influxes of immigrants from developing Third World nations, rising homeless populations, and the emergence of HIV led to an increase in reported cases in the mid-1980s, reversing a 40-year period of decline.

RISK FACTORS

Although TB can affect anyone, certain segments of the population have an increased risk of contracting the disease (Galantino and Bishop, 1994):

- Health care workers*
- Older people, who constitute nearly half of the newly diagnosed cases of TB in the United States
- Overcrowded housing most common among the economically disadvantaged; homeless, especially those people in crowded homeless shelters
- People who are incarcerated
- Immigrants from Southeast Asia, Ethiopia, Mexico, and Latin America
- Clients who are dependent on alcohol or other chemicals with resultant malnutrition, debilitation, and poor health
- Infants and children under the age of 5 years
- Clients with reduced immunity or malnutrition (e.g., anyone undergoing cancer therapy or steroid therapy) and those with HIV-positive lung cancer or head and neck cancer
- Persons with diabetes mellitus and/or end-stage renal disease
- People with a history of gastrointestinal disease (e.g., chronic malabsorption syndrome, upper gastrointestinal carcinomas, gastrectomy, intestinal bypass)

The mycobacterium is usually spread by airborne droplet nuclei, which are produced when actively infected persons sneeze, speak, sing, or cough. Once released into the atmosphere, the organisms are dispersed and can be inhaled by a susceptible host. Brief exposure to a few bacilli rarely causes an infection. More commonly, it is spread with repeated close contact with an infected person.

Drug-resistant strains of TB have developed when the full course of treatment, lasting 6 to 9 months, is not completed. Once the infected person feels better and stops taking the prescribed medication, a new drug-resistant strain is passed along. Noncompletion of treatment among inner-city residents and the homeless presents a major factor in the failure to eradicate TB.

TB most often involves the lungs, but extrapulmonary TB (XPTB) can also occur in the kidneys, bone growth plates, lymph nodes, and meninges and can be disseminated throughout the body.

Widespread dissemination throughout the body is termed *miliary tuberculosis* and is more common in people 50 years or older and very young children with unstable or underdeveloped immune systems.

On rare occasions TB will affect the hip joints and vertebrae, resulting in severe, arthritis-like damage, possibly even avascular necrosis of the hip. Tuberculosis of the spine, referred to as Pott's disease is rare but can result in compression fracture of the vertebrae.

CLINICAL SIGNS AND SYMPTOMS

Clinical signs and symptoms are absent in the early stages of TB. Many cases are found incidentally when routine chest radiographs are made for other reasons. When systemic manifestations of active disease initially appear, the clinical signs and symptoms listed here may appear.

Tuberculin skin testing is done to determine whether the body's immune response

▼ *Clinical Signs and Symptoms of*
Tuberculosis

- Fatigue
- Malaise
- Anorexia
- Weight loss
- Low-grade fevers (especially in late afternoon)
- Night sweats
- Frequent productive cough
- Dull chest pain, tightness, or discomfort
- Dyspnea

---

*Health care workers, including physical therapists, must be alert to the need to use a special mask (particulate respirator) when cough-inducing procedures are being performed. This is especially important when treating persons with HIV infection or when TB is suspected or active.

has been activated by the presence of the bacillus. A positive reaction develops 3 to 10 weeks after the initial infection. A positive skin test reaction indicates the presence of a tuberculous infection but does not show whether the infection is dormant or is causing a clinical illness. Chest x-ray films and sputum cultures are done as a follow-up to positive skin tests. All cases of active disease are treated, and certain cases of inactive disease are treated prophylactically.

Systemic Sclerosis Lung Disease

Systemic sclerosis (SS) (scleroderma) is a restrictive lung disease of unknown etiologic origin characterized by inflammation and fibrosis of many organs (see also Chapter 11). Fibrosis affecting the skin and the visceral organs is the hallmark of SS.

The lungs, highly vascularized and composed of abundant connective tissue, are a frequent target organ, ranking second only to the esophagus in visceral involvement.

The most common pulmonary manifestation of SS is interstitial fibrosis, which is clinically apparent in more than 50% of cases. Autopsy results suggest a prevalence of 75%, indicating the insensitivity of traditional tests such as pulmonary function tests and chest radiographs.

CLINICAL SIGNS AND SYMPTOMS

As discussed in Chapter 11, skin changes associated with SS generally preceded visceral alterations. Dyspnea on exertion and nonproductive cough are the most common clinical findings associated with SS. Rarely, these symptoms precede the occurrence of cutaneous changes of scleroderma.

Clubbing of the nails rarely occurs in SS because of the nearly universal presence of sclerodactyly (hardening and shrinking of connective tissues of fingers and toes). Peripheral edema may develop secondary to cor pulmonale, which occurs as the pulmonary fibrosis becomes advanced.

Pulmonary manifestations in systemic sclerosis include:

- *Common:* Interstitial pneumonitis and fibrosis and pulmonary vascular disease
- *Less common:* Pleural disease, aspiration pneumonia, pneumothorax, neoplasm, pneumoconiosis, pulmonary hemorrhage, and drug-induced pneumonitis

Pleural effusions may appear with orthopnea, edema, and paroxysmal nocturnal dyspnea if congestive heart failure occurs. Cystic changes in the parenchyma may progress to form pneumatoceles (thin-walled air-containing cysts) that may rupture spontaneously and produce a pneumothorax. Clients with SS have an increased incidence of lung cancer. Hemoptysis is usually the first signal of pulmonary malignancy.

The course of SS is unpredictable, from a mild, protracted course to rapid respiratory failure and death. Treatment of pulmonary complications, pulmonary hypertension, and interstitial lung disease remains difficult (Stone and Wigley, 1998).

▼ *Clinical Signs and Symptoms of*
Systemic Sclerosis Lung Disease

- Dyspnea on exertion
- Nonproductive cough
- Peripheral edema (secondary to cor pulmonale)
- Orthopnea
- Paroxysmal nocturnal dyspnea (congestive heart failure)
- Hemoptysis

▼ NEOPLASTIC DISEASE

Lung Cancer (Bronchogenic Carcinoma)

Lung cancer is malignancy in the epithelium of the respiratory tract. At least a dozen different cell types of tumors are included under the classification of lung cancer.

The four major types of lung cancer include small cell carcinoma (oat cell carcinoma), squamous cell carcinoma, adenocarcinoma, and large cell carcinoma. Clinically, lung cancers are grouped into two divisions: small cell lung cancer and non-small cell lung cancer.

Cancers of the lung are staged at the time of their initial presentation. The American Joint Committee for Cancer's tumor, nodes, metastasis (TNM) staging system is used (see explanation in Chapter 10).

Since the mid-1950s, lung cancer has been the most common cause of death from cancer in men. In 1987 lung cancer surpassed breast cancer to become the leading cause of cancer death in women in the United States.

Risk Factors

Smoking is the major risk factor for lung cancer, accounting for 90% of all cases. Other risk factors include (Biesalski et al, 1998):

- Low consumption of fruit and vegetables
- Genetic predisposition
- Exposure to nontobacco procarcinogens, carcinogens, and tumor promoters
- Previous lung disease (e.g., COPD, TB)
- Previous tobacco-related cancer
- Passive (environmental) smoke

Compared with nonsmokers, heavy smokers (i.e., those who smoke more than 25 cigarettes a day) have a 20-fold greater risk of developing cancer. Quitting smoking lowers the risk but the decrease is gradual and does not approach that of a nonsmoker. The risk of lung cancer is increased in the smoker who is exposed to other carcinogenic agents, such as radon, asbestos, and chemical carcinogens.

The increase of lung cancer mortality in the last decades can be entirely attributed to the trend of tobacco consumption (Takkouche and Gastal-Otero, 1996). However, there is a lag time of many years between beginning smoking and the clinical manifestation of cancer.

Metastases

Metastatic spread of pulmonary tumors is usually to the long bones, vertebral column (especially the thoracic vertebrae), liver, and adrenal glands. Brain metastasis is also common, occurring in as much as 50% of cases.

Local metastases by direct extension may involve the chest wall, pleura, pulmonary parenchyma, or bronchi. Further local tumor growth may erode the first and second ribs and associated vertebrae, causing bone pain and paravertebral pain associated with involvement of sympathetic nerve ganglia.

The respiratory system is a common site for complications associated with cancer and cancer therapy. Several factors can lead to pulmonary complications. Immunosuppression caused by the underlying disease or the cancer therapy can lead to infectious disease.

In addition, the lungs contain an enormous capillary bed through which flows the entire venous circulation, making it a common site of metastasis and pulmonary emboli. Carcinomas of the kidney, breast, pancreas, colon, and uterus are especially likely to metastasize to the lungs.

Finally, the pulmonary capillary bed is uniquely sensitive to side effects of chemotherapy and radiation therapy, leading to respiratory symptoms (Stover and Kaner, 1996).

CLINICAL SIGNS AND SYMPTOMS

Clinical signs and symptoms of lung cancer often remain silent until the disease process is at an advanced stage. In many instances lung cancer may mimic other pulmonary conditions or may initially appear as chest, shoulder, or arm pain. Chest pain is a vague aching, and depending on the type of cancer, the client may have pleuritic pain on inspiration that limits lung expansion.

Hemoptysis (coughing or spitting up blood) may occur secondary to ulceration of blood vessels. Wheezing occurs when the tumor obstructs the bronchus. Dyspnea, either unexplained or out of proportion, is a red flag indicating the need for medical screening.

Centrally located tumors cause increased cough, dyspnea, and diffuse chest pain that can be referred to the shoulder, scapulae, and upper back. This pain is the result of peribronchial or perivascular nerve involve-

▼ *Clinical Signs and Symptoms of*
Lung Cancer

- Any change in respiratory patterns
- Recurrent pneumonia or bronchitis
- Hemoptysis
- Persistent cough
- Change in cough or development of hemoptysis in a chronic smoker
- Hoarseness or dysphagia
- Sputum streaked with blood
- Dyspnea (shortness of breath)
- Wheezing
- Sharp pleuritic pain aggravated by inspiration
- Sudden, unexplained weight loss
- Chest, shoulder, or arm pain
- Atrophy and weakness of the arm and hand muscles
- See also Clinical Signs and Symptoms of Paraneoplastic Syndrome, Brain Metastasis, and Metastasis to the Spinal Cord, Chapter 10.

ment. Other symptoms may include postobstructive pneumonia with fever, chills, malaise, anorexia, hemoptysis, and fecal breath odor (secondary to infection within a necrotic tumor mass). If these tumors extend to the pericardium, the client may develop a sudden onset of arrhythmia (tachycardia or atrial fibrillation), weakness, anxiety, and dyspnea.

Peripheral tumors are most often asymptomatic until the tumor extends through visceral and parietal pleura to the chest wall. Irritation of the nerves causes localized sharp, pleuritic pain that is aggravated by inspiration.

Metastases to the mediastinum (tissue and organs between the sternum and the vertebrae, including the heart and its large vessels; trachea; esophagus; thymus; lymph nodes) may cause hoarseness or dysphagia secondary to vocal cord paralysis as a result of entrapment or local compression of the laryngeal nerve.

Apical (Pancoast's) tumors of the lung apex do not usually cause symptoms while confined to the pulmonary parenchyma. They can extend into surrounding structures and frequently involve the eighth cervical and first thoracic nerves within the brachial plexus. This nerve involvement produces sharp pleuritic pain in the axilla, shoulder, and subscapular area on the affected side, with pain down the medial aspect of the arm and hand (ulnar nerve distribution) and subsequent atrophy of the upper extremity muscles. The pain of this tumor sometimes masquerades as subcranial bursitis.

Trigger points of the serratus anterior muscle (see Fig. 12-4) also mimic the distribution of pain caused by the eighth cervical nerve root compression. Trigger points can be ruled out by palpation and lack of neurologic deficits and may be confirmed by elimination with appropriate physical therapy treatment.

Paraneoplastic syndromes (remote effects of a malignancy; see explanation in Chapter 10) occur in 10 to 20% of lung cancer clients. These usually result from the secretion of hormones by the tumor acting on target organs, producing a variety of symptoms. Occasionally, symptoms of paraneoplastic syndrome occur before detection of the primary lung tumor.

As mentioned earlier, brain metastasis is common, occurring in as much as 50% of cases. About 10% of all individuals with lung cancer have CNS involvement at the time of diagnosis. Major clinical symptoms of brain metastasis result from increased intracranial pressure and may include headache, nausea, vomiting, malaise, anorexia, weakness, and alterations in mental processes. Localized motor or sensory deficits occur, depending on the location of lesions (see discussion in Chapter 10).

Metastasis to the spinal cord produces signs and symptoms of cord compression including back pain (localized or radicular), muscle weakness, loss of lower extremity sensation, bowel and bladder incontinence, and diminished or absent lower extremity reflexes (unilateral or bilateral).

▼ GENETIC DISEASE OF THE LUNG

Cystic Fibrosis

Cystic fibrosis (CF) is an inherited disease of the exocrine ("outward-secreting") glands primarily affecting the digestive and respiratory systems.

This disease is the most common genetic disease in the United States, inherited as a recessive trait: both parents must be carriers, each having a defective copy of the CF gene. Each time two carriers conceive a child, there is a 25% chance that the child will have CF, a 50% chance that the child will be a carrier, and a 25% chance that the child will be a noncarrier. In the United States 5% of the population, or 12 million people, carry a single copy of the CF gene.

Because cysts and scar tissue on the pancreas were observed during autopsy when the disease was first being differentiated from other conditions, it was given the name *cystic fibrosis of the pancreas*. Although this term describes a secondary rather than primary characteristic, it has been retained.

In 1989 scientists isolated the cystic fibrosis gene located on chromosome 7. In healthy people a protein called cystic fibrosis transmembrane conductance regulator (CFTR) provides a channel by which chloride (a component of salt) can pass in and out of cells.

Persons with CF have a defective copy of the gene that normally enables cells to construct that channel. As a result, salt accumulates in the cells lining the lungs and digestive tissues, making the surrounding mucus abnormally thick and sticky. These secretions, which obstruct ducts in the pancreas, liver, and lungs, and abnormal secretion of sweat and saliva are the two main features of CF.

Obstruction of the bronchioles by mucous plugs and trapped air predisposes the client to infection, which starts a destructive cycle of increased mucus production with increased bronchial obstruction, infection, and inflammation with eventual destruction of lung tissue (Rosenstein and Zeitlin, 1998).

CLINICAL SIGNS AND SYMPTOMS

Pulmonary involvement is the most common and severe manifestation of CF. Obstruction of the airways leads to a state of hyperinflation and bronchiectasis. In time, fibrosis develops, and restrictive lung disease is

▼ Clinical Signs and Symptoms of Cystic Fibrosis

In early or undiagnosed stages:
- Persistent coughing and wheezing
- Recurrent pneumonia
- Excessive appetite but poor weight gain
- Salty skin/sweat
- Bulky, foul-smelling stools (undigested fats caused by a lack of amylase and tryptase enzymes)

In older child and young adult:
- Infertility
- Nasal polyps
- Periostitis
- Glucose intolerance

▼ Clinical Signs and Symptoms of Pulmonary Involvement in Cystic Fibrosis

- Tachypnea (very rapid breathing)
- Sustained chronic cough with mucous production and vomiting
- Barrel chest (caused by trapped air)
- Use of accessory muscles for respiration and intercostal retraction
- Cyanosis and digital clubbing
- Exertional dyspnea with decreased exercise tolerance

Further complications include:
- Pneumothorax
- Hemoptysis
- Right-sided heart failure secondary to pulmonary hypertension

superimposed on the obstructive disease. Over time, pulmonary obstruction leads to chronic hypoxia, hypercapnia, and acidosis. Pneumothorax, pulmonary hypertension, and eventually cor pulmonale may develop. These are poor prognostic indicators in adults and are associated with a mean survival of 8 months (Ruzal-Shapiro, 1998).

Advances in treatment, including aerosalized antibiotics, mucous thinning agents, antiinflammatory agents, chest physical therapy, enzyme supplements, and nutrition programs, have extended the average life expectancy for CF sufferers into their early 20s, with maximal survival estimated at 30 to 40 years. Because the genetic abnormality has been identified, considerable progress has been made in the development of gene therapy and preventive gene transfer for this disease (Middleton and Alton, 1998; Rosenecker et al, 1998).

The course of CF varies from one client to another depending on the degree of pulmonary involvement. Deterioration is inevitable, leading to debilitation and eventually death.

▼ OCCUPATIONAL LUNG DISEASES

Lung diseases are among the most common occupational health problems. They are caused by the inhalation of various chemicals, dusts, and other particulate matter present in certain work settings.

Not all clients exposed to occupational inhalants will develop lung disease.

During the interview process, the therapist will ask questions about occupational and smoking history to identify the possibility of an underlying pulmonary pathologic condition.

The most commonly encountered occupational lung diseases are occupational asthma, hypersensitivity pneumonitis, pneumoconioses, and acute respiratory irritation. The greatest number of occupational agents causing *asthma* are those with known or suspected allergic properties, such as plant and animal proteins (e.g., wheat, flour, cotton, flax, and grain mites). In most cases the asthma will resolve after exposure is terminated.

Hypersensitivity pneumonitis, or allergic alveolitis, is most commonly due to the inhalation of organic antigens of fungal, bacterial, or animal origin. *Pneumoconioses,* or "the dust diseases," result from inhalation of minerals, notably silica, coal dust, or asbestos. These diseases are most commonly seen in miners, construction workers, sandblasters, potters, and foundry and quarry workers. Pneumoconioses usually develop gradually over a period of years, eventually leading to diffuse pulmonary fibrosis, which diminishes lung capacity and produces restrictive lung disease.

Acute respiratory irritation results from the inhalation of chemicals such as ammonia, chlorine, and nitrogen oxides in the form of gases, aerosols, or particulate matter. If such irritants reach the lower airways, alveolar damage and pulmonary edema can result. Although the effects of these acute irritants are usually short-lived, some may cause chronic alveolar damage or airway obstruction.

CLINICAL SIGNS AND SYMPTOMS

Early symptoms of occupational-related lung disease depend on the specific exposure but may include cough and dyspnea on exertion. Chest pain, productive cough, and dyspnea at rest develop as the condition progresses. The physical therapist needs to be alert for the combination of significant past occupational and smoking history accompanied by respiratory symptoms.

▼ PLEUROPULMONARY DISORDERS

Pulmonary Embolism and Deep Venous Thrombosis

Pulmonary embolism (PE) involves pulmonary vascular obstruction by a displaced thrombus (blood clot), an air bubble, a fat globule, a clump of bacteria, amniotic fluid, vegetations on heart valves that develop with endocarditis, or other particulate matter. Once dislodged, the obstruction travels to the lungs, causing shortness of breath, tachypnea (very rapid breathing), tachycardia, and chest pain.

The most common cause of PE is deep venous thrombosis (DVT) originating in the proximal deep venous system of the lower legs. The embolism causes an area of blockage, which then results in a localized area of ischemia known as a *pulmonary infarct.* The infarct may be caused by small emboli that extend to the lung surface (pleura) and result in acute pleuritic chest pain.

Three major risk factors linked with DVT are blood stasis (e.g., immobilization because of bed rest, such as with burn clients, obstetric and gynecologic clients, and older or obese populations), endothelial injury (secondary to neoplasm, surgical procedures, trauma, or fractures of the legs or pelvis), and hypercoagulable states.

Other people at increased risk for DVT and PE include those with congestive heart failure, trauma, operation (especially hip, knee, and prostate surgery), age over 50 years, previous history of thromboembolism, malignant disease, infection, diabetes mellitus, inactivity or obesity, pregnancy, clotting abnormalities, and oral contraceptive use (see discussion in Chapter 3).

Given the mortality of PE and the difficulties involved in its clinical diagnosis, prevention of DVT and PE is critical. A careful review of the Personal/Family History form (outpatient) or hospital medical chart (inpatient) may alert the therapist to the presence of factors that predispose a client to have a PE.

Although frequent changing of position, exercise, and early ambulation are necessary to prevent thrombosis and embolism, sudden and extreme movements should be avoided. Under no circumstances should the legs be massaged to relieve "muscle cramps," especially when the pain is located in the calf and the client has not been up and about. Restrictive clothing and prolonged sitting or standing should be avoided. Ele-

vating the legs should be accomplished with caution to avoid severe flexion of the hips, which will slow blood flow and increase the risk of new thrombi.

Deep Venous Thrombosis
(See also Chapter 3)

Signs and symptoms include tenderness, leg pain, swelling (a difference in leg circumference of 1.4 cm in men and 1.2 cm in women is significant), and warmth. One may also see a positive Homans' sign,* subcutaneous venous distention, discoloration, a palpable cord, and/or pain upon placement of a blood pressure cuff around the calf (considerable pain with the cuff inflated to 160 to 180 mm Hg). Unfortunately, at least half the cases of DVT are asymptomatic, and in up to 30% of clients with clinical evidence of DVT, no DVT is demonstrable.

▼ **Clinical Signs and Symptoms of**
Deep Venous Thrombosis (DVT)

- Unilateral tenderness or leg pain
- Unilateral swelling (difference in leg circumference)
- Warmth
- Positive Homans' sign
- Subcutaneous venous distension (superficial thrombus)
- Discoloration
- Palpable cord (superficial thrombus)
- Pain with placement around calf of blood pressure cuff inflated to 160 to 180 mm Hg

---

*Physical evidence of phlebitis is *Homans' sign,* which is deep calf pain on slow dorsiflexion of the foot or gentle squeezing of the affected calf. The inflamed nerves in the veins within the muscle are stretched. Only half of all people with DVT experience pain. Homans' sign is not specific for this condition because it also occurs with Achilles tendinitis and gastrocnemius and plantar muscle injury (Jarvis, 1992).

▼ *Clinical Signs and Symptoms of*
Pulmonary Embolism (PE)

- Dyspnea
- Pleuritic (sharp, localized) chest pain
- Diffuse chest discomfort
- Persistent cough
- Hemoptysis (bloody sputum)
- Apprehension, anxiety, restlessness
- Tachypnea (increased respiratory rate)
- Tachycardia
- Fever

▼ *Clinical Signs and Symptoms of*
Cor Pulmonale

- Peripheral edema (bilateral legs)
- Chronic cough
- Central chest pain
- Exertional dyspnea or dyspnea at rest
- Distension of neck veins
- Fatigue
- Wheezing
- Weakness

Pulmonary Embolism

Signs and symptoms of PE are nonspecific and vary greatly, depending on the extent to which the lung is involved, the size of the clot, and the general condition of the client.

Clinical presentation does not differ between younger and older persons (Gisselbrecht et al, 1996). Dyspnea, pleuritic chest pain, and cough are the most common symptoms reported. Pleuritic pain is caused by an inflammatory reaction of the lung parenchyma or by pulmonary infarction or ischemia caused by obstruction of small pulmonary arterial branches. Typical pleuritic chest pain is sudden in onset and aggravated by breathing. The client may also report hemoptysis, apprehension, tachypnea, and fever (temperature as high as 39.5° C, or 103.5° F). The presence of hemoptysis indicates that the infarction or areas of atelectasis have produced alveolar damage.

Cor Pulmonale

When a PE has been sufficiently massive to obstruct 60% to 75% of the pulmonary circulation, the client may have central chest pain, and acute cor pulmonale occurs. Cor pulmonale is a serious cardiac condition and an emergency situation arising from a sudden dilatation of the right ventricle as a result of PE.

As cor pulmonale progresses, edema and other signs of right-sided heart failure develop. Symptoms are similar to those of congestive heart failure from other causes: dyspnea, edema of the lower extremities, distension of the veins of the neck, and liver distension. The hematocrit is increased as the body attempts to compensate for impaired circulation by producing more erythrocytes.

Pleurisy

Pleurisy is an inflammation of the pleura (serous membrane enveloping the lungs) and is caused by infection, injury, or tumor. The membranous pleura that encases each lung consists of two close-fitting layers: the visceral layer encasing the lungs and the parietal layer lining the inner chest wall. A lubricating fluid lies between these two layers.

If the fluid content remains unchanged by the disease, the pleurisy is said to be dry. If the fluid increases abnormally, it is a wet pleurisy or pleurisy with effusion (pleural effusion). If the wet pleurisy becomes infected with formation of pus, the condition is known as purulent pleurisy or empyema.

Pleurisy may occur as a result of many factors, including pneumonia, tuberculosis, lung abscess, influenza, systemic lupus erythematosus (SLE), rheumatoid arthritis, and pulmonary infarction. Pleurisy, with or

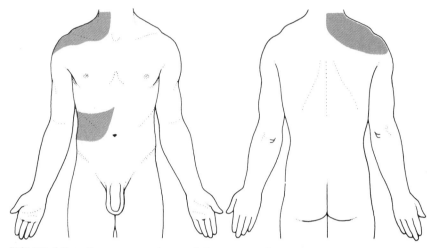

FIGURE 4-5 • Chest pain over the site of pleuritis is usually perceived by the client. Referred pain *(light red)* associated with pleuritis may occur on the same side as the pleuritic lesion affecting the shoulder, upper trapezius muscle, neck, lower chest wall, or abdomen.

▼ *Clinical Signs and Symptoms of*
Pleurisy

- Chest pain
- Cough
- Dyspnea
- Fever, chills
- Tachypnea (rapid, shallow breathing)

without effusion associated with SLE, may be accompanied by acute pleuritic pain and dysfunction of the diaphragm.

CLINICAL SIGNS AND SYMPTOMS

The chest pain is sudden and may vary from vague discomfort to an intense stabbing or knifelike sensation in the chest. The pain is aggravated by breathing, coughing, laughing, or other similar movements associated with deep inspiration.

The visceral pleura is insensitive; pain results from inflammation of the parietal pleura. Because the latter is innervated by the intercostal nerves, chest pain is usually felt over the site of the pleuritis, but pain may be referred to the lower chest wall,

abdomen, neck, upper trapezius muscle, and shoulder because of irritation of the central diaphragmatic pleura (Fig. 4-5).

Pneumothorax

Pneumothorax, or free air in the pleural cavity between the visceral and parietal pleurae, may occur secondary to pulmonary disease (e.g., when an emphysematous bulla or other weakened area on the lung ruptures) or as a result of trauma and subsequent perforation of the chest wall.

Pneumothorax is not uncommon after surgery or after an invasive medical procedure involving the chest or thorax. Spontaneous pneumothorax occasionally affects the exercising individual and occurs without preceding trauma or infection. Peak incidence for this type of pneumothorax is in adults between 20 and 40 years.

Air may enter the pleural space directly through a hole in the chest wall (open pneumothorax) or diaphragm. Air may escape into the pleural space from a puncture or tear in an internal respiratory structure (e.g., bronchus, bronchioles, or alveoli). This form of pneumothorax is called closed or spontaneous pneumothorax.

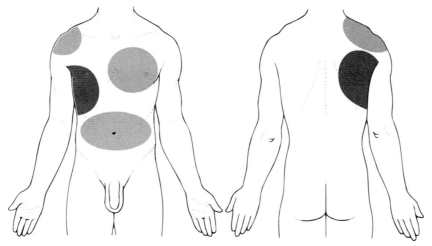

FIGURE 4-6 • Possible pain patterns associated with pneumothorax: Upper and lateral thoracic wall with referral to the ipsilateral shoulder, across the chest, or over the abdomen.

▼ *Clinical Signs and Symptoms of*
Pneumothorax

- Dyspnea
- Change in respiratory movements (affected side)
- Sudden, sharp chest pain
- Increased neck vein distension
- Weak and rapid pulse
- Fall in blood pressure
- Dry, hacking cough
- Shoulder pain
- Sitting upright is the most comfortable position

CLINICAL SIGNS AND SYMPTOMS

Symptoms of pneumothorax, whether occurring spontaneously or as a result of injury or trauma, vary depending on the size and location of the pneumothorax and on the extent of lung disease. When air enters the pleural cavity, the lung collapses, producing dyspnea and a shift of tissues and organs to the unaffected side. The client may have severe pain in the upper and lateral thoracic wall, which is aggravated by any movement and by the cough and dyspnea that accompany it.

The pain may be referred to the ipsilateral shoulder (corresponding shoulder on the same side as the pneumothorax), across the chest, or over the abdomen (Fig. 4-6). The client may be most comfortable when sitting in an upright position.

Other symptoms may include a fall in blood pressure, a weak and rapid pulse, and cessation of normal respiratory movements on the affected side of the chest.

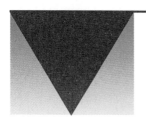

Case Example. An 18-year-old male, who was injured in a motor vehicle accident (MVA) has come into the hospital physical therapy department with orders to begin ambulation. He had a long leg cast on his left leg and has brought a pair of crutches with him. This is the first time he has been out of bed in the upright position; he has not ambulated in his room yet.

continued

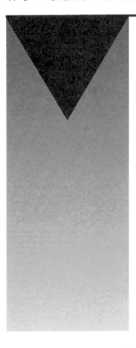

Blood pressure measurement taken while the client was sitting in the wheelchair was 110/78 mm Hg. Pulse was easily palpated and measured at 72 BPM. The therapist gave the necessary instructions and assisted the client to the standing position in the parallel bars. Immediately on standing, this young man began to experience the onset of sharp midthoracic back pain and shortness of breath. He became pale and shaky, breaking out in a cold sweat.

The therapist assisted him to a seated position and asked the client if he was experiencing pain anywhere else (e.g., chest, shoulder, abdomen) while reassessing blood pressure. His blood pressure had fallen to 90/56 mm Hg, and he was unable to respond verbally to the questions asked. A clinic staff person was asked to telephone for immediate emergency help. While waiting for a medical team, the therapist noted a weak and rapid pulse, distension of the client's neck veins, and diminished respiratory movements.

This young man was diagnosed with tension pneumothorax caused by a displaced fractured rib. Untreated, tension pneumothorax can quickly produce life-threatening shock and bradycardia. Monitoring of the client's vital signs by the physical therapist resulted in fast action to save this young man's life.

OVERVIEW   OVERVIEW PULMONARY PAIN PATTERNS

▼ PLEUROPULMONARY DISORDERS (Fig. 4-7)

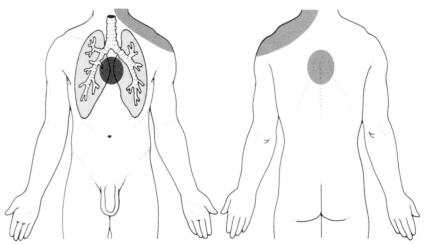

FIGURE 4-7 • Primary pain patterns *(dark red)* associated with pleuropulmonary disorders, such as pulmonary embolus, cor pulmonale, pleurisy, or spontaneous pneumothorax, may vary, but they usually include substernal or chest pain. Pain over the involved lung fields (anterior, lateral, or posterior) may occur (not shown). Pain may radiate *(light red)* to the neck, upper trapezius muscle, ipsilateral shoulder, thoracic back, costal margins, or upper abdomen (the latter two areas are not shown).

Location:	Substernal or chest over involved lung fields—anterior, side, and back
Referral:	Often well localized (client can point right to the exact site of pain) without referral
	May radiate to neck, upper trapezius muscle, shoulder, costal margins, or upper abdomen
	Thoracic back pain occurs with irritation of the posterior parietal pleura
Description:	Sharp ache, stabbing, angina-like pressure, or crushing pain with pulmonary embolism
	Angina-like chest pain with severe pulmonary hypertension
Intensity:	Moderate
Duration:	Hours to days
Associated signs and symptoms:	Preceded by pneumonia or upper respiratory infection
	Wheezing
	Dyspnea (exertional or at rest)
	Hyperventilation
	Tachypnea (increased respirations)
	Fatigue, weakness
	Tachycardia (increased heart rate)
	Fever, chills
	Edema
	Apprehension or anxiety, restlessness
	Persistent cough or cough with blood (hemoptysis)
	Dry hacking cough (occurs with the onset of pneumothorax)
	Medically determined signs and symptoms (e.g., by chest auscultation and chest radiograph)
Relieving factors:	Sitting
	Some relief when at rest, but most comfortable position varies (pneumonia)
	Pleuritic pain may be relieved by lying on the affected side
Aggravating factors:	Breathing at rest
	Increased inspiratory movement (e.g., laughter, coughing, sneezing)
	Symptoms accentuated with each breath

▼ LUNG CANCER

Location:	Anterior chest
Referral:	Scapulae, upper back, ipsilateral shoulder radiating along the

	medial aspect of the arm
	First and second ribs and associated vertebrae and paravertebral muscles (apical or Pancoast's tumors)
Description:	Localized, sharp pleuritic pain (peripheral tumors)
	Dull, vague aching in the chest
	Neuritic pain of shoulders/arm (apical or Pancoast's tumors)
	Bone pain caused by metastases to adjacent bone or to the vertebrae
Intensity:	Moderate to severe
Duration:	Constant
Associated signs and symptoms:	Dyspnea or wheezing
	Hemoptysis (coughing up or spitting up blood)
	Fever, chills, malaise, anorexia, and weight loss
	Fecal breath odor
	Tachycardia or atrial fibrillation (palpitations)
	Muscle weakness or atrophy (e.g., Pancoast's tumor may involve the shoulder and the arm on the affected side)
	Associated CNS symptoms:
	Headache
	Nausea
	Vomiting
	Malaise
	Signs of cord compression:
	Localized or radicular back pain
	Weakness
	Loss of lower extremity sensation
	Bowel/bladder incontinence
	Hoarseness, dysphagia (peripheral tumors)
Relieving factors:	None without medical intervention
Aggravating factors:	Inspiration: Deep breathing, laughing, coughing

▼ PHYSICIAN REFERRAL

It is more common for a physical therapist to be treating a client with a previously diagnosed musculoskeletal problem who now has chronic, recurrent pulmonary symptoms than to be the primary evaluator and health care provider of a client with pulmonary symptoms. In either case the physical thera-

pist needs to know what further questions to ask and which of the client's responses represent serious symptoms that require medical follow-up.

Shoulder or back pain can be referred from diseases of the diaphragmatic or parietal pleura or secondary to metastatic lung cancer. When clients have chest pain, they usually fall into two categories: those who demonstrate chest pain associated with pul-

GUIDELINES FOR PHYSICIAN REFERRAL

- Shoulder pain aggravated by respiratory movements; have the client hold his or her breath and re-assess symptoms; any reduction or elimination of symptoms with breath holding or the Valsalva maneuver suggests pulmonary or cardiac source of symptoms
- Shoulder pain that is aggravated by supine positioning; pain that is worse when lying down and improves when sitting up or leaning forward is often pleuritic in origin; abdominal contents push up against diaphragm and, in turn, against the parietal pleura; see Figs. 4-5 and 12-6)
- Shoulder or chest (thorax) pain that subsides with autosplinting (lying on the painful side)
- (For the client with asthma): Signs of asthma or bronchial activity during exercise
- Weak and rapid pulse accompanied by fall in blood pressure (pneumothorax)
- Presence of associated signs and symptoms, such as persistent cough, dyspnea (rest or exertional), or constitutional symptoms (see Systemic Signs and Symptoms Requiring Physician Referral; see also Systems Review, Chapter 1)

GUIDELINES FOR IMMEDIATE MEDICAL ATTENTION

- Weak and rapid pulse accompanied by fall in blood pressure (pneumothorax), especially following motor vehicle accident, chest injury, or other traumatic event
- Client with symptoms of inadequate ventilation or carbon dioxide retention (see Respiratory Acidosis)

monary symptoms and those who have true musculoskeletal problems, such as intercostal strains and tears, myofascial trigger points, fractured ribs, or myalgias secondary to overuse.

Clients with chronic, persistent cough, whether that cough is productive or dry and hacking, may develop sharp, localized intercostal pain similar to pleuritic pain. Both intercostal and pleuritic pain are aggravated by respiratory movements, such as laughing, coughing, deep breathing, or sneezing. Clients who have intercostal pain secondary to insidious trauma or repetitive movements, such as coughing, can benefit from physical therapy.

For the client with asthma, it is important to maintain contact with the physician if the client develops signs of asthma or any bronchial activity during exercise. The physician must be informed to help alter the dosage or the medications to maintain optimal physical performance.

The physical therapist will want to screen for medical disease through a series of questions to elicit the presence of associated systemic (pulmonary) signs and symptoms. Aggravating and relieving factors may provide further clues that can assist in making treatment or referral decision.

In all these situations, the referral of a client to a physician is based on the family/personal history of pulmonary disease, the presence of pulmonary symptoms of a systemic nature, or the absence of substantiating objective findings indicating a musculoskeletal lesion.

Systemic Signs and Symptoms Requiring Physician Referral

Anorexia
Apprehension
Anxiety
Arthralgias, myalgias
Barrel chest

Bowel/bladder incontinence
Bulky, foul-smelling stools
Chest pain
Chronic laryngitis
Cough with sputum
Cyanosis
Digital clubbing
Dysphagia
Dyspnea
Fecal breath odor
Fever, chills
Hacking cough
Headache
Hemoptysis

Hoarseness
Malaise, fatigue
Muscle weakness
Nausea, vomiting
Orthopnea
Pursed-lip breathing
Restlessness
Salty skin and sweat
Skin rash, pigmentation
Sore throat
Syncope
Tachypnea
Unexplained weight loss
Wheezing

 KEY POINTS TO REMEMBER

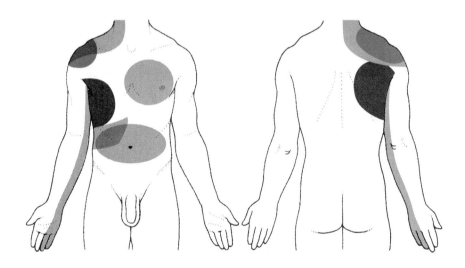

▶ Pulmonary pain patterns are usually localized in the substernal or chest region over involved lung fields, which may include the anterior chest, side, or back.

▶ Pulmonary pain can radiate to the neck, upper trapezius muscle, costal margins, thoracic back, scapulae, or shoulder.

▶ Shoulder pain caused by pulmonary involvement may radiate along the medial aspect of the arm, mimicking other neuromuscular causes of neck or shoulder pain.

▶ Pulmonary pain usually increases with inspiratory movements, such as laughing, coughing, sneezing, or deep breathing.

▶ Shoulder pain that is relieved by lying on the involved side may be "auto splinting," a sign of a pulmonary cause of symptoms.

▶ Shoulder pain that is aggravated when lying supine (arm/elbow supported) may be an indication of a pulmonary cause of symptoms.

▶ For anyone with pain patterns pictured here as presenting symptoms, especially in the absence of trauma or injury, check the client's personal medical history for previous or recurrent upper respiratory infection or pneumonia.

▶ Any client with symptoms of inadequate ventilation, pneumothorax, or CO_2 retention needs immediate medical referral.

▶ CNS symptoms, such as muscle weakness, muscle atrophy, headache, loss of lower extremity sensation, and localized or radicular back pain, may be associated with lung cancer.

▶ Any CNS symptom may be the silent presentation of a lung tumor.

▶ Posterior leg or calf pain postoperatively may be caused by a thrombus and must be reported to the physician before physical therapy begins or continues.

▶ Hemoptysis or exertional/at rest dyspnea, either unexplained or out of proportion to the situation or person, is a red-flag symptom requiring medical referral.

▶ Any client with chest pain should be evaluated for trigger points and intercostal tears.

SUBJECTIVE EXAMINATION

• SPECIAL QUESTIONS TO ASK

Past Medical History

- Have you ever had trouble with breathing or lung disease such as bronchitis, emphysema, asthma, pneumonia, or blood clots?
  - *If yes:* Describe what this problem was, when it occurred, and how it was treated.
  - *If the person indicated yes to asthma, either on the Personal/Family History form or to this question, ask:* How can you tell when you are having an asthma episode? What triggers an asthma episode for you? Do you use medications during an episode? Do you have trouble with asthma during exercise? Do you time your medications with your exercise to prevent an asthma episode during exercise?
- Have you ever had tuberculosis?
  - *If yes:* When did it occur, and how was it treated? What is your current status?
  - When was your last test for tuberculosis? What was the test result?
- Have you had a chest x-ray film taken in the last 5 years?
  - *If yes:* What were the results?
- Have you ever broken your nose, been told that you have a deviated septum (nasal passageway), nasal polyps, or sleep apnea? **(Hypoxia)**
- Have you ever had lung or heart surgery?
  - *If yes:* What and when? **(Decreased vital capacity)**

Associated Signs and Symptoms

- Are you having difficulty breathing now?

- Do you ever have shortness of breath or breathlessness or cannot quite catch your breath?
  - *If yes:* When does this happen? When you rest? When you lie flat, walk on level ground, or walk up stairs?
  - How far can you walk before you feel breathless?
  - What symptoms stop your walking (e.g., shortness of breath, heart pounding, chest tightness, or weak legs)?
  - Are these episodes associated with night sweats, cough, chest pain, or bluish color around your lips or fingernails?
  - Does your breathlessness seem to be related to food, pollen, dust, animals, season, stress, or strong emotion? **(Asthma)**
  - Do you have any breathing aids (e.g., oxygen, nebulizer, inhaler, humidifier, air cleaner, or other aid)?
- Do you have a cough? (Note whether the client smokes, for how long, and how much.)
  - *If yes to cough, separate this cough from a smoker's cough by asking:* When did it start? Is it related to smoking?
  - Do you cough anything up? *If yes:* Describe the color, amount, and frequency.
  - Are you taking anything to prevent this cough? *If yes,* does it seem to help?
  - Are there occasions when you cannot seem to stop coughing?
  - Do you ever cough up blood or anything that looks like coffee grounds? (Bright red = fresh blood; brown or black = older blood)
  - Have you strained a muscle or your lower back from coughing?
  - Does it hurt to touch your chest or take a deep breath, cough, sneeze, or laugh?
- Have you lost or gained 10 or more pounds recently? (*Gained:* **pulmonary edema, congestive heart failure, fat deposits under the diaphragm in the obese client reduces ventilation;** *lost:* **emphysema, cancer**)
- Do your ankles swell? **(Congestive heart failure)**
- Have you been unusually tired lately? **(Congestive heart failure, emphysema)**
- Have you noticed a change in your voice? **(Pathology of left hilum or trachea)**

Occupational History

- Do you work around (or have you had previous exposure to) asbestos, coal, dust, chemicals, gasses, or fumes?
  - *If yes:* Describe.
  - Do you wear a mask at work?
- If the client is a farmer, ask what kind of farming (some agricultural products may cause respiratory irritation).

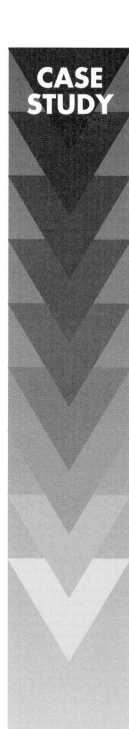

CASE STUDY

REFERRAL

A 65-year-old man has come to you for an evaluation of low back pain, which he attributes to lifting a heavy box 2 weeks ago. During the course of the medical history, you notice that the client has a persistent cough and that he sounds hoarse. After reviewing the Personal/Family History form, you note that the client smokes two packs of cigarettes each day and that he has smoked at least this amount for at least 50 years. (One pack per day for one year is considered "one pack year.") This person has smoked an estimated 100 pack years; anyone who has smoked for 20 pack years or more is considered to be at risk for the development of serious lung disease. What questions will you ask to decide for yourself whether this back pain is systemic?

PHYSICAL THERAPY INTERVIEW
Introduction to Client

It is important for me to make certain that your back pain is not caused by other health problems, such as prostate problems or respiratory infection, so I will ask a series of questions that may not seem to be related to your back pain, but I want to be very thorough and cover every possibility to obtain the best and most effective treatment for you.

Pain

From your history form I see that you associate your back pain with lifting a heavy box 2 weeks ago. When did you first notice your back pain (sudden or gradual onset)?

Have you ever hurt your back before or have you ever had pain similar to this episode in the past? (Systemic disease: recurrent and gradually increases over time)

Please describe your pain (supply descriptive terms if necessary)

How often do you have this pain?

> **FUPs** How long does it last when you have it?
>
> What aggravates your pain/symptoms?
>
> What relieves your pain/symptoms?
>
> How does rest affect your pain?
>
> Have you noticed any changes in your pain/symptoms since they first started to the present time?

Do you have any numbness in the groin or inside your legs? (Saddle anesthesia: **cauda equina)**

Pulmonary

I notice you have quite a cough and you sound hoarse to me. How long have you had this cough and hoarseness (when did it first begin)?

Do you have any back pain associated with this cough? Any other pain associated with your cough? *If yes:* Have the person describe where, when, intensity, aggravating and relieving factors.

How does it feel when you take a deep breath? Does your lower back hurt when you laugh or take a deep breath?

continued

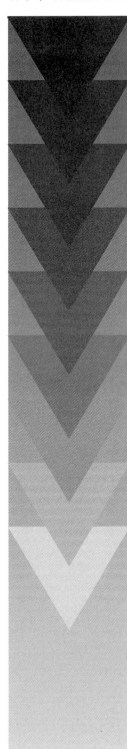

When you cough, do you produce phlegm or mucus? *If yes:* Have you ever noticed any red streaks or blood in it?

Does your coughing or back pain keep you awake at night?

Have you been examined by a physician for either your cough or your back pain?

Have you had any recent chest or spine x-rays taken? *If yes:* When and where? What were the results?

General Systemic

Have you had any night sweats, daytime fevers, or chills?

Do you have difficulty in swallowing or experience recurrent laryngitis? **(Oral cancer)**

Urologic

Have you ever been told that you have a prostate problem or prostatitis? *If yes:* Determine when this occurred, how it was treated, and whether the person had the same symptoms at that time that he is now describing to you.

Have you noticed any change in your bladder habits?

> **FUPS:** Have you had any difficulty in starting or continuing to urinate?
>
> Is there any burning or discomfort on urination?
>
> Have you noticed any blood in your urine?
>
> Have you recently had any difficulty with kidney stones or bladder or kidney infections?

Gastrointestinal

Have you noticed any change in your bowel pattern?

Have you had difficulty having a bowel movement or do you find that you have soiled yourself without even realizing it? **(Cauda equina lesion**—this would require immediate referral to a physician)

Does your back pain begin or increase when you are having a bowel movement?

Is your back pain relieved after having a bowel movement?

Have you noticed any association between when you eat and when your pain/symptoms increase or decrease?

Final Question

Is there anything about your current back pain or your general health that we have not discussed that you think is important for me to know?

(Refer to Special Questions to Ask for other questions that may be pertinent to this client, depending on the answers to these questions.)

PHYSICIAN REFERRAL

As always, correlation of findings is important in making a decision regarding medical referral. If the client has a positive family history for respiratory problems (especially lung cancer) and if clinical findings indicate pulmonary

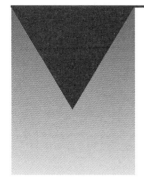

involvement, the client should be strongly encouraged to see a physician for a medical check-up. If there are positive systemic findings, such as difficulty in swallowing, persistent hoarseness, shortness of breath at rest, night sweats, fevers, bloody sputum, recurrent laryngitis, or upper respiratory infections *either in addition to or in association with* the low back pain, the client should be advised to see a physician, and the physician should receive a copy of your findings. This guideline covers the client who has a true musculoskeletal problem but also has other health problems, as well as the client who may have back pain of systemic origin that is unrelated to the lifting injury 2 weeks ago.

PRACTICE QUESTIONS

1. If a client reports that the shoulder/upper trapezius muscle pain increases with deep breathing, how can you assess whether this results from a pulmonary or musculoskeletal cause?

2. Neurologic symptoms such as muscle weakness or muscle atrophy may be the first indication of:

   a. Cystic fibrosis

   b. Bronchiectasis

   c. Neoplasm

   d. Deep vein thrombosis

3. Back pain with radiating numbness and tingling down the leg past the knee does not occur as a result of:

   a. Postoperative thrombus

   b. Bronchogenic carcinoma

   c. Pott's disease

   d. Trigger points

4. Pain associated with pleuropulmonary disorders can radiate to the:

   a. Anterior neck

   b. Upper trapezius muscle

   c. Ipsilateral shoulder

   d. Thoracic spine

   e. (a) and (c)

   f. All of the above

5. The presence of a persistent dry cough (no sputum or phlegm produced) has no clinical significance to the physical therapist. True or false?

6. Dyspnea associated with emphysema is the result of:

   a. Destruction of the alveoli

   b. Reduced elasticity of the lungs

   c. Increased effort to exhale trapped air

   d. (a) and (b)

   e. All of the above

7. What is the significance of autosplinting?

8. Which symptom has greater significance: dyspnea at rest or exertional dyspnea?

9. The presence of pain and anxiety in a client can often lead to hyperventilation. When a client hyperventilates, the arterial concentration of carbon dioxide will do which of the following?

   a. Increase

b. Decrease

c. Remain unchanged

d. Vary depending on potassium concentration

10. Common symptoms of respiratory acidosis would be most closely represented by which of the following descriptions?

a. Presence of numbness and tingling in face, hands, and feet

b. Presence of dizziness and lightheadedness

c. Hyperventilation with changes in level of consciousness

d. Onset of sleepiness, confusion, and decreased ventilation

References

Biesalski HK, deMesquita BB, Chesson A et al: European consensus statement on lung cancer: risk factors and prevention, *CA Cancer J Clin* 48:167-176, 1998.

Galantino ML, Bishop KL: The new TB, *PT Magazine* 2(2):52-61, 1994.

Gisselbrecht M, Diehl J, Meyer G: Clinical presentation and results of thrombolytic therapy in older patients with massive pulmonary embolism: a comparison with non-elderly patients, *J Am Geriatr Soc (JAGS)* 44(2):189-193, 1996.

Jarvis C: *Physical examination and health assessment,* Philadelphia, 1992, WB Saunders.

Middleton PG, Alton EW: Gene therapy for cystic fibrosis, *Thorax* 53(3):197-199, 1998.

Rosenecker J, Schmalix WA, Schindelhauer D et al: Towards gene therapy of cystic fibrosis, *Eur J Med Res* 3(3):149-156, 1998.

Rosenstein BJ, Zeitlin PL: Cystic fibrosis, *Lancet* 351:277-281, 1998.

Ruzal-Shapiro C: Cystic fibrosis: an overview, *Radiol Clin Am* 36(1):143-160, 1998.

Sandford AJ, Weir TD, Pare PD: Genetic risk factors for chronic obstructive pulmonary disease, *Eur Respir J* 10(6):1380-1391, 1997.

Stone JH, Wigley FM: Management of systemic sclerosis: the art and the science, *Semin Cutan Med Surg* 17(1):55-64, 1998.

Stover DE, Kaner RJ: Pulmonary complications in cancer patients, *CA Cancer J Clin* 46:303-320, 1996.

Takkouche B, Gastal-Otero JJ: The epidemiology of lung cancer, *Eur J Epidemiol* 12:341-349, 1996.

Overview of Hematologic Signs and Symptoms

5

The blood consists of two major components: plasma, a pale yellow or gray-yellow fluid; and formed elements, erythrocytes (red blood cells, or RBCs), leukocytes (white blood cells, or WBCs), and platelets (thrombocytes). Blood is the circulating tissue of the body; the fluid and its formed elements circulate through the heart, arteries, capillaries, and veins.

The *erythrocytes* carry oxygen to tissues and remove carbon dioxide from them. *Leukocytes* act in inflammatory and immune responses. The *plasma* carries antibodies and nutrients to tissues and removes wastes from tissues. *Platelets,* together with *coagulation factors* in plasma, control the clotting of blood.

Primary hematologic diseases are uncommon, but hematologic manifestations secondary to other diseases are common. Cancers of the blood are discussed in Chapter 10.

In the physical therapist's practice, symptoms of blood disorders are most common in relation to the use of nonsteroidal antiinflammatory drugs (NSAIDs) for inflammatory conditions, neurologic complications associated with pernicious anemia, and complications of chemotherapy or radiation.

Changes in the hands and fingernail beds; symptoms of dyspnea, weakness, fatigue, and palpitations; neurologic symptoms such as headache, drowsiness, dizziness, syncope, or polyneuropathy; and easy bruising or bleeding should alert the physical therapist to the possibility of a hematologic-based systemic disorder.

▼ CLASSIFICATION OF BLOOD DISORDERS

Erythrocyte Disorders

Erythrocytes (red blood cells or corpuscles) consist mainly of hemoglobin and a supporting framework. Erythrocytes transport oxygen and carbon dioxide; they are important in maintaining normal acid-base balance. There are many more erythrocytes than leukocytes (600 to 1). The total number is determined by gender (women have fewer erythrocytes than men), altitude (less oxygen in the air requires more erythrocytes to carry sufficient amounts of oxygen to the tissues), and physical activity (sedentary people have fewer erythrocytes, athletes have more).

Disorders of erythrocytes are classified as follows (not all of these conditions are discussed in this text):

- Anemia (too few erythrocytes)
- Polycythemia (too many erythrocytes)
- Poikilocytosis (abnormally shaped erythrocytes)
- Anisocytosis (abnormal variations in size of erythrocytes)
- Hypochromia (deficient in hemoglobin)

Anemia

Anemia is a reduction in the oxygen-carrying capacity of the blood as a result of an abnormality in the quantity or quality of erythrocytes. Anemia is not a disease but is a symptom of any number of different blood disorders. Excessive blood loss, increased destruction of erythrocytes, and decreased production of erythrocytes are the most common causes of anemia.

In the physical therapy practice, anemia-related disorders usually occur in one of four broad categories: (1) iron deficiency associated with chronic gastrointestinal (GI) blood loss secondary to NSAID use; (2) chronic diseases or inflammatory diseases, such as rheumatoid arthritis or systemic lupus erythematosus; (3) neurologic conditions (pernicious anemia); and (4) infectious diseases, such as tuberculosis or AIDS, and neoplastic disease or cancer (bone marrow failure). Anemia with neoplasia may be a common complication of chemotherapy or develop as a consequence of bone marrow metastasis (Goodman and Boissonnault, 1998).

CLINICAL SIGNS AND SYMPTOMS

Deficiency in the oxygen-carrying capacity of blood may result in disturbances in the function of many organs and tissues leading

TABLE 5-1 ▼ Changes Associated with Hematologic Disorders

Changes	Causes
Skin	
Light, lemon-yellow tint	Untreated pernicious anemia
White, waxy appearance	Severe anemia resulting from acute hemorrhage
Gray-green yellow	Chronic blood loss
Gray tint	Leukemia
Pale hands or palmar creases	Anemia
Nail Bed	
Brittle	Long-standing iron deficiency anemia
Concave (rather than convex)	Long-standing iron deficiency anemia
Oral Mucosa/Conjunctiva	
Pale or yellow color	Anemia

to various symptoms that differ from one person to another. Slowly developing anemia in young, otherwise healthy individuals is well tolerated, and there may be no symptoms until hemoglobin concentration and hematocrit fall below one half of normal (see values inside book cover).

However, rapid onset may result in symptoms of dyspnea, weakness and fatigue, and palpitations, reflecting the lack of oxygen transport to the lungs and muscles. Many people can have moderate-to-severe anemia without these symptoms. Although there is no difference in normal blood volume associated with severe anemia, there is a redistribution of blood so that organs most sensitive to oxygen deprivation (e.g., brain, heart, muscles) receive more blood than, for example, the hands and kidneys.

Changes in the hands and fingernail beds (Table 5-1; Fig. 5-1) may be observed during the inspection/observation portion of the physical therapy evaluation. The physical therapist should look for pale palms with normal-colored creases (severe anemia causes pale creases as well). Observation of the hands should be done at the level of the client's heart. In addition, the anemic client's

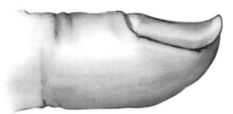

FIGURE 5-1 • Abnormal condition of the nails associated with anemia. Thin, depressed nails with lateral edges tilted up, forming a concave profile called koilonychia (spoon nails); may also be caused by a congenital or hereditary trait. (From Jarvis C: *Physical examination and health assessment*, Philadelphia, WB Saunders, 1992, p 271.)

▼ *Clinical Signs and Symptoms of*
Anemia

- Skin pallor (palms, nail beds) or yellow-tinged skin (mucosa, conjunctiva)
- Fatigue and listlessness
- Dyspnea on exertion accompanied by heart palpitations and rapid pulse (more severe anemia)
- Decreased diastolic blood pressure
- CNS manifestations (pernicious anemia):
  Headache
  Drowsiness
  Dizziness, syncope
  Slow thought processes
  Apathy, depression
  Polyneuropathy

▼ *Clinical Signs and Symptoms of*
Polycythemia

Clinical signs and symptoms of polycythemia (whether primary or secondary) are directly related to the increase in blood viscosity described earlier and may include

- Headache
- Dizziness
- Irritability
- Blurred vision
- Fainting
- Decreased mental acuity
- Feeling of fullness in the head
- Disturbances of sensation in the hands and feet
- General malaise and fatigue
- Weight loss
- Easy bruising
- Intolerable pruritus (skin itching) **(polycythemia vera)***
- Cyanosis (blue hue to the skin)
- Clubbing of the fingers
- Splenomegaly (enlargement of spleen)
- Gout
- Hypertension

*This condition of skin itching is particularly related to warm conditions, such as being in bed at night or in a bath and is called the "hot bath sign."

hands should be warm; if they are cold, the paleness is due to vasoconstriction.

Pallor in dark-skinned people may be observed by the absence of the underlying red tones that normally give brown or black skin its luster. The brown-skinned individual demonstrates pallor with a more yellowish-brown color, and the black-skinned person will appear ashen or gray.

Systolic blood pressure may not be affected, but diastolic pressure may be lower than normal, with an associated increase in the resting pulse rate. Resting cardiac output is usually normal in people with ane-

mia, but cardiac output increases with exercise more than it does in nonanemic persons. As the anemia becomes more severe, resting cardiac output increases and exercise tolerance progressively decreases until dyspnea, tachycardia, and palpitations occur at rest.

Diminished exercise tolerance is expected in the client with anemia. Exercise testing and prescribed exercise(s) in anemic clients must be instituted with extreme caution and should proceed very gradually to tolerance and/or perceived exertion levels (Painter, 1993). In addition, exercise for any anemic client should be first approved by his or her physician.

Case Example. A 72-year-old woman, status post hip fracture, was treated surgically with nails (used for the fixation of the ends of fractured bones) and was referred to physical therapy for follow-up treatment before hospital discharge. The physician's preoperative examination and surgical report were unremarkable for physical therapy precautions or contraindications.

When the therapist met with the client for the first time, she had already been ambulating alone in her room from the bed to the bathroom and back using a hospital wheeled walker. She was wearing thigh length support hose, hospital gown, and open heeled slippers from home. Although the nursing report indicated she was oriented to time and place, she seemed confused and required multiple verbal cues to follow the physical therapist's directions.

After ambulating a distance of approximately 50 feet using her wheeled walker and standby assistance from the therapist, the client reported that she could not "catch her breath" and asked to sit down. She placed her hand over her heart and commented that her heart was "fluttering." Blood pressure and pulse measurements were taken and recorded as 145/72 mm Hg (blood pressure) and 90 bpm (pulse rate).

The physical therapist consulted with nursing staff immediately regarding this episode and was given the "go ahead" to complete the therapy session. The physical therapist documented the episode in the medical record and left a note for the physician, briefly describing the incident and ending with the question: Are there any medical contraindications to continuing progressive therapy?

Result. A significant fall in hemoglobin (Hb) often occurs after hip fracture and surgical intervention secondary to the blood loss caused by the fracture and surgery. Other contributing factors may include blood transfusion and alcoholic liver cirrhosis (Lombardi et al, 1996).

In this case, although the physician did not offer a direct reply to the physical therapist, the physician's notes indicated a suspected diagnosis of anemia. Follow-up blood work was ordered and the diagnosis was confirmed. Nursing staff conferred with the physician, and the therapist was advised to work within the patient's tolerance using perceived exertion as a guide while monitoring pulse and blood pressure.

Polycythemia

Polycythemia (also known as erythrocytosis) is characterized by increases in both the number of red blood cells and the concentration of hemoglobin. People with polycythemia have increased whole blood viscosity and increased blood volume.

The increased erythrocyte production results in this thickening of the blood and an increased tendency toward clotting. The viscosity of the blood limits its ability to flow easily, diminishing the supply of blood to the brain and to other vital tissues. Increased platelets in combination with the increased blood viscosity may contribute to the formation of intravascular thrombi.

There are two distinct forms of polycythemia: primary polycythemia (also known as polycythemia vera) and secondary polycythemia. *Primary polycythemia* is a relatively uncommon neoplastic disease of the bone marrow of unknown etiology. *Secondary polycythemia* is a physiologic condition resulting from a decreased oxygen supply to the tissues. It is associated with high altitudes, heavy tobacco smoking, and chronic heart and lung disorders, especially congenital heart defects.

CLINICAL SIGNS AND SYMPTOMS

The symptoms of this disease are often insidious in onset with vague complaints. The affected individual may be diagnosed only secondary to a sudden complication (e.g., stroke or thrombosis). Increased skin coloration and elevated blood pressure may develop as a result of the increased concentration of erythrocytes and increased blood viscosity. Gout is sometimes a complication of primary polycythemia, and a typical attack of acute gout may be the first symptom of polycythemia.

Blockage of the capillaries supplying the digits of either the hands or the feet may cause a peripheral vascular neuropathy with decreased sensation, burning, numbness, or tingling. This small blood vessel occlusion can also contribute to the development of cyanosis and clubbing. If the underlying disorder is not recognized and treated, the person may develop gangrene and have subsequent loss of tissue.

Sickle Cell Anemia

Sickle cell disease is a generic term for a group of inherited, autosomal recessive disorders characterized by the presence of an abnormal form of hemoglobin, the oxygen-carrying constituent of erythrocytes. A genetic mutation resulting in a single amino acid substitution in hemoglobin causes the hemoglobin to aggregate into long chains, altering the shape of the cell. This sickled or curved shape causes the cell to lose its ability to deform and squeeze though tiny blood vessels, thereby depriving tissue of an adequate blood supply.

The two features of sickle cell disorders, chronic hemolytic anemia and vasoocclusion, occur as a result of obstruction of blood flow to the tissues and early destruction of the abnormal cells. Anemia associated with this condition is merely a symptom of the disease and not the disease itself, despite the term *sickle cell anemia.*

CLINICAL SIGNS AND SYMPTOMS

A series of "crises," or acute manifestations of symptoms, characterize sickle cell disease. Some people with this disease have only a few symptoms, whereas others are affected severely and have a short life span. Cerebrovascular accidents (CVAs) are a frequent and severe manifestation.

Stress from viral or bacterial infection, hypoxia, dehydration, emotional disturbance, extreme temperatures, fever, strenuous physical exertion, or fatigue may precipitate a crisis. Pain caused by the blockage of sickled red blood cells (RBCs) forming sickle cell clots is the most common symptom; it may in any organ, bone, or joint of the body. Painful episodes of ischemic tissue damage may last 5 or 6 days and manifest in many different ways, depending on the location of the blood clot.

Leukocyte Disorders

The blood contains three major groups of leukocytes including (1) lymphoid cells (lymphocytes, plasma cells); (2) monocytes; and (3) granulocytes (neutrophils, eosinophils, and basophils). *Lymphocytes* produce antibodies and react with antigens, thus initiating the immune response to fight infection. *Monocytes* are the largest circulating blood cells and represent an immature cell until they leave the blood and travel to the tissues where they form macrophages in response to foreign substances such as bacteria. *Granulocytes* contain lysing agents capable of digesting various foreign materials and defend the body against infectious agents by phagocytosing bacteria and other infectious substances.

Disorders of leukocytes are recognized as the body's reaction to disease processes and noxious agents. The therapist will encounter

▼ *Clinical Signs and Symptoms of*
Sickle Cell Anemia

- Pain
  - Abdominal
  - Chest
  - Headaches
- Bone and joint crises from the ischemic tissue, lasting for hours to days and subsiding gradually
  - Low-grade fever
  - Extremity pain
  - Back pain
  - Periosteal pain
  - Joint pain, especially in the shoulder and hip
- Vascular complications
  - Cerebrovascular accidents (affects children and young adults most often)
  - Chronic leg ulcers
  - Avascular necrosis of the femoral head
  - Bone infarcts
- Pulmonary crises
  - Bacterial pneumonia
  - Pulmonary infarction (less common)
- Neurologic manifestations
  - Convulsions
  - Drowsiness
- Coma
- Stiff neck
- Paresthesias
- Cranial nerve palsies
- Blindness
- Nystagmus
- Hand-foot syndrome
  - Fever
  - Pain
  - Dactylitis (painful swelling of the dorsum of hands and feet)
- Splenic sequestration crisis (occurs before adolescence)
  - Liver and spleen enlargement due to trapped erythrocytes
  - Subsequent spleen atrophy due to repeated blood vessel obstruction
- Renal complications
  - Enuresis (bed-wetting)
  - Nocturia (excessive urination at night)
  - Hematuria (blood in the urine)
  - Pyelonephritis
  - Renal papillary necrosis
  - End-stage renal failure (elderly population)

many clients who demonstrate alterations in the blood leukocyte (WBC) concentration as a result of acute infections or chronic systemic conditions. The leukocyte count also may be elevated (leukocytosis) in pregnant clients, in clients with bacterial infections, appendicitis, leukemia, uremia, or ulcers, in newborns with hemolytic disease and normally at birth. The leukocyte count may drop below normal values (*leukopenia*) in clients with viral diseases (e.g., measles), infectious hepatitis, rheumatoid arthritis, cirrhosis of the liver, and lupus erythematosus, and also after treatment with radiation or chemotherapy.

Leukocytosis

Leukocytosis characterizes many infectious diseases and is recognized by a count of more than 10,000 leukocytes/mm^3. It can be associated with an increase in circulating neutrophils (neutrophilia), which are recruited in large numbers early in the course of most bacterial infections.

Leukocytosis is a common finding and is helpful in aiding the body's response to any of the following:

- Bacterial infections
- Inflammation or tissue necrosis (e.g., infarction, myositis, vasculitis)

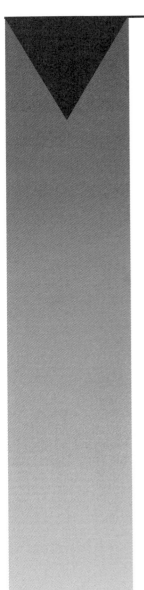

Case Example. A 20-year-old African-American woman came to physical therapy with severe right knee joint pain. She could recall no traumatic injury but reported hiking 2 days previously in the Rocky Mountains with her brother, whom she was visiting (she was from New York City).

A general screen for systemic illness revealed frequent urination over the past 2 days. She also complained of stomach pain, but she thought this was related to the stress of visiting her family. Past medical history included one other similar episode when she had acute pneumonia at the age of 11 years. She stated that she usually felt fatigued but thought it was because of her active social life and busy professional career.

On examination, the right knee was enlarged and inflamed, with joint range of motion limited by the local swelling. In fact, pain, swelling, and guarded motion in the joint prevented a complete evaluation. Given that restraint, there were no other physical findings, but not all special tests were completed. The neurologic screen was negative.

This woman was treated for local joint inflammation, but the combination of change in altitude, fatigue, increased urination, and stomach pains alerted the therapist to the possibility of a systemic process despite the client's explanation for the fatigue and stomach upset. Because the client was from out of town and did not have a local physician, the therapist telephoned the hospital emergency department for a telephone consultation. It was suggested that a blood sample be obtained for preliminary screening while the client continued to receive physical therapy. Laboratory results included the following:

Hct 30%   (normal = 35% to 47%)

Hb 10 g/dl   (normal = 12 to 15 g/dl)

WBC 20,000/mm³   (normal = 4500 to 11,000/mm³)

Based on these findings, the client was admitted to the hospital and diagnosed as having sickle cell anemia. It is likely that the change in altitude, the emotional stress of visiting family, and the physical exertion precipitated a "crisis." She received continued physical therapy treatment during her hospital stay and was discharged with further follow-up planned in her home city.

*Adapted from Jennings B: Nursing role in management: hematological problems. In Lewis S, Collier I (editors): *Medical-surgical nursing: assessment and management of clinical problems,* St Louis, 1992, Mosby, pp 664-714. Used with permission.

- Metabolic intoxications (e.g., uremia, eclampsia, acidosis, gout)
- Neoplasms (especially bronchogenic carcinoma, lymphoma, melanoma)
- Acute hemorrhage
- Splenectomy
- Acute appendicitis
- Pneumonia
- Intoxication by chemicals
- Acute rheumatic fever

▼ *Clinical Signs and Symptoms of*
Leukocytosis

These clinical signs and symptoms are usually associated with symptoms of the conditions listed earlier and may include

- Fever
- Symptoms of localized or systemic infection
- Symptoms of inflammation or trauma to tissue

▼ *Clinical Signs and Symptoms of*
Leukopenia

- Sore throat, cough
- High fever, chills, sweating
- Ulcerations of mucous membranes (mouth, rectum, vagina)
- Frequent or painful urination
- Persistent infections

Leukopenia

Leukopenia, or reduction of the number of leukocytes in the blood below 5000 per microliter, can be caused by a variety of factors. Unlike leukocytosis, leukopenia is never beneficial.

Leukopenia can occur in many forms of bone marrow failure such as that following antineoplastic chemotherapy or radiation therapy, in overwhelming infections, in dietary deficiencies, and in autoimmune diseases.

It is important for the physical therapist to be aware of the client's most recent white blood cell count prior to and during the course of physical therapy. If the client is immunosuppressed, infection is a major problem.

Nadir, or the lowest point the white blood count reaches, usually occurs 7 to 14 days after chemotherapy or radiation therapy. At this time, the client is extremely susceptible to opportunistic infections and severe complications. The importance of good hand-

washing and hygiene practices cannot be overemphasized when treating any of these people.

Leukemia

Leukemia is a disease arising from the bone marrow and involves the uncontrolled growth of blood cells; a complete discussion of this cancer is found in Chapter 10.

Platelet Disorders

Platelets (thrombocytes) function primarily in hemostasis (stopping bleeding) and in maintaining capillary integrity (see normal values listed inside book cover). They function in the coagulation (blood clotting) mechanism by forming hemostatic plugs in small ruptured blood vessels or by adhering to any injured lining of larger blood vessels.

A number of substances derived from the platelets that function in blood coagulation have been labeled "platelet factors." Platelets survive approximately 8 to 10 days in circulation and are then removed by the reticuloendothelial cells. *Thrombocytosis* refers to a condition in which the number of platelets is abnormally high, whereas *thrombocytopenia* refers to a condition in which the number of platelets is abnormally low.

Platelets are affected by anticoagulant drugs, including aspirin and heparin, by diet (presence of lecithin preventing coagulation or vitamin K from promoting coagulation), by exercise that boosts the production of chemical activators that destroy unwanted clots, and by liver disease that affects the supply of vitamin K. Platelets are also easily suppressed by radiation and chemotherapy.

Thrombocytosis

Thrombocytosis is an increase in platelet count that is usually temporary. It may occur as a compensatory mechanism after severe hemorrhage, surgery, and splenectomy; in iron deficiency and polycythemia vera; and as a manifestation of an occult (hidden) neoplasm (e.g., lung cancer).

▼ *Clinical Signs and Symptoms of*
Thrombocytosis

- Thrombosis
- Splenomegaly
- Easy bruising

▼ *Clinical Signs and Symptoms of*
Thrombocytopenia

- Bleeding after minor trauma
- Spontaneous bleeding
  - Petechiae (small red dots)
  - Ecchymoses (bruises)
  - Purpura spots (bleeding under the skin)
  - Epistaxis (nosebleed)
- Menorrhagia (excessive menstruation)
- Gingival bleeding
- Melena (black, tarry stools)

It is associated with a tendency to clot because blood viscosity is increased by the very high platelet count, resulting in intravascular clumping (or thrombosis) of the sludged platelets. Peripheral blood vessels, particularly in the fingers and toes are affected.

Thrombocytosis remains asymptomatic until the platelet count exceeds 1 million/mm^3. Other symptoms may include splenomegaly and easy bruising.

Thrombocytopenia

Thrombocytopenia, a decrease in the number of platelets (less than 150,000/mm^3) in circulating blood, can result from decreased or defective platelet production or from accelerated platelet destruction.

There are many causes of thrombocytopenia. In a physical therapy practice the most common causes seen are bone marrow failure from radiation treatment, leukemia, or metastatic cancer; cytotoxic agents used in chemotherapy; and drug-induced platelet reduction, especially among adults with rheumatoid arthritis treated with gold or inflammatory conditions treated with aspirin or other NSAIDs.

Primary bleeding sites include bone marrow or spleen; secondary bleeding occurs from small blood vessels in the skin, mucosa (e.g., nose, uterus, gastrointestinal tract, urinary tract, and respiratory tract), and brain (intracranial hemorrhage).

CLINICAL SIGNS AND SYMPTOMS

Severe thrombocytopenia results in the appearance of multiple petechiae (small, purple, pinpoint hemorrhages into the skin),

most often observed on the lower legs. Gastrointestinal bleeding and bleeding into the central nervous system associated with severe thrombocytopenia may be life-threatening manifestations of thrombocytopenic bleeding.

The physical therapist must be alert for obvious skin or mucous membrane symptoms of thrombocytopenia, which include severe bruising, external hematomas, and the presence of multiple petechiae. These symptoms usually indicate a platelet count well below 100,000/mm^3. Strenuous exercise or any exercise that involves straining or bearing down could precipitate a hemorrhage, particularly of the eyes or brain. People with undiagnosed thrombocytopenia need immediate physician referral.

Coagulation Disorders

Hemophilia

Hemophilia is a hereditary blood-clotting disorder caused by an abnormality of functional plasma-clotting proteins known as factors VIII and IX. In most cases, the hemophiliac person has normal amounts of the deficient factor circulating, but it is in a functionally inadequate state. Persons with hemophilia bleed longer than those with normal levels of functioning factors VIII or IX, but the bleeding is not any faster than

▼ *Clinical Signs and Symptoms of*
Acute Hemarthrosis

- Aura, tingling, or prickling sensation
- Stiffening into the position of comfort
- Decreased range of motion
- Pain
- Swelling
- Tenderness
- Heat

▼ *Clinical Signs and Symptoms of*
Muscle Hemorrhage

- Gradually intensifying pain
- Protective spasm of the muscle
- Limitation of movement at the surrounding joints
- Muscle assumes the position of comfort (usually shortened)
- Loss of sensation

would occur in a normal person with the same injury.

CLINICAL SIGNS AND SYMPTOMS

Bleeding into the joint spaces (hemarthrosis) is one of the most common clinical manifestations of hemophilia. It may result from an identifiable trauma or stress or may be spontaneous, most often affecting the knee, elbow, ankle, hip, and shoulder (in order of most common appearance).

Recurrent hemarthrosis results in hemophiliac arthopathy (joint disease) with progressive loss of motion, muscle atrophy, and flexion contractures. Bleeding episodes must be treated early with factor replacement and joint immobilization during the period of pain. This type of affected joint is particularly susceptible to being injured again, setting up a cycle of vulnerability to trauma and repeated hemorrhages.

Hemarthroses are not common in the first year of life but increase in frequency as the child begins to walk. The severity of the hemarthrosis may vary (depending on the degree of injury) from mild pain and swelling, which resolves without treatment within 1 to 3 days, to severe pain with an excruciatingly painful, swollen joint that persists for several weeks and resolves slowly with treatment.

Bleeding into the muscles is the second most common site of bleeding in persons with hemophilia. Muscle hemorrhages can be more insidious and massive than joint

▼ *Clinical Signs and Symptoms of*
Gastrointestinal Involvement

- Abdominal pain and distention
- Melena (blood in stool)
- Hematemesis (vomiting blood)
- Fever
- Low abdominal/groin pain due to bleeding into wall of large intestine or iliopsoas muscle
- Flexion contracture of the hip due to spasm of the iliopsoas muscle secondary to retroperitoneal hemorrhage

hemorrhages. They may occur anywhere but are common in the flexor muscle groups, predominantly the iliopsoas, gastrocnemius, and flexor surface of the forearm, and they result in deformities such as hip flexion contractures, equinus position of the foot, or Volkmann's deformity of the forearm.

When bleeding into the psoas or iliacus muscle puts pressure on the branch of the femoral nerve supplying the skin over the anterior thigh, loss of sensation occurs. Distention of the muscles with blood causes pain that can be felt in the lower abdomen, possibly even mimicking appendicitis when bleeding occurs on the right side. In an attempt to relieve the distention and reduce the pain, a position with hip flexion is preferred.

Two tests are used to distinguish an iliopsoas bleed from a hip bleed:

1. When the client flexes the trunk, severe pain is produced in the presence of *iliopsoas bleeding,* whereas only mild pain is found with a hip hemorrhage.
2. When the hip is gently rotated in either direction, severe pain is experienced with a *hip hemorrhage,* but is absent or mild with iliopsoas bleeding.

Over time, the following complications may occur:

- Vascular compression causing localized ischemia and necrosis
- Replacement of muscle fibers by nonelastic fibrotic tissue causing shortened muscles and thus producing joint contractures
- Peripheral nerve lesions from compression of a nerve that travels in the same compartment as the hematoma, most commonly affecting the femoral, ulnar, and median nerves
- Pseudotumor formation with bone erosion

▼ PHYSICIAN REFERRAL

Understanding the components of a client's past medical history that can affect hematopoiesis (production of blood cells) can provide the physical therapist with valuable insight into the client's present symptoms, which are usually already well known to the attending physician.

For example, the effects of certain drugs, exposure to radiation, or recent cytotoxic cancer chemotherapy can affect bone marrow. Whenever uncertain, the physical therapist is encouraged to contact the physician by telephone for discussion and clarification of the client's medical symptoms.

A history of excessive menses, a folate-poor diet, alcohol abuse, drug ingestion, family history of anemia, and family roots in geographic areas where red blood cell enzyme or hemoglobin abnormalities are prevalent represent some important findings. The presence of any one or more of these factors should alert the physical therapist to the need for medical referral when the client is not already under the care of a physician or when new signs or symptoms develop.

In addition, exercise for *anemic* clients must be instituted with extreme caution and should first be approved by the client's physician. Clients with undiagnosed thrombocytopenia need immediate medical referral. The physical therapist must be alert for obvious skin or mucous membrane symptoms of *thrombocytopenia.* The presence of severe bruising, hematomas, and multiple petechiae usually indicates a platelet count well below normal. With clients who have been diagnosed with *hemophilia,* medical referral should be made when any painful episode develops in the muscle(s) or joint(s). Pain usually occurs before any other evidence of bleeding. Any unexplained symptom may be a signal of bleeding.

Systemic Signs and Symptoms Requiring Physician Referral

Any client who has any of the generalized symptoms in the following list, without obvious or already known cause, should be further evaluated by a physician. At the very least, these signs and symptoms should be documented and a copy sent to the physician.

Abdominal/chest/back pain

Blurred vision

Changes in hands and fingernails

Changes in skin color

Cyanosis

Dactylitis

Decreased mental acuity

Digital clubbing

Disturbances of sensation in hands/feet

Dizziness

CLUES TO SCREENING FOR HEMATOLOGIC DISEASE

- Previous history (delayed effects) or current administration of chemotherapy or radiation therapy.
- Chronic or long-term use of aspirin or other NSAIDs (drug-induced platelet reduction).
- Spontaneous bleeding of any kind (e.g., nosebleed, vaginal/menstrual bleeding, blood in the urine or stool, bleeding gums, easy bruising, hemarthrosis), especially with a previous history of hemophilia.
- Recent major surgery or previous transplantation.
- Rapid onset of dyspnea, weakness, and fatigue with palpitations associated with recent significant change in altitude.
- Observed changes in the hands and fingernail beds (see Table 5-1 and Fig. 5-1).

GUIDELINES FOR PHYSICIAN REFERRAL

- Consultation with the physician may be necessary when establishing or progressing an exercise program for a client with known anemia
- New episodes of muscle or joint pain in a client with hemophilia; pain usually occurs before any other evidence of bleeding. Any unexplained symptom(s) may be a signal of bleeding; coughing up blood in this population group must be reported to the physician

GUIDELINES FOR IMMEDIATE MEDICAL ATTENTION

- Signs and symptoms of thrombocytopenia (decreased platelets) (e.g., excessive or spontaneous bleeding, petechiae, severe bruising) previously unseen or unreported to the physician

Dyspnea on exertion
Easy bruising
Evidence of hemarthrosis/muscle hemorrhage
Fainting
Fatigue and listlessness
Fever
Feeling of fullness in head

Headache
Irritability
Palpitations
Petechiae
Pruritus
Rapid pulse
Weakness
Weight loss

KEY POINTS TO REMEMBER

▶ Anemia may have no symptoms until hemoglobin concentration and hematocrit fall below one half of normal.

▶ Weakness, fatigue, and dyspnea are early signs of anemia.

▶ Exercise for anemic clients must be instituted gradually per tolerance and/or perceived exertion levels with physician approval.

▶ Platelet level below 20,000/mm³ (thrombocytopenia) can be lethal. Multiple bruises and petechiae may be the only sign.

▶ For clients with known thrombocytopenia, exercise programs must avoid the Valsalva (or bearing down) movement, and caution must be used to avoid further injury by bumping against objects.

▶ During the inspection/observation portion of the objective examination, screen both hands for skin or nail bed changes indicative of hematologic involvement.

▶ For the client with hemophilia, bleeding episodes must be treated early with factor replacement and joint immobilization during the period of pain. Never apply heat to a bleeding or suspected bleeding area.

▶ Pain may be the only symptom of a joint or muscle bleed for the client with hemophilia. Any painful or unexplained symptom in this population must be screened medically. Coughing up blood is not a finding with hemophilia and should be reported to the physician immediately.

▶ The National Hemophilia Foundation (NHF) publishes additional materials for physical therapists. These can be ordered by calling the NHF at (212) 328-3700.

SUBJECTIVE EXAMINATION

- ### SPECIAL QUESTIONS TO ASK

Past Medical History

- Have you recently been diagnosed as anemic?
- Have you recently had a serious blood loss (possibly requiring transfusion)? **(Anemia; also consider jaundice/hepatitis posttransfusion)**
- Have you ever been told that you have a congenital heart defect (also chronic lung/heart disorders)? **(Polycythemia: also possible with history of heavy tobacco use)**
- Do you have a history of bruising easily, nose bleeds, or excessive blood loss?* **(Polycythemia, hemophilia, thrombocytopenia)**
  - For example, do you bleed or bruise easily after minor trauma, surgery, or dental procedures?
  - Has any previous bleeding been severe enough to require a blood transfusion?
- Have you been exposed to occupational or industrial gases, such as chlorine gas, mustard gas, Agent Orange, napalm?

Associated Signs and Symptoms

- Do you experience shortness of breath or heart palpitations with slight exertion (e.g., climbing stairs) or even just at rest? **(Anemia)**

- **For persons at elevations above 3500 feet:** Have you recently moved from one geographic location to another? **(Polycythemia)**

- Do you ever have episodes of dizziness, blurred vision, headaches, fainting, or a feeling of fullness in your head? **(Polycythemia)**

- Do you have recurrent infections and low-grade fever such as colds, influenza-like symptoms, or other upper respiratory infections? **(Abnormal leukocytes)**

- Do you have black, tarry stools **(bleeding into the gastrointestinal tract)** or blood in urine **(genitourinary tract)**?

- **For women (anemia, thrombocytopenia):** Do you frequently have prolonged or excessive bleeding in association with your menstrual flow? (Excessive may be considered to be measured by the use of more than four tampons each day; prolonged menstruation usually refers to more than 5 days—both of these measures are subjective and must be considered along with other factors, such as the presence of other symptoms, personal menstrual history, placement in the life cycle [i.e., in relation to menopause].)

---

*Symptoms beginning in infancy or childhood suggest a congenital hemostatic defect, whereas symptoms beginning later in life indicate an acquired disorder, such as secondary to drug-induced defect of platelet function, a common cause of easy bruising and excessive bleeding. This bruising or bleeding occurs usually in association with trauma, menstruation, dental work, or surgical procedures. Drug-induced bruising or bleeding may also occur with use of aspirin and aspirin-containing compounds; nonsteroidal antiinflammatory agents such as ibuprofen (Motrin) and naproxen (Naprosyn) (see Table 6-3); and penicillins, because these drugs inhibit platelet function to some extent.

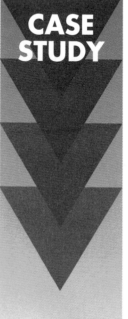

CASE STUDY

REFERRAL

You are working in a hospital setting and you have received a physician's referral to ambulate and exercise a patient who was involved in a serious automobile accident 10 days ago. The patient had internal injuries that required immediate abdominal surgery and 600 ml of blood transfused within 24 hours postoperatively. His condition is considered to be medically "stable."

CHART REVIEW

What specific medical information should you look for in the medical record before beginning your evaluation?

Name, age, and occupation

Past medical history:	Previous myocardial infarcts, history of heart disease, diabetes (type)
Surgical report:	Type of surgery, locations of scar, any current contraindications
Were there any other injuries?	If yes, what were these and what is the current status of each injury?

Body weight

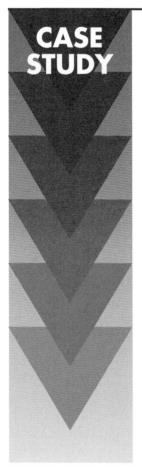

CASE STUDY

Pulmonary status:	Is the patient a cigarette or pipe smoker?
	Is the patient currently receiving oxygen or respiratory therapy?
	What was the patient's pulmonary status after the accident and postoperatively?
Laboratory report:	Hematocrit/hemoglobin levels
	Anemia?
Current status:	Nursing reports of the patient's complaints of any kind (e.g., symptoms of dyspnea or heart palpitations from rapid loss of blood)
	Has the patient been out of bed at all yet?
	If yes, when? How far did he walk? How much assistance was required? Did he have symptoms of orthostatic hypotension?
	Does the patient have any gastrointestinal symptoms?
	Is patient oriented to time, place, and person?
	Are there any dietary or fluid restrictions to be observed while the patient is in the physical therapy department? Is he on an intravenous line?
Vital signs:	Blood pressure
	Presence of fever
	Resting pulse rate
Current medications:	Be aware of the purpose for each medication and its potential side effects.

Are there any known discharge plans at this time?

PRACTICE QUESTIONS

1. If rapid onset of anemia occurs after major surgery, which of the following symptom patterns might develop?

   a. Continuous oozing of blood from the surgical site

   b. Exertional dyspnea and fatigue with increased heart rate

   c. Decreased heart rate

   d. No obvious symptoms would be seen

2. Chronic GI blood loss sometimes associated with use of nonsteroidal antiinflammatory drugs (NSAIDs) can result in which of the following problems?

   a. Increased incidence of joint inflammation

   b. Iron deficiency

   c. Decreased heart rate and bleeding

   d. Weight loss, fever, and loss of appetite

3. Under what circumstances would you consider asking a client about a recent change in altitude or elevation?

4. Preoperatively, clients cannot take aspirin or antiinflammatory medications because these:

   a. Decrease leukocytes

   b. Increase leukocytes

   c. Decrease platelets

   d. Increase platelets

   e. None of the above

5. Skin color and nail bed changes may be observed in the client with:

   a. Thrombocytopenia resulting from chemotherapy

   b. Pernicious anemia resulting from Vitamin B_{12} deficiency

   c. Leukocytosis resulting from AIDs

   d. All of the above

6. In the case of a client with hemarthrosis associated with hemophilia, what physical therapy treatment measures would be contraindicated?

7. Bleeding under the skin, nosebleeds, bleeding gums, and black stools require medical evaluation as these may be indications of:

   a. Leukopenia

   b. Thrombocytopenia

   c. Hemophilia

   d. Sickle cell anemia

8. Describe the two tests used to distinguish an iliopsoas bleed from a joint bleed.

9. What is the significance of *nadir?*

10. When exercising a client with known anemia, what two measures can be used as guidelines for frequency, intensity, and duration of the program?

References

Goodman CC, Boissonnault WG: *Pathology: implications for the physical therapist,* Philadelphia, 1998, WB Saunders.

Lombardi G, Rizzi E, Zocca N et al: Epidemiology of anemia in older patients with hip fracture, *J Am Geriatr Soc* 44(6):740-741, June 1996.

Painter P: End stage renal disease. In Skinner J, editor: *Exercise testing and exercise prescription for special cases: theoretical basis and clinical application.* ed 2, Philadelphia, 1993, Lea and Febiger, pp 351-362.

Overview of Gastrointestinal Signs and Symptoms

6

A great deal of new understanding of the enteric system and its relationship to other systems has been discovered over the last decade. For example, it is now known that the lining of the digestive tract from the esophagus through the large intestine (Fig. 6-1) is lined with cells that contain neuropeptides and their receptors. These substances, produced by nerve cells, are a key to the mind-body connection that contributes to the physical manifestation of emotions (Pert et al, 1998).

In addition to the classic hormonal and neural negative feedback loops, there are direct actions of gut hormones on the dorsal vagal complex. The person experiencing a "gut reaction" or "gut feeling" may indeed by experiencing the direct effects of gut peptides on brain function (Whitcomb and Taylor, 1992; Mayer, 1995).

The association between the enteric system, the immune system, and the brain (now a part of the research referred to as psychoneuro-immunology or PNI) has been clearly established and forms an integral part of gastrointestinal (GI) symptoms associated with immune disorders such as fibromyalgia, systemic lupus erythematosus, rheumatoid arthritis, chronic fatigue syndrome, and others.

Researchers estimate that more than two thirds of all immune activity occurs in the gut. In some people, the wall of the gut seems to have been breached, either because the network of intestinal cells develop increased permeability (a syndrome referred to as "leaky gut") or perhaps because bacteria and yeast overwhelm it and migrate into the bloodstream.

Allowing undigested food or bacteria into the bloodstream sets in motion a chain of events as the immune system reacts. The body responds as if to an illness, and expresses it in a number of ways such as a rash, diarrhea, GI upset, joint pain, migraines, and headache. The exact cause for these microscopic breaches remains unknown but food allergies, too much aspirin or ibuprofen, certain antibiotics, excessive alcohol consumption, smoking, or parasitic infections may be implicated.

All of these associations and new findings support the need for the physical therapist to assess carefully the possibility of GI symptoms

197

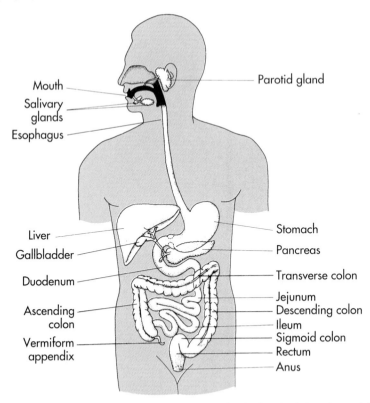

Mouth
Salivary glands
Esophagus

Parotid gland

Liver
Gallbladder
Duodenum
Ascending colon
Vermiform appendix

Stomach
Pancreas
Transverse colon
Jejunum
Descending colon
Ileum
Sigmoid colon
Rectum
Anus

FIGURE 6-1 • Organs of the digestive system. (From Guyton AC: *Textbook of medical physiology,* ed 8, Philadelphia, 1991, WB Saunders.)

present but unreported. This is especially important when considering the fact that GI tract symptoms can sometimes imitate musculoskeletal dysfunction.

GI disorders can refer pain to the sternal region, shoulder and neck, scapular region, midback, lower back, hip, pelvis, and sacrum. This pain can mimic primary musculoskeletal lesions, causing confusion for the physical therapist or for the physician assessing the client's chief complaint.

Although these musculoskeletal symptoms can occur alone and far from the actual site of the disorder, the client usually has other systemic signs and symptoms associated with GI disorders that should give the physical therapist who does a thorough investigation grounds for suspicion.

A careful interview to screen for systemic illness should include a few important questions concerning the client's history, prescribed medications, and the presence of any associated signs or symptoms that would immediately alert the physical therapist about the need for medical follow-up.

The most common intraabdominal diseases that refer pain to the musculoskletal system are those that involve ulceration or infection of the mucosal lining. Drug-induced GI symptoms (e.g., antibiotic colitis, GI "blues" of nausea, vomiting, and anorexia from digitalis toxicity, NSAID-induced ulcers) can also occur with delayed reactions as much as 6 or 8 weeks after exposure to the medication.

▼ GASTROINTESTINAL ORGAN SYMPTOMS

Any disruption of the digestive system can create symptoms such as pain, diarrhea, and constipation. The bowel is susceptible to altered patterns of normal motility caused by food, alcohol, tobacco, caffeine, drugs, physical and emotional stress, and lifestyle (e.g., lack of regular exercise). Gastrointestinal effects of chemotherapy include nausea and vomiting, anorexia, taste alteration, weight loss, oral mucositis, diarrhea, and constipation.

Symptoms, including pain, can be related to various GI organ disturbances and differ in character depending on the affected organ. The most clinically meaningful GI symptoms reported in a physical therapy practice include:

- Abdominal pain
- Dysphagia
- Odynophagia
- Melena
- Epigastric pain with radiation to the back
- Symptoms affected by food
- Early satiety with weight loss
- Constipation
- Diarrhea
- Fecal incontinence
- Arthralgia
- Referred shoulder pain
- Psoas abscess
- Tenderness over McBurney's point (see Appendicitis)

Abdominal Pain

Visceral Pain

Visceral pain (internal organs) occurs in the midline because the abdominal organs receive sensory afferents from both sides of the spinal cord (Fig. 6-2). The site of pain

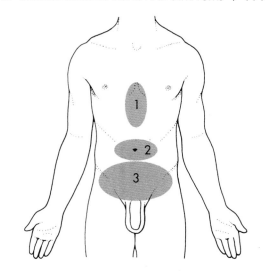

FIGURE 6-2 • Visceral pain: (1) the epigastric region; (2) the periumbilical region; and (3) the lower midabdominal region.

corresponds to dermatomes from which the diseased organ receives its innervation (see Fig. 1-2). Pain is not well localized because innervation of the viscera is multisegmental over up to eight segments of the spinal cord but with few nerve endings.

The abdominal viscera are ordinarily insensitive to many stimuli, such as cutting, tearing, or crushing, that when applied to the skin evoke severe pain. Visceral pain fibers are sensitive only to stretching or tension in the wall of the gut from neoplasm, distention, or forceful muscular contractions secondary to bowel obstruction or spasm.

The rate that tension develops must be rapid enough to produce pain; gradual distention, such as with malignant obstruction, may be painless unless ulceration occurs.

Inflammation may produce visceral pain and ischemia (deficiency of blood) that subsequently produces pain by increasing the concentration of tissue metabolites in the region of the sensory nerve. Pain associated with ischemia is steady pain, whether this ischemia is secondary to vascular disease or due to obstruction causing strangulation of tissue.

Case Example. A 66-year-old university professor consulted with a physical therapist after twisting his back while taking the garbage out. He reported experiencing ongoing, painful low back symptoms 3 weeks after the incident. The objective assessment was consistent with a strain of the right paraspinal muscles with overall diminished lumbar spinal motion consistent with this gentleman's age. Given the reported mechanism of injury and the results of the examination consistent with a musculoskeletal problem, a medical screening examination was not included in the interview. A home exercise program was initiated including stretching and conditioning components.

When the client did not return for his follow-up appointment, telephone contact was made with his family. The client had been hospitalized after collapsing at work. A medical diagnosis of colon cancer was determined. The family reported he had been experiencing digestive difficulties "off and on" and low back pain for the past 3 years, always alternately and never simultaneously. The client died 6 weeks later.

In this case, the only red flag suggesting the need for medical screening was the client's age. However, the therapist must always remember that even with a known and plausible reason for the injury, the client may wrongfully attribute symptoms to a logical event or occurrence. This man had been experiencing both abdominal symptoms and referred back pain, but since these episodes did not occur at the same time, he did not connect them.

Additionally, although the viscera experience pain, the visceral peritoneum (membrane enveloping organs) is insensitive to pain. Except in the presence of widespread inflammation or ischemia, it is possible to have extensive disease without pain until the disease progresses enough to involve the parietal peritoneum.

Referred Pain

Afferent nerve impulses transmit pain from the esophagus to the spinal cord by sympathetic nerves. Visceral afferent nerves from the liver, diaphragm, and pericardium are derived from dermatomes C3 to C5 and reach the central nervous system (CNS) via the phrenic nerve (see Fig. 1-2). The visceral pain associated with these structures is referred to the corresponding somatic area (i.e., the shoulder).

Afferent nerves from the gallbladder, stomach, pancreas, and small intestine travel through the celiac plexus (network of ganglia and nerves supplying the abdominal viscera) and the greater splanchnic nerves and enter the spinal cord from T6 to T9. Referred visceral pain from these visceral structures may be perceived in the midback and scapular regions.

Afferent stimuli from the colon, appendix, and pelvic viscera enter the 10th and 11th thoracic segments through the mesenteric plexus and lesser splanchnic nerves. Finally, the sigmoid colon, rectum, ureters, and testes are innervated by fibers that reach T11 to L1 segments through the lower splanchnic nerve and through the pelvic splanchnic nerves from S2 to S4. Referred pain may be perceived in the pelvis, flank, low back, or sacrum.

Hyperesthesia (excessive sensibility to sensory stimuli) of skin and hyperalgesia (excessive sensibility to painful stimuli) of muscle may develop in the referred pain distribution.

Referred pain can occur alone, without accompanying visceral pain, but usually vis-

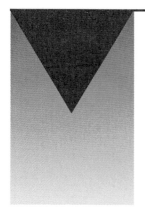

Case Example. An obese 88-year-old woman with a total knee replacement (TKR) was referred for rehabilitation because of loss of motion, joint swelling, and persistent knee pain. She was accompanied to the clinic for each session by one of her three daughters. Over a period of 2 or 3 weeks, each daughter commented on how much weight the mother had lost. When questioned, the client complained of a loss of appetite and difficulty in swallowing, but she had been evaluated and treated only for her knee pain by the orthopedist. She was encouraged to contact her family doctor for evaluation of these red flag symptoms and was subsequently diagnosed with esophageal cancer. Knowing the right questions to ask and making the referral resulted in early diagnosis of her condition.

ceral pain precedes the development of referred pain. The therapist will find that the client does not connect the two sets of symptoms or fails to report abdominal pain and GI symptoms when experiencing a painful shoulder or low back, thinking these are two separate problems.

Dysphagia

Dysphagia is the sensation of food catching or sticking in the esophagus. This sensation may occur (initially) just with coarse, dry foods and may eventually progress to include anything swallowed, even thin liquids and saliva. Achalasia is a process by which the circular and longitudinal muscular fibers of the lower esophageal sphincter do not relax. This disorder contributes to esophageal stricture. Closure *(achalasia)* of the esophageal sphincter may also create an obstruction of the esophagus.

Other possible GI causes of dysphagia include peptic esophagitis (inflammation of the esophagus) with stricture (narrowing) and neoplasm.

Dysphagia may be a symptom of many other disorders unrelated to GI disease (e.g., stroke, Alzheimer's disease, Parkinson's disease). Certain types of drugs, including antidepressants, antihypertensives, and asthma drugs, can make swallowing difficult.

The presence of dysphagia requires prompt attention by the physician. Treat-

ment is based on a subsequent endoscopic examination.

Odynophagia

Odynophagia, or pain during swallowing, can be caused by esophagitis or esophageal spasm. Esophagitis may occur secondary to the herpes simplex virus or fungus caused by the prolonged use of strong antibiotics. Pain after eating may occur with esophagitis or may be associated with coronary ischemia.

To differentiate esophagitis from coronary ischemia: *esophagitis pain* is relieved by upright positioning, whereas *cardiac pain* is relieved by nitroglycerin or by supine positioning. Both conditions require medical attention.

Melena

Melena, or black, tarry stool, occurs as a result of large quantities of blood in the stool. When asked about changes in bowel function, clients may describe black, tarry stools that have an unusual odor. The odor is caused by the presence of blood, and the black color arises as the digestive acids in the bowel oxidize red blood cells. Melena is very sticky and does not clean well. Clients may describe bowel smears on their undergarments.

Upper GI tract (e.g., esophageal, stomach, or duodenal) lesions produce melena. The lesion may be caused by a bleeding ulcer, esophageal varices, or vascular abnormalities of the stomach that break open and bleed easily. There is often a history of NSAID use.

Esophageal varices are dilated blood vessels, usually secondary to alcoholic cirrhosis of the liver. Blood that would normally be pumped back to the heart must bypass the damaged liver. The blood then "backs up" through the esophagus. Vascular abnormalities of the stomach causing bleeding may include ulcers.

The client should be asked about the presence of any blood in the stool to determine whether it is melenotic (from the upper GI tract) or bright red (from the distal colon or rectum). Bleeding from internal or external *hemorrhoids* (enlarged veins inside or outside the rectum), rectal fissures, or colorectal carcinoma can cause bright red blood in the stools.

Epigastric Pain with Radiation

Epigastric pain perceived as intense or sharp pain behind the breastbone with radiation to the back may occur secondary to long-standing ulcers. For example, the client may be aware of an ulcer but does not relate the back pain to the ulcer. Close questioning related to GI symptoms can provide the physical therapist with knowledge of underlying systemic disease processes.

Anyone with epigastric pain accompanied by a burning sensation that begins at the xiphoid process and radiates up toward the neck and throat may be experiencing heartburn. Other common symptoms may include a bitter or sour taste in the back of the throat, abdominal bloating, gas, and general abdominal discomfort. Heartburn is often associated with gastroesophageal reflux disease (GERD). It can be confused with angina or heart attack when accompanied by chest pain, cough, and shortness of breath. A physician must evaluate and diagnose the cause of epigastric pain or heartburn.

Diagnostic interviewing is especially helpful when clients have neglected medical treatment for so long that epigastric back pain may in turn have created biomechanical changes in muscular contractions and spinal movement. These changes eventually create pain of a biomechanical nature (Rose and Rothstein, 1982). The client then presents with enough true musculoskeletal findings such that a diagnosis of back dysfunction can be supported. However, the symptoms may be associated with a systemic problem. A good medical history can be a valuable tool in revealing the actual cause of the back pain.

Symptoms Affected by Food

Clients may or may not be able to relate pain to meals. Pain associated with gastric ulcers (located more proximally in the GI tract) may begin within 30 to 90 minutes after eating, whereas pain associated with duodenal or pyloric ulcers (located distally beyond the stomach) may occur 2 to 4 hours after meals (i.e., between meals). Alternatively stated, food is not likely to relieve the pain of a gastric ulcer, but it may relieve the symptoms of a duodenal ulcer.

The client with a duodenal ulcer may report pain during the night between 12 midnight and 3:00 A.M. This pain should be differentiated from the nocturnal pain associated with cancer by its intensity and duration. More specifically, the *gnawing pain of an ulcer* may be relieved by eating, but the *intense, boring pain associated with cancer* is not relieved by any measures.

Early Satiety

Early satiety occurs when the client feels hungry, takes one or two bites of food, and feels full. The sensation of being full is out of proportion with the time of the previous meal and the initial degree of hunger experienced.

Constipation

Constipation is defined clinically as being a condition of prolonged retention of fecal con-

TABLE 6-1 ▼ CAUSES OF CONSTIPATION

Neurogenic	Muscular	Mechanical	Rectal Lesions	Drugs/Diet
Cortical, voluntary, or involuntary evacuation	Atony (loss of tone)	Bowel obstruction	Thrombosed hemorrhoids	Anesthetic agents (recent general surgery)
Central nervous system lesions	Severe malnutrition	Neoplasm	Perirectal abscess	Antacids (containing aluminum or calcium)
Multiple sclerosis	Metabolic defects	Volvulus (intestinal twisting)		Anticholinergics
Cord tumors	Hypothyroidism	Diverticulitis		Anticonvulsants
Tabes dorsalis	Hypercalcemia	Extraalimentary tumors (including pregnancy)		Antidepressants
Traumatic spinal cord lesions	Potassium depletion	Colostomy		Antihistamines
	Hyperparathyroidism			Antipsychotics
	Inactivity			Barium sulfate
				Diuretics
				Iron compounds
				Narcotics
				Lack of dietary bulk
				Renal failure (due to fluid restriction, phosphate binders)
				Myocardial infarction (narcotics for pain control)

Adapted from Blacklow RS, editor: *MacBryde's signs and symptoms,* ed 6, Philadelphia, 1983, JB Lippincott.

tent in the GI tract resulting from decreased motility of the colon or difficulty in expelling stool.

Common manifestations of this problem are hard stools, stools that are difficult to expel, infrequent stools or a feeling of incomplete evacuation after defecation, and general discomfort. Intractable constipation is called *obstipation* and can result in a fecal impaction that must be removed.

Changes in bowel habit may be a response to many other factors, such as diet (decreased fluid and bulk intake), smoking, side effects of medication, acute or chronic diseases of the digestive system, extraabdominal diseases, personality, mood (depression), emotional stress, inactivity, prolonged bed rest, and lack of exercise (Table 6-1). Commonly implicated medications include narcotics, aluminum- or calcium-containing antacids, anticholinergics, tricyclic antidepressants, phenothiazines, calcium channel blockers, and iron salts.

Diets that are high in refined sugars and low in fiber discourage bowel activity. Transit time of the alimentary bolus from the mouth to the anus is influenced mainly by dietary fiber and is decreased with increased fiber intake. Additionally, motility can be decreased by emotional stress that has been correlated with personality. Constipation associated with severe depression can be improved by exercise.

People with low back pain may develop constipation as a result of muscle guarding and splinting that causes reduced bowel motility. Pressure on sacral nerves from stored fecal content may cause an *aching discomfort in the sacrum, buttocks, or thighs.*

Because there are many specific organic causes of constipation, it is a symptom that may require further medical evaluation. It is considered a red flag symptom when clients with unexplained constipation have sudden and unaccountable changes in bowel habits or blood in the stools.

Diarrhea

Diarrhea, by definition, is an abnormal increase in stool liquidity and daily stool weight associated with increased stool frequency (i.e., more than three times per

TABLE 6-2 ▼ CAUSES OF DIARRHEA

Malabsorption	Neuromuscular	Mechanical	Infectious	Nonspecific
Pancreatitis	Irritable bowel syn-	Incomplete obstruction	Viral	Ulcerative colitis
Pancreatic carcinoma	drome	Neoplasm	Bacterial	Diverticulitis
Crohn's disease	Diabetic enteropathy	Adhesions	Parasitic	Diet
	Hyperthyroidism	Stenosis	Protozoal *(Giardia)*	Laxative abuse
	Caffeine	Fecal impaction		Food allergy
		Muscular incompetency		Antibiotics
		Postsurgical effect		Lactose (milk)
		(ileal bypass)		intolerance

Adapted from Blacklow RS, editor: *MacBryde's signs and symptoms,* ed 6, Philadelphia, 1983, JB Lippincott.

day). This may be accompanied by urgency, perianal discomfort, and fecal incontinence. The causes of diarrhea vary widely from one person to another, but food, alcohol, use of laxatives ad other drugs, medication side effects, and travel may contribute to the development of diarrhea (Table 6-2).

Acute diarrhea, especially when associated with fever, cramps, and blood or pus in the stool, can accompany invasive enteric infection. Chronic diarrhea associated with weight loss is more likely to indicate neoplastic or inflammatory bowel disease. Extraintestinal manifestations such as arthritis or skin or eye lesions are often present in inflammatory bowel disease. Any of these combinations of symptoms must be reported to the physician.

Drug-induced diarrhea is associated most commonly with antibiotics. Diarrhea may occur as a direct result of antibiotic use and the GI symptom resolves when the drug is discontinued. Symptoms may also develop 6 to 8 weeks after first ingestion of an antibiotic.

For the client describing chronic diarrhea, it may be necessary to probe further about the use of laxatives as a possible contributor to this condition. Laxative abuse contributes to the production of diarrhea and begins a vicious cycle as chronic laxative users experience excessive secretion of aldosterone and resultant edema when they attempt to stop using laxatives. This edema and increased weight forces the person to continue to rely on laxatives. The abuse of laxatives is common in the eating disorder populations (e.g.,

anorexia, bulimia); affected persons may ingest up to 100 laxatives at a time.

Questions about laxative use can be asked tactfully during the Core Interview when asking about medications, including over-the-counter drugs such as laxatives. Encourage the client to discuss bowel management without drugs at the next appointment with the physician.

Fecal Incontinence

Fecal incontinence may be described as an inability to control evacuation of stool and is associated with a sense of urgency, diarrhea, and abdominal cramping. Causes include partial obstruction of the rectum (cancer), colitis, and radiation therapy, especially in the case of women treated for cervical or uterine cancer. The radiation may cause trauma to the rectum that results in incontinence and diarrhea. Anal distortion secondary to traumatic childbirth, hemorrhoids, and hemorrhoidal surgery may also cause fecal incontinence.

Arthralgia

Although dissimilar in both structure and function, the gut and locomotor system are linked by a number of clinical syndromes. Inflammatory bowel disease (ulcerative colitis and Crohn's disease) is often accompanied by rheumatic manifestations; peripheral joint arthritis and spondylitis with sacroiliitis are the most common (Orchard and Jewell, 1997).

Joint arthralgia associated with gastrointestinal infection is usually asymmetric, migratory, and oligoarticular (affecting only one or two joints). This type of joint involvement is termed *reactive arthritis* when triggered by microbial infection from the GI (and sometimes genitourinary or respiratory) tract. Other accompanying symptoms may include fever, malaise, skin rash or other skin lesions, nail bed changes (nails separate from the nail beds and become thin and discolored), iritis, or conjunctivitis.

The bowel and joint symptoms may or may not occur at the same time. Usually this type of arthralgia is preceded 1 to 3 weeks by diarrhea, urethritis, regional enteritis (Crohn's disease) or other bacterial infection. The knees, ankles, shoulders, wrists, elbows, and small joints of the hands and feet (listed in order of decreasing frequency) are the peripheral joints affected most often (Anderson and Robinson, 1996).

A large knee effusion is a common presentation, but some clients have joint pain with minimal or no signs of inflammation. Muscle atrophy occurs when a chronic condition is present, in which case, there will be a history of previous GI and joint involvement. Stiffness, pain, tenderness, and reduced range of motion may be present, but with proper medical treatment, there is no permanent deformity.

Spondylitis with sacroiliitis may present as low back pain and morning stiffness that improves with activity and restriction of chest and spinal movement. Radiographic findings are consistent with those of classic ankylosing spondylitis with bilateral sacroiliac joint involvement and bony erosion and sclerosis of the symphysis pubis, ischial tuberosities, and iliac crests. Ultimately "bamboo spine" (see Fig. 11-3) will result.

Inflammation involving the sites of bony insertion of tendons and ligaments termed *enthesitis* is a classic sign of reactive arthritis. Tendon sheaths and bursae may also become inflamed. Ligaments along the spine and sacroiliac joints and around the ankle and midfoot may also show evidence of inflammation.

Heel pain is a frequent complaint, with swelling and tenderness located either posteriorly at the Achilles tendon insertion site or inferiorly where the plantar fascia attaches to the calcaneus. Plantar fasciitis is common. Enthesopathy can also occur around the knee, ischial tuberosities, greater femoral trochanter, and costovertebral and manubriosternal joints (Mustafa and Khan, 1996).

Pain in the Left Shoulder

Pain in the left shoulder (Kehr's sign) can occur as a result of free air or blood in the abdominal cavity, such as a ruptured spleen causing distention. The Core Interview may help the client recall any precipitating trauma or injury, such as a sharp blow during an athletic event, a fall, or perhaps an automobile accident. The client may not connect these seemingly unrelated events with the present shoulder pain.

Psoas Abscess

Psoas abscess is usually the consequence of spread of inflammation or infection from an adjacent structure. It is usually confined to the psoas fascia but can spread to the hip, upper thigh, or buttock. Psoas abscesses most commonly result from direct extension of intraabdominal infections such as diverticulitis, Crohn's disease, pelvic inflammatory disease (PID), and appendicitis (see also McBurney's point).

The iliacus muscle joins with the lower portion of the psoas muscle. Osteomyelitis of the ilium or septic arthritis of the sacroiliac joint can penetrate the muscle sheath of either muscle producing an abscess.

Clinical manifestations of a psoas or iliacus abscess include fever, night sweats, lower abdominal pain or back pain, or pain referred to the hip, medial thigh or groin (femoral triangle area), or knee. The right side is affected most often when associated with appendicitis. Both sides can be involved with generalized peritonitis, but

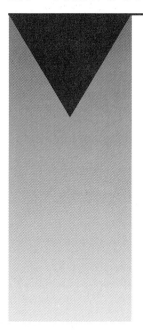

Case Example. A 23-year-old soccer player sustained a blow from the side as he was moving down the soccer field. He fell on his left side with the full force of his own body weight and the weight of the other player on top of him. He reported having "the wind knocked out of me" and sat out on the sidelines for 20 minutes. He resumed playing and completed the game. The next morning, he woke up with severe left shoulder pain and stopped by the office of a physical therapist located in the same building as his office. The objective examination was unremarkable for shoulder movement dysfunction, which was inconsistent with the client's complaint of "constant pain." The client was treated symptomatically and instructed in pendulum exercises to maintain the joint motion.

He made a follow-up appointment with the therapist for the next day, but before noon, he collapsed at work and was taken to a hospital emergency department. A diagnosis of ruptured spleen was made during emergency surgery. A ruptured spleen would have sent the typical adult for medical care much sooner, but this client was in excellent physical condition with a high tolerance for pain. Physical therapy treatment was not appropriate in this situation; an immediate medical referral was indicated given the history of trauma, sudden onset of symptoms, left shoulder pain (Kehr's sign), and constancy of pain.

usually that person has a clear systemic presentation and seeks medical evaluation.

Antalgic gait may develop secondary to a reflex spasm pulling the leg into internal rotation causing a functional hip flexion contracture. Often a tender mass can be palpated in the groin. The physical therapist must assess for trigger points of the iliopsoas muscle. A psoas minor syndrome can be mistaken for appendicitis (Travell and Simons, 1992).

Four tests can be performed to assess the possibility of systemic origin of painful hip or thigh symptoms. Gently pick up the client's leg on the involved side and tap the heel. A painful expression and report of right lower quadrant pain may accompany peritoneal inflammation. If the client is willing and able, have him or her hop on one leg. The person with an inflamed peritoneum will clutch that side unable to complete the movement. The *iliopsoas muscle test* (Fig. 6-3) is performed when acute abdominal pain is a possible cause of hip or thigh pain. When the iliopsoas muscle is inflamed by an inflamed or perforated appendix or inflamed peritoneum, the iliopsoas muscle test causes pain felt in the right lower abdominal quad-

▼ *Clinical Signs and Symptoms of* Psoas Abscess

- Fever ("hectic" fever pattern: up and down)
- Night sweats
- Abdominal pain
- Loss of appetite or other GI upset
- Back, pelvic, abdominal, hip, and/or knee pain
- Antalgic gait
- Palpable, tender mass

rant.* Alternately, the client lies on the pain-free side, and the therapist gently hyperextends the involved leg to stretch the psoas major muscle. Additionally, palpate the iliopsoas muscle by placing the client in a supine position with hips and knees flexed and fully supported in a 90-degree position (Fig. 6-4).

---

*Pain and tenderness in the lower left side of the abdomen may be caused by bowel perforation associated with diverticulitis.

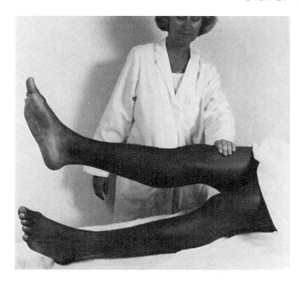

FIGURE 6-3 • Iliopsoas muscle test. In the supine position, have the client actively perform a straight leg raise; apply resistance to the distal thigh as the client tries to hold the leg up. Alternately, ask the client to turn onto the left side. Extend the person's right leg at the hip. Increased abdominal, flank, or pelvic pain on either maneuver constitutes a positive sign, suggesting irritation of the psoas muscle by an inflamed appendix or peritoneum. From Jarvis C: *Physical examination and health assessment*, Philadelphia, 1992, WB Saunders.

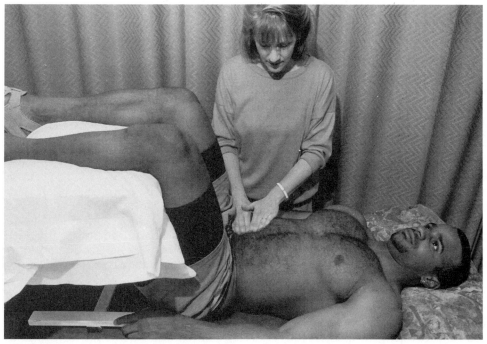

FIGURE 6-4 • Palpating the iliopsoas muscle. Place the client in a supine position with the hips and knees both flexed and supported at a 90-degree angle. Slowly press fingers into abdomen approximately one third the distance form the anterior superior iliac spine (ASIS) toward the umbilicus. It may be necessary to ask the client to initiate slight hip flexion to help isolate the muscle and avoid palpating the bowel. Reproducing or causing right lower quadrant, pelvic, or abdominal pain is considered a positive sign for iliopsoas abscess. Palpation may produce back pain or local muscular pain from shortened or contracted muscle. (From Goodman CC, Boissonnault WG: *Pathology: special implications for the physical therapist*, Philadelphia, 1998, WB Saunders.)

Palpate one third of the distance between the anterior superior iliac spine (ASIS) and the umbilicus. The client is asked to flex the hip gently to assist in isolating the iliopsoas muscle. Muscular tightness in the iliopsoas may result in radiating pain to the low back region during palpation, whereas inflammation or abscess will bring on painful symptoms in the right lower abdominal quadrant.

The *obturator muscle test* (Fig. 6-5) is also performed when the appendix could be the cause of referred pain to the hip. A perforated appendix or inflamed peritoneum irritates the obturator muscle, producing right lower quadrant abdominal pain during the obturator test.

▼ GASTROINTESTINAL DISORDERS

Peptic Ulcer

Peptic ulcer is a loss of tissue lining the lower esophagus, stomach, and duodenum. Gastric and duodenal ulcers are considered together in this section. Acute lesions that do not extend through the mucosa are called erosions. Chronic ulcers involve the muscular coat, destroying musculature and replacing it with permanent scar tissue at the site of healing.

Originally, all ulcers in the upper GI tract were believed to be caused by the aggressive action of hydrochloric acid and pepsin on the mucosa. They thus became known as "peptic ulcers," which is actually a misnomer.

It is now known that 9 of 10 gastric and duodenal ulcers are caused by infection with *H. Pylori,* a corkscrew-shaped bacterium that bores through the layer of mucus that protects the stomach cavity from stomach acid. Ten percent of ulcers are induced by chronic use of nonsteroidal anti-inflammatory drugs (NSAIDs), such as aspirin, ibuprofen, and naproxen, commonly taken by people with arthritis (Margolis, 1998).

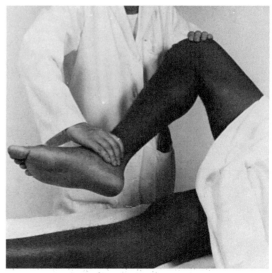

FIGURE 6-5 • Obturator muscle test. In the supine position, perform active assisted motion, flexing at the hip and 90 degrees at the knee. Hold the ankle and rotate the leg internally and externally. A negative or normal response is no pain. A positive test for muscle affected by peritoneal infection or inflammation reproduces right lower quadrant abdominal or pelvic pain. (From Jarvis C: *Physical examination and health assessment,* Philadelphia, 1992, WB Saunders.)

H. Pylori ulcers are primarily located in the lining of the duodenum (upper portion of the small intestine that connects to the stomach) (Fig. 6-6). NSAID-induced ulcers occur primarily in the lining of the stomach, most frequently on the posterior wall, which accounts for back pain as an associated symptom.

Ulcers can be dangerous if left untreated, eroding into the stomach arteries and causing life-threatening bleeding or perforating the stomach and spreading infection. Any suspicion of back or shoulder pain associated with peptic ulcers must be reported to the physician.

CLINICAL SIGNS AND SYMPTOMS

The cardinal symptom of peptic ulcer is epigastric pain that may be described as "heartburn" or as burning, gnawing, cramping, or aching located over a small area near the midline in the epigastrium near the xiphoid. Gastric ulcer pain often occurs in

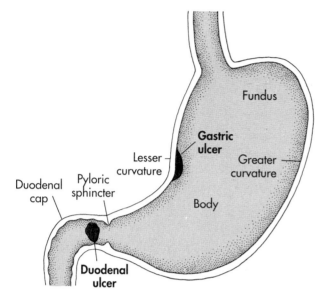

FIGURE 6-6 • Most common sites for peptic ulcers. (Adapted from Ignatavicius DD, Bayne MV: *Medical-surgical nursing,* Philadelphia, 1991, WB Saunders.)

▼ Clinical Signs and Symptoms of
Peptic Ulcer

- "Heartburn" or epigastric pain aggravated by food (gastric ulcer); relieved by food, milk, antacids, or vomiting (duodenal ulcer)
- Night pain (12 midnight to 3:00 A.M.)—same relief as for epigastric pain (duodenal ulcer)
- Radiating back pain
- Stomach pain
- Right shoulder pain (rare)
- Lightheadedness or fainting
- Nausea
- Vomiting
- Anorexia
- Weight loss
- Bloody stools
- Black, tarry stools

the upper epigastrium with localization to the left of the midline, whereas duodenal pain is in the right epigastrium.

The pain comes in waves that last several minutes (rather than hours) and may radi-ate below the costal margins into the back, or rarely, to the right shoulder. The daily pattern of pain is related to the secretion of acid and the presence of food in the stomach to act as a buffer.

Pain associated with duodenal ulcers is prominent when the stomach is empty, such as between meals and in the early morning. The pain may last from minutes to hours and may be relieved by antacids. Gastric ulcers are more likely to cause pain associated with the presence of food. Symptoms often appear for 3 or 4 days or weeks and then subside, reappearing weeks or months later.

Other symptoms of uncomplicated peptic ulcer include nausea, vomiting, loss of ap-petite, sometimes weight loss, and occasion-ally back pain. In duodenal ulcers, steady pain near the midline of the back (see Fig. 6-9) between T6 and T10 with radiation to the right upper quadrant may indicate per-foration of the posterior duodenal wall.

Back pain may be the first and only symptom. Complications of hemorrhage, per-foration, and obstruction may lead to addi-tional symptoms that the client does not re-late to the back pain. Bleeding may occur when the ulcer erodes through a blood ves-sel. It may present as vomited bright red blood or coffee-ground vomitus and by dark tarry stools (melena). The bleeding may vary from massive hemorrhage to occult (hidden) bleeding that occurs over a long period of time.

Gastrointestinal Complications of NSAIDs

NSAIDs (Table 6-3) have become increasingly popular by virtue of their analgesic, antiinflammatory, antipyretic, and antithrombotic (platelet-inhibitory) actions. NSAIDs have deleterious effects on the entire GI tract from the esophagus to the colon, although the most obvious clinical effect is on the gastroduodenal mucosa.

GI effects of NSAIDs are responsible for approximately 40 percent of hospital admissions among clients with arthritis. NSAID-induced GI bleeding is a major cause of morbidity and mortality among the elderly (Hirschowitz, 1997).

Gastrointestinal complications of NSAID use include ulcerations, hemorrhage, perforation, stricture formation, and exacerbation of inflammatory bowel disease. Each NSAID has its own pharmacodynamic characteristics, and clients' responses to each drug may vary greatly.

Other possible adverse side effects of NSAIDs may include suppression of cartilage repair and synthesis, fluid retention and kidney damage, liver damage, skin reactions (e.g., itching, rashes, acne), and impairment of the nervous system such as headache, depression, confusion or memory loss, mood changes, and ringing in the ears.

Many people diagnosed with painful musculoskeletal conditions, especially arthritis, rely on NSAIDs to relieve pain and improve function. Anyone with a history of NSAID use presenting with back or shoulder pain, especially when accompanied by any of the associated signs and symptoms listed for peptic ulcer, must be evaluated by a physician. The therapist should remain alert for the client taking multiple NSAIDs and simultaneously combining prescription and over-the-counter (OTC) drugs.

TABLE 6-3 ▼ NONSTEROIDAL ANTI-INFLAMMATORY DRUGS (NSAIDS)

Generic	Brand Name
Over-the-Counter (OTC)	
aspirin	Anacin, Ascriptin*, Bayer*, Bufferin*, Ecotrin*, Excedrin*
ibuprofen	Advil, Motrin, Nuprin, Ibuprofen, various generic store brands
ketoprofen	Actron, Orudis KT
naproxen sodium	Aleve, various generic store brands
Prescription	
diclofenac sodium	Voltaren
etodolac	Lodine
ibuprofen	Motrin (prescription strength)
indomethacin	Indocin
ketoprofen	Orudis, Oruvail
nabumetone	Relafen
naproxen	Anaprox, Anaprox DS, EC, Naprosyn
oxaprozin	Daypro
piroxicam	Feldene
sulindac	Clinoril
ketorolac	Toradol (short-term use only)

*These all have "extras" in them besides aspirin but are known as aspirin products.

Diverticular Disease

The terms *diverticulosis* and *diverticulitis* are used interchangeably although they have distinct meanings. *Diverticulosis* is a benign condition in which the mucosa (lining) of the colon balloons out through weakened areas in the wall. Up to 60% of people over age 65 have these sac-like protrusions diagnosed typically when screening for colon cancer or other problems (Apstein, 1998).

Diverticulitis describes the infection and inflammation that accompany a microperforation of one of the diverticula. Diverticulosis is very common, whereas complications resulting in diverticulitis occur in only 10 to 25 percent of people with diverticulosis. There may be an association between the use of NSAIDs or acetaminophen and diverticular disease (Mold, 1998).

▼ *Clinical Signs and Symptoms of*
Diverticulitis

- Left lower abdominal pain and tenderness
- Left pelvic pain
- Bloody stools

There is some controversy regarding whether diverticulosis is symptomatic, but perforation and subsequent infection causes symptoms of left lower abdominal or pelvic pain and tenderness in diverticulitis. For the physical therapist performing the iliopsoas and obturator tests, abdominal pain in the left lower quadrant may be caused by diverticular disease and should be reported to the physician. The diagnosis of diverticulitis is confirmed by accompanying fever, bloody stools, and elevated white blood cell count.

Appendicitis

Appendicitis is an inflammation of the vermiform appendix that occurs most commonly in adolescents and young adults. It is a serious disease usually requiring surgery. When the appendix becomes obstructed, inflamed, and infected, rupture may occur, leading to peritonitis.

Diseases that can be mistaken for appendicitis include Crohn's disease (regional enteritis), perforated duodenal ulcer, gallbladder attacks, and kidney infection on the right side, and for women, ruptured ectopic pregnancy, twisted ovarian cyst, or a hemorrhaging ovarian follicle at the middle of the menstrual cycle. Right lower lobe pneumonia sometimes is associated with prominent right lower quadrant pain.

CLINICAL SIGNS AND SYMPTOMS

The classic symptoms of appendicitis are pain preceding nausea and vomiting and low-grade fever in adults. Children tend to have higher fevers. Other symptoms may include coated tongue and bad breath.

The pain usually begins in the umbilical region and eventually localizes in the right lower quadrant of the abdomen over the site of the appendix. In retrocecal appendicitis, the pain may be referred to the thigh or right testicle. The pain comes in waves, becomes steady, and is aggravated by movement, causing the client to bend over and tense the abdominal muscles or to lie down and draw the legs up to relieve abdominal muscle tension.

Generalized peritonitis, whether caused by appendicitis or some other abdominal or pelvic inflammatory condition, results in a "boardlike" abdomen due to the spasm of the rectus abdominis muscles. Lean muscle mass deteriorates with aging, especially evident in the abdominal muscles of the aging population. The very old person may not present with this classic sign of generalized peritonitis because of the lack of toned abdominal muscles.

For this reason, the nursing home, skilled care facility, or home health physical therapist must evaluate the aging client who presents with hip or thigh pain for possible systemic origin (see specific tests for iliopsoas or obturator abscess and McBurney's point).

▼ *Clinical Signs and Symptoms of*
Appendicitis

- Periumbilical and/or epigastric pain
- Right lower quadrant or flank pain
- Right thigh or testicle pain
- Abdominal muscular rigidity
- Positive McBurney's point
- Rebound tenderness (peritonitis)
- Nausea and vomiting
- Anorexia
- Dysuria (painful/difficult urination)
- Low-grade fever
- Coated tongue and bad breath

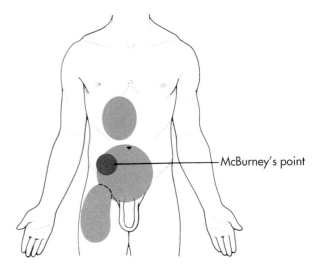

McBurney's point

FIGURE 6-7 • Primary *(dark red)* and referred *(light red)* pain patterns associated with the appendix. Gentle palpation of McBurney's point produces pain or exquisite tenderness. Rebound tenderness should also be assessed (see text).

McBURNEY'S POINT

Parietal pain caused by inflammation of the peritoneum in acute appendicitis or peritonitis may be located at McBurney's point (Fig. 6-7). McBurney's point is located by palpation with the client in a fully supine position.

Isolate the ASIS and the umbilicus: palpate for tenderness halfway between these two surface anatomic points. This method differs from palpitation of the iliopsoas muscle, because the position used to locate the iliopsoas muscle is that of the client in a supine position, with hips and knees flexed in a 90-degree position, whereas McBurney's point is palpated with the client in the fully supine position. The palpation point for the iliopsoas muscle is one third the distance between the ASIS and the umbilicus, whereas McBurney's point is halfway between these two points.

Both McBurney's point and the iliopsoas muscle are palpated for reproduction of symptoms to rule out appendicitis or iliopsoas abscess associated with appendicitis or peritonitis. One final test may be used to assess for the possibility of hip, pelvic, or flank pain from peritonitis. When palpating for McBurney's point, press the fingers in firmly and slowly, and then quickly withdraw them. Pain induced or increased by quick withdrawal results from rapid movement of inflamed peritoneum and is called *rebound tenderness*. If tenderness or pain is felt elsewhere, that area may be the real source of the pain.

Pancreatitis*

Pancreatitis is an inflammation of the pancreas that may result in autodigestion of the pancreas by its own enzymes. Pancreatitis can be acute or chronic, but the physical therapist is most likely to see acute pancreatitis.

Acute pancreatitis can arise from a variety of etiologic factors, but in most instances, the specific cause is unknown. Chronic alcoholism or toxicity from some other agent, such as glucocorticoids, thiazide diuretics, or acetaminophen, can bring on an acute attack of pancreatitis. A mechanical obstruction of the biliary tract may be present, usu-

*The pancreas is both an exocrine gland and an endocrine gland. Its function in digestion is primarily an exocrine activity. This chapter focuses on digestive disorders associated with the pancreas. See Chapter 9 for pancreatic disorders associated with endocrine function.

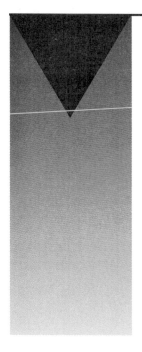

Case Example. Remember the 32-year-old female university student featured in Figure 1-5? She had been referred to physical therapy with the provisional diagnosis: *Possible right oblique abdominis muscle tear/possible right iliopsoas muscle tear.* Her history included the sudden onset of "severe pain" in the right lower quadrant with accompanying nausea and abdominal distention. Aggravating factors included hip flexion, sit-ups, fast walking, and movements such as reaching, turning, and bending. Painful symptoms could be reproduced by resisted hip or trunk flexion, and tenderness/tightness was elicited on palpation of the right iliopsoas muscle as compared with the left. A neurologic screen was negative. Screening questions for general health revealed constitutional symptoms including fatigue, night sweats, nausea, and repeated episodes of severe, progressive pain in the right lower abdominal quadrant.

Although she presented with a musculoskeletal pattern of symptoms at the time of her initial evaluation with the physician, by the time she entered the physical therapy clinic her symptoms had taken on a definite systemic pattern. She was returned for further medical follow-up, and a diagnosis of appendicitis complicated by peritonitis was established. This client recovered fully from all her symptoms following emergency appendectomy surgery.

ally because of gallstones in the bile ducts. Viral infections (e.g., mumps, herpesviruses, hepatitis) also may cause an acute inflammation of the pancreas.

Chronic pancreatitis is caused by long-standing alcohol abuse in more than 90% of adult cases. Chronic pancreatitis is characterized by the progressive destruction of the pancreas with accompanying irregular fibrosis and chronic inflammation.

CLINICAL SIGNS AND SYMPTOMS

The clinical course of most clients with *acute pancreatitis* follows a self-limited pattern. Symptoms can vary from mild, nonspecific abdominal pain to profound shock with coma and, ultimately, death. Abdominal pain begins abruptly in the midepigastrium, increases in intensity for several hours, and can last from days to more than a week. The pain has a penetrating quality and radiates to the back. Pain is made worse by walking and lying supine and is relieved by sitting and leaning forward.

Symptoms associated with *chronic pancreatitis* include persistent or recurrent epi-

▼ *Clinical Signs and Symptoms of*
Acute Pancreatitis

- Epigastric pain radiating to the back
- Nausea and vomiting
- Fever and sweating
- Tachycardia
- Malaise
- Weakness
- Jaundice

sodes of epigastric and left upper quadrant pain with referral to the upper left lumbar region. Anorexia, nausea, vomiting, constipation, flatulence, and weight loss are common. Attacks may last only a few hours or as long as 2 weeks: pain may be constant.

In clients with alcohol-associated pancreatitis, the pain often begins 12 to 48 hours after an episode of inebriation. Clients with gallstone-associated pancreatitis typically experience pain after a large meal. Nausea and vomiting accompany the pain. Other

▼ *Clinical Signs and Symptoms of*
Chronic Pancreatitis

- Epigastric pain radiating to the back
- Upper left lumbar region pain
- Nausea and vomiting
- Constipation
- Flatulence
- Weight loss

▼ *Clinical Signs and Symptoms of*
Pancreatic Carcinoma

- Epigastric/upper abdominal pain radiating to the back
- Low back pain may be the only symptom
- Jaundice
- Anorexia and weight loss
- Light-colored stools
- Constipation
- Nausea and vomiting
- Weakness

symptoms include fever, tachycardia, jaundice, and malaise.

Pancreatic Carcinoma

Pancreatic carcinoma is the fifth most common cause of death from cancer, exceeded only by lung, colorectal, breast, and prostate cancer. The majority of pancreatic cancers (70%) arise in the head of the gland and only 20% to 30% occur in the body and tail. The latter usually have grown to a large size by the time the diagnosis is made, due to the absence of symptoms.

CLINICAL SIGNS AND SYMPTOMS

The clinical features of pancreatic cancer initially are nonspecific and vague, contributing to a delay in diagnosis. The most common symptoms of pancreatic cancer are anorexia and weight loss, epigastric/upper abdominal pain with radiation to the back, and jaundice secondary to obstruction of the bile duct. Epigastric pain is often vague and diffuse. Radiation of pain into the lumbar region is common and sometimes is the only symptom.

Sitting up and leaning forward may provide some relief, and this usually indicates that the lesion has spread beyond the pancreas and is inoperable. Other signs and symptoms include light-colored stools, constipation, nausea, vomiting, and weakness.

Inflammatory Bowel Disease

Inflammatory bowel disease (IBD) refers to two inflammatory conditions:

- Ulcerative colitis (UC)
- Crohn's disease (CD) (also referred to as regional enteritis or ileitis)

Crohn's disease and ulcerative colitis are disorders of unknown etiology involving genetic and immunologic influences on the GI tract. Evidence to suggest increased intestinal permeability allowing increased exposure to foreign antigens has been discovered (Ma, 1997). These two diseases share many epidemiologic, clinical, and therapeutic features. Both are chronic, medically incurable conditions.

Extraintestinal manifestations occur frequently in clients with inflammatory bowel disease and complicate its management. Manifestations involve the joints most commonly (see previous discussion of *Arthralgia*). Skin lesions may occur as either erythema nodosum (red bumps/purple knots over the ankles and shins) or pyoderma (deep ulcers or canker sores) of the shins, ankles, and calves. Uveitis may cause red and painful eyes that are sensitive to light, but this condition does not affect the person's vision.

Nutritional deficiencies are the most common complications of IBD. Inflammation alone and the decrease in functioning surface area of the small intestine, increases food requirements, causing poor absorption.

Nutritional problems associated with the medical treatment of IBD may occur. The use of prednisone decreases vitamin D metabolism, impairs calcium absorption, decreases potassium supplies, and increases the nutritional requirement for protein and calories. Decreased vitamin D metabolism and impaired calcium absorption subsequently result in bone demineralization and osteoporosis.

Crohn's Disease

Crohn's disease (CD) is an inflammatory disease that most commonly attacks the terminal end (or distal portion) of the small intestine (ileum) and the colon. However, it can occur anywhere along the alimentary canal from the mouth to the anus. It occurs more commonly in young adults and adolescents but can appear at any age.

CLINICAL SIGNS AND SYMPTOMS

CD may have acute manifestations, but the condition is usually slow and nonaggressive. The client may present with mild intermittent symptoms months before the diagnosis is made. Fever may occur, with acute inflammation, abscesses, or rheumatoid manifestations.

Terminal ileum involvement produces pain in the periumbilical region with possible referred pain to the corresponding segment of the low back. Pain of the ileum is intermittent and felt in the lower right quadrant with possible associated iliopsoas abscess causing hip pain (see previous discussion of *Psoas abscess*). The client may experience relief of discomfort after passing stool or flatus. For this reason, it is important to ask whether low back pain is relieved after passing stool or gas.

Twenty-five percent of people with CD may present with arthritis or migratory arthralgias (joint pain). The person may present with monoarthritis (i.e., asymmetric pattern affecting one joint at a time), usually involving an ankle or knee, although elbows and wrists can be included. Polyarthritis (involving more than one joint) or sacroiliitis (arthritis of the lower spine and pelvis) is common and may lead to ankylosing spondylitis in rare cases. Whether monoarthritic or polyarthritic, this condition comes and goes with the disease process and may precede repeat episodes of bowel symptoms by 1 to 2 weeks. With proper medical treatment, there is no permanent joint deformity.

Ulcerative Colitis

By definition, UC is an inflammation and ulceration of the inner lining of the large intestine (colon) and rectum. When inflammation is confined to the rectum only, the condition is known as ulcerative proctitis. UC is not the same as irritable bowel syndrome (IBS) or spastic colitis (another term for IBS).

Cancer of the colon is more common among clients with UC than among the general population. The incidence is greatly increased among those who develop UC before the age of 16 years and those who have had the condition for more than 30 years.

CLINICAL SIGNS AND SYMPTOMS

The predominant symptom of UC is rectal bleeding; mainly the left colon is involved; the small intestine is never involved. Clients often experience diarrhea, possibly 20 or more stools per day. Nausea, vomiting, anorexia, weight loss, and decreased serum potassium may occur with severe disease. The development of anemia depends on the degree of blood loss, severity of the illness, and dietary iron intake. Ankylosing spondylitis, anemia, and clubbing of the fingers are occasional findings.

▼ *Clinical Signs and Symptoms of*

Ulcerative Colitis and Crohn's Disease

- Diarrhea
- Constipation
- Fever
- Abdominal pain
- Rectal bleeding
- Night sweats
- Decreased appetite, nausea, weight loss
- Skin lesions
- Uveitis (inflammation of the eye)
- Arthritis
- Migratory arthralgias
- Hip pain (iliopsoas abscess)

Fever is present during acute disease. Nocturnal diarrhea is usually present when daytime diarrhea is prominent.

Medical testing and diagnosis are required to differentiate between these inflammatory conditions. Most often, the physical therapist is faced with clients presenting complaints of pain located in the shoulder, back, or groin that may have a GI origin and not be true musculoskeletal dysfunction at all.

Irritable Bowel Syndrome

Irritable bowel syndrome (IBS) has been called the "common cold of the stomach"; it is a functional disorder of motility in the small and large intestines.

IBS is classified as a "functional" disorder because the abnormal muscle contraction identified in people with IBS cannot be attributed to any identifiable abnormality of the bowel. Chronic visceral hypersensitivity present in the majority of people with functional bowel disorders is manifested as lowered perception threshold and/or altered visceromatic referral (Mertz et al, 1994). In other words, affected individuals perceive unpleasant or inappropriate sensory experiences in the absence of any physiologic or pathophysiologic event. IBS rarely progresses and is never fatal.

Other descriptive names for this condition are spastic colon, irritable colon, nervous indigestion, functional dyspepsia, pylorospasm, spastic colitis, intestinal neuroses, and laxative or cathartic colitis.

IBS is the most common gastrointestinal disorder in Western society and accounts for 50% of subspecialty referrals. It is often linked with psychologic stress; a history of physical or sexual abuse is common (Drossman et al, 1990). IBS is most common in women in early adulthood and there is a well-documented association between IBS and dysmenorrhea (Crowell et al, 1994). It is unclear whether this correlation represents diagnostic confusion or whether dysmenorrhea and IBS have a common physiologic basis.

As mentioned earlier in this chapter, emotional or psychologic responses to stress have a profound effect on brain chemistry, which in turn influences the enteric nervous system (Mayer, 1995; Mayer and Gebhart, 1994). Conversely, messages from the central nervous system are processed in the intestines by an elaborate neural network.

CLINICAL SIGNS AND SYMPTOMS

There is a highly variable complex of intermittent gastrointestinal symptoms, including nausea and vomiting, anorexia, foul breath, sour stomach, flatulence, cramps, and constipation or diarrhea. Nocturnal diarrhea, awakening the client from a sound sleep, is more often a result of organic disease of the bowel and is less likely to occur in IBS.

Pain may be steady or intermittent, and there may be a dull deep discomfort with sharp cramps in the morning or after eating. The typical pain pattern consists of lower left quadrant abdominal pain, constipation, and diarrhea.

These primary symptoms occur when the natural motility of the bowel (rhythmic peristalsis) is disrupted by stress, smoking, eating, and drinking alcohol. Rapid alterations in the speed of bowel movement create an obstruction to the natural flow of stool and

▼ **Clinical Signs and Symptoms of**
Irritable Bowel Syndrome

- Painful abdominal cramps
- Constipation
- Diarrhea
- Nausea and vomiting
- Anorexia
- Flatulence
- Foul breath

▼ **Clinical Signs and Symptoms of**
Colorectal Cancer

Early stages
- Rectal bleeding, hemorrhoids
- Abdominal, pelvic, back, or sacral pain
- Back pain that radiates down the legs
- Changes in bowel patterns

Advanced stages
- Constipation progressing to obstipation
- Diarrhea with copious amounts of mucus
- Nausea, vomiting
- Abdominal distention
- Weight loss
- Fatigue and dyspnea
- Fever (less common)

gas. The resultant pressure build-up in the bowel produces pain and spasm.

Colorectal Cancer

Colorectal cancer is the third most commonly diagnosed cancer and second most common cause of death from malignant disease for both men and women in the Western world. Incidence increases with age, beginning around 40 years of age, and is higher in men than women.

Mortality can be significantly reduced by population screening by means of a simple fecal occult blood test (FOBT) (Hardcastle, 1997). Screening is particularly applicable to individuals belonging to high-risk groups, particularly those with a previous history of chronic inflammatory bowel disease (e.g., Crohn's disease, ulcerative colitis) or adenomatous polyps; previous history of breast, ovarian, or endometrial carcinoma; and a family history of colorectal cancer, especially if diagnosed before age 45 (Jessup et al, 1997).

CLINICAL SIGNS AND SYMPTOMS

The presentation of colorectal carcinoma is related to the location of the neoplasm within the colon. Individuals are asymptomatic in the early stages, then develop minor changes in their bowel patterns (e.g., increased frequency of morning evacuation,

sense of incomplete evacuation), and experience occasional rectal bleeding. When vague cramping pain or an aching-pressure sensation occurs, it is usually associated with a palpable abdominal mass, although these symptoms are experienced before the identification of the mass. Acute pain is often indistinguishable from that of cholecystitis or acute appendicitis.

Fatigue and shortness of breath may occur secondary to the iron deficiency anemia that develops with chronic blood loss. Mahogany-colored stools may be present when there is blood mixed with the stool.* Bleeding with bright red blood is more common with a carcinoma of the left side of the colon. Pencil-thin stool may be described with cancer of the rectum.

When rectal tumors enlarge and invade the perirectal tissue, a sensation of rectal fullness develops and may progress to a dull, aching, perineal or sacral pain that can radiate down the legs when peripheral nerves are involved.

---

*The reddish-mahogany color associated with bleeding in the lower GI/colon differs from the melena or dark, tarry stools that occur when blood loss in the upper GI tract is oxidized before being excreted.

OVERVIEW	GASTROINTESTINAL PAIN PATTERNS

▼ ESOPHAGEAL PAIN (Fig. 6-8)

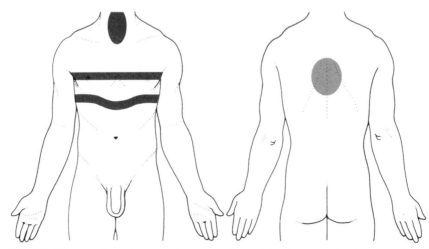

FIGURE 6-8 • Esophageal pain may be projected around the chest at any level corresponding to the esophageal lesion. Only two of the possible bands of pain around the chest are shown here.

Location: Substernal discomfort at the level of the lesion

Lesion of upper esophagus: pain in the (anterior) neck

Lesion of lower esophagus: pain originating from the xiphoid process, radiating around the thorax

Referral: Severe esophageal pain: pain referred to the middle of the back

Back pain may be the only symptom or may be the earliest symptom of esophageal cancer

Description: Sharp, sticking, knifelike, stabbing

Strong burning pain (esophagitis)

Intensity: Varies from mild discomfort to severe pain

Duration: May be constant; associated with meals

Associated Signs and Symptoms: Dysphagia, odynophagia, melena

Possible Etiology: Obstruction of the esophagus (neoplasm)

Esophageal stricture secondary to acid reflux (peptic esophagitis)

Esophageal stricture of unknown cause

Achalasia

Esophagitis or esophageal spasm

Esophageal varices (usually asymptomatic except bleeding)

▼ STOMACH AND DUODENAL PAIN (Fig. 6-9)

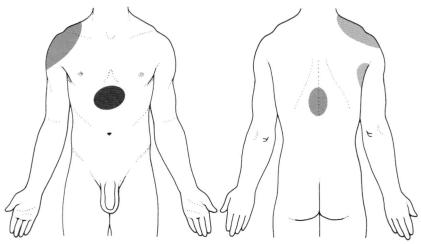

FIGURE 6-9 • Stomach or duodenal pain *(dark red)* may occur anteriorly in the midline of the epigastrium or upper abdomen just below the xiphoid process. Referred pain *(light red)* to the back may occur at the level of the abdominal lesion (T6 to T10). Other patterns of referred pain *(light red)* may include the right shoulder and upper trapezius or the lateral border of the right scapula.

Location:	Pain in the midline of the epigastrium
	Upper abdomen just below the xiphoid process
Referral:	Common referral pattern to the back at the level of the lesion (T6 to T10)
	Right shoulder/upper trapezius
	Lateral border of the right scapula
Description:	Aching, burning, gnawing, cramplike pain (true visceral pain)
Intensity:	Can be mild or severe
Duration:	Comes in waves
Associated Signs and Symptoms:	Early satiety
	Melena
	Symptoms may be associated with meals
Possible Etiology:	Peptic ulcers: gastric, pyloric, duodenal (history of NSAIDs)
	Stomach carcinoma
	Kaposi's sarcoma (most common malignancy associated with acquired immunodeficiency syndrome [AIDS])

▼ SMALL INTESTINE PAIN (Fig. 6-10)

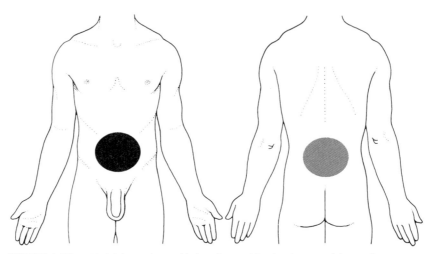

FIGURE 6-10 • Midabdominal pain *(dark red)* caused by disturbances of the small intestine is centered around the umbilicus and may be referred *(light red)* to the low back area at the same level.

Location:	Midabdominal pain (about the umbilicus)
Referral:	Pain referred to the back if the stimulus is sufficiently intense or if the individual's pain threshold is low
Description:	Cramping pain
Intensity:	Moderate to severe
Duration:	Intermittent (pain comes and goes)
Associated Signs and Symptoms:	Nausea, fever, diarrhea
	Pain relief may not occur after passing stool or gas
Possible Etiology:	Obstruction (neoplasm)
	Increased bowel motility
	Crohn's disease (regional enteritis)

▼ LARGE INTESTINE AND COLON PAIN (Fig. 6-11)

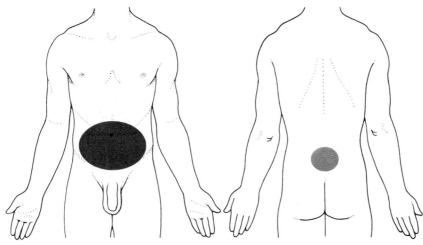

FIGURE 6-11 • Pain associated with the large intestine and colon *(dark red)* may occur in the lower midabdomen across either or both abdominal quadrants. Pain may be referred to the sacrum *(light red)* when the rectum is stimulated.

Location:	Lower midabdomen (across either or both quadrants)
	Poorly localized
Referral:	Pain may be referred to the sacrum when the rectum is stimulated
Description:	Cramping
Intensity:	Dull
Duration:	Steady
Associated Signs and Symptoms:	Bloody diarrhea, urgency
	Constipation
	Pain relief may occur after defecation or passing gas
Possible Etiology:	Ulcerative colitis
	Crohn's disease (regional enteritis)
	Carcinoma of the colon
	Long-term use of antibiotics
	Irritable bowel syndrome (IBS)

▼ PANCREATIC PAIN (Fig. 6-12)

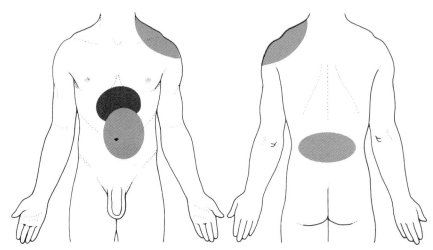

FIGURE 6-12 • Pancreatic pain *(dark red)* occurs in the midline or left of the epigastrium, just below the xiphoid process, but may be referred *(light red)* to the left shoulder or to the middle or low back.

Location:	Midline or to the left of the epigastrium, just below the xiphoid process
Referral:	Referred pain in the middle or lower back is typical with pancreatic disease
	Somatic pain felt in the left shoulder may result from activation of pain fibers in the left diaphragm by an adjacent inflammatory process in the tail of the pancreas
Description:	Burning, or gnawing abdominal pain
Intensity:	Severe
Duration:	Constant pain, sudden onset

Associated Signs and Symptoms:

Sudden weight loss

Jaundice

Nausea and vomiting

Light-colored stools (carcinoma)

Weakness

Fever

Malaise

Constipation

Flatulence

Tachycardia

Symptoms may be unrelated to digestive activities (carcinoma)

Symptoms may be related to digestive activities (pancreatitis)

Aggravating Factors:	Malaise
Relieving Factors:	Walking and lying supine (pancreatitis)
	Alcohol, large meals

Possible Etiology: Sitting and leaning forward (pancreatitis, pancreatic carcinoma)

Pancreatitis

Pancreatic carcinoma (primarily disease of men, occurs during the 6th to 7th decade)

▼ APPENDICEAL PAIN (see Fig. 6-7)

Location:

Right lower quadrant pain

Referral: Well localized

First referred to epigastric or periumbilical area

Description: Referred pain pattern to the right hip and/or right testicle

Intensity: Aching, comes in waves

Duration: Moderate to severe

Steadily progresses over time (usually 12 hours with acute appendicitis)

Associated Signs
and Symptoms: Positive McBurney's point for tenderness

Iliopsoas abscess may occur; positive iliopsoas muscle test or positive obturator test

Anorexia, nausea, vomiting, low-grade fever

Coated tongue and bad breath

Dysuria (painful/difficult urination)

▼ PHYSICIAN REFERRAL

A 67-year-old man is seeing you through home health care for a home program after discharge from the hospital 2 weeks ago for a total hip replacement. His recovery has been slowed by chronic diarrhea. A 25-year-old woman who is diagnosed as having a sacroiliac pain and joint dysfunction asks you what exercises she can do for constipation. A 44-year-old man with biceps tendinitis reports several episodes of fever and chills, diarrhea, and abdominal pain, which he contributes to "the stress of meeting deadlines on the job."

These are common examples of symptoms of a GI nature that are described by clients and are unrelated to current physical ther-apy treatment. These people may be seeking the physical therapist's advice as the only medical person with whom they have contact. Knowing the pain patterns associated with GI involvement and which follow-up questions to ask can assist the physical therapist in deciding when to suggest that the client return to a physician for a medical examination and treatment.

The client may not associate GI symptoms or already diagnosed GI disease with his or her musculoskeletal pain, which makes it necessary for the physical therapist to initiate questions to determine the presence of such GI involvement.

Taking the client's temperature and vital signs during the initial evaluation is recommended for any person who has musculoskeletal pain of unknown origin. Fever,

GUIDELINES FOR PHYSICIAN REFERRAL

- Clients who chronically rely on laxatives should be encouraged to discuss bowel management without drugs with their physician.
- Joint involvement accompanied by skin or eye lesions may be reflective of inflammatory bowel disease and should be reported to the physician if the physician is unaware of these extraintestinal manifestations.
- Anyone with a history of NSAID use presenting with back or shoulder pain, especially when accompanied by any of the associated signs and symptoms listed for peptic ulcer must be evaluated by a physician.
- Back pain associated with meals or relieved by a bowel movement (especially if accompanied by rectal bleeding) or with back pain and abdominal pain at the same level requires medical evaluation.
- Back pain of unknown cause that does not fit a musculoskeletal pattern, especially in a person with a previous history of cancer.

GUIDELINES FOR IMMEDIATE MEDICAL ATTENTION

- Anytime appendicitis or iliopsoas/obturator abscess is suspected (positive McBurney's and/or iliopsoas/obturator test).

CLUES TO SCREENING FOR GASTROINTESTINAL DISEASE

- Age over 45
- Previous history of NSAID-induced GI bleeding; NSAID use, especially chronic or multiple prescription and over-the-counter NSAIDs taken simultaneously
- Symptoms increase within 2 hours after taking NSAIDs or other medication
- Presence of abdominal or GI symptoms occurring within 4 to 6 weeks of musculoskeletal symptoms, especially recurring or cyclical symptoms (systemic pattern)
- Back pain and abdominal pain at the same level, simultaneously or alternately, especially when accompanied by constitutional symptoms
- Shoulder, back, pelvic, or sacral pain:
  - Of unknown origin, especially with a past history of cancer
  - Affected by food, milk, antacids, or vomiting
  - Accompanied by constitutional symptoms
- Back, pelvic, or sacral pain that is relieved or reduced by a bowel movement or accompanied by rectal bleeding
- Shoulder pain within 24 to 48 hours of laparoscopy, ruptured ectopic pregnancy, or traumatic blow or injury to the left side (Kehr's sign; see Chapter 12)
- Positive iliopsoas or obturator sign; positive McBurney's point; right (or left) lower quadrant abdominal or pelvic pain produced when palpating the iliopsoas muscle or tapping the heel of the involved side
- Joint pain or arthralgias preceded by skin rash
- When evaluated during early onset of referred pain, there is usually full and painless range of motion but, as time goes on, muscle splinting and guarding secondary to pain will produce altered movements as well

low-grade fever over a long period (even if cyclic), or night sweats is indicative of systemic disease.

When appendicitis is suspected because of the client's symptoms, a physician should be notified immediately. The client should lie down and remain as quiet as possible. It is best to give her or him nothing by mouth because of the danger of aggravating the condition, possibly causing rupture of the appendix, or in case surgery is needed. Applications of heat are contraindicated for the same reason.

On the other hand, the physical therapist may be evaluating a client who presents with shoulder, back, or groin pain and limitations that are not caused by true musculoskeletal lesions but rather the result of GI involvement. The presence of associated GI symptoms in the absence of conclusive musculoskeletal findings will alert the physical therapist to the possible need for medical referral. Correlate the *history* with *pain patterns* and any *unusual findings* that may indicate systemic disease.

Systemic Signs and Symptoms Requiring Physician Referral

Bloody diarrhea
Boring, stabbing pain
Chills
Constant pain
Cutting, knifelike pain
Dark urine
Dysphagia
Early satiety
Fecal incontinence
Fever
Gnawing, burning pain
Iliopsoas muscle test (positive)
Jaundice
Kehr's sign (positive)
Light stools
McBurney's point (positive)
Melena
Migratory arthralgias
Night pain
Night sweats
Obturator test (positive)
Odynophagia
Skin lesions
Sudden weight loss
Uveitis
Vomiting

 KEY POINTS TO REMEMBER

▶ Gastrointestinal disorders can refer pain to the sternum, neck, shoulder, scapula, low back, and hip.

▶ When evaluated during early onset of referred pain, there is usually full and painless range of motion, but as time goes on, muscle splinting and guarding secondary to pain will produce altered movements as well.

▶ The membrane that envelops organs (visceral peritoneum) is insensitive to pain so that, except in the presence of inflammation/ischemia, it is possible to have extensive disease without pain.

▶ Clients may not relate known GI disorders to current (or new) musculoskeletal symptoms.

▶ Sudden and unaccountable changes in bowel habits, blood in the stool, or vomiting red blood or coffee-ground vomitus are red flag symptoms requiring medical follow-up.

▶ Antibiotics and NSAIDs are the drugs that most commonly induce GI symptoms.

▶ Kehr's sign (left shoulder pain) occurs as a result of free air or blood in the abdominal cavity causing distention (e.g., trauma, ruptured spleen, laparoscopy).

▶ Epigastric pain radiating to the upper back or upper back pain alone can be the primary symptom of peptic ulcer, pancreatitis, or pancreatic carcinoma.

▶ Appendicitis and diseases of the intestines such as Crohn's disease and ulcerative colitis can cause abscess of the iliopsoas muscle, resulting in hip, thigh, or groin pain.

▶ Arthritis and migratory arthalgias occur in 25% of Crohn's disease cases.

Figures 6-13 and 6-14 provide a summary of all the GI pain patterns described that can mimic the pain and dysfunction usually associated with musculoskeletal lesions.

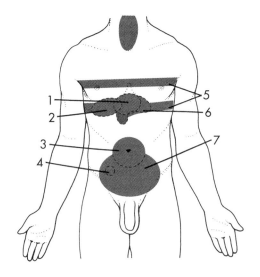

FIGURE 6-13 • Full-figure **primary pain pattern:** (1) stomach/duodenum; (2) liver/gallbladder/common bile duct; (3) small intestine; (4) appendix; (5) esophagus; (6) pancreas; and (7) large intestine/colon.

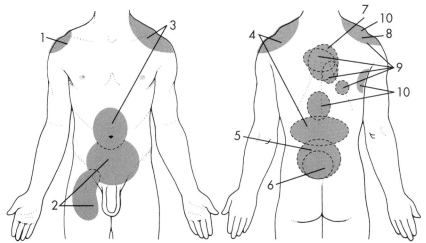

FIGURE 6-14 • Full-figure **referred pain patterns:** (1) liver/gallbladder/common bile duct; (2) appendix; (3) pancreas; (4) pancreas; (5) small intestine; (6) colon; (7) esophagus; (8) stomach/duodenum; (9) liver/gallbladder/common bile duct; and (10) stomach/duodenum.

SUBJECTIVE EXAMINATION

- ### SPECIAL QUESTIONS TO ASK

After completing the initial intake interview, if there is cause to suspect GI involvement, include the following additional questions. It may be helpful to let the client know you will be asking some questions about overall health issues that may seem unrelated to their current symptoms but that are nevertheless important.

When asking questions about medications, look for long-term use of antibiotics, corticosteroids such as prednisone, or other hepatotoxic drugs. See Table 6-1 for a list of medications that cause constipation.

Past Medical History

- **(For the client with left shoulder pain):** Have you sustained any injuries in the last week during a sports activity, fall, or automobile accident? Were you pushed down or pushed against something hard (assault)? **(Ruptured spleen: positive Kehr's sign)**
- Have you experienced any abdominal or intestinal problems, nausea, vomiting, episodes of night sweats or fever?
  - *If yes,* have you seen a physician about these problems or reported them to your physician?
  - For further follow-up questions related to this area, see *Associated Signs and Symptoms* below.
- Have you ever had an upset stomach or heartburn while taking NSAID pain relievers like ibuprofen, naproxen, or the like?
- Have you ever been treated for an ulcer or internal bleeding while taking nonsteroidal antiinflammatory drug (NSAID) pain relievers?
  - *If so,* when?
  - Do you still have any pain from your ulcer? Please describe.
- Have you ever had a colonoscopy, proctoscopy, or endoscopy? *If yes,* why and how long ago?
- Have you ever been diagnosed with cancer of any kind? *If yes,* what, when, and has there been any follow-up?
- Have you ever had abdominal surgery?
  - *If yes,* when and what type was it?
- Do you have hemorrhoids?
  - *If yes,* have you had surgery for your hemorrhoids? **(Most common cause of bright red blood coating stools)**

Associated Signs and Symptoms: Effects of eating/drinking

- Do you have any problems chewing or swallowing food? Do you have any pain when swallowing food or liquids? **(Dysphagia, odynophagia)**
- Have you been vomiting? **(Esophageal varices, ulcers)**

- *If so,* how often?

- Is your vomitus ever dark brown or black or look like it has coffee grounds in it? **(Blood)**

- Have you ever vomited, coughed up, or spit up blood?

- Have you experienced any loss of appetite or sudden weight loss in the last few weeks? (i.e., 10 to 15 pounds in 2 weeks without trying)

- Does eating relieve your symptoms? **(Duodenal or pyloric ulcer)**

  - *If yes,* how soon after eating?

- Does eating aggravate your symptoms? **(Gastric ulcer, gallbladder inflammation)**

- Does your pain occur 1 to 3 hours after eating or between meals? **(Duodenal or pyloric ulcers, gallstones, pancreatitis)**

  - Have you ever had gallstones?

- Have you noticed any change in your symptoms after drinking alcohol? **(Alcohol-associated pancreatitis)**

- Have you ever awakened at night with pain? **(Duodenal ulcer, cancer)**

  - Approximately what time does this occur? **(12 midnight to 3:00 a.m.: ulcer)**

  - Can you relieve the pain in any way and get back to sleep. *If yes,* how? **(Ulcer: eating and antacids relieve/Cancer: nothing relieves)**

- Do you have a feeling of fullness after only one or two bites of food? **(Early satiety: esophagus, stomach and duodenum, or gallbladder)**

Associated Signs and Symptoms: Change in bowel habits

- Have you had any changes in your bowel movements (Normal frequency varies from three times a day to once every 3 or more days)? **(Constipation/bowel obstruction)**

  - *If yes to constipation* (see Table 6-1), do you use laxative or stool softeners? How often?

- Do you have diarrhea? **(Ulcerative colitis, Crohn's disease, long-term use of antibiotics, colonic obstruction, amebic colitis, angiodysplasia)**

  - Do you have more than two loose stools a day? *If so,* do you take medication for this problem? What kind of medication do you use?

  - Have you traveled outside of the United States within the last 6 months to 1 year? **(Amebic colitis associated with bloody diarrhea)**

- Do you have a sense of urgency so that you have to find a bathroom immediately without waiting?

- Do you ever have any blood in your stool, reddish Mahogany-colored stools, or dark, tarry stools that are hard to wipe clean? **(Bleeding ulcer, esophageal varices, colon or rectal cancer, hemorrhoids or rectal fissures)**

  - *If yes,* how often?

  - Is the blood mixed in with the stool or does it coat the surface? **(Distal colon or rectum versus melena)**

- Do you ever have gray-colored stools? **(Lack of bile or caused by biliary obstruction such as hepatitis, gallstones, cirrhosis, pancreatic carcinoma, hepatotoxic drugs)**
- Are your stools ever pencil thin? **(Indicates bowel obstruction such as tumor or rectocele (prolapsed rectum) in women after childbirth)**
- Is your pain relieved after passing stool or gas? **(Yes: large intestine and colon; No: small intestine)**

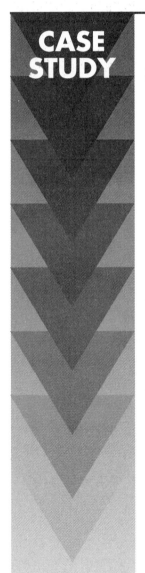

CASE STUDY

REFERRAL

A 21-year-old woman comes to you with complaints of pain on hip flexion when she lifts her right foot off the brake in the car. There are no other aggravating factors, and she is unaware of any way to relieve the pain when she is driving her car. Before the onset of symptoms, she jogged 5 to 6 miles/day, but could not recall any injury or trauma that might contribute to this pain. The Family/Personal History form indicates no personal illness but shows a complex, positive family history for heart disease, diabetes, ulcerative colitis, stomach ulcers, stomach cancer, and alcoholism.

PHYSICAL THERAPY INTERVIEW

It is suggested that the physical therapist use the physical therapy interview to assess the client's complaints today and follow up with appropriate additional questions, such as those noted here.

Introduction to Client

From your family history form, I notice that a number of your family members have reportedly been diagnosed with various diseases.

Do you have any other medical or health-related problems?

Have you sustained any injuries to the lower back, side, or abdomen in the last week—for example, during a sports activity, fall, automobile accident, or assault of any kind?

Although the symptoms that you have described appear to be a musculoskeletal problem, I would like to check out the possibility of a urologic, abdominal, or gynecologic source of this irritation. I will ask you some additional questions that may seem to be unrelated to the problem with your hip, but which will help me put together the whole picture of the history, symptoms, and actual physical results from my examination today.

General Systemic

What other symptoms have you had with this problem? (After allowing the client to answer, you may prompt her by asking: For example, have you had any . . .)

- Numbness
- Fatigue

continued

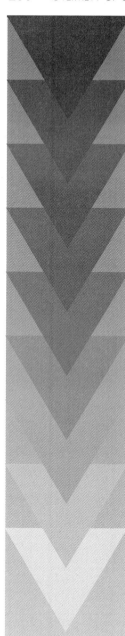

- Legs giving out from under you
- Burning, tingling sensation
- Weakness

Gastrointestinal

- Nausea
- Diarrhea
- Loss of appetite
- Feeling of fullness after only one or two bites of a meal
- Unexpected weight gain or loss (10 to 15 pounds without trying)
- Vomiting
- Constipation
- Blood in your stool

(If yes to any of these, follow-up with *Special Questions to Ask* from this chapter.)

Have you noticed any association between when you eat and your symptoms? (After allowing the client to respond, you may want to prompt her by asking whether eating relieves the pain or aggravates the pain.)

Is your pain relieved or aggravated during or after you have a bowel movement?

Gynecologic

Since your hip/groin/thigh symptoms started, have you been examined by a gynecologist to rule out any gynecologic causes of this problem?

If no:

- Have you ever been told that you have ovarian cysts, uterine fibroids, retroverted uterus, endometriosis, an ectopic pregnancy, or any other gynecologic problem?
- Are you pregnant or have you recently terminated a pregnancy either by miscarriage or abortion?
- Are you using an intrauterine contraceptive device (IUD)?
- Are you having any unusual vaginal discharge?

(If yes to any of these questions, see the follow-up questions for women in Chapter 2.)

Urologic

Have you had any problems with your kidneys or bladder? *If yes,* please describe.

Have you noticed any changes in your ability to urinate since your pain or symptoms started? (If no, it may be necessary to provide examples of what changes you are referring to; for example, difficulty in starting or continuing

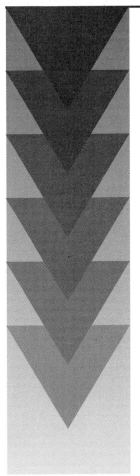

the flow of urine, numbness or tingling in the groin or pelvis, painful urination, urinary incontinence, blood in the urine.)

Have you had burning with urination during the last 1 to 3 weeks?

OBJECTIVE EXAMINATION

Your objective examination reveals tenderness or palpation over the right anterior upper thigh muscles into the groin, with reproduction of the pain on resisted trunk flexion only. This woman attends daily ballet classes, stretches daily, and seems to be very active physically. All tests for flexibility were negative for tightness, including the Thomas' test for tight hip flexors. Other special tests for hip and a neurologic screen had negative results. The client's temperature was normal when it was taken today during the intake screen of vital signs, but during the physical therapy interview, when specifically asked about fevers and night sweats, she indicated several recurrent episodes of night sweats during the last 3 months.

RESULTS

Although the client's complaints are primarily musculoskeletal, the absence of trauma, positive family history for systemic disease, limited musculoskeletal findings, and the client's remark concerning the presence of night sweats will alert the physical therapist to the need for a medical referral to rule out the possibility of a systemic origin of symptoms.

The client's condition gradually worsened during a 3-week period and reexamination by the physician led to an eventual diagnosis of Crohn's disease (regional gastroenteritis). The client was treated with medications that reduce abdominal inflammation and eliminated subjective reports of pain on active hip flexion. Performing the special tests for iliopsoas abscess may have provided valuable information and earlier medical referral if assessed during the initial evaluation.

PRACTICE QUESTIONS

1. Explain the different ways bleeding in the GI tract can be manifested and the possible causes.

2. What is the significance of Kehr's sign?

3. What areas of the body can gastrointestinal (GI) disorders refer pain to?

4. What are the most common GI pathologies to refer pain to the musculoskeletal system?

5. Name two of the most common medications likely to induce GI signs and symptoms.

6. What is the significance of the psoas sign?

7. Which of the following are clues to the possible involvement of the GI system?

   a. Abdominal pain alternating with shoulder pain within a 2-week period

b. Abdominal pain at the same level as back pain, occurring either simultaneously or alternately

c. Shoulder pain alleviated by a bowel movement

d. All of the above

8. Aching pain of the sacrum that radiates can be caused by:

a. Pressure on sacral nerves from stored fecal content in the constipated client

b. Rectal tumors impinging peripheral nerves

c. Crohn's disease manifested as sacroiliitis

d. (a) and (b)

e. (a) and (c)

f. (b) and (c)

g. (a), (b), and (c)

9. A 64-year old woman with chronic rheumatoid arthritis fell and broke her hip. Six months after her total hip replacement, she is still using a walker and complains of continued loss of strength and function. Her family practice physician has referred her to physical therapy for a home program to "improve gait and increase strength."

The client reports frequent episodes of lightheadedness when her legs feel rubbery and weak. She is taking a prescription NSAID along with an OTC NSAID 3 times each day and has been taking NSAIDs 3 years continuously. There are no reported GI complaints or associated signs and symptoms, but after completing the intake interview and objective examination, you think there may be weakness associated with blood loss and anemia secondary to chronic NSAID use. How would you handle a case like this?

10. Body temperature should be taken as part of vital sign assessment:

a. For every client evaluated

b. For any client who has musculoskeletal pain of unknown origin

c. For any client reporting the presence of constitutional symptoms, especially fever or night sweats

d. (b) and (c)

References

Anderson M, Robinson M: Watching for—and managing—joint problems in inflammatory bowel disease, *J Musculoskel Med* 13(11):28-34, November 1996.

Apstein M: Diverticulosis: is conventional wisdom right—or wrong? *Women's Health Advocate* 5(1):7, March 1998.

Crowell MD, Dubin NH, Robinson JC et al: Functional bowel disorders in women with dysmenorrhea, *Am J Gastroenterol* 89:1973, 1994.

Drossman DA, Leserman J, Nachman G: Sexual and physical abuse in women with functional or organic gastrointestinal disorders, *Ann Intern Med* 113:828-833, 1990.

Hardcastle JD: Colorectal cancer, *CA Cancer Clin* 47(2):66-69, March/April 1997.

Hirschowitz BI: NSAIDs and the gut: understanding and preventing problems, *J Musculoskeletal Med* 14(6):38-49, 1997.

Jessup JM, Menck HR, Fremgen A et al: Diagnosing colorectal carcinoma: clinical and molecular approaches, *CA Cancer Clin* 47(2):70-92, March/April, 1997.

Ma TY: Intestinal epithelial barrier dysfunction in Crohn's disease, *Proc Soc Exp Biol Med* 214(4):318-327, April 1997.

Margolis S, editor: Getting the right cure for ulcers, *Johns Hopkins Medical Letter* 10(1):1-2, March 1998.

Mayer EA: Gut feelings: what turns them on? *Gastroenterology* 108(3):927-931, March 1995.

Mayer EA, Gebhart GF: Basic and clinical aspects of visceral hyperalgesia, *Gastroenterology* 107(1):271-293, 1994.

Mertz H, Munakata J, Niazi N et al: Evidence for the alteration of splanchnic afferent pathways in IBS patients, *Gastroenterology* 106:A539, 1994.

Mold JW: Analgesics and symptomatic diverticular disease, *Archives Fam Med* 7(3):262-263, May/June 1998.

Mustafa K, Khan MA: Recognizing and managing reactive arthritis, *J Musculoskeletal Med* 13(6):28-41, 1996.

Orchard T, Jewell DP: Review article: pathophysiology of the intestinal mucosa in inflammatory bowel disease and arthritis: similarities and dissimilarities in clinical findings, *Alimentary Pharmacol Ther* 11 Suppl 3:10-15, December 1997.

Pert CB, Dreher HE, Ruff MR: The psychosomatic network: foundations of mind-body medicine, *Altern Ther Health Med* 4(4):30-41, July 1998.

Rose SJ, Rothstein JM: Muscle mutability: general concepts and adaptations to altered patterns of use, *Physical Therapy* 62:1773, 1982.

Travell JG, Simons DG: *Myofascial pain and dysfunction: the trigger point manual,* Vol 2, Baltimore, 1992, Williams and Wilkins.

Whitcomb DC, Taylor IL: A new twist in the brain-gut axis, *Am J Med Sci* 304(5):334-338, November 1992.

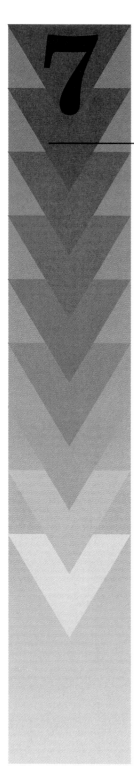

Overview of Renal and Urologic Signs and Symptoms

A 40-year-old athletic man comes to your clinic for an evaluation of back pain that he attributes to a very hard fall on his back while he was alpine skiing 3 days ago. His chief complaint is a dull, aching costovertebral pain on the left side, which is unrelieved by a change in position or by treatment with ice, heat, or aspirin. He stated that "even the skin on my back hurts." He has no previous history of any medical problems.

After further questioning, the client reveals that inspiratory movements do not aggravate the pain, and he has not noticed any change in color, odor, or volume of urine output. However, percussion of the costovertebral angle (see Fig. 7-5) results in the reproduction of the symptoms. This type of symptom complex may suggest renal involvement even without obvious changes in urine.

Whether secondary to trauma or of insidious onset, a client's complaints of flank pain, low back pain, or pelvic pain may be of renal or urologic origin and should be screened carefully through the subjective and objective examinations. Medical referral may be necessary.

This chapter is intended to guide the physical therapist in understanding the origins and relationships of renal, ureteral, bladder, and urethral symptoms. The urinary tract, consisting of kidneys, ureters, bladder, and urethra (Fig. 7-1), is an integral component of human functioning that disposes of the body's toxic waste products and unnecessary fluid and expertly regulates extremely complicated metabolic processes.

Formation and excretion of urine is the primary function of the renal nephron (the functional unit of the kidney) (Fig. 7-2). Through this process the kidney is able to maintain a homeostatic environment in the body. Besides the excretory function of the kidney, which includes the removal of wastes and excessive fluid, the kidney plays an integral role in the balance of various essential body functions, including:

- Acid base balance
- Electrolyte balance
- Control of blood pressure with renin

234

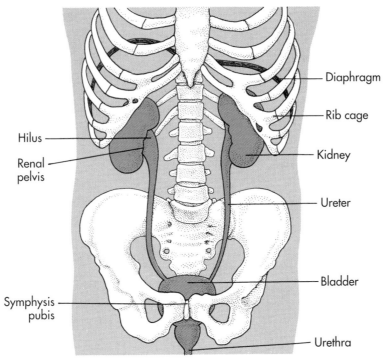

FIGURE 7-1 • Urinary tract structures. The upper portion of each kidney is protected by the rib cage, and the bladder is partially protected by the symphysis pubis.

- Formation of red blood cells (RBCs)
- Activation of vitamin D and calcium balance

The failure of the kidney to perform any of these functions results in severe alteration and disruption in homeostasis.

▼ URINARY TRACT

The upper urinary tract consists of the kidneys and ureters. The kidneys are located in the posterior upper abdominal cavity in a space behind the peritoneum (retroperitoneal space). Their position is in front of and on both sides of the vertebral column at the level of T12 to L2. The upper portion of the kidney is in contact with the diaphragm and moves with respiration. The kidneys are protected by the rib cage and abdominal organs anteriorly and by large back muscles and ribs posteriorly. The lower portions of the kidney and the ureters extend below the ribs and are separated from the abdominal cavity by the peritoneal membrane.

The lower urinary tract consists of the bladder and urethra. From the renal pelvis, urine is moved by peristalsis to the ureters and into the bladder. The bladder, which is a muscular, membranous sac, is located directly behind the symphysis pubis and is used for storage and excretion of urine. The urethra is connected to the bladder and serves as a channel through which urine is passed from the bladder to the outside of the body.

Voluntary control of urinary excretion is based on learned inhibition of reflex pathways from the walls of the bladder. Release of urine from the bladder occurs

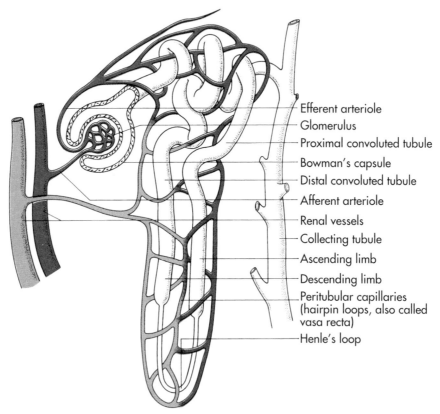

Efferent arteriole
Glomerulus
Proximal convoluted tubule
Bowman's capsule
Distal convoluted tubule
Afferent arteriole
Renal vessels
Collecting tubule
Ascending limb
Descending limb
Peritubular capillaries
(hairpin loops, also called
vasa recta)
Henle's loop

FIGURE 7-2 • Components of the nephron. The afferent arteriole carries blood to the glomerulus for filtration through Bowman's capsule and the renal tubular system. (From Foster RL, Hunsberger MM, Anderson JJ: *Family-centered nursing care of children*, Philadelphia, 1989, WB Saunders.

under voluntary control of the urethral sphincter.

In males the posterior portion of the urethra is surrounded by the prostate gland, a gland approximately 3.5 cm long by 3 cm wide (about the size of two almonds) (Fig. 7-3). The prostate gland is commonly divided into five lobes. This gland can cause severe urethral obstruction if it enlarges. Prostate carcinoma usually affects the posterior lobe of the gland; the middle and lateral lobes typically are associated with the nonmalignant process called benign prostatic hypertrophy.

▼ RENAL AND UROLOGIC PAIN

Upper Urinary Tract (Renal/Ureteral)

The kidneys and ureters are innervated by both sympathetic and parasympathetic fibers. The kidneys receive sympathetic innervation from the lesser splanchnic nerves through the renal plexus, which is located next to the renal arteries. Renal vasoconstriction and increased renin release are associated with sympathetic stimulation.

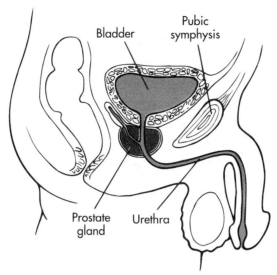

FIGURE 7-3 • The prostate is located at the base of the bladder, surrounding a part of the urethra. As the prostate enlarges, the urethra can become obstructed, interfering with the normal flow of urine.

Parasympathetic innervation is derived from the vagus nerve, and the function of this innervation is not known.

Renal sensory innervation is not completely understood, even though the capsule (covering of the kidney) and the lower portions of the collecting system seem to cause pain with stretching (distension) or puncture. Information transmitted by renal and ureteral pain receptors is relayed by sympathetic nerves that enter the spinal cord at T10 to L1 (see Fig. 1-2).

Because visceral and cutaneous sensory fibers enter the spinal cord in close proximity and actually converge on some of the same neurons, when visceral pain fibers are stimulated, concurrent stimulation of cutaneous fibers also occurs. The visceral pain is then felt as though it is skin pain (hyperesthesia), similar to the condition of the alpine skier who stated that "even the skin on my back hurts." Renal and urethral pain can be felt throughout the T10 to L1 dermatomes.

Renal pain (Fig. 7-4) is typically felt in the posterior subcostal and costovertebral re-gions. To assess the kidney, the test for costovertebral angle tenderness can be included in the objective examination (Fig. 7-5).

Ureteral pain is felt in the groin and genital area (Fig. 7-6). With either renal pain or ureteral pain, radiation forward around the flank into the lower abdominal quadrant and abdominal muscle spasm with rebound tenderness can occur on the same side as the source of pain.

The pain can also be generalized throughout the abdomen. Nausea, vomiting, and impaired intestinal motility (progressing to intestinal paralysis) can occur with severe, acute pain. Nerve fibers from the renal plexus are also in direct communication with the spermatic plexus, and because of this close relationship, testicular pain may also accompany renal pain. Neither renal nor urethral pain is altered by changing body position.

The typical renal pain sensation is aching and dull in nature but can occasionally be a severe, boring type of pain. The constant dull and aching pain usually accompanies distension or stretching of the renal capsule, pelvis,

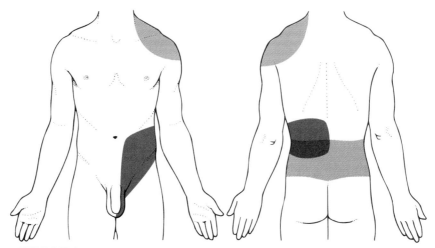

FIGURE 7-4 • Renal pain is typically felt in the posterior subcostal and costovertebral region *(dark red)*. It can radiate across the low back *(light red)* and/or forward around the flank into the lower abdominal quadrant. Ipsilateral testicular pain may also accompany renal pain. Pressure from the kidney on the diaphragm may cause ipsilateral shoulder pain.

or collecting system. This stretching can result from intrarenal fluid accumulation, such as inflammatory edema, inflamed or bleeding cysts, and bleeding or neoplastic growths. Whenever the renal capsule is punctured, a dull pain can also be felt by the client. Ischemia of renal tissue caused by blockage of blood flow to the kidneys results in a *constant* dull or a *constant* sharp pain.

Pseudorenal pain may occur secondary to radiculitis or irritation of the costal nerves caused by mechanical derangements of the costovertebral or costotransverse joints. Disorders of this sort are common in the cervical and thoracic areas, but the most common sites are T10 and T12 (Smith and Raney, 1976). Irritation of these nerves causes costovertebral pain that often radiates into the ipsilateral lower abdominal quadrant.

The onset is usually acute with some type of traumatic history, such as lifting a heavy object, sustaining a blow to the costovertebral area, or falling from a height onto the buttocks. The pain is affected by body position, and although the client may be awakened at night when assuming a certain position (e.g., sidelying on the affected side), the pain is usually absent on awakening and increases gradually during the day. It is also aggravated by prolonged periods of sitting, especially when driving on rough roads in the car, and again it is relieved by changing to another position.

Radiculitis may mimic ureteral colic or renal pain, but true renal pain is seldom affected by movements of the spine. Exerting pressure over the costovertebral angle (CVA) with the thumb may elicit local tenderness of the involved peripheral nerve at its point of emergence, whereas gentle percussion over the angle may be necessary to elicit renal pain, indicating a deeper, more visceral sensation. Fig. 7-5 illustrates percussion over the CVA (Murphy's percussion).

Ureteral obstruction (e.g., from a urinary calculus or "stone" consisting of mineral salts) results in distension of the ureter and causes spasm that produces intermittent or constant severe colicky pain until the stone is passed. Pain of this origin usually starts in the CVA and radiates to the ipsilateral lower abdomen, upper thigh, testis, or labium (see Fig. 7-6). Movement of a stone down a ureter can cause *renal colic,* an excruciating pain that radiates to the region just described and usually increases in intensity in waves of colic or spasm.

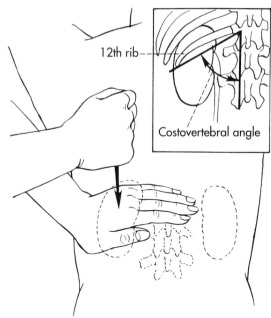

FIGURE 7-5 • Murphy's percussion to test for costoverte-bral angle tenderness. Indirect fist percussion causes the tis-sues to vibrate. To assess the kidney, position the client prone or sitting, and place one hand over the rib at the costoverte-bral angle on the back. Thump that hand with the ulnar edge of your other fist. The person normally feels a thud but no pain. (From Black JM, Matassarin-Jacobs E, editors: *Luck-mann and Sorensen's medical-surgical nursing*, ed 4, Philadelphia, 1993, WB Saunders.)

Chronic ureteral pain and renal pain tend to be vague, poorly localized, and easily confused with many other problems of abdominal or pelvic origin. There are also areas of *referred pain* related to renal or ureteral lesions. For example, if the diaphragm becomes irritated because of pressure from a renal lesion, shoulder pain may be felt. If a lesion of the ureter occurs *outside* the ureter, pain may occur on movement of the adjacent iliopsoas muscle (see Fig. 6-8). Abdominal rebound tenderness results when the adjacent peritoneum becomes inflamed.

Active trigger points along the upper rim of the pubis and the lateral half of the inguinal ligament may lie in the lower internal oblique muscle and possibly in the lower rectus abdominis. These trigger points can cause increased irritation and spasm of the detrusor and urinary sphincter muscles, producing urinary frequency, retention of urine, and groin pain (Travell and Simons, 1983).

Lower Urinary Tract (Bladder/Urethra)

Bladder innervation occurs through sympathetic, parasympathetic, and sensory nerve pathways. Sympathetic bladder innervation assists in the closure of the bladder neck during seminal emission. Afferent sympathetic fibers also assist in providing awareness of bladder distension, pain, and abdominal distension caused by bladder distension. This input reaches the cord at T9 or higher. Parasympathetic bladder innervation is at S2, S3, and S4 and provides motor coordination for the act of voiding. Afferent parasympathetic fibers assist in sensation of the desire to void, proprioception (position sensation), and perception of pain.

Sensory receptors are present in the mucosa of the bladder and in the muscular bladder walls. These fibers are more plentiful near the bladder neck and the junctional area between the ureters and bladder.

Urethral innervation, also at the S2, S3, and S4 level, occurs through the pudendal nerve. This is a mixed innervation of both sensory and motor nerve fibers. This innervation controls the opening of the external urethral sphincter (motor) and an awareness of the imminence of voiding and heat (thermal) sensation in the urethra.

Bladder or urethral pain is felt above the pubis (suprapubic) or low in the abdomen. The sensation is usually characterized as one of urinary urgency, a sensation to void, and dysuria (painful urination). Irritation of the neck of the bladder or of the urethra can result in a burning sensation localized to these areas, probably caused by the urethral thermal receptors (Fig. 7-7).

Other causes of pain similar to upper or lower urinary tract pain of either an acute or chronic nature may include:

- Perforated viscus (any large internal organ)
- Intestinal obstruction
- Cholecystitis (inflammation of the gallbladder)

- Pelvic inflammatory disease
- Tuboovarian abscess
- Ruptured ectopic pregnancy
- Twisted ovarian cyst

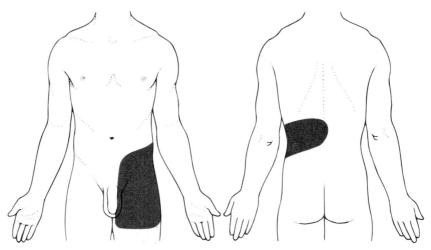

FIGURE 7-6 • *Ureteral pain may begin posteriorly in the costovertebral angle. It may then radiate anteriorly to the ipsilateral lower abdomen, upper thigh, testes, or labium.*

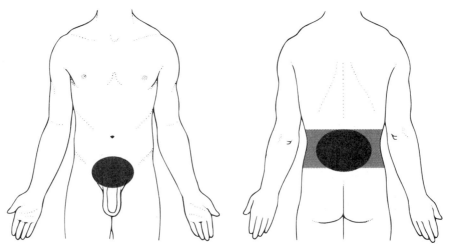

FIGURE 7-7 • *Left,* Bladder or urethral pain is usually felt suprapubically or ipsilaterally in the lower abdomen. *Right,* Bladder or urethral pain may also be perceived in the low back area (*dark red:* primary pain center; *light red:* referred pain). Low back pain may occur as the first and only symptom associated with bladder/urethral pain, or it may occur along with suprapubic or abdominal pain or both.

▼ RENAL AND URINARY TRACT PROBLEMS

Pathologic conditions of the upper and lower urinary tracts can be categorized according to primary causative factors. Three general categories—inflammatory/infectious, obstructive, and mechanical (neuromuscular)—are used for discussion and classification of clinical symptoms in this text.

Inflammatory/Infectious Disorders

Inflammatory disorders of the kidney and urinary tract can be caused by bacterial infection, by changes in immune response, and by toxic agents such as drugs and radiation. Common infections of the urinary tract de-velop in either the upper or lower urinary tract (Table 7-1). Lower urinary tract infections include cystitis (bladder infection) or urethritis (urethra). Symptoms of urinary tract infection (UTI) depend on the location of the infection in either the upper or lower urinary tract (although, rarely, infection could occur in both simultaneously).

Disorders of the Upper Urinary Tract

Infections or inflammations of the upper urinary tract (kidney and ureters) are considered to be more serious because these lesions can be a direct threat to renal tissue itself.

The more common conditions include pyelonephritis (inflammation of the renal parenchyma) and acute and chronic glomerulonephritis (inflammation of the glomeruli of both kidneys). Less common conditions include renal papillary necrosis and renal tuberculosis.

Symptoms of upper urinary tract inflammations and infections are shown in Table 7-2. If the diaphragm is irritated, ipsilateral shoulder pain may occur. Signs and symptoms of renal impairment are also shown in Table 7-2 and, if present, are significant symptoms of impending kidney failure.

Disorders of the Lower Urinary Tract

Both the bladder and urine have a number of defenses against bacterial invasion. These defenses are mechanisms such as voiding, urine acidity, osmolality, and the bladder

---

TABLE 7-1 ▼ Urinary Tract Infections

Upper Urinary Tract Infection	Lower Urinary Tract Infection
Renal infections, such as pyelonephritis (renal parenchyma, i.e., kidney tissue)	Cystitis (bladder infection)
Acute or chronic glomerulonephritis (glomeruli)	Urethritis (urethra infection)
Renal papillary necrosis	
Renal tuberculosis	

TABLE 7-2 ▼ Clinical Symptoms of Infectious/Inflammatory Urinary Tract Problems

Upper Urinary Tract	Lower Urinary Tract	Renal Impairment
Costovertebral tenderness	Urinary frequency	Decreased urinary output
Flank pain	Urinary urgency	Hypertension
Ipsilateral shoulder pain	Dysuria	Dependent edema
Fever and chills	Hematuria	Weakness
Hyperesthesia of dermatomes	Pyuria	Anorexia
Hematuria	Bacteriuria	Shortness of breath
Pyuria	Low back pain	Mild headache
Bacteriuria	Pelvic/lower abdominal pain	Proteinuria
	Dyspareunia	Abnormal blood serum values
		Anemia

▼ *Clinical Signs and Symptoms of*

Upper Urinary Tract Infections
(see Table 7-2)

Symptoms of upper urinary tract infection, particularly renal infection, can be categorized according to urinary tract manifestations or systemic manifestations caused by renal impairment. Clinical signs and symptoms of urinary tract involvement can include:

- Unilateral costovertebral tenderness
- Flank pain
- Ipsilateral shoulder pain
- Fever and chills
- Skin hypersensitivity
- Hematuria (blood in urine)
- Pyuria (pus in urine)
- Bacteriuria (presence of bacteria in urine)

▼ *Clinical Signs and Symptoms of*

Renal Impairment
(see Table 7-2)

- Hypertension
- Decreased urinary output
- Dependent edema
- Weakness
- Anorexia (loss of appetite)
- Dyspnea
- Mild headache
- Proteinuria (protein in urine, urine may be foamy)
- Abnormal blood serum level, such as elevated blood urea nitrogen (BUN) and creatinine
- Anemia

mucosa itself, which is thought to have antibacterial properties.

Urine in the bladder and kidney is normally sterile, but urine itself is a good medium for bacterial growth. Interferences in the defense mechanisms of the bladder, such as the presence of residual or stagnant urine, changes in urinary pH or concentration, or obstruction of urinary excretion, can promote bacterial growth.

Routes of entry of bacteria into the urinary tract can be *ascending* (most commonly up the urethra into the bladder and then into the ureters and kidney), *bloodborne* (bacterial invasion through the bloodstream), or *lymphatic* (bacterial invasion through the lymph system, the least common route).

A lower UTI occurs most commonly in women because of the short female urethra and the proximity of the urethra to the vagina and rectum. The rate of occurrence increases with age and sexual activity. Chronic health problems, such as diabetes mellitus, gout, hypertension, and obstructive urinary tract problems, are also predisposing risk factors for the development of these infections.

Persons with diabetes are prone to complications associated with urinary tract infections. Staphylococcus infection of the urinary tract may be a source of osteomyelitis, an infection of a vertebral body resulting from hematogenous spread or spread from a local abscess into the vertebra. The infected vertebral body may gradually undergo degeneration and destruction, with collapse and formation of a segmental scoliosis (Cailliet, 1995).

This condition is suspected from the onset of nonspecific low back pain, unrelated to any specific motion. Local tenderness can be elicited, but the initial x-ray finding is negative. Usually, a low-grade fever is present but undetected, or it develops as the infection progresses. This is why anyone with low back pain of unknown origin should have his or her temperature taken, even in a physical therapy setting.

Cystitis (inflammation with infection of the bladder), *interstitial cystitis* (inflammation without infection), and *urethritis* (inflammation and infection of the urethra) appear with a similar symptom progression.

Clients with any of these symptoms at presentation should be referred promptly to a physician for further diagnostic work-

Clinical Signs and Symptoms of
Cystitis and Urethritis
(see Table 7-2)

Lower urinary tract symptoms are directly related to irritation of the bladder and urethra. The intensity of symptoms depends on the severity of the infection. These symptoms include:

- Urinary frequency
- Urinary urgency
- Dysuria (discomfort, such as pain or burning during urination)
- Hematuria (presence of RBCs in the urine: may be gross to slight)
- Pyuria (presence of WBCs in the urine)
- Bacteriuria
- Low back pain
- Pelvic/lower abdominal pain
- Pain during intercourse (dyspareunia)

up and possible treatment. Infections of the lower urinary tract are potentially very dangerous because of the possibility of upward spread and resultant damage to renal tissue. Some individuals, however, are asymptomatic, and routine urine culture and microscopic examination are the most reliable methods of detection and diagnosis.

Obstructive Disorders

Urinary tract obstruction can occur at any point in the urinary tract and can be the result of *primary* urinary tract obstructions (obstructions occurring within the urinary tract) or *secondary* urinary tract obstructions (obstructions resulting from disease processes outside the urinary tract). A primary obstruction might include problems such as acquired or congenital malformations, strictures, renal or ureteral calculi (stones), polycystic kidney disease, or neoplasms of the urinary tract (e.g., bladder, kidney).

Secondary obstructions produce pressure on the urinary tract from outside and might be related to conditions such as prostatic enlargement (benign or malignant); abdominal aortic aneurysm; gynecologic conditions such as pregnancy, pelvic inflammatory disease, and endometriosis; or neoplasms of the pelvic or abdominal structures.

Obstruction of any portion of the urinary tract results in a backup or collection of urine behind the obstruction. The result is dilation or stretching of the urinary tract structures that are positioned behind the point of blockage. Muscles near the affected area contract in an attempt to push urine around the obstruction. Pressure accumulates above the point of obstruction and can eventually result in severe dilation of the renal collecting system (hydronephrosis) and renal failure. The greater the intensity and duration of the pressure, the greater is the destruction of renal tissue.

Because urine flow is decreased with obstruction, urinary stagnation and infection or stone formation can result. Stones are formed because urine stasis permits clumping or precipitation of organic matter and minerals. Lower urinary tract obstruction can also result in constant bladder distension, hypertrophy of bladder muscle fibers, and formation of herniated sacs of bladder mucosa. These herniated sacs result in a large, flaccid bladder that cannot empty completely. In addition, these sacs retain stagnant urine, which causes infection and stone formation.

Disorders of the Upper Urinary Tract

Obstruction of the upper urinary tract may be sudden (acute) or slow in development. Tumors of the kidney or ureters may develop slowly enough that symptoms are totally absent or very mild initially, with eventual progression to pain and signs of impairment. *Acute* ureteral or renal blockage by a stone (calculus consisting of mineral salts), for example, may result in excruciating, spasmodic, and radiating pain accompanied by severe nausea and vomiting.

Calculi form primarily in the kidney. This process is called *nephrolithiasis*. The

Case Example. A 55-year-old woman came to the clinic with back pain associated with paraspinal muscle spasms. Pain was of unknown cause (insidious onset), and the client reported that she was "just getting out of bed" when the pain started. The pain was described as a dull aching that was aggravated by movement and relieved by rest (musculoskeletal pattern).

No numbness, tingling, or saddle anesthesia was reported, and the neurologic screening examination was negative. Sacroiliac (SI) testing was negative. Spinal movements were slow and guarded, with muscle spasms noted throughout movement and at rest. Because of her age and the insidious onset of symptoms, further questions were initiated to screen for medical disease.

This client was midmenopausal and undergoing no hormone replacement therapy (HRT). She had had a bladder infection a month ago that was treated with antibiotics; tests for this were negative when she was evaluated and referred by her physician for back pain. Two weeks ago she had had an upper respiratory infection (a "cold") and had been "coughing a lot." There was no previous history of cancer.

Local treatment to reduce paraspinal muscle spasms was initiated, but the client did not respond as expected over the course of five treatment sessions. Because of her recent history of upper respiratory and bladder infections, questions related to the presence of constitutional symptoms and changes in bladder function/urine color, force of stream, burning on urination, and so on were repeated. Occasional "sweats" (present sometimes during the day, sometimes at night) was the only red flag present. The combination of recent infection, failure to respond to treatment, and the presence of sweats suggested referral to the physician for early reevaluation.

The client did not return to the clinic for further treatment, and a follow-up telephone call indicated that she did indeed have a recurrent bladder infection that was treated successfully with antibiotics. Her back pain and muscle spasm were eliminated after only 24 hours of taking a different antibiotic.

stones can remain in the kidney (renal pelvis) or travel down the urinary tract and lodge at any point in the tract.* The most characteristic symptom of renal or ureteral stones is sudden, sharp, severe pain. If the pain originates deep in the lumbar area and radiates around the side and down toward the testicle in the male and the bladder in the female, it is termed *renal colic. Ureteral colic* occurs if the stone becomes trapped in the ureter. Ureteral colic is characterized by radiation of painful symptoms toward the genitalia and thighs.†

---

*Strictly speaking, the term *kidney stones* refers to stones that are in the kidney. Once they move into the ureter, they become ureteral stones; these are the stones that cause the most pain.

†The testicles and ovaries form in utero (where the kidneys are at full term) and then migrate, following the pathways of the ureters. For this reason kidney stones moving down the pathway of the ureters cause pain in the flank, radiating to the scrotum (male) and the labia (female). For the same reason ovarian or testicular cancer can refer pain to the back at the level of the kidneys.

CAUSES OF URINARY TRACT OBSTRUCTION

URETHRA AND BLADDER NECK

- Benigh prostatic hypertrophy
- Urethral stricture
- Urethral valves
- Meatal stenosis
- Phimosis

BLADDER

- Neurogenic bladder
- Blood clot
- Calculus
- Carcinoma of bladder

URETER

- Intrinsic obstruction (calculus, blood clot, renal papilla, carcinoma of ureter)
- Extrinsic obstruction (retroperitoneal or pelvic tumors, strictures, retroperitoneal fibrosis, uterine prolapse, ureterocele)
- Reflux (vesicoureteral reflux, megaloureter)

URETEROPELVIC JUNCTION

- Intrinsic obstruction (calculus, blood clot, renal papilla)
- Extrinsic obstruction (stricture, aberrant vessels, fibrous band)

RENAL PELVIS

- Calculus
- Blood clot
- Papilla
- Carcinoma of renal pelvis, carcinoma of kidney
- Tuberculosis

From Fang LST: Renal diseases. In Ramsey PG, Larson EB: *Medical therapeutics*, Philadelphia, 1993, WB Saunders.

Renal tumors may also be detected as a flank mass combined with unexplained weight loss, fever, pain, and hematuria. The presence of any amount of blood in the urine is always grounds for referral to a physician for further diagnostic evaluation because this is a primary symptom of urinary tract neoplasm.

Disorders of the Lower Urinary Tract

Common conditions of obstruction of the lower urinary tract are bladder tumors (bladder cancer is the most common site of urinary tract cancer) and prostatic enlargement, either benign (benign prostatic hypertrophy [BPH]) or malignant (cancer of the prostate). An enlarged prostate

Clinical Signs and Symptoms of
Obstruction of the Upper Urinary Tract

- Pain (depends on the rapidity of onset and on the location)
  - Acute, spasmodic, radiating
  - Mild and dull flank pain
  - Lumbar discomfort with some renal diseases or renal back pain with ureteral obstruction
- Hyperesthesia of dermatomes (T10 through L1)
- Nausea and vomiting
- Palpable flank mass
- Hematuria
- Fever and chills
- Urge to urinate frequently
- Abdominal muscle spasms
- Renal impairment indicators (see inside front cover: Renal Blood Studies; see also Table 7-2)

gland can occlude the urethra partially or completely.

Benign prostatic hypertrophy is a common complaint in men older than 50. Because of the prostate's position around the urethra (see Fig. 7-3), enlargement of the prostate quickly interferes with the normal passage of urine from the bladder.

Urination becomes increasingly difficult, and the bladder never feels completely empty. If left untreated, continued enlargement of the prostate eventually obstructs the bladder completely, and emergency measures become necessary to empty the bladder.

If the prostate is greatly enlarged, chronic constipation may result. Prostatitis is a relatively common inflammation of the prostate and may be acute or chronic.

Cancer of the prostate usually occurs in men older than 50. It is often diagnosed when the man seeks medical assistance because of symptoms of urinary obstruction or low back, hip, or leg pain. These symptoms can be caused by metastasis of the cancer to the bones of the pelvis, lumbar spine, or femur. (See the Case Study at the end of this chapter.)

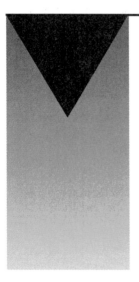

Case Example. A 66-year-old man with low back pain was evaluated by a female physical therapist but treated by a male physical therapy aide. By the end of the third session, the client reports some improvement in his painful symptoms. During the second week there is no improvement and even a possible slight setback. During the treatment session he comments to the aide that he is impotent.

Given this man's age, inconsistent response to therapy, and report of impotency, a medical referral was necessary. A brief note was sent to the physician relating this information and requesting medical follow-up. (The therapist was careful to use the word *follow-up* rather than *medical reevaluation* since the impotency was present at the time of the initial medical evaluation.)

Result. A medical diagnosis of testicular cancer was established, and appropriate treatment was initiated. Physical therapy was discontinued until medical treatment was completed and systemic origin of the back pain could be ruled out.

▼ *Clinical Signs and Symptoms of*
Obstruction of the Lower Urinary Tract

Lower urinary tract symptoms of blockage are most commonly related to bladder or urethral pressure (e.g., prostate enlargement). This pressure results in bladder distension and subsequent pain. Common symptoms of lower urinary tract obstruction include:

- Bladder palpable above the symphysis pubis
- Suprapubic or pelvic pain
- Difficulty in voiding
- Hesitancy: Difficulty in initiating urination or an interrupted flow of urine
- Small amounts of urine with voiding
- Lower abdominal discomfort with a feeling of the need to void
- Nocturia (unusual voiding during the night)
- Hematuria (RBCs in the urine)
- Low back, pelvic, and/or thigh pain

▼ *Clinical Signs and Symptoms of*
Prostatitis

- Sudden moderate-to-high fever
- Chills
- Low back and perineal pain
- Urinary frequency and urgency
- Nocturia
- Dysuria (painful or difficult urination)
- Weak or interrupted urine stream
- General malaise
- Arthralgia
- Myalgia

Mechanical (Neuromuscular) Disorders

Mechanical problems of the urinary tract relate specifically to difficulty with emptying urine from the bladder. Improper emptying of the bladder results in urinary retention and impairment of voluntary bladder control (incontinence). Several possible causes of mechanical bladder dysfunction include mechanical stress (stress incontinence), spinal cord injury, central nervous system disease (e.g., multiple sclerosis and Guillain-Barré syndrome), UTI, partial urethral obstruction, trauma, and removal of the prostate gland.

Incontinence

The Clinical Practice Guideline Update (1996) for urinary incontinence (UI) in adults identifies four primary types of urinary incontinence: (1) stress, (2) urge, (3) mixed (combination of urge and stress), and (4) overflow. Causes of incontinence can range from urologic/gynecologic to neurologic, psychologic, pharmacologic, or environmental. Disruptions in the cycle of micturition (urination) may occur for many different physiologic reasons and are beyond the scope of this text. The reader is referred to the Clinical Practice Guideline Update (1996) for more detailed information.

Incontinence is not a normal part of the aging process. When confronted with urinary incontinence in an older adult, consider some of the following causes of this disorder: infection, endocrine disorders, atrophic urethritis or vaginitis, restricted mobility, stool impaction (especially in smokers)*, alcohol or caffeine intake, and medications. Medications commonly involved with alterations in urinary continence include anticholinergic agents, calcium channel blockers, diuretics, sedatives, α-antagonists, and α-agonists (Yim and Peterson, 1996).

Overflow incontinence is an overdistension of the bladder. It may be caused by

---

*Smoking contributes to constipation and is often accompanied by chronic cough, which stresses the bladder. Chronic constipation leads to frequent straining to defecate, causing damage to tissue in the lower pelvis. Additionally, obesity places excess pressure on the bladder.

an acontractile detrusor (bladder) muscle, a hypotonic or underactive detrusor muscle secondary to drugs, fecal impaction, diabetes, lower spinal cord injury, or disruption of the motor innervation of the detrusor muscle (e.g., multiple sclerosis). In men, overflow incontinence is most often secondary to obstruction caused by prostatic hyperplasia, prostatic carcinoma, or urethral stricture. In women, this type of incontinence occurs as a result of obstruction caused by severe genital prolapse or surgical overcorrection of urethral detachment.

Stress incontinence occurs when pressure applied to the bladder from coughing, sneezing, laughing, lifting, exercising, or other physical exertion increases abdominal pressure and the pelvic floor musculature cannot counteract the urethral/bladder pressure. This type of incontinence causes 75% of all cases of urinary incontinence in women and is primarily related to urethral sphincter weakness, pelvic floor weakness, and ligamentous and fascial laxity.

Risk factors for women include pregnancy followed by a long and difficult vaginal delivery, postmenopause without hormone replacement, frequent high-impact aerobics, heavy lifting, chronic constipation, obesity, and smoking.

Urge incontinence is the involuntary loss of urine associated with a strong desire to void (urgency). The bladder involuntarily contracts or is unstable, or there may be involuntary sphincter relaxation. Alcohol, certain medications, bladder infections, and nerve damage can cause urge incontinence.

With any kind of incontinence, the onset of cervical spine pain at the same time that urinary incontinence develops is a red flag. These two findings would suggest that there is a protrusion pressing on the spinal cord. If a medical diagnosis for cervical disk protrusion has been established, referral would not be necessary. However, in such a case, the physician should be made aware of this information. Cervical spinal manipulation is considered contraindicated.

Renal Failure

A person is unlikely to seek treatment for renal problems from the physical therapist. However, renal patients/clients may receive treatment for primary musculoskeletal lesions in both inpatient and outpatient clinics.

Renal failure exists when the kidneys can no longer maintain the homeostatic balances within the body that are necessary for life. Renal failure is classified as acute or chronic in origin and progression.

Acute renal failure refers to the abrupt cessation of kidney activity, usually occurring over a period of hours to a few days. Acute renal failure is often reversible, with return of kidney function in 3 to 12 months.

Chronic renal failure, or irreversible renal failure, is defined as a state of progressive reduction of renal functioning resulting in eventual permanent loss of kidney function. It can develop slowly over a period of years or can result from an episode of acute renal failure that does not resolve. Diabetes mellitus and hypertension are the most common causes of chronic renal failure.

CLINICAL SIGNS AND SYMPTOMS

Failure of the filtering and regulating mechanisms of the kidney can be either acute (sudden in onset and potentially reversible) or chronic (called uremia, which develops gradually and is usually irreversible). Individuals with either type of renal failure develop signs and symptoms characteristic of impaired fluid and waste excretion and altered renal regulation of other body metabolic processes, such as pH regulation, RBC production, and calcium-phosphorus balance.

Signs of renal impairment are shown in Table 7-2. The signs of actual renal failure are the same but more pronounced. In most cases of renal failure, urine volume is significantly decreased or absent. Edema becomes severe and can result in heart failure. Renal anemia is usually associated with extreme fatigue and intolerance to normal daily activities.

TABLE 7-3 ▼ Systemic Manifestations of Renal Failure

Systemic Symptoms	Probable Causes
Urinary System	
Decreased urinary output	Damaged renal tissue
Abnormal urinary constituents (blood cells, protein, casts)	
Cardiopulmonary	
Hypertension	Fluid overload
Congestive heart failure	
Pulmonary edema	
Pericarditis	Uremic toxins irritate pericardial sac
Gastrointestinal Tract	
Bleeding	Irritation of gastric mucosa by uremic toxins combined with platelet changes
Nausea and vomiting	
Uremic breath	Uremic toxins change saliva
Anorexia	
Nervous System	
Central (CNS)	
Irritability	Effect of uremic toxins on brain cells (usually resolve with dialysis treatment)
Impaired judgment	
Inability to concentrate	
Seizures	
Lethargy/coma	
Sleep disturbances	
Peripheral (PNS)	
Loss of vibratory sense and deep tendon reflexes	Effect of uremic toxins on peripheral nerves
Impairment of motor nerve conduction velocity	
Burning, tingling, paresthesias	
Tremors	Electrolyte imbalances (calcium, sodium, potassium)
Muscle cramps, muscle twitching	
Foot drop	
Weakness	
Integumentary (Skin)	
Pruritus (itching)/excoriation (scratching)	Skin calcifications related to calcium/phosphorus imbalances
Hyperpigmentation	Retained uremic pigments
Pallor	Anemia
Bruising	Platelet dysfunction
Eyes	
Band keratopathy	Corneal calcifications related to calcium/phosphorus imbalance
Visual blurring	
Red eyes	Conjunctival calcifications related to calcium/phosphorus imbalance
Endocrine	
Fertility and sexual dysfunction	Effect of uremic toxins on menstrual cycles, ovulation, and sperm production
Hyperparathyroidism	Result of calcium/phosphorus imbalance
Hematopoietic	
Anemia	Decreased production of erythropoietin by kidney
	Destruction of RBCs by dialysis
Platelet dysfunction	Uremic toxins interfere with platelet aggregation
Skeletal	
Renal osteodystrophy (demineralization of bones)	Related to decreased calcium absorption and resultant calcium/phosphorus imbalance
Joint pain	Joint calcifications

In addition, the continuous presence of toxic waste products in the bloodstream (urea, creatinine, uric acid) results in damage to many other body systems, including the central nervous system, peripheral nervous system, eyes, gastrointestinal tract, integumentary system, endocrine system, and cardiopulmonary system (Table 7-3).

Treatment of renal failure involves several elements designed to replace the lost excretory and metabolic functions of this organ. Treatment options include dialysis, dietary changes, and medications to regulate blood pressure and assist in replacement of lost metabolic functions, such as calcium balance and RBC production.

The choice of treatment options, such as dialysis, transplantation, or no treatment, depends on many factors, including the person's age, underlying physical problems, and availability of compatible organs for transplantation. Untreated or chronic renal failure eventually results in death.

OVERVIEW RENAL AND UROLOGIC PAIN PATTERNS

▼ KIDNEY (see Fig. 7-4)

Location:
Posterior subcostal and costovertebral region

Usually unilateral

Referral:
Radiates forward, around the flank or the side into the lower abdominal quadrant (T11 to T12), along the pelvic crest and into the groin

Pressure from the kidney on the diaphragm may cause ipsilateral shoulder pain

Description:
Dull aching, boring

Intensity:
Acute: Severe, intense

Chronic: Vague and poorly localized

Duration:
Constant

Associated Signs and Symptoms:
Fever, chills

Increased urinary frequency

Blood in urine

Hyperesthesia of associated dermatomes (T9 and T10)

Ipsilateral or generalized abdominal pain

Spasm of abdominal muscles

Nausea and vomiting when severely acute

Testicular pain may occur in men

Unrelieved by a change in position

▼ URETER* (see Fig. 7-6)

Location: Costovertebral angle
                       Unilateral or bilateral
Referral: Radiates to the lower abdomen, upper thigh, testis, or labium on the same side (groin and genital area)
Description: Described as crescendo waves of colic
Intensity: Excruciating, severe
Duration: Ureteral pain caused by calculus is intermittent or constant without relief until treated or until the stone is passed
Associated Signs and Symptoms:
                       Rectal tenesmus (painful spasm of anal sphincter with urgent desire to evacuate the bowel/bladder; involuntary straining with little passage of urine or feces)
                       Nausea, abdominal distension, vomiting
                       Hyperesthesia of associated dermatomes (T10 to L1)
                       Tenderness over the kidney or ureter
                       Unrelieved by a change in position
                       Movement of iliopsoas may aggravate symptoms associated with a lesion outside the ureter (see Fig. 6-8)

▼ BLADDER/URETHRA (see Fig. 7-7)

Location: Suprapubic or low abdomen, low back
Referral: Pelvis
                       Can be confused with gas
Description: Sharp, localized
Intensity: Moderate to severe
Duration: Intermittent; may be relieved by emptying the bladder
Associated Signs and Symptoms:
                       Great urinary urgency
                       Tenesmus
                       Dysuria
                       Hot or burning sensation during urination

*NOTE: Ureteral pain is commonly acute and caused by a calculus (kidney stone). Lesions outside the ureter are usually painless until advanced progression of the disease occurs.

CLUES SUGGESTING PAIN OF RENAL/UROLOGIC ORIGIN

- Men 45 years old or older
- In men, back pain accompanied by burning on urination, difficulty in urination, or fever may be associated with prostatitis; usually in such a case there is no limitation of back motion and no muscle spasm (until symptoms progress, causing muscle guarding and splinting)
- Blood in urine
- Presence of constitutional symptoms, especially fever and chills
- Change in urinary frequency, flow of urine stream
- Pain is constant (may be dull or sharp, depending on the cause)
- Pain is unchanged by altering body position; sidebending to the involved side and pressure at that level is "more comfortable" (may reduce pain but does not eliminate it)
- Straight leg–raising test is negative with renal colic appearing as back pain
- Back pain at the level of the kidneys in a woman with previous breast or uterine cancer (ovarian cancer)
- Assess for pseudorenal pain
  - Usually traumatic history (e.g., fall, assault, blow, lifting)
  - Pain is affected by change of position (e.g., lying on the involved side increases pain, prolonged sitting increases pain, symptoms are reproduced with movements of the spine)
  - Check for costovertebral angle tenderness (see Fig. 7-5)
  - No associated signs and symptoms present

▼ DIAGNOSTIC TESTING

Screening of the composition of the urine is called *urinalysis* (UA), and UA is the commonly used method of determining various properties of urine. This analysis is actually a series of several tests of urinary components and is a valuable aid in the diagnosis of urinary tract or metabolic disorders. Normal urinary constituents are shown (see inside front cover: Urine Analysis). Urine cultures are also very important studies in the diagnosis of UTIs.

Various *blood studies* can be done to assess renal function (see inside front cover: Renal Blood Studies). These studies examine both the serum and cellular components of the blood for specific changes characteristic of renal performance. Substances that must be examined in the serum are those that are a *direct* reflection of renal function, such as creatinine, and others that are more *indirect* in renal evaluation, such as BUN, pH-related substances, uric acid, various

ions, electrolytes, and cellular components (RBCs).*

▼ PHYSICIAN REFERRAL

Pain related to a urinary tract pathologic condition is often similar to pain felt from an injury to the back, flank, abdomen, or upper thigh. Further diagnostic testing and medical examination must be performed by the physician to differentiate urinary tract conditions from musculoskeletal problems. The proximity of the kidneys, ureters, bladder, and urethra to the ribs, vertebrae, diaphragm, and accompanying muscles and tendinous

---

*Understanding laboratory values has become necessary for the physical therapist in the acute care or nursing home setting. For an in-depth discussion, the reader is referred to Goodman and Boissonnault, 1998; Polich and Faynor, 1996.

GUIDELINES FOR IMMEDIATE MEDICAL ATTENTION

- Presence of cervical spine pain at the same time that urinary incontinence develops: If a diagnosis of cervical disk prolapse has been made, the physician should be notified of these findings and referral is not necessary.
- Client with bowel/bladder incontinence and/or saddle anesthesia secondary to cauda equina lesion.

insertions often can make it difficult to identify the client's problems accurately.

The physical therapist must be able to recognize the systemic origin of urinary tract symptoms that mimic musculoskeletal pain. Many conditions that produce urinary tract pain also include an elevation in temperature, abnormal urinary constituents, and changes in color, odor, or amount of urine.

The presence of any amount of blood in the urine always requires a referral to a physician. However, the presence of abnormalities in the urine may not be obvious, and thus a thorough diagnostic analysis of the urine may be needed. Careful questioning of the client regarding urinary tract history, urinary patterns, urinary characteristics, and pain patterns may elicit valuable information relating to potential urinary tract symptoms.

Referral by a physical therapist to the physician is recommended when the client has any combination of systemic signs and symptoms presented in this chapter. Damage to urinary tract structures can occur concurrently with trauma and damage to musculoskeletal structures, which are in the same anatomic location.

For example, the alpine skier discussed at the beginning of the chapter had a dull, aching costovertebral pain on the left side that was unrelieved by a change of position or by ice, heat, or aspirin. His pain is related directly to a traumatic episode, and musculoskeletal injury is a definite possibility in his case. He has no medical history of urinary tract problems and denies any urine changes. Because the pain is constant and is unrelieved by usual measures and the location of the pain is approximate to the renal structures, a medical follow-up and urinalysis would be recommended.

When making a medical referral, the physical therapist should review the signs and symptoms listed in the next section, the findings of the objective examination combined with the medical history, and the current symptom complex.

Systemic Signs and Symptoms Requiring Physician Referral

The physical therapist is advised to question the client further whenever any of the following signs and symptoms are reported or observed:

Abdominal muscle spasms

Anorexia

Anuria (totally absent urine)

Decreased urinary output

Dependent edema

Dyspnea

Dysuria

Fever and chills

Flank pain

Foul odor to urine

Headache

Hematuria (change in urine color: black, brown, gray, or red)

Hypertension

Incontinence

Low back and perineal pain

Nausea and vomiting

Proteinuria

Pyuria (cloudy urine)

Shoulder pain (result of pressure from the kidney on the diaphragm)

Skin hyperesthesia (T9-L1)
Small amounts of urine with voiding
Spasmodic radiating pain to the testis, labia, thigh, suprapubic or pelvic area
Unilateral costovertebral tenderness

Unusual nocturia
Urinary frequency
Urinary hesitancy
Urinary urgency
Weakness

GUIDELINES FOR PHYSICIAN REFERRAL

- Presence of any amount of blood in the urine always requires a referral to a physician.
- Damage to the urinary tract structures can occur with accident, injury, assault, or other trauma to the musculoskeletal structures surrounding the kidney and urinary tract and may require medical evaluation if the clinical presentation or response to physical therapy treatment suggests it.
- Back or shoulder pain accompanied by abnormal urinary constituents (e.g., change in color, odor, amount, flow of urine).
- Positive Murphy's percussion test, especially with a recent history of renal or urologic infection.

COMMON SYMPTOMS OF GENITOURINARY DISEASE

WOMEN

- Abnormal vaginal bleeding
- Painful menstruation (dysmenorrhea)
- Pelvic masses or lesions
- Vaginal itching or discharge
- Abdominal, low back, or pelvic pain
- Pain during intercourse (dyspareunia)
- Changes in urinary pattern
- Pain with urination
- Changes in menstrual pattern
- Infertility

MEN

- Urinary tract, pelvic, low back, or leg pain
- Painful burning on urination
- Changes in urinary pattern or urine flow
- Red urine
- Discharge
- Penile lesions
- Enlargement of scrotal contents
- Swelling or mass in groin
- Impotence
- Infertility

Modified from Swartz M: *Textbook of physical diagnosis*, Philadelphia, 1989, WB Saunders.

KEY POINTS TO REMEMBER

▶ Renal and urologic pain can be referred to the shoulder or low back.

▶ Lesions outside the ureter can cause pain on movement of the adjacent iliopsoas muscle.

▶ Radiculitis can mimic ureteral colic or renal pain, but true renal pain is seldom affected by movements of the spine.

▶ Low-back, pelvic, or femur pain may be the first symptom of prostate cancer.

▶ Inflammatory pain may be relieved by a change in position. Renal colic remains unchanged by a change in position.

▶ Urinary incontinence is not a normal part of aging and should be evaluated carefully. Incontinence concomitant with cervical spine pain contraindicates the use of cervical spinal manipulation.

▶ All the possible pain patterns discussed in this chapter are presented as follows:

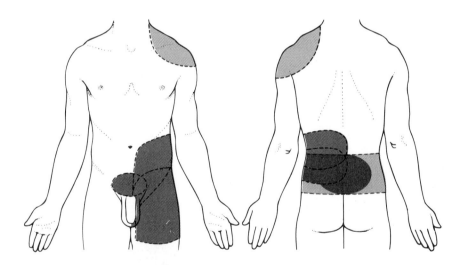

SUBJECTIVE EXAMINATION

● SPECIAL QUESTIONS TO ASK

Clients may be reluctant to answer the physical therapist's questions concerning bladder and urinary function. The physical therapist is advised to explain the need to rule out possible causes of pain related to the kidneys and bladder and to give the client time to respond if answers seem to be uncertain. For example, the physical therapist may ask the client to observe urinary function over the next 2 days. These questions should be reviewed again at the next appointment.

Past Medical History

● Have you had any problems with your prostate (for men), kidneys, or bladder? *If so,* describe.

- Have you ever had kidney or bladder stones? *If so,* when? How were these stones treated?

- Have you had an injury to your bladder or kidneys? *If so,* when? How was this treated? (**Be aware of unreported domestic abuse/assault.**)

- Have you had any kidney or bladder infections in the past 6 months? How were these infections treated? Were they related to any specific circumstances (**e.g., pregnancy, intercourse, after strep throat or strep skin infections**)?

- Have you ever had surgery on your bladder or kidneys? *If so,* when and what?

- Have you had any hernias? *If yes,* when and how was this treated?

Associated Signs and Symptoms*

- Have you had any side (flank) pain (**kidney or ureter**) or pain just above the pubic area (**suprapubic: bladder or urethra**)?

    - *If so,* what relieves this pain? Does a change in position affect it? (**Inflammatory pain** may be relieved by a change in position. **Renal colic** remains unchanged by a change in position.)

- During the last 2 to 3 weeks have you noticed a change in the amount or number of times that you urinate? (**Infection**)

    - Have you had to urinate during the night during the last 2 to 3 weeks? *If yes,* is this a change in pattern or unusual for you?

    - Does this happen every night or just when you drink a large amount of fluid before bedtime? (**Nocturia can be a sign of systemic disease but may also indicate a diminished bladder capacity or inability to empty the bladder completely.**)

- When you urinate, do you have trouble starting or continuing the flow of urine? (**Urethral obstruction**)

    - (Alternately): Do you urinate in a steady stream, or do you start and stop the flow of urination?

- Has your urine stream changed in size? *If so,* describe. (**Urethral obstruction**); early symptoms of enlarging prostate may be ignored or unreported by the client

- When you are finished urinating, do you feel like your bladder is completely empty? (**Bladder dysfunction; enlarged prostate**)

- Do you ever have pain or a burning sensation when you urinate? (**Lower urinary tract irritation; venereal disease**)

- Do you ever dribble urine, leak urine, or have trouble holding your urine?

    - Do you accidentally leak when you sneeze, laugh, cough, or bear down? (**Stress incontinence;** may be caused by weakness or medications such as antihistamines, antispasmodics, sedatives, diuretics, and psychotropic drugs.)

For men: Before asking these detailed and specific questions, make sure that you have asked about a past history of prostate problems. If yes, follow-up questions flow accordingly with comparisons made between symptoms then and symptoms now.

- Does your urine look brown, red, or black? (**Hematuria** or may be normal with some medications and foods such as beets or rhubarb.)

- Is your urine clear or cloudy? If not clear, describe. How often does this happen? (Could indicate **upper or lower urinary tract infection.**)

- Have you noticed an unusual or foul odor coming from your urine? (**Infection, secondary to medication;** may be normal after eating asparagus.)

Questions for Women

- Have you noticed any unusual vaginal discharge during the time that you had pain (pubic, flank, thigh, back, labia)? (**Infection**)

Questions for Men

- Have you noticed any unusual discharge from your penis during the time that you had pain (especially pain above the pubic area)? (**Infection**)

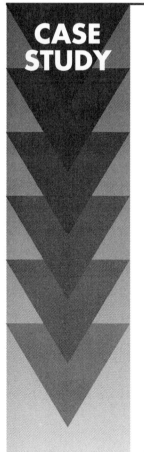

CASE STUDY

REFERRAL

The client is self-referred and states that he has been to your hospital-based outpatient clinic in the past. He has a very extensive chart containing his entire medical history for the last 20 years.

BACKGROUND INFORMATION

He is a 44-year-old man who describes his current occupation as "errand boy/gopher," which requires minimal lifting, bending, or strenuous physical activity. His chief complaint today is pain in the lower back, which comes and goes and seems to be aggravated by sitting. The pain is poorly described, and the client is unable to specify any kind of descriptive words for the type of pain, intensity, or duration.

SPECIAL QUESTIONS TO ASK

See Chapter 12 for Special Questions to Ask about the back. The client's answer to any questions related to bowel and bladder functions is either "I don't know" or "Well, you know," which makes a complete interview impossible.

SUBJECTIVE/OBJECTIVE FINDINGS

There are radiating symptoms of numbness down the left leg to the foot. The client denies any saddle anesthesia. Deep tendon reflexes are intact bilaterally, and the client stands with an obvious scoliotic list to one side. He is unable to tell you whether his symptoms are relieved or alleviated on performing a lateral shift to correct the curve. There are no other positive neuromuscular findings or associated systemic symptoms.

RESULT

After 3 days of treatment over the course of 1 week, the client has had no subjective improvement in symptoms. Objectively, the scoliotic shift has not

continued

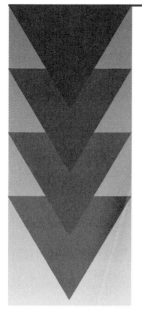

changed. A second opinion is sought from two other staff members, and the consensus is to refer the client to his physician. The physician performs a rectal examination and confirms a positive diagnosis of prostatitis based on the results of laboratory tests. These test were consistent with the client's physical findings and previous history of prostate problems 1 year ago. The client was reluctant to discuss bowel or bladder function with the female therapist but readily suggested to his physician that his current symptoms mimicked an earlier episode of prostatitis.

It is not always possible to elicit thorough responses from clients concerning matters of genitourinary function. If the client hesitates or is unable to answer questions satisfactorily, it may be necessary to present the questions again at a later time (e.g., next treatment session), to ask a colleague of the client's sex to confer with the client, or to refer the client to his or her physician for further evaluation. Occasionally, the client will answer negatively to any questions regarding observed changes in urinary function and will then report back at the next session that there was some pathologic condition that was not noted earlier.

In this case a close review of the extensive medical records may have alerted the physical therapist to the client's previous treatment for the same problem, which he was reluctant to discuss.

PRACTICE QUESTIONS

1. Percussion of the costovertebral angle that results in the reproduction of symptoms:

   a. Signifies radiculitis

   b. Signifies pseudorenal pain

   c. Has no significance

   d. Requires medical referral

2. Renal pain is aggravated by:

   a. Spinal movement

   b. Palpatory pressure over the costovertebral angle

   c. Lying on the involved side

   d. All of the above

   e. None of the above

3. Important functions of the kidney include all the following *except:*

   a. Formation and excretion of urine

   b. Acid-base and electrolyte balance

   c. Stimulation of red blood cell production

   d. Production of glucose

4. Who should be screened for possible renal/urologic involvement?

5. What do the following terms mean?

   • Dyspareunia

   • Dysuria

   • Hematuria

   • Urgency

6. What is the difference between urge incontinence and stress incontinence?

7. What is the significance of "skin pain" over the T9/T10 dermatomes?

8. How do you screen for possible prostate involvement in a man with pelvic/low-back pain of unknown cause?

9. Explain why renal/urologic pain can be felt through the T9 to L1 dermatomes.

10. What is the mechanism of referral for urologic pain to the shoulder?

References

Cailliet R: *Low back pain syndrome,* ed 5, Philadelphia, 1995, FA Davis.

Clinical practice guideline update: managing acute and chronic urinary incontinence, Rockville, Md, 1996, U.S. Department of Health and Human Services, Publ. No. 96-0686.

Goodman CC, Boissonnault WG: *Pathology: implications for the physical therapist,* Philadelphia, 1998, WB Saunders.

Polich S, Faynor S: Interpreting lab test values, *PT Magazine* 4(1):76-88, 1996.

Smith DR, Raney FL Jr: Radiculitis distress as a mimic of renal pain, *J Urol* 116:269, 1976.

Travell JG, Simons DG: *Myofascial pain and dysfunction: The Trigger Point Manual,* vol 1, Baltimore, 1983, Williams & Wilkins.

Yim PS, Peterson AS: Urinary incontinence, *Postgrad Med* 99(5):137-150, 1996.

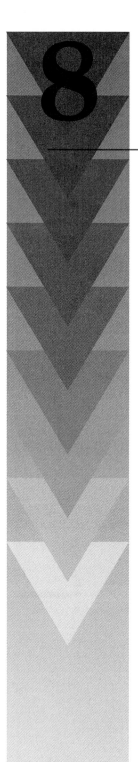

Overview of Hepatic and Biliary Signs and Symptoms

8

As with many of the organ systems in the human body, the hepatic and biliary organs (liver, gallbladder, and common bile duct) (Fig. 8-1) can develop diseases that mimic primary musculoskeletal lesions. The musculoskeletal symptoms associated with hepatic and biliary pathologic conditions are generally confined to the midback, scapular, and right shoulder regions. These musculoskeletal symptoms can occur alone (as the only presenting symptom) or in combination with other systemic signs and symptoms discussed in this chapter.

▼ HEPATIC AND BILIARY SYMPTOMS

The major causes of acute hepatocellular injury include hepatitis, drug-induced hepatitis, and ingestion of toxins. The physical therapist is most likely to encounter liver or gallbladder diseases manifested by a variety of signs and symptoms outlined in this section.

Taking a careful history and making close observations of the client's physical condition and appearance can detect telltale signs of hepatic disease. Medical diagnosis of liver or gallbladder disease is made by x-ray examination or ultrasonic scanning of the gallbladder and computed tomography (CT) scanning of the abdomen, including the liver. Laboratory tests useful in the diagnosis and treatment of liver and biliary tract disease are listed inside the front cover.

Skin Changes

Skin changes associated with the hepatic system include *jaundice,* pallor, and orange or green skin. In some situations jaundice may be the first and only manifestation of disease. It is first noticeable in the sclera of the eye as a yellow hue when bilirubin reaches levels of 2 to 3 mg/dl. When the bilirubin level reaches 5 to 6 mg/dl, the skin becomes yellow.

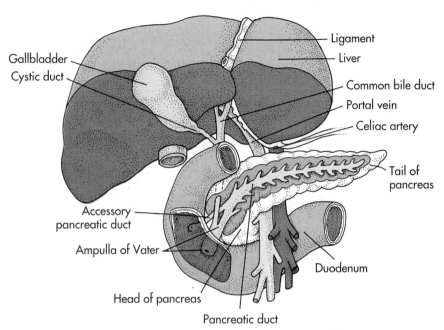

FIGURE 8-1 ● Anatomy of the liver, gallbladder, common bile duct, and pancreas.

Skin changes accompanied by dark urine and hepatitis, gallbladder disease, and/or pancreatic cancer blocking the bile duct, hepatotoxic medications, or cirrhosis may cause associated light stools. Normally, bile that is converted from bilirubin causes the stool to assume a brown color. Light-colored (almost white) stools and urine the color of tea or cola indicate an inability of the liver or biliary system to excrete bilirubin properly. Other skin changes may include bruising, spider angiomas, and palmar erythema.

Spider angiomas (arterial spider, spider telangiectasis, vascular spider), branched dilations of the superficial capillaries resembling a spider in appearance, may be vascular manifestations of increased estrogen levels (hyperestrogenism). Spider angiomas and palmar erythema both occur in the presence of liver impairment as a result of increased estrogen levels normally detoxified by the liver. *Palmar erythema* (warm redness of the skin over the palms, also called *liver palms*) especially affects the hypothenar and thenar emi-nences and pulps of the finger. The soles of the feet may be similarly affected. The person may complain of throbbing, tingling palms.

Musculoskeletal Pain

Musculoskeletal pain associated with the hepatic and biliary systems includes thoracic pain between the scapulae, right shoulder, right upper trapezius, right interscapular, or right subscapular areas (Fig. 8-2 and Table 8-1).

Referred shoulder pain may be the only presenting symptom of hepatic or biliary disease. Sympathetic fibers from the biliary system are connected through the celiac (abdominal) and splanchnic (visceral) plexuses to the hepatic fibers in the region of the dorsal spine.

These connections account for the intercostal and radiating interscapular pain that accompanies gallbladder disease. Although the innervation is bilateral, most of the biliary fibers reach the cord through the

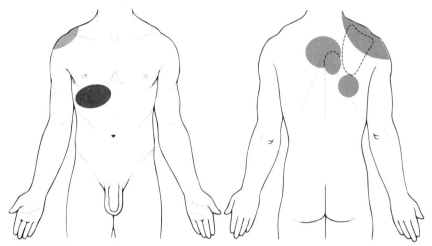

FIGURE 8-2 • Pain from the liver, gallbladder, and common bile duct *(dark red)* occurs typically in the midepigastrium or right upper quadrant of the abdomen, with referred pain *(light red)* to the right shoulder, interscapular, or subscapular area.

TABLE 8-1 ▼ Referred Pain Patterns: Liver, Gallbladder, Common Bile Duct

Systemic Causes	Location
Upper Back/Scapulae Area	
Gallbladder	Midback between scapulae; right upper trapezius; right subscapular area
Biliary colic	Right upper back; midback between scapulae; right interscapular or subscapular areas
Shoulder Area	
Liver disease (abscess, cirrhosis, tumors, hepatitis)	Right shoulder; right subscapular area
Gallbladder disease irritating diaphragm	Right upper trapezius; right shoulder; between scapulae; right subscapular area

right splanchnic nerves, synapsing with adjacent phrenic nerve fibers innervating the diaphragm and producing pain in the right shoulder.

Hepatic osteodystrophy, abnormal development of bone, can occur in all forms of cholestasis (bile flow suppression) and hepatocellular disease, especially in the alcoholic person. Either osteomalacia or, more often, osteoporosis frequently accompanies bone pain. Vertebral wedging, vertebral crush fractures, and kyphosis can be severe; decal-cification of the ribcage and pseudofractures* occur frequently.

Osteoporosis associated with primary biliary cirrhosis and primary sclerosing chol-

---

*Pseudofractures, or Looser's zones, are narrow lines of radiolucency (areas of darkness on x-ray film) usually oriented perpendicular to the bone surface. This may represent a stress fracture that is repaired by laying down inadequately mineralized osteoid, or these sites may occur as a result of mechanical erosion caused by arterial pulsations since arteries frequently overlie sites of pseudofractures (Key and Bell, 1998).

angitis parallels the severity of liver disease rather than its duration. Painful osteoarthropathy may develop in the wrists and ankles as a nonspecific complication of chronic liver disease.

Neurologic Symptoms

Neurologic symptoms such as confusion, sleep disturbances, muscle tremors, hyperreactive reflexes, and asterixis may occur. When liver dysfunction results in increased serum ammonia and urea levels, peripheral nerve function can be impaired.

Ammonia from the intestine (produced by protein breakdown) is normally transformed by the liver to urea, glutamine, and asparagine, which are then excreted by the renal system. When the liver does not detoxify ammonia, ammonia is transported to the brain, where it reacts with glutamate (excitatory neurotransmitter), producing glutamine.

The reduction of brain glutamate impairs neurotransmission, leading to altered central nervous system metabolism and function. Asterixis and numbness/tingling (misinterpreted as carpel tunnel syndrome) can occur as a result of this ammonia abnormality, causing an intrinsic nerve pathologic condition. There are many potential causes of carpel tunnel syndrome, both musculoskeletal and systemic (see Table 9-2). Careful evaluation is required.

Asterixis (also called *flapping tremors* or *liver flap*) is a motor disturbance, specifically, the inability to maintain wrist extension with forward flexion of the upper extremities. Asterixis can be tested for by asking the client to dorsiflex the hand with the rest of the arm supported on a firm surface or with the arms held out in front of the body. Observe for quick, irregular extensions and flexions of the wrist and fingers. Altered neurotransmission, specifically, impaired inflow of joint and other afferent information to the brainstem reticular formation, results in this movement dysfunction.

▼ **Clinical Signs and Symptoms of Liver Disease**

- Sense of fullness of the abdomen
- Anorexia, nausea, and vomiting
- Skin changes
  Jaundice
  Bruising
  Spider angioma
  Palmar erythema
- Dark urine and light-colored or clay-colored feces
- Ascites (abnormal accumulation of serous fluid in the peritoneal cavity)
- Edema and oliguria (reduced urine secretion in relation to fluid intake)
- Right upper quadrant (RUQ) abdominal pain
- Musculoskeletal pain, especially right shoulder pain
- Neurologic symptoms
  - Confusion
  - Sleep disturbances
  - Muscle tremors
  - Hyperactive reflexes
  - Asterixis (motor disturbance resembling body or extremity flapping)
  - Bilateral carpal/tarsal tunnel
- Pallor (often linked to cirrhosis or carcinoma)
- Gynecomastia (enlargement of breast tissue in men)

A careful history and close observation of the client are important in determining whether a person may need a medical referral for possible liver disease. Jaundice in the postoperative client is not uncommon, but it may be a potentially serious complication of surgery and anesthesia. Clues to screening for hepatic disease (see Clues to Screening for Hepatic Disease, p. 280) should be taken into consideration when evaluating the clinical history and observations.

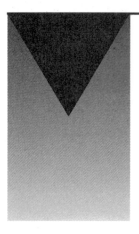

Case Example. A 45-year-old truck driver was diagnosed by a hand surgeon as having bilateral carpal tunnel syndrome (CTS) and was referred to physical therapy. During the course of treatment, the client commented that he was seeing an acupuncturist, who had told him that liver disease was the cause of his bilateral CTS.

Further questioning at that time indicated the absence of any other associated symptoms to suggest liver or hepatic involvement. However, because his symptoms were bilateral and there is a known correlation between liver disease and CTS, the referring physician was notified of these findings.

The client was referred for evaluation, and a diagnosis of liver cancer was confirmed. Physical therapy for CTS was appropriately discontinued.

▼ *Clinical Signs and Symptoms of*
Gallbladder Disease

- Right upper abdominal and epigastric pain
- Jaundice (result of blockage of the common bile duct)
- Fever, chills
- Indigestion
- Nausea
- Intolerance of fatty foods
- Sudden, excruciating pain in the mid-epigastrium with referral to the back and right shoulder (acute cholecystitis)

▼ HEPATIC AND BILIARY PATHOPHYSIOLOGY

Liver Diseases

Hepatitis

Hepatitis is an acute or chronic inflammation of the liver. It can be caused by a virus, a chemical, a drug reaction, or alcohol abuse. In addition, hepatitis can be secondary to disease conditions, such as an infection with other viruses (e.g., Epstein-Barr virus or cytomegalovirus).

VIRAL HEPATITIS

Viral hepatitis is an acute infectious inflammation of the liver caused by one of the following identified viruses: A, B, C, D, E, and G* (Table 8-2).

Hepatitis is a major uncontrolled public health problem for several reasons: not all the causative agents have been identified, there are limited specific drugs for its treatment, its incidence has increased in relation to illicit drug use, and it can be communicated before the appearance of observable clinical symptoms.

Viral hepatitis is spread easily to others and usually results in an extended period of convalescence with loss of time from school or work. It is estimated that 60% to 90% of viral hepatitis cases are unreported because many cases are subclinical or involve mild symptoms.

Hepatitis affects people in three stages: the initial or preicteric stage, the icteric or jaundiced stage, and the recovery period (Table 8-3). During the *initial* or *preicteric*

---

*Hepatitis G (HGV) has been identified as the causative agent in approximately 20% of posttransfusion cases and approximately 15% of community-acquired hepatitis cases that are not caused by hepatitis A virus (HAV). Since HGV is a distant relative of HCV, it is not handled separately but combined with information on HCV (see Table 8-2).

TABLE 8-2 ▼ Comparison of Major Types of Viral Hepatitis

Factor	Hepatitis A	Hepatitis B	Hepatitis C	Hepatitis D (Delta Agent)	Hepatitis E
Incidence	Endemic in areas of poor sanitation; common in fall and early winter	Worldwide, especially in drug addicts, homosexuals, people exposed to blood and blood products; occurs all year	Posttransfusion; those working around blood and blood products; occurs all year	Causes hepatitis only in association with hepatitis B and only in presence of HbsAg; endemic in Mediterranean area	Parts of Asia, Africa, and Mexico, where sanitation is poor
Incubation period	2-6 wk	6 wk-6 mo	6-7 wk	Same as hepatitis B	2-9 wk
Risk factors	Close personal contact or by handling feces-contaminated food or water	Health care workers in contact with body secretions, blood, and blood products; hemodialysis and posttransfusion clients; homosexually active males and drug abusers; morticians; those receiving tattoos	Similar to hepatitis B; health care workers in contact with blood and body fluids; blood transfusion recipients	Same as hepatitis B	Traveling or living in areas where incidence is high
Transmission	Infected feces, fecal-oral route*; may be airborne (if copious secretions); shellfish from contaminated water; also rarely parenteral; no carrier state	Parenteral, sexual contact, and fecal-oral route; carrier state	Contact with blood and body fluids; source of infection uncertain in many clients; carrier state	Coinfects with hepatitis B, close personal contact; carrier state	Fecal-oral route, food-borne or waterborne; no carrier state
Severity	Mortality low; rarely causes fulminating hepatic failure	More serious; may be fatal; mortality rate is up to 60%	Can lead to chronic hepatitis	Similar to hepatitis B; more severe if occurs with chronic active hepatitis B	Illness self-limiting; mortality rate in pregnant women is 10% to 20%
Prophylaxis and active or passive immunity	Hygiene; HAV vaccine; immune globulin	Hygiene; avoidance of risk factors; immune globulin (passive); hepatitis B vaccine (active)	Hygiene; immune globulin (passive); treatment: Interferon alfacon-1 (Infergen)	Hygiene; hepatitis B vaccine (active)	Hygiene; sanitation; no immunity

Modified Black JM, Matassarin-Jacobs E: *Medical-surgical nursing: clinical management for continuity of care,* ed 5, Philadelphia, 1997, WB Saunders, Table 65-2, p 1862.

*The oral-fecal route of transmission is primarily from poor or improper handwashing and personal hygiene, particularly after using the bathroom and then handling food for public consumption. This route of transmission may also occur through shared use of razors and oral utensils such as straws, silverware, and toothbrushes.

stage, which lasts for 1 to 3 weeks, the person experiences vague gastrointestinal (GI) and general body symptoms. Fatigue, malaise, lassitude, weight loss, and anorexia are common. Many people develop an aversion to food, alcohol, and cigarette smoke. Nausea, vomiting, diarrhea, arthralgias,* and influenza-like symptoms may occur. The liver becomes enlarged and tender, and intermittent itching (pruritus) may develop. From 1 to 14 days before the icteric stage, the urine darkens and the stool lightens as less bilirubin is conjugated and excreted.

The *icteric stage* is characterized by the appearance of jaundice, which peaks in 1 to 2 weeks and persists for 6 to 8 weeks. During this stage the acuteness of the inflammation subsides. The GI symptoms begin to disappear, and after 1 to 2 weeks of jaundice the liver decreases in size and becomes less tender. During the icteric stage the postcervical lymph nodes and spleen are enlarged. Persons who have been treated with human immune serum globulin (ISG) may not develop jaundice.

The *recovery stage* lasts for 3 to 4 months, during which time the person generally feels well but fatigues easily.

People with mild-to-moderate acute hepatitis rarely require hospitalization. The emphasis is on preventing the spread of infectious agents and avoiding further liver damage when the underlying cause is drug-induced or toxic hepatitis. People with fulminant (severe, sudden intensity, sometimes fatal) hepatitis require special management

---

*There is a strong association between arthralgia and age with increasing incidence of joint involvement with increased age; arthralgia in children is much less common.

TABLE 8-3 ▼ Stages of Hepatitis

Initial/Preicteric (1-3 wk)	Icteric (6-8 wk)	Recovery (3-4 mo)
Dark urine	Jaundice	Easily fatigued
Light stools	GI symptoms subside	
Vague GI symptoms	Liver decreases in size and tenderness	
Constitutional symptoms	Enlarged spleen	
Fatigue	Enlarged postcervical lymph nodes	
Malaise		
Weight loss		
Anorexia		
Nausea/vomiting		
Diarrhea		
Aversion to food, alcohol, cigarette smoke		
Enlarged and tender liver		
Intermittent pruritus (itching)		
Arthralgias		

Modified from Goodman CC, Boissonnault WG: *Pathology: implication for the physical therapist,* Philadelphia, 1998, WB Saunders, p 502.

▼ ***Clinical Signs and Symptoms of***
Hepatitis A

Hepatitis A is often acquired in childhood as a mild infection with symptoms similar to the "flu" and may be misdiagnosed or ignored. It does not usually cause lasting damage to the liver, although the following symptoms may persist for weeks:

- Extreme fatigue
- Anorexia
- Fever
- Arthralgias and myalgias (generalized aching)
- Right upper abdominal pain
- Clay-colored stools
- Dark urine
- Icterus (jaundice)
- Headache
- Pharyngitis
- Alterations in the senses of taste and smell
- Loss of desire to smoke cigarettes or drink alcohol
- Low-grade fever
- Indigestion (varying degrees of nausea, heartburn, flatulence)

because of the rapid progression of their disease and the potential need for urgent liver transplantation.

An entire spectrum of rheumatic diseases can occur concomitantly with hepatitis B and hepatitis C, including transient arthralgias, vasculitis, polyarteritis nodosa, rheumatoid arthritis (RA), fibromyalgia, lymphoma, Sjögren's syndrome, and persistent synovitis. Some conditions, such as RA and fibromyalgia, occur only in association with HCV, whereas others, such as polyarteritis nodosa, are observed in association with

▼ *Clinical Signs and Symptoms of*
Hepatitis B

Hepatitis B may be asymptomatic but can include:
- Jaundice (changes in skin and eye color)
- Arthralgias
- Rash (over entire body)
- Dark urine
- Anorexia, nausea
- Painful abdominal bloating
- Fever

both forms of hepatitis (Lovy and Wener, 1996; Rull et al., 1998).

Rheumatic manifestations of hepatitis are varied early in the course of disease and can be indistinguishable from mild RA. The therapist should be suspicious of anyone with risk factors for hepatitis (e.g., injection drug use; previous blood transfusion, especially before 1991; hemodialysis; or other exposure to blood products/body fluids, such as a health care worker [see "Risk Factors for Hepatitis" box below]) or a past history of hepatitis that currently appears with arthralgias.

Other red-flag symptoms include joint or muscle pain that is disproportionate to the physical findings and the presence of palmar tendinitis in someone with RA and positive risk factors for hepatitis.

CHRONIC HEPATITIS

Chronic hepatitis is the term used to describe an illness associated with prolonged inflammation of the liver after unresolved viral hepatitis or associated with *chronic active hepatitis* (CAH) of unknown cause. *Chronic* is defined as inflammation of the liver for 6 months or more. The symptoms and biochemical abnormalities may continue for months or years. It is divided by

RISK FACTORS FOR HEPATITIS

- Injection drug use
- Acupuncture
- Tattoo inscription or removal
- Ear or body piercing
- Recent operative procedure
- Blood or plasma transfusion before 1991
- Hemodialysis
- Health care worker exposed to blood products or body fluids
- Exposure to certain chemicals or medications
- Homosexual/bisexual activity
- Severe alcoholism
- Consumption of raw shellfish

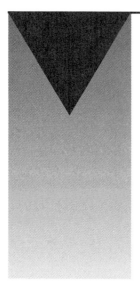

Case Example. A 43-year-old man, 1 year following traumatic injury to the right forearm, underwent surgery to transplant his great toe to function as a thumb. The surgery took place in another state, and the man, who had been a client in our facility before surgery, returned for postoperative rehabilitation.

Complaints of hives of the involved forearm, fatigue, depression, and increased perspiration were documented but attributed by his physician to recovery from the traumatic injury and the multiple operations. Medical records from the hospital consisted of therapy notes only.

Eventually, the client developed a yellowing of the sclerae (white outer coat of the eyeballs). Medical referral was requested, and the client was evaluated by an internal medicine specialist.

Hepatitis C was diagnosed, and full medical records then obtained revealed that although the man had donated his own blood in advance for the surgery, he was short by one unit of blood, which he received through a blood bank.

Clinical Signs and Symptoms of
Chronic Active Hepatitis

The clinical signs and symptoms of chronic active hepatitis may range from asymptomatic to the person who is bedridden with cirrhosis and advanced hepatocellular failure. In the latter the prominent signs and symptoms may reflect multisystem involvement, including:

- Fatigue
- Jaundice
- Abdominal pain
- Anorexia
- Arthralgia
- Fever
- Splenomegaly and hepatomegaly
- Weakness
- Ascites
- Hepatic encephalopathy

Clinical Signs and Symptoms of
Chronic Persistent Hepatitis

- Right upper quadrant pain
- Anorexia
- Mild fatigue
- Malaise

---

findings on liver biopsy into CAH and *chronic persistent hepatitis* (CPH).

Chronic Active Hepatitis. This type of hepatitis refers to seriously destructive liver disease that can result in cirrhosis. CAH is often a result of viral infection (HBV, HCV, and HDV), but it can also be secondary to drug sensitivity (e.g., methyldopa [Aldomet], an antihypertensive medication, and isoniazid [INH], an antitubercular drug). Steroid therapy is sometimes recommended for clients with evidence of aggressive liver inflammation and necrosis (identified by liver biopsy) as a result of these drugs.

If CAH is left untreated, its course is unpredictable and may range from progressive deterioration of liver function to spontaneous remissions and exacerbations.

Steroids may be used to treat CAH. They are usually prescribed for a period of 3 to 5 years. In addition, recombinant interferon-alpha-2b injections in low doses over a 6-month period have been shown to improve hepatic function in persons with CAH. Treatment of hepatitis C is relatively new and consists of the use of interferons (IFNs). Infergen (interferon alfacon-1) is an interferon that was recently approved for the treatment of chronic hepatitis C viral infections (Davis, 1997).

Metabolic Disease. The most common metabolic diseases that can cause chronic hepatitis and are of interest to a physical therapist are Wilson's disease and hematochromatosis, also termed *hemochromatosis*. Both these diseases are dealt with in greater detail as metabolic disorders in Chapter 9.

Wilson's disease is an autosomal recessive disorder in which biliary excretion of copper is impaired, and, as a consequence, total body copper is progressively increased. There may be mild-to-severe neurologic dysfunction, depending on the rate of hepatocyte injury.

Hemochromatosis is the most common genetic disorder (autosomal recessive defect in iron absorption) causing liver failure. Excessive iron is stored in various parenchymal organs with subsequent development of fibrosis. Arthralgias and arthropathy may develop and are often confused with RA or osteoarthritis. The second and third metacarpophalangeal joints are usually involved first. Knees, hips, shoulders, and lower back may be affected. Acute synovitis with pseudogout of the knees has been observed.

NONVIRAL HEPATITIS

Nonviral hepatitis is considered to be a toxic or drug-induced form of liver inflammation. This type of hepatitis occurs secondary to exposure to alcohol, certain chemicals, or drugs such as antiinflammatories, anticonvulsants, antibiotics, cytotoxic drugs for the treatment of cancer, antituberculars, radiographic contrast agents for diagnostic testing, antipsychotics, and antidepressants.

The mechanism by which these agents induce overt injury may be dose-related and predictable or idiosyncratic and unpredictable, with the latter caused by an unusual susceptibility of the individual. Some drugs (e.g., oral contraceptives) may impair liver function and produce jaundice without caus-

▼ *Clinical Signs and Symptoms of*
Toxic and Drug-Induced Hepatitis

These vary with the severity of liver damage and the causative agent. In most individuals symptoms resemble those of acute viral hepatitis:

- Anorexia, nausea, vomiting
- Fatigue and malaise
- Jaundice
- Dark urine
- Clay-colored stools
- Headache, dizziness, drowsiness (carbon tetrachloride poisoning)
- Fever, rash, arthralgias, epigastric or right upper quadrant pain (halothane anesthetic)

ing necrosis, fatty infiltration of liver cells, or a hypersensitivity reaction.

Cirrhosis

Cirrhosis is a chronic hepatic disease characterized by the destruction of liver cells and by the replacement of connective tissue by fibrous bands. As the liver becomes more and more scarred (fibrosed), blood and lymph flow becomes impaired, causing hepatic insufficiency and increased clinical manifestations. The causes of cirrhosis can be varied, although alcohol abuse is the most common cause of liver disease in the United States.

The activity level of the client with cirrhosis is determined by the symptoms. Because hepatic blood flow diminishes with moderate exercise, rest periods are advised and are adjusted according to the level of fatigue experienced by the client both during the exercise and afterward at home. The person may return to work with medical approval but is advised to avoid straining, such as lifting heavy objects, if portal hypertension and esophageal varices are a problem. Because stress decreases hepatic blood flow, any reduction of stress at home, at work, or during treatment is therapeutic.

▼ *Early Clinical Signs and Symptoms of*

Cirrhosis

- Mild right upper quadrant pain (progressive)
- GI symptoms
  - Anorexia
  - Indigestion
  - Weight loss
  - Nausea and vomiting
  - Diarrhea or constipation
- Dull abdominal ache
- Ease of fatigue (with mild exertion)
- Weakness
- Fever

▼ *Clinical Signs and Symptoms of*

Portal Hypertension

- Ascites (abnormal collection of fluid in the peritoneal cavity)
- Dilated collateral veins
  - Esophageal varices (upper GI)
  - Hemorrhoids (lower GI)
- Splenomegaly (enlargement of the spleen)
- Thrombocytopenia (decreased number of blood platelets for clotting)

▼ *Clinical Signs and Symptoms of*

Hemorrhage Associated with Esophageal Varices

- Restlessness
- Pallor
- Tachycardia
- Cooling of the skin
- Hypotension

PROGRESSION OF CIRRHOSIS

As the cirrhosis progresses and hepatic insufficiency develops, a series of conditions emerge, including portal hypertension, ascites, and esophageal varices. Late symptoms affecting the entire body develop (Table 8-4).

Portal hypertension is elevated pressure in the portal vein (through which blood passes from the GI tract and spleen to the liver), occurring as portal blood meets increased resistance to flow in the fibrotic liver. The blood then backs up into esophageal, stomach, and splenic structures and bypasses the liver through collateral vessels.

Ascites is an abnormal accumulation of fluid in the peritoneal cavity as a result of portal backup and loss of proteins. For the physical therapist, abdominal hernias and lumbar lordosis observed in clients with ascites may present symptoms that mimic musculoskeletal involvement, such as groin or low-back pain.

Esophageal varices are dilated veins of the lower esophagus that occur as a result of portal vein blood backup. These varices are thin-walled and can rupture, causing severe hemorrhage and sometimes death.

Hepatic Encephalopathy (Hepatic Coma)

Hepatic coma is a neurologic disorder resulting from the inability of the liver to detoxify ammonia (produced from protein breakdown) in the intestine. Increased serum levels of ammonia are directly toxic to central and peripheral nervous system function, causing an array of neurologic symptoms. Flapping tremors (asterixis) and numbness/tingling (misinterpreted as carpal/tarsal tunnel syndrome) are common resultant symptoms of this ammonia abnormality.

CLINICAL SIGNS AND SYMPTOMS

Clinical manifestations of hepatic encephalopathy vary, depending on the severity of neurologic involvement, and develop in

TABLE 8-4 ▼ Clinical Manifestations of Cirrhosis

Body System	Clinical Manifestations
Respiratory	Limited thoracic expansion (caused by ascites)
	Hypoxia
	Dyspnea
	Cyanosis
	Clubbing
Central nervous system (progressive to hepatic coma)	Subtle changes in mental acuity (progressive)
	Mild memory loss
	Poor reasoning ability
	Irritability
	Paranoia and hallucinations
	Slurred speech
	Asterixis (tremor of outstretched hands)
	Peripheral neuritis
	Peripheral muscle atrophy
Hematologic	Impaired coagulation/bleeding tendencies
	Nosebleeds
	Easy bruising
	Bleeding gums
	Anemia (usually caused by GI blood loss from esophageal varices)
Endocrine (caused by liver's inability to metabolize hormones)	Testicular atrophy
	Menstrual irregularities
	Gynecomastia (excessive development of breasts in men)
	Loss of chest and axillary hair
Integument (cutaneous and skin)	Severe pruritus (itching)
	Extreme dryness
	Poor tissue turgor
	Abnormal pigmentation
	Prominent spider angiomas (benign tumor made up of blood vessels)
	Palmar erythema (redness caused by extensive collection of arteriovenous anastomoses)
	Jaundice
Hepatic	Hepatomegaly (enlargement of the liver)
	Ascites
	Edema of the legs
	Hepatic encephalopathy
Gastrointestinal (GI)	Anorexia
	Nausea
	Vomiting
	Diarrhea

four stages as the ammonia level increases in the serum. The accompanying clinical features are presented in the box.

For the physical therapist, the inpatient with impending hepatic coma has difficulty in ambulating and is unsteady. Protection from falling and seizure precautions must be taken. Skin breakdown in a client who is malnourished because of liver disease, immobile, jaundiced, and edematous can occur in less than 24 hours. Careful attention to skin care, passive exercise, and frequent changes in position are required.

Liver Abscess

A liver abscess occurs when bacteria or protozoa destroy hepatic tissue and produce a cavity that fills with infectious organisms, liquefied liver cells, and leukocytes. Necrotic tissue then isolates the cavity from the rest of the liver.

Even though liver abscess is relatively uncommon, it carries a mortality of 30% to 50%. This rate rises to more than 80% with multiple abscesses or other complications.

▼ *Clinical Signs and Symptoms of*
Hepatic Encephalopathy

Prodromal Stage (Stage I) (subtle symptoms that may be overlooked)
- Slight personality changes
  - Disorientation, confusion
  - Euphoria or depression
  - Forgetfulness
  - Slurred speech
- Slight tremor
- Muscular incoordination
- Impaired handwriting

Impending Stage (Stage II)
- Tremor progresses to asterixis
- Resistance to passive movement (increased muscle tone)
- Lethargy
- Aberrant behavior
- Apraxia*
- Ataxia
- Facial grimacing and blinking

Stuporous Stage (Stage III) (client can still be aroused)
- Hyperventilation
- Marked confusion
- Abusive and violent
- Noisy, incoherent speech
- Asterixis (liver flap)
  - Muscle rigidity
  - Positive Babinski reflex†
  - Hyperactive deep tendon reflexes

Comatose Stage (Stage IV) (client cannot be aroused, responds only to painful stimuli)
- No asterixis
- Positive Babinski reflex
- Hepatic fetor (musty, sweet odor to the breath caused by the liver's inability to metabolize the amino acid methionine)

*This type of motor apraxia can be best observed by keeping a record of the client's handwriting and drawings of simple shapes, such as a circle, square, triangle, rectangle. Check for progressive deterioration.
†A reflex action of the toes that is normal during infancy but abnormal after 12 to 18 months. It is elicited by a firm stimulus (usually scraping with the handle of a reflex hammer) on the sole of the foot from the heel along the lateral border of the sole to the little toe, across the ball of the foot to the big toe. Normally such a stimulus causes all the toes to flex downward. A positive Babinski reflex occurs when the great toe flexes upward and the smaller toes fan outward.

▼ *Clinical Signs and Symptoms of*
Liver Abscess

Clinical signs and symptoms of liver abscess depend on the degree of involvement; some people are acutely ill, others are asymptomatic. Depending on the type of abscess, the onset may be sudden or insidious. The most common signs include:
- Right abdominal pain
- Right shoulder pain
- Weight loss
- Fever, chills
- Diaphoresis
- Nausea and vomiting
- Anemia

Liver Cancer

Metastatic tumors to the liver occur 20 times more often than primary liver tumors. The liver is one of the most common sites of metastasis from other primary cancers (e.g., colorectal, stomach, pancreas, esophagus, lung, breast).

Primary liver tumors (hepatocellular carcinoma [HCC]) are usually associated with cirrhosis but can be linked to other predisposing factors, such as fungal infection (common in moldy foods of Africa), viral hepatitis, excessive use of anabolic steroids, trauma, nutritional deficiencies, and exposure to hepatotoxins.

Several types of benign and malignant hepatic neoplasms can result from the admin-

▼ *Clinical Signs and Symptoms of*

Liver Neoplasm

If clinical signs and symptoms of liver neoplasm do occur (whether of primary or metastatic origin), these may include:
- Jaundice (icterus)
- Progressive failure of health
- Anorexia and weight loss
- Overall muscular weakness
- Epigastric fullness and pain or discomfort
- Constant ache in the epigastrium or mid-back
- Early satiety (cystic tumors)

istration of chemical agents. For example, adenoma (a benign tumor) can occur in recipients of oral contraceptives. Regression of the tumor occurs after withdrawal of the drug.

In most instances interference with liver function does not occur until approximately 80% to 90% of the liver is replaced by metastatic carcinoma or primary carcinoma.

Gallbladder and Duct Diseases

Cholelithiasis

Gallstones are stonelike masses called calculi (singular: calculus) that form in the gallbladder possibly as a result of changes in the normal components of bile.

Although there are two types of stones, pigment and cholesterol stones, most types of gallstone disease in the United States, Europe, and Africa are associated with cholesterol stones.

Cholelithiasis, the presence or formation of gallstones, is the fifth leading cause of hospitalization among adults and accounts for 90% of all gallbladder and duct diseases. The incidence of gallstones increases with age, occurring in more than 40% of people older than 70.

The risk factors to look for in a client's history that correlate with the incidence of gallstones include the following:

- Age: Incidence increases with age
- Sex: Women are affected more than men
- Elevated estrogen levels
  - Pregnancy
  - Oral contraceptives
  - Postmenopausal therapy
  - Multiparity (woman who has had two or more pregnancies resulting in viable offspring)
- Obesity
- Diet: High cholesterol, low fiber
- Diabetes mellitus
- Liver disease

Biliary stasis leads to stagnation of bile, excessive resorption of water by the gallbladder, and subsequent mixed stone formation. Situations of delayed gallbladder emptying, such as obstructions caused by pathologic conditions of the liver, hormonal influences, and pregnancy, can facilitate biliary stasis.

Inflammation of the biliary system causes the bile constituents to become altered, with stone formation occurring from these changes.

Clients with gallstones may be asymptomatic or may have symptoms of a gallbladder attack described in the next section. The prognosis is usually good with medical treatment, depending on the severity

▼ *Clinical Signs and Symptoms of*

Acute Cholecystitis

- Chills, low-grade fever
- Jaundice
- GI symptoms
  - Nausea
  - Anorexia
  - Vomiting
- Tenderness over the gallbladder
- Severe pain in the right upper quadrant and epigastrium (increases on inspiration and movement)
- Pain radiating into the right shoulder and between the scapulae

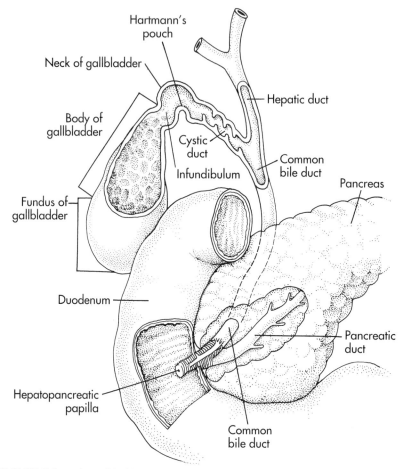

Hartmann's pouch

Neck of gallbladder

Hepatic duct

Body of gallbladder

Cystic duct

Common bile duct

Infundibulum

Pancreas

Fundus of gallbladder

Duodenum

Pancreatic duct

Hepatopancreatic papilla

Common bile duct

FIGURE 8-3 • The gallbladder and its divisions: fundus, body, infundibulum, and neck. Obstruction of either the hepatic or common bile duct by stone or spasm blocks the exit of bile from the liver, where it is formed, and prevents bile from ejecting into the duodenum.

of disease, presence of infection, and response to antibiotics.

Cholecystitis

Cholecystitis, or inflammation of the gallbladder, may be acute or chronic and occurs as a result of impaction of gallstones in the cystic duct (Fig. 8-3), causing painful distension of the gallbladder. Other causes of acute cholecystitis may be typhoid fever or a malignant tumor obstructing the biliary tract. Whatever the cause of the obstruction, the normal flow of bile is interrupted

and the gallbladder becomes distended and ischemic.

Gallstones may also cause chronic cholecystitis (persistent gallbladder inflammation), in which the gallbladder atrophies and becomes fibrotic, adhering to adjacent organs. It is not unusual for affected clients to have repeated episodes before seeking medical attention.

CLINICAL SIGNS AND SYMPTOMS

The typical pain of gallbladder disease has been described as colicky pain that oc-

▼ *Clinical Signs and Symptoms of*

Chronic Cholecystitis

These may be vague or a sense of indigestion and abdominal discomfort after eating, unless a stone leaves the gallbladder and causes obstruction of the common duct (called choledocholithiasis), causing:

- Biliary colic: Severe, steady pain for 3 to 4 hours in the right upper quadrant
- Pain: May radiate to the midback between the scapulae (caused by splanchnic fibers synapsing with phrenic nerve fibers)
- Nausea (intolerance of fatty foods: decreased bile production results in decreased fat digestion)
- Abdominal fullness
- Heartburn
- Excessive belching
- Constipation and diarrhea

curs in the right upper quadrant of the abdomen after the person has eaten a meal that is high in fat (although food that provokes an attack of pain does not need to be "fatty"). However, the pain is not necessarily limited to the right upper quadrant, and more likely than not, it is constant, not colicky.

Primary Biliary Cirrhosis

Primary biliary cirrhosis (PBC) is a chronic, progressive, inflammatory disease of the liver that involves primarily the intrahepatic bile ducts and results in impairment of bile secretion. The disease, which often affects middle-aged women, begins with pruritus or biochemical evidence of cholestasis and progresses at a variable rate to jaundice, portal hypertension, and liver failure. The cause of PBC is unknown, although various factors are being investigated.

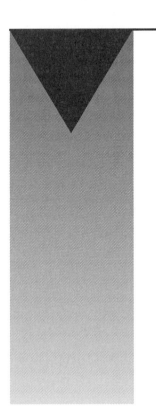

Case Example. A 48-year-old schoolteacher was admitted to the hospital following an episode of intense, sharp pain that started in the epigastric region and radiated around her thorax to the interscapular area. Her gallbladder had been removed 2 years ago, but she remarked that her current symptoms were "exactly like a gallbladder attack." The client was referred to physical therapy for "back care/education" on the day of discharge.

On examination, the client was in acute distress, unable to tolerate a full examination. She had not been able to transfer or ambulate independently. She was instructed in relaxation and breathing techniques to reduce her extreme level of anxiety associated with pain and given supportive reassurance. Instruction and assistance were provided in all transfers to minimize pain and maximize independent function. Given her discharge status, outpatient physical therapy was recommended for follow-up.

She returned to physical therapy as planned and was provided with a back care program. She was also treated locally for scar tissue adhesion at the site of the gallbladder removal. Symptomatic relief was obtained in the first two sessions without recurrence of symptoms.

This case example is included to demonstrate how scar tissue associated with organ removal can reproduce visceral symptoms that are actually of musculoskeletal origin—the opposite concept of what is presented in this text.

▼ *Clinical Signs and Symptoms of*
Primary Biliary Cirrhosis

- Pruritus
- Jaundice
- GI bleeding
- Ascites
- Fatigue
- Right upper quadrant pain (posterior)
- Sensory neuropathy of hands/feet (rare)
- Osteoporosis (decreased bone mass)
- Osteomalacia (softening of the bones)
- Burning, pins and needles, prickling of the eyes
- Muscle cramping

Many clients have associated autoimmune features, particularly Sjögren's syndrome, autoimmune thyroiditis, and renal tubular acidosis. The most significant clinical problem for clients with PBC is bone disease characterized by impaired osteoblastic activity and accelerated osteoclastic activity. Calcium and vitamin D should be carefully monitored and appropriate replacement instituted. Physical activity following an osteoporosis protocol should be encouraged.

No specific treatment has been established yet for PBC other than liver transplantation or supportive measures for the clinical symptoms described.

Text continues on p. 279

OVERVIEW LIVER/BILIARY PAIN PATTERNS

▼ LIVER PAIN (see Fig. 8-2)

Location:	Pain in the midepigastrium or right upper quadrant (RUQ) of abdomen
Referral:	Pain over the liver, especially after exercise (hepatitis)
	RUQ pain may be associated with right shoulder pain
	Both RUQ and epigastrium pain may be associated with back pain between the scapulae
	Pain may be referred to the right side of the midline in the interscapular or subscapular area
Description:	Dull abdominal aching
	Sense of fullness of the abdomen or epigastrium
Intensity:	Mild at first, then increases steadily
Duration:	Constant
Associated signs and symptoms:	Nausea, anorexia (viral hepatitis)
	Early satiety (cystic tumors)
	Aversion to smoking for smokers (viral hepatitis)
	Aversion to alcohol (hepatitis)
	Arthralgias and myalgias (hepatitis A, B, or C)
	Headaches (hepatitis A, drug-induced hepatitis)

Dizziness/drowsiness (drug-induced hepatitis)
Low-grade fever (hepatitis A)
Pharyngitis (hepatitis A)
Extreme fatigue (hepatitis A, cirrhosis)
Alterations in the sense of taste and smell (hepatitis A)
Rash (hepatitis B)
Jaundice
Dark urine, light- or clay-colored stools
Ascites
Edema and oliguria
Neurologic symptoms (hepatic encephalopathy)
   Confusion, forgetfulness
   Muscle tremors
   Asterixis
   Slurred speech
   Impaired handwriting
Pallor (often linked with cirrhosis or carcinoma)
Bleeding disorders
   Purpura
   Ecchymosis
Spider angiomas
Palmar erythema
Diaphoresis (liver abscess)
Overall muscular weakness (cirrhosis, liver carcinoma)

Possible etiology: Peripheral neuropathy (chronic liver disease)
Any liver disease
   Hepatitis
   Cirrhosis
   Metastatic tumors
Pancreatic carcinoma
Liver abscess
Medications: Use of hepatotoxic drugs

▼ GALLBLADDER PAIN (see Fig. 8-2)

Location:
Pain in the midepigastrium (heartburn)

Referral: RUQ of abdomen
RUQ pain may be associated with right shoulder pain
Both may be associated with back pain between the scapulae

	Pain may be referred to the right side of the midline in the interscapular or subscapular area
Description:	Dull aching
	Deep visceral pain (gallbladder suddenly distends)
	Biliary carcinoma is more persistent and boring
Intensity:	Mild at first, then increases steadily to become severe
Duration:	2 to 3 hours
Aggravating factors:	Respiratory inspiration
	Upper body movement
	Lying down
Associated signs and symptoms:	Dark urine, light stools
	Jaundice
	Skin: Green hue (prolonged biliary obstruction)
	Persistent pruritus (cholestatic jaundice)
	Pain and nausea occur 1 to 3 hours after eating (gallstones)
	Pain immediately after eating (gallbladder inflammation)
	Intolerance of fatty foods or heavy meals
	Indigestion, nausea
	Excessive belching
	Flatulence (excessive intestinal gas)
	Anorexia
	Weight loss (gallbladder cancer)
	Bleeding from skin and mucous membranes (late sign of gallbladder cancer)
	Vomiting
	Feeling of fullness
	Low-grade fever, chills
Possible etiology:	Gallstones (cholelithiasis)
	Gallbladder inflammation (cholecystitis)
	Neoplasm
	Medications: Use of hepatotoxic drugs

▼ COMMON BILE DUCT PAIN (see Fig. 8-2)

Location: Pain in midepigastrium or RUQ of abdomen

Referral: Epigastrium: Heartburn (choledocholithiasis)

RUQ pain may be associated with right shoulder pain

Both may be associated with back pain between the scapulae

Pain may be referred to the right side of the midline in the interscapular or subscapular area

Description: Dull aching

Vague discomfort (pressure within common bile duct increasing)

Severe, steady pain in RUQ (choledocholithiasis)

Biliary carcinoma is more persistent and boring

Intensity: Mild at first, increases steadily

Duration: Constant

3 to 4 hours (choledocholithiasis)

Associated signs and symptoms:

Dark urine, light stools

Jaundice

Nausea after eating

Intolerance of fatty foods or heavy meals

Feeling of abdominal fullness

Skin: Green hue (prolonged biliary obstruction)

Low-grade fever, chills

Excessive belching (choledocholithiasis)

Constipation and diarrhea (choledocholithiasis)

Sensory neuropathy (primary biliary cirrhosis)

Osteomalacia (primary biliary cirrhosis)

Osteoporosis (primary biliary cirrhosis)

Possible etiology: Common duct stones

Common duct stricture (previous gallbladder surgery)

Pancreatic carcinoma (blocking the bile duct)

Medications: Use of hepatotoxic drugs

Neoplasm

Primary biliary cirrhosis

Choledocholithiasis (obstruction of common duct)

CLUES TO SCREENING FOR HEPATIC DISEASE

- Right shoulder/scapular and/or upper midback pain of unknown cause (see also Clues to Screening Shoulder Pain, Chapter 12)
- Shoulder motion is not limited by painful symptoms; client is unable to localize or pinpoint pain or tenderness
- Presence of GI symptoms, especially if there is any correlation between eating and painful symptoms
- Bilateral carpal/tarsal tunnel syndrome, especially of unknown origin
- Personal history of cancer, liver, or gallbladder disease
- Personal history of hepatitis, especially with joint pain associated with rheumatoid arthritis or fibromyalgia accompanied by palmar tendinitis
- Recent operative procedure (possible postoperative jaundice)
- Recent (within last 6 months) injection drug use, tattoo (receiving or removal), acupuncture, ear or body piercing, dialysis, blood or plasma transfusion, active homosexual activity, heterosexual sexual activity with homosexuals, consumption of raw shellfish (hepatitis)
- Changes in skin (yellow hue, spider angiomas, palmar erythema) or eye color (jaundice)
- Employment or lifestyle involving alcohol consumption (jaundice)
- Contact with jaundiced persons (health care worker handling blood or body fluids, dialysis clients, injection drug users, active homosexual sexual activity, heterosexual sexual activity with homosexuals)

GUIDE TO PHYSICIAN REFERRAL

- Obvious signs of hepatic disease, especially with a history of previous cancer or risk factors for hepatitis (see "Risk Factors" box on p. 267).
- Presence of bilateral carpal tunnel syndrome accompanied by bilateral tarsal tunnel syndrome unknown to the physician, asterixis, or other associated hepatic signs and symptoms
- Development of arthralgias of unknown cause in anyone with a previous history of hepatitis or risk factors for hepatitis (see "Risk Factors" box on p. 267).

▼ PHYSICIAN REFERRAL

A careful history and close observation of the client are important in determining whether a person may need a medical referral for possible hepatic or biliary involvement. Any client with midback, scapular, or right shoulder pain (see Table 8-1) without a history of trauma (e.g., forceful movement of the spine, repetitive movements of the shoulder or back, or easy lifting) should be screened for possible systemic origin of symptoms.

For the physical therapist treating the inpatient population, jaundice in the post-operative individual is not uncommon and may be a potentially serious complication of surgery and anesthesia. Clinical management of jaundice is complicated by anything capable of damaging the liver, including stress (emotional or physical), hypoxemia, blood loss, infection, and administration of multiple drugs.

When making the referral, it is important to report to the physician the results of your objective findings, especially when there is a lack of physical evidence to support a musculoskeletal lesion. The Special Questions to Ask may assist in assessing the client's overall health status.

Systemic Signs and Symptoms Requiring Physician Referral

Whenever the client reports any of the following accompanying systemic signs or symptoms that have not been evaluated or treated, the physician should be notified.

Alterations in sense of smell/taste

Anorexia

Arthralgias

Ascites

Asterixis

Aversion to cigarettes, alcohol

Changes in skin color (yellow, green)

Chills, fever

Constipation

Dark urine

Diaphoresis

Diarrhea

Dizziness

Drowsiness

Early satiety

Ecchymosis

Edema

Excessive belching

Fatigue

Feeling of abdominal fullness

Fever, chills

Flatulence

Headaches

Heartburn

Intolerance to fatty foods

Jaundice

Light-colored stools

Malaise

Mental confusion

Muscle tremors

Myalgias

Nausea, especially after eating

Oliguria (reduced urine secretion)

Pallor

Palmar erythema

Pharyngitis

Pruritus (itching)

Purpura (subcutaneous bleeding)

Restlessness

Skin rash

Slurred speech

Spider angiomas

Tachycardia

Vomiting

Weakness

See also Table 8-3

 KEY POINTS TO REMEMBER

▶ Primary signs and symptoms of liver diseases vary and can include GI symptoms, edema/ascites, dark urine, light-colored or clay-colored feces, and right upper abdominal pain.

▶ Neurologic symptoms, such as confusion, muscle tremors, and asterixis, may occur.

▶ Skin changes associated with the hepatic system include jaundice, pallor, orange or green skin, bruising, spider angiomas, and palmar erythema.

▶ Active, intense exercise should be avoided when the liver is compromised (jaundice or other active disease).

▶ Antiinflammatory and minor analgesic agents can cause drug-induced hepatitis. Nonviral hepatitis may occur postoperatively.

▶ When liver dysfunction results in increased serum ammonia and urea levels, peripheral nerve function is impaired. Flapping tremors (asterixis) and numbness/tingling (misinterpreted as carpal/tarsal tunnel syndrome) can occur.

▶ Musculoskeletal locations of pain associated with the hepatic and biliary systems include thoracic spine between scapulae, right shoulder, right upper trapezius, right interscapular, or right subscapular areas.

▶ Referred shoulder pain may be the only presenting symptom of hepatic or biliary disease.

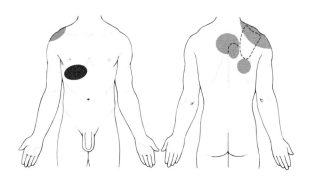

SUBJECTIVE EXAMINATION

• SPECIAL QUESTIONS TO ASK

Past Medical History

- Have you ever had an ulcer, gallbladder disease, your spleen removed, or hepatitis/jaundice?

    – *If yes to hepatitis or jaundice:* When was this diagnosed? How did you get this?

- Has anyone in your family ever been diagnosed with Wilson's disease **(excessive copper retention)** or hemochromatosis **(excessive iron absorption)**? **(Hereditary)**

- Do you work in a clinical laboratory or with dialysis clients? **(Hepatitis)**

- Have you been out of the United States in the last 6 to 12 months? **(parasitic infection, country where hepatitis is endemic)**

- Have you had any recent contact with hepatitis or with a jaundiced person?

- Have you eaten any raw shellfish recently? **(Viral hepatitis)**

- Have you had any recent blood or plasma transfusion, blood tests, acupuncture, ear or body piercing, tattoos (including removal), or dental work done? **(Viral hepatitis)**

- Have you had any kind of injury or trauma to your abdomen? **(Possible liver damage)**

For women: Are you currently using oral contraceptives? **(Hepatitis, adenoma)**

For the therapist:

    – When asking about drug history, keep in mind that oral contraceptives may cause cholestasis (suppression of bile flow) or liver tumors. Some common over-the-counter drugs (e.g., acetaminophen) and some antibiotics, antitubercular drugs, anticonvulsants, cytotoxic drugs for cancer, antipsychotics, and antidepressants may have hepatotoxic effects.

– Use questions from Chapter 2 to determine possible consumption of alcohol as a hepatotoxin.

Associated Signs and Symptoms

- Have you noticed a recent tendency to bruise or bleed easily? **(Liver disease)**
- Have you noticed any change in the color of your stools or urine? **(Dark urine, the color of cola and light- or clay-colored stools associated with jaundice)**
- Has your weight fluctuated 10 or 15 pounds or more recently without a change in diet? **(Cancer, cirrhosis, ascites, but also congestive heart failure)**
  - *If no,* have you noticed your clothes fitting tighter around the waist from abdominal swelling or bloating? **(Ascites)**
- Do you have a feeling of fullness after only one or two bites of food? **(Early satiety: stomach and duodenum, cystic tumors, or gallbladder)**
- Does your stomach feel swollen or bloated after eating? **(Abdominal fullness)**
- Do you have any abdominal pain? (Abdominal pain may be *visceral* from an internal organ [dull, general, poorly localized], *parietal* from inflammation of overlying peritoneum [sharp, precisely localized, aggravated by movement], or *referred* from a disorder in another site.)
- How does eating affect your pain? **(When eating aggravates symptoms: gastric ulcer, gallbladder inflammation)**
  - Are there any particular foods you have noticed that aggravate your symptoms?
  - *If yes,* which ones? **(Gallbladder: intolerance to fatty foods)**
- Have you noticed any unusual aversion to odors, food, alcohol, or (for people who smoke) smoking? **(Jaundice)**
- *For clients with only shoulder or back pain:* Have you noticed any association between when you eat and when your symptoms increase or decrease?

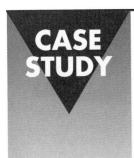

CASE STUDY

REFERRAL

A 29-year-old male law student has come to you (self-referral) with headaches that developed after a motor vehicle accident 18 months ago.

The headaches occur two to three times each week, starting at the base of the occiput and progressing up the back of his head to localize in the forehead bilaterally. The client has a sedentary lifestyle with no regular exercise, and he describes his stress level as being 6 on a scale from 0 to 10. The Family/Personal History form indicates that he has had hepatitis.

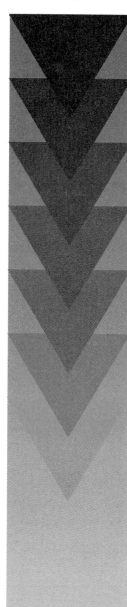

PHYSICAL THERAPY INTERVIEW

What follow-up questions will you ask this client related to the hepatitis?

- Introductory remarks: I see from your History form that you have had hepatitis.
- When did you have hepatitis?

(Remember the three stages when trying to determine whether this person may still be contagious, requiring handwashing and hygiene precautions, including avoidance of any body fluids on your part through the use of protective gloves. This is especially true when treating a person with diabetes requiring fingerstick blood testing, when performing needle electromyograms, or providing open wound care, especially with debridement.

- Do you know how you initially came in contact with hepatitis?

(In this person's case, the only possible cause he can postulate is a shot he received for influenza when he was traveling with a singing group in a rural area of the United States. This information is inconclusive in assisting the physician to establish a direct causative factor.) Other considerations requiring further questioning may include:

- Illicit or recreational drug use
- Poor sanitation in close quarters with travel companion
- Ingestion of contaminated food, water, milk, or seafood
- Recent blood transfusion or contact with blood/blood products
- *For type B:* Modes of sexual transmission
- What type of hepatitis did you have?

Give the client a chance to respond, but you may need to prompt with "type A," "type B," or "types C or D." (Remember that hepatitis A is communicable before the appearance of any observable clinical symptoms [i.e., during the initial and icteric stages that usually last from 1 to 6 weeks]. Hepatitis B can persist in body fluids indefinitely, requiring necessary precautions by you.)

MEDICAL TREATMENT

- Did you receive any medical treatment? (In this case the client and the members of his traveling group received gamma globulin shots.)
- How soon after you were diagnosed did you receive the gamma globulin shots?

(Gamma globulin shots are considered most effective in producing passive immunity for 3 to 4 months when administered as soon as possible after exposure to the hepatitis virus, but within 2 weeks after the onset of jaundice.)

- Are you currently receiving follow-up care for your hepatitis through a local physician?

(This information will assist you in determining the appropriate medical source for further information if you need it and, in a case like this, assist you in choosing further follow-up questions that may help you determine

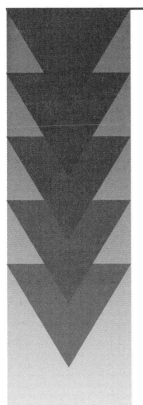

whether this person requires additional medical follow-up. If the client is receiving no further medical follow-up [especially if no gamma globulin was administered initially*], consider these follow-up questions):

ASSOCIATED SYMPTOMS

- What symptoms did you have with hepatitis?
- Do you have any of those symptoms now?
- Are you experiencing any unusual fatigue or muscle or joint aches and pains?
- Have you noticed any unusual aversion to foods, alcohol, or cigarettes/smoke that you did not have before?
- Have you had any problems with diarrhea, vomiting, or nausea?
- Have you noticed any change in the color of your stools or urine?

(One to 4 days before the icteric stage, the urine darkens and the stool lightens.)

- Have you noticed any unusual skin rash developing recently?
- When did you notice the headaches developing?

(Try to correlate this with the onset of hepatitis because headaches can be persistent symptoms of hepatitis A.)

*Persons who have been treated with human immune serum globulin (ISG) may not develop jaundice, but those who have not received the gamma globulin usually develop jaundice.

PRACTICE QUESTIONS

1. Referred pain patterns associated with hepatic and biliary pathologic conditions produce musculoskeletal symptoms in the:

   a. Left shoulder

   b. Right shoulder

   c. Midback or upper back, scapular, and right shoulder areas

   d. Thorax, scapulae, right or left shoulder

2. What is the mechanism for referred right shoulder pain from hepatic or biliary disease?

3. Why does someone with liver dysfunction develop numbness and tingling that is sometimes labeled carpal tunnel syndrome?

4. When a client with bilateral carpal tunnel syndrome is being evaluated, how do you screen for the possibility of a pathologic condition of the liver?

5. What is the first most common sign associated with liver disease?

6. You are treating a 53-year-old woman who has had an extensive medical history that includes bilateral kidney disease with kidney removal on one side and transplantation on the other. The client is 10 years posttransplant and has now developed multiple problems as a

result of the long-term use of immuno-suppressants (cyclosporine to prevent organ rejection) and corticosteroids (prednisone). For example, she is extremely osteoporotic and has been diagnosed with cytomegalovirus and corticosteroid-induced myopathy. The client has fallen and broken her vertebra, ankle, and wrist on separate occasions. You are seeing her at home to implement a strengthening program and to instruct her in a falling prevention program, including home modifications. You notice the sclerae of her eyes are yellow-tinged. How do you tactfully ask her about this?

7. Clients with significant elevations in serum bilirubin levels caused by biliary obstruction will have which of the following associated signs?

   a. Dark urine, clay-colored stools, jaundice

   b. Yellow-tinged sclera

   c. Decreased serum ammonia levels

   d. *a* and *b* only

8. Preventing falls and trauma to soft tissues would be of utmost importance in the client with liver failure. Which of the following laboratory parameters would give you the most information about potential tissue injury?

   a. Decrease in serum albumin levels

   b. Elevated liver enzyme levels

   c. Prolonged coagulation times

   d. Elevated serum bilirubin levels

9. Decreased level of consciousness, impaired function of peripheral nerves, and asterixis (flapping tremor) would probably indicate an increase in the level of:

   a. AST (aspartate aminotransferase)

   b. Alkaline phosphatase

   c. Serum bilirubin

   d. Serum ammonia

10. A decrease in serum albumin is common with a pathologic condition of the liver since albumin is produced in the liver. The reduction in serum albumin results in some easily identifiable signs. Which of the following signs might alert the therapist to the condition of decreased albumin?

    a. Increased blood pressure

    b. Peripheral edema and ascites

    c. Decreased level of consciousness

    d. Exertional dyspnea

References

Davis G: Treatment of acute and chronic hepatitis C, *Clin Liver Dis* 1(3):615-630, 1997.

Key LL, Bell NH: Osteomalacia and disorders of vitamin D metabolism. In Stein JH, editor: *Internal medicine*, ed 5, St Louis, 1998, Mosby.

Lovy MR, Wener MH: Rheumatic disease: when is hepatitis C the culprit? *J Musculoskel Med* 13(4):27-35, 1996.

Rull M, Zonay L, Schumacher HR: Hepatitis C and rheumatic diseases, *J Musculoskel Med* 15(11):38-44, 1998.

Overview of Endocrine and Metabolic Signs and Symptoms

9

Endocrinology is the study of ductless (endocrine) glands that produce hormones. A hormone acts as a chemical agent that is transported by the bloodstream to target tissues, where it regulates or modifies the activity of the target cell.

The endocrine system cannot be understood fully without consideration of the effects of the nervous system on the endocrine system. The endocrine system works with the nervous system to regulate metabolism, water and salt balance, blood pressure, response to stress, and sexual reproduction.

The endocrine system is slower in response and takes longer to act than the nervous system in transferring biochemical information. The pituitary (hypophysis), thyroid, parathyroids, adrenals, and pineal are glands of the endocrine system whose functions are solely endocrine* (Fig. 9-1). The hypothalamus controls pituitary function and thus has an important indirect influence on the other glands of the endocrine system. Feedback mechanisms exist to keep hormones at normal levels.

The endocrine system meets the nervous system at the hypothalamic-pituitary interface. The hypothalamus and the pituitary form an integrated axis† that maintains control over much of the endocrine system. The hypothalamus exerts direct control over both the anterior and posterior portions of the pituitary gland and can synthesize and release hormones from its axon terminals directly into the blood circulation. These *neurosecretory cells* are so called because the neurons have a hormone-secreting function.

Although neurons can have a hormone-secreting function, the opposite pathway is also present. Hormones that can stimulate the

---

*Other glands in the body have dual functions. For example, the pancreas produces the hormone insulin from its islet cells, but it also produces digestive enzymes, which are carried by ducts and are thus exocrine.

†The concept of two systems meeting at an interface and forming an axis is a gross oversimplification and an outdated way to view this phenomenon. We now know that the body systems interface in a complex series of interactions that has linked behavior-neural-endocrine-immunologic responses. The study of this new concept, labeled psychoneuroimmunology (PNI), has identified major links between these systems; with this discovery a new understanding of interactive biologic signaling has begun.

287

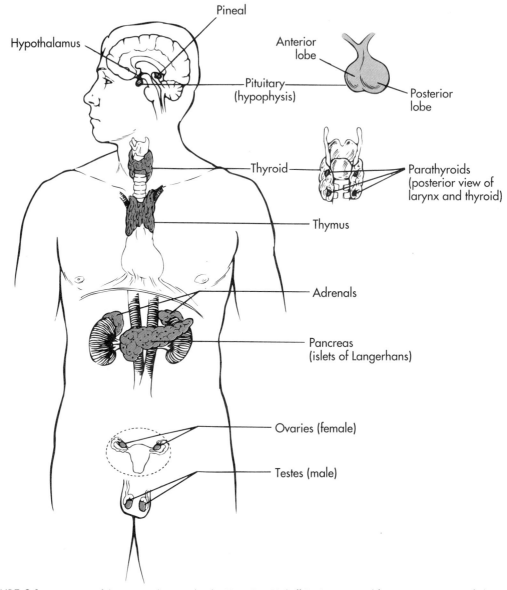

FIGURE 9-1 • Location of the nine endocrine glands. (From Butts-Krakoff D: Structure and function: assessment of clients with metabolic disorders. In Black JM, Matassarin-Jacobs E, editors: *Luckmann and Sorensen's medical-surgical nursing*, ed 4, Philadelphia, 1993, WB Saunders, p. 1759.)

neural mechanism are called *neurohormones*. For example, acetylcholine (a neurotransmitter that is released at synapses to allow messages to pass along a nerve network, resulting in the release of hormones and chemicals) is considered a neurohormone.

ASSOCIATED NEUROMUSCULOSKELETAL SIGNS AND SYMPTOMS

The musculoskeletal system is composed of a variety of connective tissue structures

TABLE 9-1 ▼ Signs and Symptoms of Endocrine Dysfunction

Neuromusculoskeletal	Systemic
Signs and symptoms associated with rheumatoid arthritis	Excessive or delayed growth
Muscle weakness	Polydipsia
Muscle atrophy	Polyuria
Myalgia	Mental changes (nervousness, confusion, depression)
Fatigue	Changes in hair (quality and distribution)
Carpal tunnel syndrome	Changes in skin pigmentation
Synovial fluid changes	Changes in distribution of body fat
Periarthritis	Changes in vital signs (elevated body temperature,
Adhesive capsulitis (diabetes)	pulse rate, increased blood pressure)
Chondrocalcinosis	Heart palpitations
Spondyloarthropathy	Increased perspiration
Osteoarthritis	Kussmaul's respirations (deep, rapid breathing)
Hand stiffness	Dehydration or excessive retention of body water
Arthralgia	

From Goodman CC, Boissonnault WG: *Pathology: implications for the physical therapist,* Philadelphia, 1998, WB Saunders, p 222.

in which normal growth and development are influenced strongly and sometimes controlled by various hormones and metabolic processes.

Alterations in these control systems can result in structural changes and altered function of various connective tissues, producing systemic and musculoskeletal signs and symptoms (Table 9-1).

Muscle Weakness, Myalgia, and Fatigue

Muscle weakness, myalgia, and fatigue may be early manifestations of thyroid or parathyroid disease, acromegaly, diabetes, Cushing's syndrome, and osteomalacia. In endocrine disease most proximal muscle weakness is usually painless and unrelated to either the severity or the duration of the underlying disease.

Bilateral Carpal Tunnel Syndrome

Bilateral carpal tunnel syndrome (CTS), resulting from median nerve compression at the wrist, is a common finding in a variety of systemic and neuromusculoskeletal conditions but especially with certain endocrine and metabolic disorders* (Atcheson et al, 1998) (Table 9-2).

Thickening of the transverse carpal ligament itself may be sufficient to compress the median nerve in certain systemic disorders (e.g., acromegaly, myxedema), and any condition that increases the volume of the contents of the carpal tunnel compresses the median nerve (e.g., neoplasm, calcium, and gouty tophi deposits).

The fact that the majority of persons with CTS are women at or near menopause suggests that the soft tissues about the wrist may be affected in some way by hormones (Grossman et al, 1961; Phalen, 1966).

Bilateral median nerve neuritis has long been recognized as the first symptom of multiple myeloma, rheumatoid arthritis, and amyloid disease, both primary and secondary (Grokoest and Demartini, 1954).

Periarthritis and Calcific Tendinitis

Periarthritis (inflammation of periarticular structures, including the tendons, ligaments,

---

*It should be noted that bilateral tarsal syndrome affecting the feet can also occur either alone or in conjunction with the carpal tunnel syndrome, although the incidence of this occurring is not great. Always assess for other systemic signs and symptoms.

TABLE 9-2 ▼ Causes of Carpal Tunnel Syndrome

Neuromusculoskeletal	Systemic
Amyloidosis	Arthritis (rheumatoid, gout, polymyalgia rheumatica)
Anatomic sequelae of medical or surgical procedures	Benign tumors (lipoma, hemangioma, ganglia)
Cervical disk lesions	
Cervical spondylosis	*Endocrine*
Congenital anatomic differences	Acromegaly
Cumulative trauma disorders (CTD)	Diabetes mellitus
Peripheral neuropathy	Hormonal imbalance (menopause; posthysterectomy)
Poor posture (may also be associated with TOS)	Hyperparathyroidism
Repetitive strain injuries (RSI)	Hyperthyroidism (Graves' disease)
Tendinitis	Hypocalcemia
Trigger points	Hypothyroidism (myxedema)
Tenosynovitis	Gout (deposits of tophi and calcium)
Thoracic outlet syndrome (TOS)	
Wrist trauma (e.g., Colles' fracture)	*Infectious Disease*
	Atypical mycobacterium
	Histoplasmosis
	Rubella
	Sporotrichosis
	Leukemia (tissue infiltration)
	Liver disease
	Multiple myeloma (amyloidosis deposits)
	Obesity
	Pregnancy
	Use of oral contraceptives
	Hemochromatosis
	Vitamin deficiency (especially vitamin B_6)

Modified from Goodman CC, Boissonnault WG: *Pathology: implications for the physical therapist,* Philadelphia, 1998, WB Saunders, Table 34-6, p 818.

and joint capsule) and calcific tendinitis occur most often in the shoulders of people who have endocrine disease.

Chondrocalcinosis

Chondrocalcinosis (deposition of calcium salts in the cartilage of joints; when accompanied by attacks of goutlike symptoms, it is called *pseudogout*) is commonly seen on x-ray films as calcified hyaline or fibrous cartilage. In 5% to 10% of individuals with chondrocalcinosis, there is an associated underlying endocrine or metabolic disease (Table 9-3).

Spondyloarthropathy and Osteoarthritis

Spondyloarthropathy (disease of joints of the spine) and osteoarthritis occur in indi-

TABLE 9-3 ▼ Endocrine and Metabolic Disorders Associated With Chondrocalcinosis

Endocrine	Metabolic
Hypothyroidism	Hemochromatosis
Hyperparathyroidism	Hypomagnesemia
Acromegaly	Hypophosphatasia
	Ochronosis
	Oxalosis
	Wilson's disease

Modified from Louthrenoo W, Schumacher HR: Musculoskeletal clues to endocrine or metabolic disease, *J Musculoskel Med,* 7(9):41, 1990.

viduals with various metabolic or endocrine diseases, including hemochromatosis (disorder of iron metabolism with excess deposition of iron in the tissues; also known as bronze diabetes and iron storage disease), ochronosis (metabolic disorder resulting in discoloration of body tissues caused by deposits of alkapton bodies), acromegaly, and diabetes mellitus.

Hand Stiffness and Hand Pain

Hand stiffness and hand pain, as well as arthralgias of the small joints of the hand, can occur with endocrine and metabolic diseases. In persons with hypothyroidism, flexor tenosynovitis with stiffness is a common finding. This condition often accompanies CTS.

▼ ENDOCRINE PATHOPHYSIOLOGY

Disorders of the endocrine glands can be classified as primary (dysfunction of the gland itself) or secondary (dysfunction of an outside stimulus to the gland) and are a result of either an excess or insufficiency of hormonal secretions.

Secondary dysfunction may also occur (iatrogenically) as a result of chemotherapy, surgical removal of the glands, therapy for a nonendocrine disorder (e.g., the use of large doses of corticosteroids resulting in Cushing's syndrome), or excessive therapy for an endocrine disorder.

Pituitary Gland

Diabetes Insipidus

Diabetes insipidus is caused by a lack of secretion of vasopressin (antidiuretic hormone [ADH]). This hormone normally stimulates the distal tubules of the kidneys to reabsorb water. Without ADH, water moving through the kidney is not reabsorbed but is lost in the urine, resulting in severe water loss and dehydration through diuresis.

Central or neurogenic diabetes insipidus, which is the most common type, can be familiar or idiopathic (primary), or it can be related to other causes (secondary), such as pituitary trauma, head injury, infections

▼ *Clinical Signs and Symptoms of* Diabetes Insipidus

- Polyuria (increased urination)
- Polydipsia (increased thirst, which occurs subsequent to polyuria in response to the loss of fluid)
- Dehydration
- Decreased urine specific gravity (1.001 to 1.005)
- Nocturia, fatigue, irritability
- Increased serum sodium (>145 mEq/dl; resulting from concentration of serum from water loss)

such as meningitis or encephalitis, pituitary neoplasm, and vascular lesions such as aneurysms.

If the person with diabetes insipidus is unconscious or confused and is unable to take in necessary fluids to replace those fluids lost, rapid dehydration, shock, and death can occur. Because sleep is interrupted by the persistent need to void (nocturia), fatigue and irritability result.

Syndrome of Inappropriate Secretion of Antidiuretic Hormone

Syndrome of inappropriate secretion of ADH (SIADH) is an excess or inappropriate secretion of vasopressin that results in marked retention of water in excess of sodium in the body. Urine output decreases dramatically as the body retains large amounts of water. Almost all the excess water is distributed within body cells, causing intracellular water gain and cellular swelling (water intoxication).

Causative factors for the development of SIADH include pituitary damage caused by infection, trauma, or neoplasm; secretion of vasopressin-like substances from some types of malignant tumors (particularly pulmonary malignancies); and thoracic pressure changes from compression of pulmonary or cardiac pressure receptors, or both.

▼ *Clinical Signs and Symptoms of*

Syndrome of Inappropriate Secretion of Antidiuretic Hormone

- Headache, confusion, lethargy (most significant, early indicators)
- Decreased urine output
- Weight gain without visible edema
- Seizures
- Muscle cramps
- Vomiting, diarrhea
- Increased urine specific gravity (>1.03)
- Decreased serum sodium (<135 mEq/dl; caused by dilution of serum from water)

▼ *Clinical Signs and Symptoms of*

Acromegaly

- Bony enlargement (face, jaw, hands, feet)
- Amenorrhea
- Diabetes mellitus
- Profuse sweating (diaphoresis)
- Hypertension
- Carpal tunnel syndrome
- Hand pain and stiffness
- Back pain (thoracic and/or lumbar

CLINICAL SIGNS AND SYMPTOMS

Symptoms of SIADH are the clinical opposite of symptoms of diabetes insipidus. They are the result of water retention and the subsequent dilution of sodium in the blood serum and body cells. Neurologic and neuromuscular signs and symptoms predominate and are directly related to the swelling of brain tissue and sodium changes within neuromuscular tissues.

Acromegaly

Acromegaly is an abnormal enlargement of the extremities of the skeleton resulting from hypersecretion of growth hormone (GH) from the pituitary gland. This condition is relatively rare and occurs in adults, most often owing to a tumor of the pituitary gland. In children, overproduction of GH stimulates growth of long bones and results in gigantism, in which the child grows to exaggerated heights. With adults, growth of the long bones has already stopped, so the bones most affected are those of the face, jaw, hands, and feet. Other signs and symptoms include amenorrhea, diabetes mellitus, profuse sweating, and hypertension.

CLINICAL SIGNS AND SYMPTOMS

Degenerative arthropathy may be seen in the peripheral joints of a client with acromegaly, most frequently attacking the large joints. On x-ray studies, osteophyte formation may be seen, along with widening of the joint space because of increased cartilage thickness. In late-stage disease joint spaces become narrowed, and occasionally chondrocalcinosis may be present.

Stiffness of the hand, typically of both hands, is associated with a broad enlargement of the fingers from bony overgrowth and with thickening of the soft tissue. X-ray findings of soft tissue thickening and widening of the phalangeal tufts are typical. In clients with these x-ray findings, much of the pain and stiffness is believed to be due to premature osteoarthritis.

CTS is seen in up to 50% of people with acromegaly. The CTS that occurs with this growth disorder is thought to be caused by compression of the median nerve at the wrist from soft tissue hypertrophy or bony overgrowth or by hypertrophy of the median nerve itself.

About half the individuals with acromegaly have back pain. X-ray studies demonstrate increased intervertebral disk spaces and large osteophytes along the anterior longitudinal ligament (ALL), mimicking diffuse idiopathic skeletal hyperostosis (DISH).

DISH is characterized by abnormal ossification of the ALL, resulting in an x-ray image of large osteophytes seemingly "flowing" along the anterior border of the spine. DISH is particularly common in the thoracic spine and has been reported to be more prevalent among persons with diabetes than among the nondiabetic population.

Adrenal Glands

The adrenals are two small glands located on the upper part of each kidney. Each adrenal gland consists of two relatively discrete parts: an outer cortex and an inner medulla.

The outer cortex is responsible for the secretion of mineralocorticoids (steroid hormones that regulate fluid and mineral balance), glucocorticoids (steroid hormones responsible for controlling the metabolism of glucose), and androgens (sex hormones).

The centrally located adrenal medulla is derived from neural tissue and secretes epinephrine and norepinephrine. Together, the adrenal cortex and medulla are major factors in the body's response to stress.

Adrenal Insufficiency

PRIMARY ADRENAL INSUFFICIENCY

Chronic adrenocortical insufficiency (hyposecretion by the adrenal glands) may be primary or secondary. Primary adrenal insufficiency is also referred to as Addison's disease (hypofunction), named after the physician who first studied and described the associated symptoms. It can be treated by the administration of exogenous cortisol (one of the adrenocortical hormones).

Primary adrenal insufficiency occurs when a disorder exists within the adrenal gland itself. This adrenal gland disorder results in decreased production of cortisol and aldosterone, two of the primary adrenocortical hormones.

The most common cause of primary adrenal insufficiency is an autoimmune process that causes destruction of the adrenal cortex.

▼ **Clinical Signs and Symptoms of**
Adrenal Insufficiency

- Dark pigmentation of the skin, especially mouth and scars (primary only: Addison's disease)
- Hypotension (low blood pressure causing orthostatic symptoms)
- Progressive fatigue (improves with rest)
- Hyperkalemia (generalized weakness and muscle flaccidity)
- GI disturbances
  - Anorexia and weight loss
  - Nausea and vomiting
- Arthralgias, myalgias (secondary only)
- Tendon calcification
- Hypoglycemia

The most striking physical finding in the person with primary adrenal insufficiency is the increased pigmentation of the skin and mucous membranes. This may vary in the white population from a slight tan or a few black freckles to an intense generalized pigmentation, which has resulted in persons being mistakenly considered to be of a darker-skinned race. Members of darker-skinned races may develop a slate-gray color that may be obvious only to family members.

Melanin, the major product of the melanocyte, is largely responsible for the coloring of skin. In primary adrenal insufficiency, the increase in pigmentation is initiated by the excessive secretion of melanocyte-stimulating hormone (MSH) that occurs in association with increased secretion of ACTH. ACTH is increased in an attempt to stimulate the diseased adrenal glands to produce and release more cortisol.

Most commonly, pigmentation is visible over extensor surfaces, such as the backs of the hands, elbows, knees, creases of the hands, lips, and mouth. Increased pigmentation of scars formed after the onset of the disease is common. However, it is possible for the person with primary adrenal insufficiency to demonstrate no significant increase in pigmentation.

SECONDARY ADRENAL INSUFFICIENCY

Secondary adrenal insufficiency refers to a dysfunction of the gland because of insufficient stimulation of the cortex owing to a lack of pituitary ACTH. Causes of secondary disease include tumors of the hypothalamus or pituitary, removal of the pituitary, or rapid withdrawal of corticosteroid drugs.

Clinical manifestations of secondary disease do not occur until the adrenals are almost completely nonfunctional and are primarily related to cortisol deficiency only.

Cushing's Syndrome

Cushing's syndrome (hyperfunction of the adrenal gland) is a general term for increased secretion of cortisol by the adrenal cortex. When corticosteroids are administered externally, a condition of hypercortisolism called Cushing's syndrome occurs, producing a group of associated signs and symptoms.

Hypercortisolism caused by excess secretion of ACTH (e.g., from pituitary stimulation) is called *Cushing's disease,* and symptoms are the same as those associated with Cushing's syndrome. Physical therapists often treat people who have developed Cushing's syndrome after these clients have received large doses of cortisol (also known as hydrocortisone) or cortisol derivatives (e.g., dexamethasone) for a number of inflammatory disorders.

It is important to remember that whenever corticosteroids are administered externally, the increase in serum cortisol levels triggers a negative feedback signal to the anterior pituitary gland to stop adrenal stimulation. Adrenal atrophy occurs during this time, and adrenal insufficiency will result if external corticosteroids are abruptly withdrawn. Corticosteroid medications must be reduced gradually so that normal adrenal function can return.

Because cortisol suppresses the inflammatory response of the body, it can mask early signs of infection. *Any unexplained*

▼ **Clinical Signs and Symptoms of**
Cushing's Syndrome (see Fig. 9-2)

- "Moon" face (very round)
- Buffalo hump at the neck (fatty deposits)
- Protuberant abdomen with accumulation of fatty tissue and stretch marks
- Muscle wasting and weakness
- Decreased density of bones (especially spine)
- Kyphosis and back pain (secondary to bone loss)
- Easy bruising
- Psychiatric or emotional disturbances
- Impaired reproductive function (e.g., decreased libido and changes in menstrual cycle)
- Diabetes mellitus
- Slow wound healing
- *For women:* Masculinizing effects (e.g., hair growth, breast atrophy, voice changes)

fever without other symptoms should be a warning to the physical therapist of the need for medical follow-up.

EFFECTS OF CORTISOL ON CONNECTIVE TISSUE

Overproduction of cortisol or closely related glucocorticoids by abnormal adrenocortical tissue leads to a protein catabolic state. This overproduction causes liberation of amino acids from muscle tissue. The resultant weakened protein structures (muscle and elastic tissue) cause a protuberant abdomen, poor wound healing, generalized muscle weakness, and marked osteoporosis (demineralization of bone causing reduced bone mass), which is made worse by an excessive loss of calcium in the urine.

Excessive glucose resulting from this protein catabolic state is transformed mainly into fat and appears in characteristic sites, such as the abdomen, supraclavicular fat pads, and facial cheeks. The change in facial

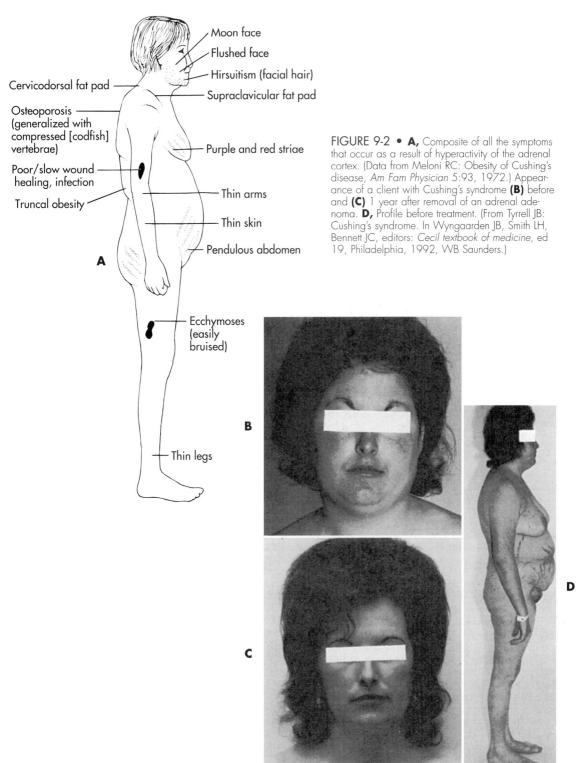

Moon face

Flushed face

Hirsuitism (facial hair)

Supraclavicular fat pad

Cervicodorsal fat pad

Osteoporosis (generalized with compressed [codfish] vertebrae)

Poor/slow wound healing, infection

Truncal obesity

Purple and red striae

Thin arms

Thin skin

Pendulous abdomen

Ecchymoses (easily bruised)

Thin legs

A

B

C

D

FIGURE 9-2 • **A,** Composite of all the symptoms that occur as a result of hyperactivity of the adrenal cortex. (Data from Meloni RC: Obesity of Cushing's disease, *Am Fam Physician* 5:93, 1972.) Appearance of a client with Cushing's syndrome **(B)** before and **(C)** 1 year after removal of an adrenal adenoma. **D,** Profile before treatment. (From Tyrrell JB: Cushing's syndrome. In Wyngaarden JB, Smith LH, Bennett JC, editors: *Cecil textbook of medicine*, ed 19, Philadelphia, 1992, WB Saunders.)

appearance may not be readily apparent to the client or to the physical therapist, but pictures of the client taken over a period of years may provide a visual record of those changes.

The effect of increased circulating levels of cortisol on the muscles of clients varies from slight to very marked. There may be so much muscle wasting that the condition simulates muscular dystrophy. Marked weakness of the quadriceps muscle often prevents affected clients from rising out of a chair unassisted. Those with Cushing's syndrome of long duration almost always demonstrate demineralization of bone. In severe cases this condition may lead to pathologic fractures but results more commonly in wedging of the vertebrae, kyphosis, bone pain, and back pain.

Poor wound healing characteristic of this syndrome becomes a problem when any surgical procedures are required. Inhibition of collagen formation with corticosteroid therapy is responsible for the frequency of wound breakdown in postsurgical clients.

Thyroid Gland

The thyroid gland is located in the anterior portion of the lower neck below the larynx, on both sides of and anterior to the trachea. The chief hormones produced by the thyroid are thyroxine (T_4), triiodothyronine (T_3), and calcitonin. Both T_3 and T_4 regulate the metabolic rate of the body and increase protein synthesis. Calcitonin has a weak physiologic effect on calcium and phosphorus balance in the body.

Thyroid function is regulated by the hypothalamus and pituitary feedback controls, as well as by an intrinsic regulator mechanism within the gland itself.

Basic thyroid disorders of significance to physical therapy practice include goiter, hyperthyroidism, hypothyroidism, and cancer. Alterations in thyroid function produce changes in hair, nails, skin, eyes, gastrointestinal (GI) tract, respiratory tract, heart and blood vessels, nervous tissue, bone, and muscle.

▼ **Clinical Signs and Symptoms of**
Goiter

- Increased neck size
- Pressure on adjacent tissue (e.g., trachea and esophagus)
- Difficulty in breathing
- Dysphagia
- Hoarseness

Goiter

Goiter, an enlargement of the thyroid gland, occurs in areas of the world where iodine (necessary for the production of thyroid hormone) is deficient in the diet. It is believed that when factors (e.g., a lack of iodine) inhibit normal thyroid hormone production, hypersecretion of TSH occurs because of a lack of a negative feedback loop. The TSH increase results in an increase in thyroid mass.

Pressure on the trachea and esophagus causes difficulty in breathing, dysphagia, and hoarseness. With the use of iodized salt, this problem has almost been eliminated in the United States. Although the younger population in the United States may be goiter-free, older adults may have developed goiter during their childhood or adolescent years and may still have clinical manifestations of this disorder.

Thyroiditis

Thyroiditis is an inflammation of the thyroid gland. Causes can include infection and autoimmune processes. The most common form of this problem is a chronic thyroiditis called Hashimoto's thyroiditis. This condition affects women more frequently than men and is most often seen in the 30- to 50-year-old age group. Destruction of the thyroid gland from this condition can cause eventual hypothyroidism.

Usually, both sides of the gland are enlarged, although one side may be larger

▼ **Clinical Signs and Symptoms of**
Thyroiditis

- Painless thyroid enlargement
- Dysphagia or choking

than the other. Other symptoms are related to the functional state of the gland itself. Early involvement may cause mild symptoms of hyperthyroidism, whereas later symptoms cause hypothyroidism.

Hyperthyroidism

Hyperthyroidism (hyperfunction), or thyrotoxicosis, refers to those disorders in which the thyroid gland secretes excessive amounts of thyroid hormone.

Graves' disease is a common type of excessive thyroid activity characterized by a generalized enlargement of the gland (or goiter leading to a swollen neck) and, often, protruding eyes caused by retraction of the eyelids and inflammation of the ocular muscles.

CLINICAL SIGNS AND SYMPTOMS

Excessive thyroid hormone creates a generalized elevation in body metabolism. The effects of thyrotoxicosis occur gradually and are manifested in almost every system (Fig. 9-3; Table 9-4).

In more than 50% of adults older than 70, three signs are found: tachycardia, fatigue, and weight loss. In clients younger than 50, 12 clinical signs are found most often: tachycardia, hyperactive reflexes, increased sweating, heat intolerance, fatigue, tremor, nervousness, polydipsia, weakness, increased appetite, dyspnea, and weight loss (Trivalle et al, 1996).

Chronic periarthritis is also associated with hyperthyroidism. Inflammation that involves the periarticular structures, including the tendons, ligaments, and joint capsule, is termed periarthritis. The syndrome is associated with pain and reduced range of motion. Calcification, whether periarticular or tendinous, may be seen on x-ray studies. Both periarthritis and calcific tendinitis occur most often in the shoulder, and both are common findings in clients who have endocrine disease.

Painful restriction of shoulder motion associated with periarthritis has been widely described among clients of all ages with hyperthyroidism. The involvement can be unilateral or bilateral and can worsen progressively to become adhesive capsulitis (frozen shoulder). Acute calcific tendinitis of the wrist also has been described in such clients. Although antiinflammatory agents may be needed for the acute symptoms, chronic periarthritis usually responds to treatment of the underlying hyperthyroidism.

Proximal muscle weakness (most marked in the pelvic girdle and thigh muscles), accompanied by muscle atrophy known as myopathy, occurs in up to 70% of people with hyperthyroidism.

Muscle strength returns to normal in about 2 months after medical treatment, whereas muscle wasting resolves more slowly. In severe cases normal strength may not be restored for months.

The incidence of myasthenia gravis is increased in clients with hyperthyroidism, which in turn can aggravate muscle weakness. If the hyperthyroidism is corrected, improvement of myasthenia gravis follows in about two thirds of clients.

Hypothyroidism

Hypothyroidism (hypofunction) results from insufficient thyroid hormone and creates a generalized depression of body metabolism. The condition may be classified as either primary or secondary. *Primary hypothyroidism* results from reduced functional thyroid tissue mass or impaired hormonal synthesis or release (e.g., iodine deficiency, loss of thyroid tissue, autoimmune thyroiditis).

Hypothyroidism in fetal development and infants is usually a result of absent thyroid tissue and hereditary defects in thyroid hormone synthesis. Untreated congenital hypothyroidism is referred to as *cretinism*.

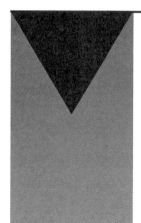

Case Example. A 38-year-old woman with right-sided groin pain was referred to physical therapy by her physician. She says that the pain came on suddenly without injury. The pain is worse in the morning and hurts at night, waking her up when she changes position. The woman's symptoms are especially acute after sitting when she tries to stand up, with weight bearing impossible for the first 5 to 10 minutes.

The woman is athletic looking and reports that before the onset of this problem, she was running 5 miles every other day without difficulty. The x-ray finding is reportedly within normal limits for structural abnormalities. Sed rate was 16 mm/hr.* The woman has chronic sinusitis and has had two surgeries for that condition in the last 3 years. She is not a smoker and drinks only occasionally on a social basis.

This client has been seen by one physical therapist so far, who tried ultrasound and stretching without improvement in symptoms or function.

The physical therapy evaluation today revealed a positive Thomas test for right hip flexion contracture. However, it was difficult to assess whether there was a true muscle contracture or only loss of motion as a result of muscle splinting and guarding. Patrick's test (FABER's) and the iliopsoas test were both negative. Joint accessory motions appeared to be within normal limits, given that the movements were tested in the presence of some residual muscle tension from protective splinting. A neurologic screen failed to demonstrate the presence of any neurologic involvement. Symptoms could be reproduced with deep palpation of the right groin area. There were no active or passive movements that could alter, provoke, change, or eliminate the pain. There were no trigger points in the abdomen or right lower quadrant that could account for the symptomatic presentation.

A definitive physical therapy diagnosis was not reached immediately after the examination. Treatment with soft tissue mobilization and proprioceptive neuromuscular facilitation techniques was initiated and used as a diagnostic tool. There was no change in the symptoms. The therapist continued trying a series of physical therapy techniques over a period of 3 weeks with no change in the clinical presentation.

Result: In a young and otherwise healthy adult, a lack of measurable, reportable, or observable progress becomes a red flag for further medical follow-up. The results of the physical therapy examination and lack of response to treatment constitute a valuable medical diagnostic tool. Further laboratory results revealed a medical diagnosis of Hashimoto's thyroiditis. Treatment with thyroxine (T_4) resulted in resolution of the musculoskeletal symptoms. The correlation between groin pain and loss of hip extension with Hashimoto's remains unclear. Still, response to the red flag here resulted in a correct medical diagnosis.

---

*The sedimentation (SED) rate (an indication of possible infection or inflammation) was within normal limits for an adult woman.

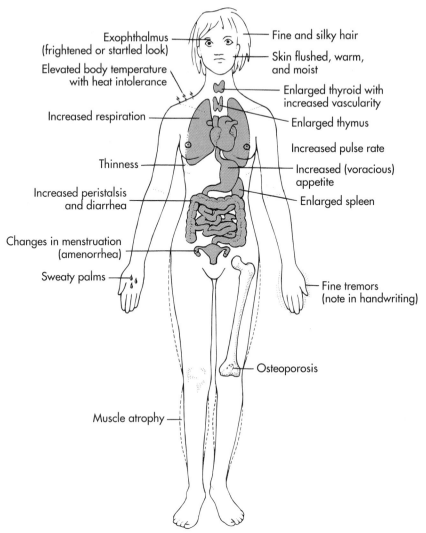

FIGURE 9-3 • Various parts of the body are affected by the symptoms and pathophysiologic complex of hyperthyroidism. (Modified from Muthe NC: *Endocrinology: a nursing approach*, Boston, 1981, Little, Brown, p 93.)

Secondary hypothyroidism (which accounts for a small percentage of all cases of hypothyroidism) occurs as a result of inadequate stimulation of the gland because of pituitary disease.

CLINICAL SIGNS AND SYMPTOMS

As with all disorders affecting the thyroid and parathyroid glands, clinical signs and symptoms affect many systems of the body (Table 9-5).

Because the thyroid hormones play such an important role in the body's metabolism, lack of these hormones seriously upsets the balance of body processes. Among the primary symptoms associated with hypothyroidism are intolerance to cold, excessive fatigue and drowsiness, headaches, weight gain, dryness of the skin, and increasing thinness and

TABLE 9-4 ▼ Systemic Manifestations of Hyperthyroidism

CNS Effects	Cardiovascular and Pulmonary Effects	Joint and Integumentary Effects	Ocular Effects	GI Effects	GU Effects
Tremors Hyperkinesis (abnormally increased motor function or activity) Nervousness Emotional lability Weakness and muscle atrophy Increased deep tendon reflexes	Increased pulse rate/tachycardia/palpitations Arrhythmias (palpitations) Weakness of respiratory muscles (breathlessness, hypoventilation) Increased respiratory rate	Chronic periarthritis Capillary dilation (warm, flushed, moist skin) Heat intolerance Oncholysis (separation of the fingernail from the nail bed) Easily broken hair and increased hair loss Hard, purple area over the anterior surface of the tibia with itching, erythema, and occasionally pain	Weakness of the extraocular muscles (poor convergence, poor upward gaze) Sensitivity to light Visual loss Spasm and retraction of the upper eyelids, lid tremor	Hypermetabolism (increased appetite with weight loss) Diarrhea, nausea, and vomiting Dysphagia	Polyuria (frequent urination) Amenorrhea (absence of menses) Female infertility

Case Example. A 73-year-old woman who has rheumatoid arthritis has just joined the Physical Therapy Aquatic Program. Despite the climate-controlled facility, she becomes flushed, demonstrates an increased respiratory rate that is inconsistent with her level of exercise, and begins to perspire profusely. She reports muscle cramping of the arms and legs and sudden onset of a headache.

Questions
• How would you handle this situation?
• Can this client resume the aquatic program when her symptoms have resolved?

Result: The client was quickly escorted from the pool. Her vital signs were taken and recorded for future reference. Later, the therapist reviewed the client's health history and noted that the "thyroid medication" she reported taking was actually an antithyroid medication for Graves' disease.

The heat intolerance associated with the Graves' disease (hyperthermia secondary to accelerated metabolic rate) presents a potential contraindication for aquatic or pool therapy. Heat intolerance contributes to exercise intolerance, and the client was exhibiting signs and symptoms of heat stroke, even when exercising in a climate-controlled facility. The physician was notified of the symptoms and how quickly the onset occurred (after only 5 minutes of warm-up exercises). Strenuous exercise or a conditioning program should be delayed until symptoms of heat intolerance, tachycardia, or arrhythmias are under medical control.

TABLE 9-5 ▼ Systemic Manifestations of Hypothyroidism

CNS Effects	Musculoskeletal Effects	Pulmonary Effects	Cardiovascular Effects	Hematologic Effects	Integumentary Effects	GI Effects
Slowed speech and hoarseness	Proximal muscle weakness	Dyspnea	Bradycardia	Anemia	Myxedema (periorbital	Anorexia
Slow mental function (loss	Myalgias	Respiratory muscle	Congestive heart failure	Easy bruising	and periph-	Constipation
of interest in	Trigger points	weakness	Poor peripheral		eral)	Weight gain dispropor-
daily activities,	Stiffness		circulation		Thickened, cool,	tionate to
poor short-term	Carpal tunnel syn-		(pallor, cold		and dry skin	caloric in-
memory)	drome		skin, intoler-		Scaly skin (es-	take
Fatigue and	Prolonged deep		ance to cold,		pecially el-	Decreased ab-
increased	tendon reflexes		hypertension)		bows and	sorption of
sleep	(especially		Severe athero-		knees)	nutrients
Headache	Achilles)		sclerosis		Carotenosis	Decreased pro-
Cerebellar	Subjective report of		Angina		(yellowing of	tein metabo-
ataxia	paresthesias				the skin)	lism (re-
	without support-				Coarse, thin-	tarded
	ive objective				ning hair	skeletal and
	findings				Intolerance to	soft tissue
	Muscular and joint				cold	growth)
	edema				Nonpitting	Delayed glu-
	Back pain				edema of	cose uptake
	Increased bone				hands and	Decreased glu-
	density				feet	cose absorp-
	Decreased bone				Poor wound	tion
	formation and				healing	
	resorption				Thin, brittle	
					nails	

brittleness of the nails. In women, menstrual bleeding may become irregular.

A characteristic sign of hypothyroidism is *myxedema* (often used synonymously with hypothyroidism). Myxedema is a result of an alteration in the composition of the dermis and other tissues, causing connective tissues to be separated by increased amounts of mucopolysaccharides and proteins.

This mucopolysaccharide-protein complex binds with water, causing a nonpitting, boggy edema especially around the eyes, hands, and feet and in the supraclavicular fossae. In addition, the binding of this protein-mucopolysaccharide complex causes thickening of the tongue and the laryngeal and pharyngeal mucous membranes. This results in hoarseness and thick, slurred speech, which are also characteristic of hypothyroidism.

In addition, persons who have myxedematous hypothyroidism demonstrate synovial fluid that is highly distinctive. The fluid's high viscosity results in a slow fluid wave that creates a sluggish "bulge" sign visible at the knee joint. Often the fluid contains calcium pyrophosphate dihydrate (CPPD) crystal deposits that may be associated with chondrocalcinosis (deposit of calcium salts in joint cartilage). Thus a finding of a highly viscous, "noninflammatory" joint effusion containing CPPD crystals may suggest to the physician possible underlying hypothyroidism.

When such clients with hypothyroidism have been treated with thyroid replacement, some have experienced attacks of acute pseudogout, caused by CPPD crystals remaining in the synovial fluid.

Neuromuscular symptoms are among the most common manifestations of hypothyroidism. Flexor tenosynovitis with stiffness often accompanies CTS in people with hypothyroidism. CTS can develop before other signs of hypothyroidism become evident. It is thought that this CTS arises from deposition of myxedematous tissue in the carpal tunnel area. Acroparesthesias may occur as a result of median nerve compression at the wrist. The paresthesias are almost always located bilaterally in the hands. Most clients do not require surgical treatment because the symptoms respond to thyroid replacement.

Proximal muscle weakness is common in clients who have hypothyroidism and is sometimes accompanied by pain. As mentioned earlier, muscle weakness is not always related to either the severity or the duration of hypothyroidism and can be present several months before the diagnosis of hypothyroidism is made. Muscle bulk is usually normal; muscle hypertrophy is rare. Deep tendon reflexes are characterized by slowed muscle contraction and relaxation (prolonged reflex).

Characteristically, the muscular complaints of the client with hypothyroidism are aches and pains and cramps or stiffness. Involved muscles are particularly likely to develop persistent myofascial trigger points (TPs). Of particular interest to the physical therapist is the concept that clinically any compromise of the energy metabolism of muscle aggravates and perpetuates TPs.

Treatment of the underlying hypothyroidism is essential in eliminating the TPs, but new research also supports the need for soft tissue treatment to achieve full recovery (Lowe and Lowe, 1998).

The correlation between hypothyroidism and *fibromyalgia syndrome (FMS)* is being investigated (Lowe et al, 1997; Lowe et al, 1998a). An underlying neuromuscular molecular abnormality in some individuals with FMS may be helped by supraphysiologic doses of T_3* (Lowe et al, 1998b). Per-

---

*When tested, blood levels of T_3 are apparently within normal limits, but transport of T_3 into the cell for use does not occur and cannot be measured by blood levels. More information on this topic can be found in the referenced articles by Lowe and colleagues. Additional information can be found at http://members.aol.com/jlowe55555/drlowe.htm or www.wilsonssyndrome.com.

▼ **Clinical Signs and Symptoms of**
Thyroid Carcinoma

- Presence of asymptomatic nodule or mass in thyroid tissue
- Nodule is firm, irregular, painless
- Hoarseness
- Hemoptysis
- Dyspnea
- Elevated blood pressure

---

sons with FMS and clients with undiagnosed myofascial symptoms may benefit from a medical referral for evaluation of thyroid function.

Neoplasms†

Cancer of the thyroid is a relatively uncommon, slow-growing neoplasm that rarely metastasizes. It is often the incidental finding in persons being treated for other disorders (e.g., musculoskeletal disorders involving the head and neck).

The initial manifestation in adults and especially in children is a palpable lymph node or nodule in the neck lateral to the sternocleidomastoid muscle in the lower portion of the posterior triangle overlying the scalene muscles (Gagel et al, 1996) (Fig. 9-4).

A physician must evaluate any client with a palpable nodule because a palpable nodule is often clinically indistinguishable from a mass associated with a benign condition. The presence of new-onset hoarseness, hemoptysis, or elevated blood pressure is a red-flag symptom for systemic disease.

Parathyroid Glands

Two parathyroid glands are located on the posterior surface of each lobe of the thyroid

---

†Primary cancers of other endocrine organs are rare and are unlikely to be encountered by the clinical therapist.

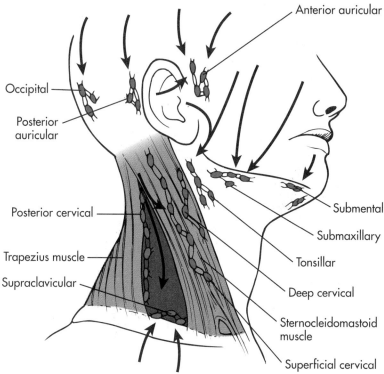

FIGURE 9-4 • Lymph node regions of the head and neck. Palpable nodal disease associated with thyroid carcinoma is commonly located lateral to the sternocleidomastoid muscle in the lower portion of the posterior triangle overlying the scalene muscles (dark red triangle). (Modified from Swartz MH: *Textbook of physical diagnosis*, Philadelphia, 1989, WB Saunders.)

gland. These glands secrete parathyroid hormone (PTH), which regulates calcium and phosphorus metabolism. Parathyroid disorders include hyperparathyroidism and hypoparathyroidism.

If damage or removal of these glands occurs, the resulting hypoparathyroidism (temporary or permanent) causes hypocalcemia, which can result in cardiac arrhythmias and neuromuscular irritability(tetany).

Disorders of the parathyroid glands may produce periarthritis and tendinitis. Both types of inflammation may be crystal-induced and can be associated with periarticular or tendinous calcification.

The physical therapist will see clients with parathyroid disorders in acute care settings and postoperatively because these disorders can result from diseases and operations.

Hyperparathyroidism

Hyperparathyroidism (hyperfunction), or the excessive secretion of PTH, disrupts calcium, phosphate, and bone metabolism. The primary function of PTH is to maintain a normal serum calcium level. Elevated PTH causes release of calcium by the bone and accumulation of calcium in the bloodstream. Symptoms of hyperparathyroidism are related to this release of bone calcium into the bloodstream. This causes demineralization of bone and subsequent loss of bone strength and density. At the same time the increase of calcium in the bloodstream can cause many other problems within the body.

The major cause of primary hyperparathyroidism is a tumor of a parathyroid gland, which results in the autonomous secretion of PTH. Renal failure, another common cause of hyperparathyroidism, causes hypocalcemia

TABLE 9-6 ▼ Systemic Manifestations of Hyperparathyroidism

Early CNS Symptoms	Musculoskeletal Effects	GI Effects	GU Effects
Lethargy, drowsiness, paresthesia	Mild-to-severe proximal muscle weakness of the extremities	Peptic ulcers	Renal colic associated with kidney stones
Slow mentation, poor memory	Muscle atrophy	Pancreatitis	Hypercalcemia (polyuria, polydipsia, constipation)
Depression, personality changes	Bone decalcification (bone pain, especially spine; pathologic fractures; bone cysts)	Nausea, vomiting, anorexia	Kidney infections
Easily fatigued	Gout and pseudogout	Constipation	
Hyperactive deep tendon reflexes	Arthralgias involving the hands		
Occasionally glove-and-stocking distribution of sensory loss	Myalgia and sensation of heaviness in the lower extremities		
	Joint hypermobility		

and stimulates PTH production. Hyperplasia of the gland occurs as it attempts to raise the blood serum calcium levels.

CLINICAL SIGNS AND SYMPTOMS

Many systems of the body are affected by hyperparathyroidism (Table 9-6). Proximal muscle weakness and fatigability are common findings and may be secondary to a peripheral neuropathic process. Myopathy of respiratory muscles with associated respiratory involvement often goes unnoticed. Striking reversal of muscle weakness and atrophy occur with successful treatment of the underlying hyperparathyroidism.

Hyperparathyroidism can also cause GI problems, pancreatitis, bone decalcification, and psychotic paranoia (Fig. 9-5). A chief concern in hyperparathyroidism is damage to the kidneys from calcium deposits, which can result in extensive renal damage.

The classic bone disease affecting persons with primary or renal hyperparathyroidism, *osteitis fibrosa cystica,* has declined in frequency for reasons unknown at this time. This condition is characterized by demineralization, subperiosteal bone resorption, bone pain, fracture, and cystlike bone lesions called brown tumors.

Bone erosion, bone resorption, and subsequent bone destruction most often affect the middle phalanx and the clavicle. Other affected areas may include the skull, wrists, shoulders, knees, and the axial skeleton. Although this condition is now unusual, the therapist may yet encounter cases of ruptured tendons caused by bone resorption in clients with hyperparathyroidism.

Currently, skeletal manifestations of primary hyperparathyroidism are more likely to include bone pain secondary to osteopenia, especially diffuse osteopenia of the spine with possible vertebral fractures. In addition, a number of articular and periarticular disorders have been recognized in association with primary hyperparathyroidism.

Inflammatory erosive polyarthritis may be associated with chondrocalcinosis and CPPD deposits in the synovial fluid. This erosion is called *osteogenic synovitis.* Concurrent illness and surgery (most often parathyroidectomy) are recognized inducers of acute arthritic episodes.

Hypoparathyroidism

Hypoparathyroidism (hypofunction), or insufficient secretion of PTH, most commonly results from accidental removal or injury of the parathyroid gland during thyroid or anterior neck surgery. A less common form of the disease can occur from a genetic autoimmune destruction of the gland. Hypofunction of the parathyroid gland results in insufficient secretion of PTH and subsequent hypocalcemia, hyperphosphatemia, and pronounced neuromuscular and cardiac irritability.

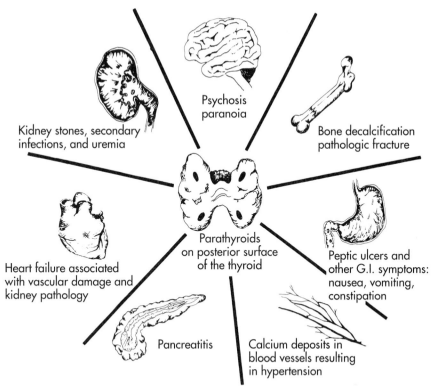

FIGURE 9-5 • The pathologic processes of body structures as a result of excess parathyroid hormone. (From Muthe NC: *Endocrinology: a nursing approach*, Boston, 1981, Little, Brown, p 115.)

TABLE 9-7 ▼ Systemic Manifestations of Hypoparathyroidism

CNS Effects	Musculoskeletal Effects*	Cardiovascular Effects*	Integumentary Effects	GI Effects
Personality changes (irritability, agitation, anxiety, depression)	Hypocalcemia (neuromuscular excitability and muscular tetany, especially involving flexion of the upper extremity)	Cardiac arrhythmias	Dry, scaly, coarse, pigmented skin	Nausea and vomiting
	Spasm of intercostal muscles and diaphragm compromising breathing	Eventual heart failure	Tendency to have skin infections	Constipation or diarrhea
	Positive Chvostek's sign (twitching of facial muscles with tapping of the facial nerve in front of the ear)		Thinning of hair, including eyebrows and eyelashes	Neuromuscular stimulation of the intestine (abdominal pain)
			Fingernails and toenails become brittle and form ridges	

*The most common and important effects for the physical therapist to be aware of are the musculoskeletal and cardiovascular effects.

CLINICAL SIGNS AND SYMPTOMS

Muscle weakness and pain have been reported along with hypocalcemia in clients with hypoparathyroidism.

Hypocalcemia occurs when the parathyroids become inactive. The resultant deficiency of calcium in the blood alters the function of many tissues in the body. These altered functions are described by the systemic manifestations of signs and symptoms associated with hypoparathyroidism (Table 9-7). The most significant clinical consequence of hypocalcemia is neuromuscular irritability. This irritability results in muscle spasms, paresthesias, tetany, and life-threatening cardiac arrhythmias.

Hypoparathyroidism is primarily treated through pharmacologic management with intravenous calcium gluconate, oral calcium salts, and vitamin D. Acute hypoparathyroidism is a life-threatening emergency and is treated rapidly with calcium replacement, anticonvulsants, and prevention of airway obstruction.

Pancreas

The pancreas is a fish-shaped organ that lies behind the stomach. Its head and neck are located in the curve of the duodenum, and its body extends horizontally across the posterior abdominal wall.

The pancreas has dual functions. It acts as both an *endocrine gland,* secreting the hormones insulin and glucagon, and an *exocrine gland,* producing digestive enzymes. Disorders of endocrine function are included in this chapter, whereas disorders of exocrine function affecting digestion are included in Chapter 6.

Diabetes Mellitus

Diabetes mellitus (DM) is a chronic disorder caused by deficient insulin or defective insulin action in the body. It is characterized by hyperglycemia (excess glucose in the blood) and disruption of the metabolism of carbohydrates, fats, and proteins. Over time it results in serious small vessel and large vessel vascular complications and neuropathies.

Type 1 diabetes mellitus* is a condition in which little or no insulin is produced. It occurs in about 10% of all cases and usually occurs in children or young adults. Type 2 diabetes mellitus commonly occurs after age 40 and is a condition of defective insulin and/or impaired cell receptor binding of insulin. Altered glucose tolerance (AGT) is another classification and includes nondiabetic persons with transiently abnormal elevations in serum glucose.

This text focuses primarily on the type 1 and type 2 classifications because these types of DM are more common and more likely to be encountered by the physical therapist in the clinical setting. Table 9-8 depicts the major differences between type 1 and type 2 in presentation and treatment.

PATHOLOGY

Specific physiologic changes occur when insulin is lacking or ineffective. Normally, after a meal the blood glucose level rises. A large amount of this glucose is taken up by the liver for storage or for use by other tissues, such as skeletal muscle and fat. When insulin function is impaired, the glucose in the general circulation is not taken up or removed by these tissues; thus it continues to accumulate in the blood. Because new glucose has not been "deposited" into the liver, the liver synthesizes more glucose and releases it into the general circulation, which increases the already elevated blood glucose level.

---

*It is important to note that the classification of DM has changed several times in the last decade. At one time DM was classified as type I (juvenile-onset diabetes) and type II (adult-onset diabetes). This nomenclature was later modified to insulin-dependent diabetes mellitus (IDDM) and non-insulin-dependent diabetes mellitus (NIDDM) without reference to types I and II. In 1997 the American Diabetes Association issued a summary of classification recommendations that eliminated the use of IDDM and NIDDM and returned to the use of type 1 and type 2, with arabic rather than roman numerals used.

TABLE 9-8 ▼ Primary Differences Between Type 1 and Type 2 Diabetes

Factors	Type 1	Type 2
Age of onset	Usually younger than 30	Usually older than 35
Type of onset	Abrupt	Gradual
Endogenous (own) insulin production	Little or none	Below normal or above normal
Incidence	10%	90%
Ketoacidosis	May occur	Unlikely
Insulin injections	Required	Needed in 20% to 30% of clients
Body weight at onset	Normal or thin	80% are obese
Management	Diet, exercise, insulin	Diet, exercise, oral hypoglycemic agents or insulin
Etiology	Possible viral/autoimmune, resulting in destruction of islet cells	Obesity-associated insulin receptor resistance
Hereditary	Yes	Yes

Modified from Birch C, Greer KH: Nursing care of clients with endocrine disorders of the pancreas. In Black JM, Matassarin-Jacobs E, editors: *Luckmann and Sorenson's medical-surgical nursing*, ed. 5, Philadelphia, 1997, WB Saunders, p. 1961.

Protein synthesis is also impaired because amino acid transport into cells requires insulin. The metabolism of fats and fatty acids is altered, and instead of fat formation, fat breakdown begins in an attempt to liberate more glucose. The oxidation of these fats causes the formation of ketone bodies. Because the formation of these ketones can be rapid, they can build quickly and reach very high levels in the bloodstream. When the renal threshold for ketones is exceeded, the ketones appear in the urine as acetone (ketonuria).

The accumulation of high levels of glucose in the blood creates a hyperosmotic condition in the blood serum. This highly concentrated blood serum then "pulls" fluid from the interstitial areas, and fluid is lost through the kidneys (osmotic diuresis). Because large quantities of urine are excreted (polyuria), serious fluid losses occur, and the conscious individual becomes extremely thirsty and drinks large amounts of water (polydipsia). In addition, the kidney is unable to resorb all the glucose, so glucose begins to be excreted in the urine (glycosuria).

Certain medications can cause or contribute to hyperglycemia. Corticosteroids taken orally have the greatest glucogenic effect. Any diabetic person taking corticosteroid medications needs to be monitored for changes in blood glucose levels.

Other hormones produced by the body also affect blood glucose levels and can have a direct influence on the severity of diabetic symptoms. Epinephrine, glucocorticoids, and growth hormone can cause significant elevations in blood glucose levels by mobilizing stored glucose to blood glucose during times of physical or psychologic stress.

When persons with DM are under stress, such as during surgery, trauma, pregnancy, puberty, or infectious states, blood glucose levels can rise and result in the need for increased amounts of insulin. If these insulin needs cannot be met, a hyperglycemic emergency such diabetic ketoacidosis can result.

It is essential to remember that clients with DM who are under stress will have increased insulin requirements and may become symptomatic even though their disease is usually well controlled in normal circumstances.

PHYSICAL COMPLICATIONS

At presentation, the client with DM may have a variety of serious physical problems. Infection and atherosclerosis are the two primary long-term complications of this disease and are the usual causes of severe illness and death in the diabetic person.

▼ *Clinical Signs and Symptoms of*
Untreated or Uncontrolled Diabetes Mellitus

The classic clinical signs and symptoms of untreated or uncontrolled diabetes mellitus usually include one or more of the following:

- Polyuria: Increased urination caused by osmotic diuresis
- Polydipsia: Increased thirst in response to polyuria
- Polyphagia: Increased appetite and ingestion of food (usually only in type 1)
- Weight loss in the presence of polyphagia: Weight loss caused by improper fat metabolism and breakdown of fat stores (usually only in type 1)
- Hyperglycemia: Increased blood glucose level (fasting level >126 mg/dl)*
- Glycosuria: Presence of glucose in the urine
- Ketonuria: Presence of ketone bodies in the urine (by-product of fat catabolism)
- Fatigue and weakness
- Blurred vision
- Irritability
- Recurring skin, gum, bladder, or other infections
- Numbness/tingling in hands and feet
- Cuts/bruises that are difficult and slow to heal

---

*To be diagnosed with diabetes, a person must have fasting plasma glucose (FPG) readings of 126 mg/dl or higher on two different days. The previous cutoff, set in 1979, was 140 mg/dl. This change occurred as a result of research showing that individuals with readings as low as the mid-120s have already started developing tissue damage from diabetes. A value >110 mg/dl is a risk factor for future diabetes and cardiovascular disease.

▼ *Clinical Signs/Symptoms and Physical Complications of*
Diabetes Mellitus

- Atherosclerosis
  Macrovascular disease
    Cerebrovascular disease (CVD)
    Coronary artery disease (CAD)
    Renal artery stenosis
    Peripheral vascular disease (PVD)
  Microvascular disease
    Nephropathy
    Retinopathy
    Decreased microcirculation to skin/body organs
- Infection/impaired wound healing
- Neuropathy
  Autonomic (gastroparesis, diarrhea, incontinence, postural hypotension, decreased heart rate)
  Peripheral (polyneuropathy, diabetic foot)
  Diabetic amyotrophy
  Carpal tunnel syndrome (ischemia of median nerve)
  Charcot's joint (diabetic arthropathy)
- Periarthritis
- Hand stiffness
  Limited joint mobility (LJM) syndrome
  Flexor tenosynovitis
  Dupuytren's contracture
  Reflex sympathetic dystrophy (RSD)

Blood vessels and nerves sustain major pathologic changes in the person affected by DM. Atherosclerosis in both large vessels (macrovascular changes) and small vessels (microvascular changes) develops at a much earlier age and progresses much faster in the individual with DM. The blood vessel changes result in decreased blood vessel lumen size, compromised blood flow, and resultant tissue ischemia. The pathologic end-products are cerebrovascular disease (CVD), coronary artery disease (CAD), renal artery stenosis, and peripheral vascular disease.

Microvascular changes, characterized by the thickening of capillaries and damage to the basement membrane, result in diabetic nephropathy (kidney disease) and diabetic retinopathy (disease of the retina).

Poorly controlled DM can lead to various tissue changes that result in impaired would healing. Decreased circulation to the skin can further delay or diminish healing.

Diabetic Neuropathy. Neuropathy is the most common chronic complication of long-term DM. Neuropathy in the client with DM is thought to be related to the accumulation in the nerve cells of sorbitol, a by-product of improper glucose metabolism. This accumulation then results in abnormal fluid and electrolyte shifts and nerve cell dysfunction. The combination of this metabolic derangement and the diminished vascular perfusion to nerve tissues contributes to the severe problem of diabetic neuropathy.

Neuropathy may affect the central nervous system, peripheral nervous system, or autonomic nervous system. The most common form of diabetic neuropathy is polyneuropathy, which affects peripheral nerves in distal lower extremities, causing burning and numbness in the feet. It can result in muscle weakness, atrophy, and foot drop.

Diabetic neuropathy can produce a syndrome of bilateral but asymmetric proximal muscle weakness called *diabetic amyotrophy*. Although the muscle enzyme levels are usually normal, muscle biopsy reveals atrophy of type II muscle fibers.

CTS is also a common finding in persons with DM; it represents one form of diabetic neuropathy. As many as 5% to 16% of people with CTS have underlying diabetes. The mechanism is thought to be ischemia of the median nerve resulting from diabetes-related microvascular damage. This ischemia then causes increased sensitivity to even minor pressure exerted in the carpal tunnel area.

Charcot's joint, or neuropathic arthropathy, is a well-known complication of diabetes mellitus. This condition is due, at least in part, to the loss of proprioceptive sensation that marks diabetic neuropathy. Severe degenerative arthritis similar to Charcot's joint has been noted in clients with CPPD crystal deposition disease.

The large- and small-vessel changes that occur with DM contribute to the changes in the feet of diabetic persons. Sensory neuropathy, which may lead to painless trauma and ulceration, can progress to infection. Neuropathy can result in drying and cracking of the skin, which creates more openings for bacteria to enter. The combination of all these factors can ultimately lead to gangrene and eventually require amputation. Prevention of these problems by meticulous care of the diabetic foot can reduce the need for amputation by 50% to 75%.

Whether a poorly controlled blood glucose level is a causative factor in the development of the long-term physical complications of diabetes is still controversial, but it does seem clear that these complications increase with the duration of the disease.

Periarthritis. Periarthritis of the shoulder is five times as common in this group as among nondiabetic persons. The condition most often affects insulin-dependent people, and involvement is typically bilateral.

The mechanism of this association is unclear, but it is believed to be related to fibroblast proliferation in the connective tissue structures around joints or to microangiopathy (disorder involving small blood vessels) involving the tendon sheaths. This periarthritic condition can behave unpredictably: it may regress spontaneously, remain stable, or progress to adhesive capsulitis.

Hand Stiffness. Diabetic stiff hand, limited joint mobility (LJM) syndrome, cheirarthritis (inflammation of the hand and finger joints), and diabetic contractures are common in both types of DM in direct relation to the presence and duration of microvascular complications.

Flexor tenosynovitis, caused by accumulation of excessive dermal collagen in the fingers, results in thickening and induration of the skin around the joints. This condition can lead to sclerodactyly (hardening and shrinking of fingers and toes), which in turn can mimic scleroderma.

Dupuytren's contracture has a strong association with DM. The syndrome is characterized by nodular thickening of the palmar fascia and flexion contracture of the digits. Clients usually have pain in the palm and digits, with decreased mobility and contracture of the fingers. In clients with diabetes, Dupuytren's contracture must be differentiated from LJM, which may involve the entire hand and is frequently bilateral, and

TABLE 9-9 ▼ Insulin Action (Average For Classifications)

Type	Onset (Hr)	Peak (Hr)	Duration (Hr)
Rapid-acting (e.g., regular insulin, Semilente)	0.5-1	2-6	5-12
Intermediate-acting (e.g., NPH, Lente)	1-3	6-12	16-24
Long-acting (e.g., Ultralente, protamine zinc)	4-8	16-18	36+

from flexor tenosynovitis, which is marked by trigger finger.

Individuals with DM may develop reflex sympathetic dystrophy (RSD) syndrome, which is characterized by pain, hyperesthesia, vasomotor and dystrophic skin changes, and tenderness and swelling around the hands and feet.

TREATMENT

Medical management of the client with diabetes is directed primarily toward maintenance of blood glucose values within the range of 80 to 120 mg/dl. The three primary treatment modalities used in the management of DM are diet, exercise, and medication (insulin and oral hypoglycemic agents) (Table 9-9).

EXERCISE-RELATED COMPLICATIONS

Exercise for the person with DM must be planned and instituted cautiously and monitored carefully because significant complications can result from strenuous exercise.

Exercise-related complications can be prevented by careful monitoring of the client's blood glucose level before, during, and after strenuous exercise sessions (safe levels are individually determined but usually fall between 100 and 250 mg/dl). If the blood glucose level is greater than 250 mg/dl, the session should be postponed until the blood glucose level is under better control. If the blood glucose level is less than 100 mg/dl, a 10 to 15 g carbohydrate snack should be given and the glucose retested in 15 minutes to ensure an appropriate level.

Clients with active retinopathy and nephropathy should avoid high-intensity exercise that causes significant increases in blood pressure because such increases can cause further damage to the retinas and kidneys. Any exercise that places the head below the waist also can aggravate retinal problems (Leon, 1993).

In addition, it is very important to have the client avoid insulin injection to active extremities within 1 hour of exercise because insulin is absorbed much more quickly in an active extremity. It is important to know the type, dose, and time of the client's insulin injections so that exercise is not planned for the peak activity times of the insulin.

Clients with type 1 diabetes may need to reduce the insulin dose or increase food intake when initiating an exercise program. During prolonged activities, a 10 to 15 g carbohydrate snack is recommended for each 30 minutes of activity. Activities should be promptly stopped with the development of any symptoms of hypoglycemia, and blood glucose should be tested. In addition, diabetic clients should not exercise alone. Partners, teammates, and coaches must be educated regarding the possibility of hypoglycemia and the way to manage it (Leon, 1993).

Severe Hyperglycemic States

The two primary life-threatening metabolic conditions that can develop if uncontrolled or untreated DM progresses to a state of severe hyperglycemia (>400 mg/dl) are diabetic ketoacidosis and hyperglycemic, hyperosmolar, nonketotic coma (HHNC) (Table 9-10).

Diabetic ketoacidosis (DKA) occurs with severe insulin deficiency caused either by undiagnosed DM or a situation in which the insulin needs of the person become greater than usual (e.g., infection, trauma, emotional upsets). It is most often seen in the client with type 1 diabetes but can, in rare situations, occur in the client with type 2 diabetes. Medical treatment is necessary.

TABLE 9-10 ▼ Clinical Symptoms of Life-Threatening Glycemic States

	Hyperglycemia		Hypoglycemia
Diabetic Ketoacidosis (DKA)	Hyperglycemic, Hyperosmolar, Nonketotic Coma (HHNC)		Insulin Shock
Gradual Onset	*Gradual Onset*		*Sudden Onset*
Thirst	Thirst		Sympathetic activity
Hyperventilation	Polyuria leading quickly to decreased		Pallor
Fruity odor to breath	urine output		Perspiration
Lethargy/confusion	Volume loss from polyuria leading		Increased heart rate
Coma	quickly to renal insufficiency		Palpitation
Muscle and abdominal cramps	Severe dehydration		Irritability/nervousness
(electrolyte loss)	Lethargy/confusion		Weakness
Polyuria, dehydration	Seizures		Hunger
Flushed face, hot/dry skin	Coma		Shakiness
Elevated temperature	Abdominal pain and distension		CNS activity
Blood glucose level >300 mg/dl	Blood glucose level >300 mg/dl		Headache
Serum pH <7.3			Double/blurred vision
			Slurred speech
			Fatigue
			Numbness of lips/tongue
			Confusion
			Convulsion/coma
			Blood glucose level <70 mg/dl

Hyperglycemic, hyperosmolar, nonketotic coma occurs most commonly in the older adult with type 2 diabetes. This complication is extremely serious and, in many cases, is fatal. Factors that can precipitate this crisis are infections (e.g., pneumonia), medications that elevate the blood glucose level (e.g., corticosteroids), and procedures, such as dialysis, surgery, or total parenteral nutrition (TPN).

There are specific clinical features that identify HHNC. Some of these are similar to those of DKA, such as severe hyperglycemia (1000 to 2000 mg/dl) and dehydration. The major differentiating feature between DKA and HHNC, however, is the absence of ketosis in HHNC.

Because it is likely that the physical therapist will work with diabetic clients in the clinical setting, it is imperative that the clinical symptoms of DM and its potentially life-threatening metabolic states be understood. *If any diabetic client arrives for a clinical appointment in a confused or lethargic state or exhibiting changes in mental function, fingerstick glucose testing should be performed. Immediate physician referral is necessary.*

Hypoglycemia

Hypoglycemia (blood glucose of <70 mg/dl) is a major complication of the use of insulin or oral hypoglycemic agents. Hypoglycemia is usually the result of a decrease in food intake or an increase in physical activity in relation to insulin administration. It is a potentially lethal problem. The hypoglycemic state interrupts the oxygen consumption of nervous system tissue. Repeated or prolonged attacks can result in irreversible brain damage and death.

HYPOGLYCEMIA ASSOCIATED WITH DIABETES MELLITUS

Hypoglycemia during or after exercise can be a problem for any diabetic person. This condition results as glucose is used by the working muscles and/or if the circulating level of injected insulin is too high. The degree of hypoglycemia depends on such factors as preexercise blood glucose levels, duration and intensity of exercise, and blood insulin concentration.

CLINICAL SIGNS AND SYMPTOMS

The severity and number of signs and symptoms depend on the individual client and the rapidity of the drop in blood glucose.

It is important to note that clients can exhibit signs and symptoms of hypoglycemia when their elevated blood glucose level drops rapidly to a level that is still elevated (e.g., 400 to 200 mg/dl). The *rapidity* of the drop is the stimulus for sympathetic activity; even though a blood glucose level appears elevated, clients may still have hypoglycemia.

Clients receiving beta-adrenergic blockers (e.g., propranolol) can be at special risk for hypoglycemia by the actions of this medication. These beta-blockers inhibit the normal physiologic response of the body to the hypoglycemic state or block the appearance of the sympathetic manifestations of hypoglycemia. Clients may also have hypoglycemia during nighttime sleep (most often related to the use of intermediate- and long-acting insulins given more than once a day), with the only symptoms being nightmares, sweating, or headache.

Treatment. Hypoglycemia can be treated in the conscious client by immediate administration of sugar. It is always safer to give the sugar, even when there is doubt concerning the origin of symptoms (DKA and HHNC can also have similar CNS symptoms at presentation). Most often 10 to 15 g of carbohydrate are sufficient to reverse the episode of hypoglycemia. Immediate-acting glucose sources should be kept in every physical therapy department (e.g., $\frac{1}{2}$ cup of fruit juice or sugared cola, 2 packets of sugar, 2-ounce tube of honey or cake-decorating gel).

Most diabetic persons carry a rapid-acting source of carbohydrate so that it is readily available for use if a hypoglycemic episode occurs. Intramuscular glucagon is also used by some diabetic individuals. If the client loses consciousness, emergency personnel will need to be notified, and glucose will be administered intravenously.

Any episode or suspected episode of hypoglycemia must be treated promptly and must be reported to the client's physician. It is important to question each diabetic client regarding his or her individual response to hypoglycemia. Information regarding individual symptoms, frequency of episodes, and precipitating factors may be invaluable to the physical therapist in preventing or minimizing a hypoglycemic attack.

OTHER HYPOGLYCEMIC STATES

Other conditions that can cause hypoglycemic states are usually related to hormonal deficiencies (e.g., cortisol, glucagon, ACTH) or overproduction of insulin or insulin-like material from tumors.

Reactive hypoglycemia, also known as functional hypoglycemia, occurs after the intake of a meal and usually results from stomach or duodenal surgery. This condition involves rapid stomach emptying with rapid rises of glucose levels. Glucose then rapidly falls to below normal levels as an exaggerated response of insulin secretion develops. The cause of reactive hypoglycemia is unknown.

CLINICAL SIGNS AND SYMPTOMS

Clinical signs and symptoms of non–diabetes-related hypoglycemic states are the same as those described earlier for hypoglycemia related to DM. The client is warned to avoid fasting and simple sugars.

▼ INTRODUCTION TO METABOLISM

As noted earlier, the endocrine system works with the nervous system to regulate and integrate the body's metabolic activities. Although acid-base metabolism is not in itself a sign or a symptom, the consequences of an acid-base metabolism disorder can result in many signs and symptoms.

The rate of metabolism can be increased by exercise, by elevated body temperature (e.g., high fever), by hormonal activity (e.g.,

TABLE 9-11 ▼ Fluid Imbalances

Imbalance	Symptoms

Fluid Deficit (Dehydration)
Increased Solutes, Decreased H_2O/
   Decreased Solutes, Decreased H_2O
	Thirst
	Weight loss
	Dryness of mouth, throat, face
	Poor skin turgor
	Decreased urine output
	Absence of sweat
	Postural changes from lying to standing
	   Increased pulse (10 beats/min)
	   Decreased blood pressure (10 mm Hg systolic when standing;
	   20 mm Hg systolic or diastolic when moving from supine to
	   sitting)
	Dizziness when standing
	Confusion

Fluid Excess (Water Intoxication)
Increased H_2O, Decreased Solutes
	Decreased mental alertness
	Sleepiness
	Anorexia
	Poor motor coordination
	Confusion
	Convulsions
	Sudden weight gain
	Hyperventilation
	Warm, moist skin
	Increased intracerebral pressure
	   Decreased pulse
	   Increased systolic blood pressure
	   Decreased diastolic blood pressure
	Mild peripheral edema

Fluid Excess (Edema)
Increased H_2O, Increased Solutes
	Weight gain
	Dependent edema
	Pitting edema
	Increased blood pressure
	Neck vein engorgement
	Effusions
	   Pulmonary
	   Pericardial
	   Peritoneal
	Congestive heart failure

thyroxine, insulin, epinephrine), and by specific dynamic action that occurs after ingestion of a meal. All metabolic functions require proper fluid and acid-base balance.

Physical therapists are unlikely to evaluate someone with a primary musculoskeletal lesion that reflects an underlying metabolic disorder. However, many inpatients in hospitals and some outpatients may be affected by disturbances in acid-base metabolism and other specific metabolic disorders. Only those conditions that are likely to be encountered by a physical therapist are included in this text.

Fluid Imbalances (Table 9-11)

Fluid Deficit

Fluid deficit can occur as a result of two primary types of imbalance. There is either a loss of water without loss of solutes or a loss of both water and solutes.

The loss of body water without solutes results in the excess concentration of body solutes within the interstitial and intravascular compartments. To preserve equilibrium, water will then be forced to shift by osmosis from inside cells to these outside compartments.

If this state persists, large amounts of body water will be shifted and excreted (osmotic diuresis), and severe cellular dehydration will result. This type of imbalance can occur as a result of several conditions:

- Decreased water intake (e.g., unavailability, unconsciousness)
- Water loss without proportionate solute loss (e.g., prolonged hyperventilation, diabetes insipidus)
- Increased solute intake without proportionate water intake (tube feeding)
- Excess accumulation of solutes (e.g., high glucose levels such as in DM)

The second type of fluid imbalance results from a loss of *both* water and solutes. Causes of the loss of both water and solutes include hemorrhage, profuse perspiration (as in marathon runners), loss of GI tract secretions (vomiting, diarrhea, draining fistulas, ileostomy).

Severe losses of water and/or solutes can lead to hypovolemic shock. It is important for the physical therapist to be aware of possible fluid losses or water shifts in any client who is already compromised by advanced age or by a situation, such as an ileostomy or tracheostomy, that results in a continuous loss of fluid. Because the response to fluid loss is highly individual, it is important to recognize the early clinical symptoms of fluid loss and to carefully monitor clients who are at risk.

Athletes and normal adults may experience orthostatic hypotension when slightly dehydrated, especially when intense exercise increases the core body temperature. The normal vascular system can accommodate this effectively.

▼ *Clinical Signs and Symptoms of*
Dehydration or Fluid Loss

Early clinical signs and symptoms:
- Thirst
- Weight loss

As the condition worsens, other symptoms may include:
- Poor skin turgor
- Dryness of the mouth, throat, and face
- Absence of sweat
- Increased body temperature
- Low urine output
- Postural hypotension (increased heart rate by 10 beats/min and decreased systolic or diastolic blood pressure by 20 mm Hg when moving from a supine to a sitting position)
- Dizziness when standing
- Confusion
- Increased hematocrit

Fluid Excess

Fluid excess can occur in two major forms: water intoxication (excess of water without an excess of solutes) or edema (excess of both solutes and water).

Because the etiologic complex, symptoms, and outcomes related to these problems are substantially different, these fluid imbalances are discussed separately.

WATER INTOXICATION

Water intoxication is an excess of extracellular water in relationship to solutes. The extracellular fluid (ECF) becomes diluted and water must then move into cells to equalize solute concentration on both sides of the cell membrane.

Water excess can be caused by an accumulation of solute-free fluid. An increase in solute-free fluid usually occurs because of excess ADH (tumors, endocrine disorders) or in-

▼ *Clinical Signs and Symptoms of*
Water Intoxication

- Decreased mental alertness

Other accompanying symptoms:

- Sleepiness
- Anorexia
- Poor motor coordination
- Confusion

In a severe imbalance, other symptoms may include:

- Convulsions
- Sudden weight gain
- Hyperventilation
- Warm, moist skin
- Signs of increased intracerebral pressure
  - Slow pulse
  - Increased systolic blood pressure (>10 mm Hg)
  - Decreased diastolic blood pressure (>10 mm Hg)
- Mild peripheral edema
- Low serum sodium
- Low hematocrit

▼ *Clinical Signs and Symptoms of*
Edema

- Weight gain (primary symptom)
- Excess fluid (several liters may accumulate before edema is evident)
- Dependent edema (collection of fluid in lower parts of the body)
- Pitting edema (finger pressed into edematous area leaves a persistent indentation in tissues)

take of large amounts of only tap water without balanced solute ingestion. The latter situation occurs most often in older adults who drink additional water after having the flu with its associated vomiting and diarrhea.

Symptoms of water intoxication are largely neurologic in nature because of the shifting of water into brain tissues.

EDEMA

An excess of solutes and water is called an isotonic volume excess. The excess fluid is retained in the extracellular compartment and results in fluid accumulation in the interstitial spaces (*edema*). Edema can be produced by many different situations, most commonly including vein obstruction, decreased cardiac output, endocrine imbalances, and loss of serum proteins (e.g., burns, liver disease, allergic reactions).

Diuretic medications are used frequently to treat volume excess. Various diuretic medications may be used depending on the underlying cause of the problem and the desired effect of the drug. The most commonly used are the thiazide diuretics (e.g., chlorothiazide, hydrochlorothiazide).

These medications inhibit sodium and water resorption by the kidneys. Potassium is usually also lost with the sodium and water, so continuous replacement of potassium is a major concern for anyone receiving non–potassium-sparing diuretics. It is essential to monitor clients who take diuretics for signs and symptoms of potassium depletion.

It is also very important to check laboratory data for the potassium level in any client taking diuretics, particularly before exercise. Any value below the normal range (<3.5 mEq/L) could be potentially dangerous and could result in a lethal cardiac arrhythmia even with moderate cardiovascular exercise.

In addition, it is important to assess clients who take diuretic therapy for potential fluid loss and dehydration by observing for clinical symptoms of both.

Questions concerning the correlation of potassium levels with exercise and possible appearance of symptoms consistent with dehydration should be discussed with a physician before physical therapy treatment.

▼ **Clinical Signs and Symptoms of**
Potassium Depletion

- Muscle weakness
- Fatigue
- Cardiac arrhythmias
- Abdominal distension
- Nausea and vomiting

▼ **Clinical Signs and Symptoms of**
Metabolic Alkalosis

- Nausea
- Prolonged vomiting
- Diarrhea
- Confusion
- Irritability
- Agitation, restlessness
- Muscle twitching and muscle cramping
- Muscle weakness
- Paresthesias
- Convulsions
- Eventual coma
- Slow, shallow breathing

▼ METABOLIC DISORDERS

Metabolic Alkalosis

Metabolic alkalosis results from metabolic disturbances that cause either an increase in available bases or a loss of nonrespiratory body acids. Blood pH rises to a level greater than 7.45 (Table 9-12).

Common causes of metabolic alkalosis include excessive vomiting or upper GI suctioning, diuretic therapy or ingestion of large quantities of base substances such as antacids.

Decreased respirations may occur as the respiratory system attempts to compensate by buffering the basic environment. The lungs attempt to retain carbon dioxide (CO_2) and thus hydrogen ions (H^+).

It is important for the physical therapist to ask clients about the use of antacids because symptoms of alkalosis can affect muscular function by causing muscle fasciculation and cramping. Prevention of problems related to alkalosis may be accomplished by education of the client regarding antacid use.

Metabolic Acidosis

Metabolic or nonrespiratory acidosis is an accumulation of fixed (nonvolatile) acids or a deficit of bases. Blood pH decreases to a level below 7.35 (see Table 9-12).

Common causes of metabolic acidosis include diabetic ketoacidosis, lactic acidosis, renal failure, severe diarrhea, and drug or chemical toxicity.

Ketoacidosis occurs because insufficiency of insulin for the proper use of glucose results in increased breakdown of fat. This accelerated fat breakdown produces ketones and other acids. These acids accumulate to high levels. While the body attempts to neutralize these increased acids, the plasma bicarbonate (HCO_3) is used up.

Renal failure results in acidosis because the failing kidney not only is unable to rid the body of excess acids but also cannot produce necessary bicarbonate.

Lactic acidosis occurs as excess lactic acid is produced during strenuous exercise or when oxygen is insufficient for proper use of carbohydrate (CHO), glucose, and water (H_2O).

Intestinal and pancreatic secretions are highly alkaline so that *severe diarrhea* depletes the body of these necessary bases. Metabolic acidosis can result from ingestion of large quantities of acetylsalicylic acid (salicylates), and symptoms of possible metabolic acidosis should be carefully assessed in clients undergoing high-dose aspirin therapy.

Hyperventilation may occur as the respiratory system attempts to rid the body of excess acid by increasing the rate and depth of respiration. The result is an increase in the

TABLE 9-12 ▼ Laboratory Values: Uncompensated and Compensated Metabolic Alkalosis and Acidosis

| | Arterial Blood | | | |
	pH (7.35-7.45)	PCO_2 (35-45 mm Hg)	HCO_3 (22-36 mEq/L)	Signs/Symptoms
Metabolic Alkalosis				
Uncompensated	>7.45	Normal	>26	Nausea
				Vomiting
				Diarrhea
				Confusion
				Irritability
				Agitation
				Muscle twitch
				Muscle cramp
				Muscle weakness
				Paresthesias
				Convulsions
				Slow breathing
Compensated	Normal	>45	>26	Decreased respiratory rate
Metabolic Acidosis				
Uncompensated	<7.35	Normal	<22	Headache
				Fatigue
				Nausea, vomiting
				Diarrhea
				Muscular twitching
				Convulsions, coma
				Hyperventilation
Compensated	Normal	<35	<22	Increased respiratory rate

▼ *Clinical Signs and Symptoms of*
Metabolic Acidosis

- Headache
- Fatigue
- Drowsiness, lethargy
- Nausea, vomiting
- Diarrhea
- Muscular twitching
- Convulsions
- Coma (severe)
- Rapid, deep breathing (hyperventilation)

amount of carbon dioxide and hydrogen excreted through the respiratory system.

Gout

Primary gout is the manifestation of an inherited inborn error of purine metabolism characterized by an elevated serum uric acid (hyperuricemia).

Increased serum uric acid levels are associated with middle age, obesity, white race, stress (including surgery, medical illness), and high dietary intake of purine-rich foods. A variety of medications (e.g., penicillin, insulin, or thiazide diuretics) may increase the serum uric acid level, as may a number of acute or chronic disorders other than gout (Table 9-13).

Uric acid is usually dissolved in the blood until it is passed into the urine through the kidneys. In individuals with gout the uric acid changes into crystals (urate) that deposit in joints (causing gouty arthritis) and other tissues such as the kidneys, causing renal disease.

Gout may occur as a result of another disorder or of its therapy. This is referred to as *secondary gout*. Secondary gout may be associated with neoplasm, renal disease, or other metabolic disorders, such as DM and hyperlipidemia (excess serum lipids).

TABLE 9-13 ▼ Causes of Secondary Hyperuricemia

Hematopoietic	Renal
Hemolytic anemia	Hemodialysis
Myeloproliferative disorders	Renal insufficiency
Polycythemia vera	
Myeloma	**Drugs**
	Low-dose aspirin
Neoplastic	Diuretics
Leukemia	Antineoplastic agents
Lymphoma	Alcohol
Multiple myeloma	
	Other
Endocrine	Chondrocalcinosis
Hypoparathyroidism	Psoriasis
Hyperparathyroidism	Sarcoidosis
Hypothyroidism	Obesity
Diabetes mellitus	Hyperlipidemia
	Starvation

From Wade JP, Liang MH: Avoiding common pitfalls in the diagnosis of gout, *J Musculoskel Med* 5(8):16-27, 1988.

Gout affects men predominantly, and the usual form of primary gout is uncommon before the third decade, with its peak incidence in the forties and fifties. After menopause the frequency of gout in women approaches that in men (Gilliland and Gardner, 1993).

Pseudogout is an arthritic condition caused by calcium pyrophosphate dihydrate (CPPD) crystals. It occurs about one eighth as often as gout and may be hereditary or secondary to other disease processes (hyperparathyroidism is the most common one).

Pseudogout is marked by attacks of gout-like symptoms, usually affecting a single joint (particularly the knee) and associated with chondrocalcinosis (deposition of calcium salts in joint cartilage).

Case Example. A 69-year-old man in previously good health complained of steadily increasing pain that had developed in his hands over the past several months. There was no history of occupational or accidental trauma.

Although the pain was present bilaterally, the pain in the left hand was more severe than in the right. The gentleman was right-hand dominant. There was a pattern of symptoms of increasing pain (described as deep aching) from morning to evening with a corresponding decrease in function.

Objective findings included reduced wrist range of motion in all directions bilaterally. There was no observed edema, warmth, or redness of the forearms, wrists, or hands. Although there were no reported symptoms at the elbow, left elbow extension and left forearm supination were also decreased by 25% as compared to the right side. Grip strength was reduced by 50% bilaterally for age and sex.

Neurologic screening was without significant findings. There were no trigger points corresponding to the pain pattern present. No constitutional symptoms were reported, and vital signs were unremarkable.

Result. This man was treated by a hand therapist without significant changes in symptoms or function. In fact, he reported an increased inability to write with his right hand. The therapist suggested a medical evaluation with possible inclusion of x-ray examination. Physician assessment resulted in a diagnosis of CPPD arthropathy (pseudogout) of unknown cause. Medical treatment included a prescription nonsteroidal antiinflammatory drug and return to physical therapy for continued symptomatic treatment addressing the loss of function.

Although a medical condition existed, physical therapy treatment was still warranted. In this case a medical differential diagnosis provided the client with necessary medical treatment and the physical therapist with information necessary to treat the client more specifically.

▼ *Clinical Signs and Symptoms of*

Gout

- Tophi: Lumps under the skin or actual eruptions through the skin of chalky urate crystals
- Joint pain and swelling (especially first metatarsal joint)
- Fever and chills
- Malaise
- Redness

In persons with pseudogout, routine x-ray studies of the knee and wrist frequently demonstrate cartilage calcification, or chondrocalcinosis. Because these changes are found in up to 10% of older adults, diagnosis must be made through aspiration of synovial fluid to identify the crystals.

CLINICAL SIGNS AND SYMPTOMS

Gouty arthritis results in periarticular and subcutaneous deposits of sodium urate (or urate salts), referred to as tophus (tophi).

The formation of tophi is directly related to the elevation of serum urate; the higher the client's serum urate concentration, the higher the rate of urate deposition in soft tissue.*

The peripheral joints of the hands and feet are involved, with 90% of gouty clients having attacks in the metatarsophalangeal joint of the great toe. Other typical sites of initial involvement (in order of frequency) are the instep, ankle, heel, knee, and wrist, although any joint in the body may be involved.

These deposits produce an acute inflammatory response that then leads to acute arthritis and later to chronic arthritis. Enlarged tophi on the joints of the hands and

feet may erupt and discharge chalky masses of urate crystals.

Many diseases have a presentation similar to that of acute gouty arthritis. Gout and septic arthritis occasionally occur together. The diagnosis of gout must be based on the demonstration of monosodium urate crystals by synovial fluid analysis rather than on the clinical presentation alone.

Onset of pain is sudden and severe and increases in intensity in one or more joints. The pain usually reaches its maximal intensity within 12 hours after its onset. Exquisite tenderness is accompanied by swelling of the inflamed joint, and any pressure (even the touch of clothes or bedsheets) on the joint is intolerable. Untreated, the attack lasts from 10 days to 2 weeks.

Hemochromatosis

Hemochromatosis, also termed *hematochromatosis,* is an inborn error of iron metabolism. It is an inherited disorder characterized by excessive GI absorption and body retention of iron, with progressive tissue damage in parenchymal organs.

Hemochromatosis is found five to ten times more often in men than in women because women lose blood through menstruation and pregnancy. Men seldom have symptoms until after 50 years of age and are rarely symptomatic before 30 years of age. Because of menstrual blood loss, women display symptoms 10 years later than men (median age: 60 years).

Ascorbic acid (vitamin C) and alcohol seem to accelerate the absorption of dietary iron. The high incidence of alcoholism among clients with hemochromatosis (40%) supports this concept.

The cardinal defect in hemochromastosis is the lack of regulation of iron absorption, but the exact mechanism is unknown. The intestinal tract absorbs more iron than is required, thus producing an excess.

In its early stages hemochromatosis produces no symptoms because it takes many years of iron accumulation to produce warning

---

*Before urate-lowering agents became available, 30% to 50% of people with acute gouty arthritis developed tophi. Today, chronic tophaceous gout is rarely seen.

▼ **Clinical Signs and Symptoms of**
Hemochromatosis

- Arthropathy (joint disease)*
- Arthralgias
- Myalgias
- Progressive weakness
- Bilateral pitting edema (lower extremities)
- Vague abdominal pain
- Hypogonadism (lack of menstrual periods, impotence)*
- Congestive heart failure
- Hyperpigmentation of the skin (gray/blue to yellow)
- Loss of body hair
- Diabetes mellitus

*Unfortunately, even with treatment (removal of accumulated iron) arthritis, impotency, and sterility are not reversed.

signs or symptoms. Unfortunately, when the disease becomes evident, it is often too late because iron accumulation has caused irreversible tissue or end-organ damage in the heart, liver, endocrine glands, skin, joints, bone, and pancreas. About half the clients with hemochromatosis will develop arthritis.

CLINICAL SIGNS AND SYMPTOMS

For many years hemochromatosis was identified by a classic clinical triad of enlarged liver, skin hyperpigmentation, and diabetes. The term *bronze diabetes* was used to describe this presentation. Hyperpigmentation is caused by an increased number of melanocytes and a thinning of the epidermis. However, hemochromatosis may have many different signs and symptoms, confusing early diagnosis.

Hemochromatosis has a well-known association with chondrocalcinosis (deposition of calcium salts in the cartilage of joints).

Acute attacks of synovitis can occur, which may resemble a rheumatoid flare. A biopsy of synovial tissue reveals iron deposition in the cells of the synovial lining that is non-inflammatory.

Arthritis may be the presenting symptom of hemochromatosis, but it usually occurs after diagnosis and is more severe in adults older than 50. Arthritic manifestations are diverse, and joint damage occurs not from iron but from deposition of calcium pyrophosphate dihydrate (CPPD) crystals.

The distribution of joint involvement may resemble rheumatoid arthritis, affecting the metacarpophalangeal (MCP) joints, in particular the second and third MCP joints. However, reduced MCP flexion is not accompanied by ulnar deviation. The arthritis can progress, and large joints may become involved, particularly the hips, knees, and shoulders.

Metabolic Bone Disease

Of the numerous metabolic disorders involving connective tissue, only the most commonly occurring diseases that would appear in a physical therapy setting are discussed in this text. These include osteoporosis, osteomalacia, and Paget's disease.

Osteoporosis

Osteoporosis, meaning "porous bone" and defined as a decreased mass per unit volume of normally mineralized bone compared with age- and sex-matched controls, is the most prevalent bone disease in the world. After the age of 30 years, human bone tissue begins to diminish gradually, owing to an imbalance between bone resorption and formation during the remodeling cycle. The body excretes more calcium than it retains, resulting in reduction of bone mass. Intestinal absorption of calcium becomes less efficient with age; older persons need more, rather than less, dietary calcium to maintain a positive calcium balance.

Osteoporosis is classified as *primary* or *secondary*. Idiopathic, postmenopausal, and senile osteoporosis are included in the primary osteoporosis classification. Secondary osteoporosis is associated with other disorders, such as endocrine conditions (e.g., hyperthyroidism, hyperparathyroidism, hypogonadism, Cushing's disease, and diabetes mellitus), chronic renal failure, rheumatoid arthritis, malabsorption syndromes related to GI and hepatic disease, chronic respiratory disease, malignancies, and chronic chemical dependency (alcohol).

Medications such as thyroid supplements, corticosteroids,* anticoagulants, lithium, and anticonvulsants can contribute to the development of secondary osteoporosis (Goodman and Simon, 1997).

Postmenopausal osteoporosis is associated with accelerated bone loss in the perimenopausal period, accompanied by high fracture rates, particularly involving the vertebrae (Sinnett, 1993).

Bone mass maintenance is related to estrogen levels because estrogen has a protective effect on the bone by suppressing resorption. Estrogen stimulates the production of calcitonin, which prevents removal of calcium from the bone. Estrogen improves calcium absorption in the intestinal tract and decreases calcium losses in the urine. After menopause, when estrogen secretion diminishes, bone becomes increasingly sensitive to parathyroid hormone, and bone resorption increases.

More than half the women in the United States who are 50 years of age or older are likely to have radiologically detectable evidence of abnormally decreased bone mass (osteopenia) in the spine. More than a third of these women develop major orthopedic problems related to osteoporosis. Most fractures sustained by women older than 50 are secondary to osteoporosis.

Senile osteoporosis, or *age-related osteoporosis,* increases with advancing age; it is caused by the bone loss that normally accompanies aging.

---

*Most common when used long term for rheumatoid arthritis, systemic lupus erythematosus, and other autoimmune diseases.

Clinical Signs and Symptoms of
Osteoporosis

- Back pain: Episodic, acute low thoracic/high lumbar pain
- Compression fracture of the spine (postmenopausal osteoporosis)
- Bone fractures (age-related osteoporosis)
- Decrease in height (more than 1 inch shorter than maximum adult height)
- Kyphosis
- Dowager's hump
- Decreased activity tolerance
- Early satiety

Many risk factors are associated with osteoporosis (see Risk Factors for Osteoporosis), but osteoporosis is the most common bone disease in older Caucasian women of northern European descent who have inadequate dietary calcium intakes and who lead sedentary lifestyles.

Inactivity results in calcium excretion, which is a bone mineral loss. Osteoporosis associated with aging involves fractures of the proximal femur and vertebrae as well as the hip, pelvis, proximal humerus, distal radius, and tibia.

Men can be affected, especially those who smoke, drink alcohol moderately, fail to maintain a calcium-rich diet, have a sedentary lifestyle, have a family history of fractures, or those undergoing dialysis or long-term steroid administration.

The Appendix at the end of this chapter presents a questionnaire to assess risk factors in clients.

Additionally, researchers are beginning to examine the environmental influences associated with industrialized countries such as the United States. For example, although menopause is universal, and the resulting estrogen deficiency is presumably similar for all women, differences in the occurrence of osteoporosis among countries cannot be explained only on the basis of estrogen deficiency (Simmons, 1996). Countries with the

RISK FACTORS FOR OSTEOPOROSIS

WOMEN

- Caucasian
- Gender: Women more than men
- Age: Postmenopausal (older than 65)
- Lifestyle: Smoking; excessive dietary intake of protein, salt, alcohol, caffeine*; vitamin D/calcium deficiency; lactose intolerance; sedentary or inactive lifestyle
- Prolonged exposure to thyroid medications, corticosteroids, antiinflammatories, or seizure medications; certain cancer treatments; aluminum-containing antacids
- Family history of osteoporosis
- Early or surgically induced menopause; menstrual dysfunction (amenorrhea)
- Thin, small-boned frame
- Chronic diseases that affect the kidneys, lungs, stomach, and intestines or alter hormones; dialysis

MEN

- Caucasian
- Gender: Increasing incidence among men
- Advancing age
- Lifestyle: Same as for women
- Prolonged exposure to medications (same as for women)
- Family history of osteoporosis
- Undiagnosed low levels of testosterone
- Chronic diseases (as listed for women)

---

*At least one study (Orwoll et al, 1996) reports that caffeine and antacid use have no probable affect on bone mass in older women. The investigators also emphasized that it is weight, not body mass index, that is important. A 10 kg increase in weight reportedly implied a 6% increase in bone mineral density.

TABLE 9-14 ▼ Endocrine and Metabolic Causes of Secondary Osteoporosis

Diabetes mellitus
Glucocorticoid excess
  Iatrogenic Cushing's syndrome
  Hyperadrenalism
Hyperparathyroidism
Hyperthyroidism
Hypocystinuria (inborn error of amino acid metabolism)
Hypogonadism
Marfan's syndrome
Premature ovarian failure
Testicular insufficiency

highest incidence of osteoporosis also have a high incidence of heart disease and the highest consumption of carbohydrates, fat, protein, salt, and caffeine.

Endocrine-mediated bone loss can produce osteoporosis because numerous endocrine hormones affect skeletal remodeling and hence skeletal mass. Secondary osteoporosis may accompany various endocrine and metabolic disorders that can produce associated osteopenia (Table 9-14).

Early osteoporosis has no visible signs or symptoms. Mild-to-severe back pain and loss of height may be the only early signs

CLUES TO RECOGNIZING OSTEOPOROSIS

- Pain is usually severe and localized to the site of fracture (usually midthoracic, lower thoracic, and lumbar spine vertebrae)
- Pain may radiate to the abdomen or flanks
- Aggravating factors: Prolonged sitting, standing, bending, or performing Valsalva's maneuver
- Alleviating factors: Sidelying with hips and knees flexed
- Sitting up from supine requires rolling to the side first
- Not usually accompanied by sciatica or chronic pain from nerve root impingement
- Tenderness to palpation over the fracture site
- Rib or spinal deformity, dowager's hump (cervical kyphosis)
- Loss of height

observed. Changes in bone density do not show up on x-ray films until they reach a 30% loss (National Osteoporosis Foundation, 1991). The cardinal features of established osteoporosis are bone fracture, pain, and deformity.

Osteomalacia

Osteomalacia is a softening of the bones resulting from impaired mineralization in bone matrix. This failure in mineralization results in a reduced rate of bone formation.

Osteomalacia is caused by a vitamin D deficiency in adults. The deficiency may be due to lack of exposure to ultraviolet rays, inadequate intake of vitamin D in the diet, failure to absorb or use vitamin D, increased catabolism of vitamin D, a renal tubular defect, or a pathologically reduced number of vitamin D receptor sites in tissues.

The disease is characterized by decalcification of the bones, particularly those of the spine, pelvis, and lower extremities. X-ray examination reveals transverse, fracture-like lines in the affected bones and areas of demineralization in the matrix of the bone. These pseudofractures, known as Looser's transformation zones, are bilateral. The most common sites are the ribs, long bones, lateral scapular margin, upper

▼ **Clinical Signs and Symptoms of**
Osteomalacia

- Bone pain
- Skeletal deformities
- Fractures
- Severe muscle weakness
- Myalgia

femur, and pubic rami. As the bones soften, they become bent, flattened, or otherwise deformed. Looser's zones are believed to result from pressure on the softened bone by the nutrient arteries of its blood supply.

Severe bone pain, skeletal deformities, fractures, and severe muscle weakness and pain are common in people with osteomalacia. Clients typically complain of muscle weakness and pain that sometimes mimic polymyositis or muscular dystrophy.

A similar condition in children, occurring before epiphyseal plate closure, is called rickets.

In children with rickets, x-ray findings include the well-known bowing of the long bones, in addition to widening, fraying, and clubbing of the areas of active bone growth. These areas especially include the metaphyseal ends of the long bones and the sternal ends of the ribs, the so-called rachitic rosary.

Paget's Disease

Paget's disease (osteitis deformans), named after Sir James Paget from the mid-1880s, is a focal inflammatory condition of the skeleton that produces disordered bone remodeling. Bone is resorbed and formed at an increased rate and in a haphazard fashion. As a result, the new bone is larger, less compact, more vascular, and more susceptible to fracture than normal bone (Wallach, 1997).

Paget's disease is the most common skeletal disorder after osteoporosis, affecting men more often than women in a 3:2 ratio. Although Paget's disease affects 2% to 5% of the population older than 50, it is most commonly seen in people older than 70, most of whom are asymptomatic (Papapoulos, 1997).

Although the cause of this condition remains unknown, available evidence points to a slow viral infection in genetically predisposed individuals. Evidence for a major genetic component is supported by 40% of affected individuals having affected first-degree relatives (Cody et al, 1997).

CLINICAL SIGNS AND SYMPTOMS

The severity of involvement and associated clinical characteristics vary greatly. Although some people are asymptomatic, with very limited bone involvement, others manifest a disabling, painful form of Paget's disease that is characterized by skeletal pain and bones that are extremely deformed and easily fractured (Wallach, 1997). The bones most commonly involved include (in decreasing order) the pelvis, lumbar spine, sacrum, femur, tibia, skull, shoulders, thoracic spine, cervical spine, and ribs.

Bone pain associated with Paget's disease is described as aching, deep and boring,

▼ **Clinical Signs and Symptoms of Paget's Disease**

These depend on the location and severity of the bone lesions and may include:
- Pain and stiffness
- Fatigue
- Headaches and dizziness
- Bone fractures
- Vertebral compression and collapse
- Deformity
  - Bowing of long bones
  - Increased size and abnormal contour of clavicles
  - Osteoarthritis of adjacent joints
  - Acetabular protrusion
  - Head enlargement
- Periosteal tenderness
- Increased skin temperature over long bones*
- Decreased auditory acuity (if skull is affected)
- Compression neuropathy
  - Spinal stenosis
  - Paresis
  - Paraplegia
  - Muscle weakness

*Increased skin temperature over affected long bones is a typical finding and is explained by soft tissue vascularity surrounding the bones.

worse at night, and diminishing but not disappearing with physical activity. Muscular pain may be referred from involved bony structures or as a result of mechanical changes caused by joint deformities.

Other complications include a variety of nerve compression syndromes, secondary osteoarthritis, and vertebral compression and collapse. Rarely, Paget's disease converts to a malignant neoplasm (osteogenic sarcoma of the femur or humerus) in which case the disease is usually fatal.

CLUES TO SYMPTOMS OF ENDOCRINE OR METABOLIC ORIGIN*

- Identified trigger points are not eliminated or relieved by trigger point therapy. Observe for signs and symptoms of hypothyroidism.
- Palpable lymph node(s) or nodule(s) in the scalene triangle (see Fig. 9-4), especially when accompanied by new-onset hoarseness, hemoptysis, or elevated blood pressure.
- Anyone with muscle weakness and fatigue who is taking diuretics may be experiencing symptoms of potassium depletion. Assess for cardiac arrhythmias, and ask about nausea and vomiting.
- Muscle fasciculation and cramping may be associated with antacid use (metabolic alkalosis).

PAST MEDICAL HISTORY

- Previous diagnosis of endocrine or metabolic disease. Bilateral carpal tunnel syndrome, proximal muscle weakness, and periarthritis of the shoulder(s) are common in persons with certain endocrine and metabolic diseases. Look for other associated signs and symptoms of endocrine or metabolic disease (see Systemic Signs and Symptoms Requiring Physician Referral, pp. 325-326).
- Long-term use of corticosteroids can result in classic symptoms referred to as Cushing's syndrome.

ASSOCIATED SIGNS AND SYMPTOMS

- Watch for anyone with arthralgias, hand pain and stiffness, or muscle weakness with an accompanying cluster of signs and symptoms of endocrine or metabolic disorders.

*See also Clues to Recognizing Osteoporosis (p. 323).

▼ PHYSICIAN REFERRAL

Disorders of the endocrine and metabolic systems may appear with recognizable clinical signs and symptoms but almost always require a combination of clinical and laboratory findings for accurate identification.

The physical therapist is encouraged to complete a thorough Family/Personal History form, augmented by the interview with the client and careful clinical observations, to provide the physician with as much information as possible when making a referral. When appropriate, the Osteoporosis Screening Evaluation in the Appendix may be helpful.

In most cases the client who has suffered from an endocrine disorder has already been diagnosed and may have been referred for physical therapy for some other musculoskeletal complaint. Such clients may have musculoskeletal problems that can be affected by symptoms associated with hormone imbalances (see Tables 9-4 through 9-7).

Any diabetic client demonstrating signs of confusion, lethargy, or changes in mental alertness and function should undergo an immediate fingerstick glucose test with a follow-up visit to the physician on the same day. Likewise, any episode or suspected episode of hypoglycemia must be treated promptly and reported to the diabetic client's physician.

It is important to monitor any client taking diuretics for signs or symptoms of potassium depletion or fluid dehydration before exercising the individual. Consultation with the physician is advised.

Systemic Signs and Symptoms Requiring Physician Referral

Diseases of the endocrine-metabolic system account for some of the most common disorders encountered in humans—diabetes, obesity, and thyroid abnormalities. In recent years new laboratory techniques have greatly enhanced the physician's ability to diagnose these diseases.

Nevertheless, in many cases the disorder remains unrecognized until relatively late in its course; signs and symptoms may be attributed to some other disease process or musculoskeletal disorder (e.g., weakness may be the major complaint in Addison's disease). Thus any client who has any of the following generalized signs and symptoms without obvious or already known cause should be further evaluated by a physician.

Abdominal cramps
Abdominal distension
Absence of sweat
Acroparesthesias
Arthralgias
Buffalo hump
Carpal tunnel syndrome
Changes in appetite
Changes in body or skin temperature
Changes in skin pigmentation
Coarse, dry skin
Confusion/lethargy
Constipation
Deep, rapid respirations
Dependent edema
Diarrhea
Dizziness
Dry mouth, throat, face
Dysphagia
Dyspnea
Ecchymosis
Excessive sweating
Fatigue
Fever and chills
Fruity breath odor
Headaches
Heart palpitations
Hoarseness
Low urine output
Myalgias
Myoedema
Myokymia
Nausea
Night sweats
Nightmares
Nocturia
Numbness (lips, tongue)
Peripheral neuropathy
Pitting edema
Polydipsia
Polyphagia
Polyuria
Postural hypotension
Prolonged reflexes
Proximal muscle weakness
Shakiness/trembling
Striae
Tachycardia/palpitations
Trigger points
Weakness
Weight loss or gain

GUIDE TO PHYSICIAN REFERRAL

- Any unexplained fever without other symptoms in a person taking corticosteroids may be an indication of infection and should be evaluated by a physician.
- Palpable nodules and/or a palpable mass in the supraclavicular area or the scalene triangle (see Fig. 9-4), especially if accompanied by new-onset hoarseness, hemoptysis, or elevated blood pressure, must be evaluated by a physician.
- Any episode (especially a series of episodes) of hypoglycemia in the client with diabetes should be reported to the physician.
- Signs of fluid loss or dehydration in anyone taking diuretics should be reported to the physician.

GUIDELINES FOR IMMEDIATE MEDICAL ATTENTION

- Any person with diabetes who is confused, lethargic, exhibiting changes in mental function, or demonstrating signs of diabetic ketoacidosis should receive medical attention. (Perform a fingerstick glucose test to help evaluate the situation.)
- Signs of potassium depletion (e.g., muscle weakness, fatigue, cardiac arrhythmias, abdominal distension, nausea and vomiting) in a client who is taking non–potassium-sparing diuretics requires medical attention.

 # KEY POINTS TO REMEMBER

▶ Clients with a variety of endocrine and metabolic disorders commonly complain of fatigue, muscle weakness, and occasionally muscle or bone pain.

▶ Muscle weakness associated with endocrine and metabolic disorders usually involves proximal muscle groups.

▶ Periarthritis and calcific tendinitis of the shoulder is common in endocrine clients. Symptoms usually respond to treatment of the underlying endocrine pathologic condition and are not likely to respond to physical therapy treatment.

▶ Carpal tunnel syndrome (CTS), hand stiffness, and hand pain can occur with endocrine and metabolic diseases.

▶ There is a correlation between hypothyroidism and fibromyalgia syndrome (FMS), which is being investigated. Any compromise of muscle energy metabolism aggravates and perpetuates trigger points (TPs). Treatment of the underlying endocrine disorder is necessary to eliminate the TPs, but myofascial treatment must be part of the recovery process to restore full function.

▶ Exercise for the client with diabetes must be carefully planned because significant

complications can result from strenuous exercise.

▶ Exercise for the client with insulin-dependent diabetes should be coordinated to avoid peak insulin dosage whenever possible. Any diabetic client who appears confused or lethargic must be tested immediately by fingerstick for glucose level. Immediate medical attention may be necessary. Other precautions regarding diabetes mellitus for the physical therapist are covered in the text.

▶ When it is impossible to differentiate between ketoacidosis and hyperglycemia, administration of some source of sugar (glucose) is the immediate action to take.

▶ Early osteoporosis has no visible signs and symptoms. History and risk factors are important clues.

▶ Cortisol suppresses the body's inflammatory response, masking early signs of infection. Any unexplained fever without other symptoms should be a warning to the physical therapist of the need for medical follow-up.

▶ Excessive use of antacids can result in muscle fasciculation and cramping (see Alkalosis).

SUBJECTIVE EXAMINATION

• SPECIAL QUESTIONS TO ASK

Endocrine and metabolic disorders may produce subtle symptoms that progress so gradually that the person may be unaware of the significance of such findings. This requires careful interviewing to screen for potential physical and psychologic changes associated with hormone imbalances or other endocrine or metabolic disorders.

As always, it is important to be aware of client medications (whether over-the-counter or prescribed), the intended purpose of these drugs, and any potential side effects.

Past Medical History

- Have you ever had head/neck radiation or cranial surgery? **(Thyroid cancer, pituitary dysfunction)**
- Have you ever had a head injury? **(Pituitary dysfunction)**
- Have you ever been told you are a diabetic or that you have "sugar" in your blood?

Associated Signs and Symptoms

- Have you noticed any changes in your vision, such as blurred vision, double vision, loss of peripheral vision, or sensitivity to light? **(Thyrotoxicosis, hypoglycemia, diabetes mellitus)**
- Have you had an increase in your thirst or the number of times you need to urinate? **(Aldosteronism, diabetes mellitus, diabetes insipidus)**
- Have you had an increase in your appetite? **(diabetes mellitus, hyperthyroidism)**
- Do you bruise easily? **(Cushing's syndrome, excessive secretion of cortisol causes capillary fragility; small bumps/injuries produce bruising)**
- When you injure yourself, do your wounds heal slowly? **(growth hormone excess, ACTH excess, Cushing's syndrome)**
- Have you noticed any decrease in your muscle strength recently? **(growth hormone imbalance, ACTH imbalance, Addison's disease, hyperthyroidism, hypothyroidism)**
- Have you had any muscle cramping or twitching? **(Metabolic alkalosis)**
  - *If yes*, do you take antacids on a daily basis? How much and how often?
- Do you frequently have unexplained fatigue? **(Hyperparathyroidism, hypothyroidism, growth hormone deficiency, ACTH imbalance, Addison's disease)**
  - *If yes*, what activities seem to be too difficult or tiring? **(Muscle weakness caused by cortisol and aldosterone hypersecretion and adrenocortical insufficiency, hypothyroidism)**
- Have you noticed any increase in your collar size (goiter growth), difficulty in breathing or swallowing? **(Goiter, Graves' disease, hyperthyroidism)**

    – *To the physical therapist:* Observe also for hoarseness.

- Have you noticed any changes in skin color? **(Addison's disease, hemochromatosis)** (e.g., overall skin color has become a darker shade of brown or bronze; occurrence of black freckles; darkening of palmar creases, tongue, mucous membranes)

For the Client Known to Be Taking Corticosteroids

- Have you ever been told that you have osteoporosis or brittle bones, fractures, or back problems? **(Wasting of bone matrix in Cushing's syndrome, osteoporosis)**
- Have you ever been told that you have Cushing's syndrome?
- Do you have any difficulty in going up stairs or getting out of chairs? **(Muscle wasting secondary to large doses of cortisol)**

For the Client with Diagnosed Diabetes Mellitus

- What type of insulin do you take? (see Table 9-9)
- What is your schedule for taking your insulin?

    – *To the physical therapist:* Coordinate exercise programs according to the time of peak insulin action. Do not schedule exercise during peak times.

- Do you ever have episodes of hypoglycemia or insulin reaction?

    – *If yes,* describe the symptoms that you experience.

- Do you carry a source of sugar with you in case of an emergency?

    – *If yes,* what is it, and where do you keep it in case I need to retrieve it?

- Have you ever had diabetic ketoacidosis ("diabetic coma")?

    – *If yes,* describe any symptoms you may have had that I can recognize if this occurs during therapy.

- Do you use the fingerstick method for testing your own blood glucose levels?

    – *To the physical therapist:* You may want to ask the person to bring the test kit for use before or during exercise.

- Do you have difficulty in maintaining your blood glucose levels within acceptable ranges (70 to 110 mg/dl)?

    – *If yes, to the physical therapist:* You may want to take a baseline of blood glucose levels before initiating an exercise program.

- Do you ever have burning, numbness, or a loss of sensation in your hands or feet? **(Diabetic neuropathy)**

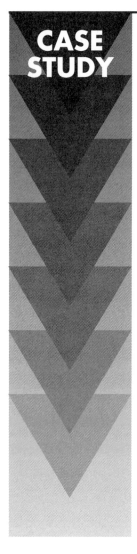

CASE STUDY

REFERRAL

Paul Martin, a 45-year-old client with type 1 diabetes mellitus, has been receiving whirlpool therapy for a foot ulcer during the last 2 weeks. Today, when he came to the clinic, he appeared slightly lethargic and confused. He indicated to you that he has had a "case of the flu" since early yesterday and that he had vomited once or twice the day before and once that morning before coming to the clinic. His wife, who had driven him to the clinic, said that he seemed to be "breathing fast" and urinating more frequently than usual. He has been thirsty, so he has been drinking "7-Up" and water, and those fluids "have stayed down okay."

PHYSICAL THERAPY INTERVIEW

When did you last take your insulin? (Client may have forgotten because of his illness, forgetfulness, confusion, or just being afraid to take it while feeling sick with the "flu.")

What type of insulin did you take?

Do you have a source of sugar with you? If *yes,* where do you keep it? (This question should be asked during the initial physical therapy interview.)

Have you contacted your physician about your condition?

Have you done a recent blood glucose level (fingerstick)? If *yes,* when was the last time that this test was done?

What were the results?

   To his wife: Your husband seems to be confused and is not himself. How long has he been like this? Have you observed any strong breath odor since this "flu" started? (Make your own observations regarding breath odor at this time.)

   If possible, have the client perform a fingerstick blood glucose test on himself. This type of client should be sent immediately to his physician without physical therapy treatment. If he is hypoglycemic (unlikely under these circumstances), this condition should be treated immediately. It is more likely that this client is hyperglycemic and may have diabetic ketoacidosis. In either situation, he should not be driving, and arrangements should be made for transport to the physician's office.

PRACTICE QUESTIONS

1. What are the most common musculoskeletal symptoms associated with endocrine disorders?

2. What systemic conditions can cause carpal tunnel syndrome?

3. What are the mechanisms by which carpal tunnel syndrome occurs?

4. Disorders of the endocrine glands can be caused by:
   a. Dysfunction of the gland
   b. External stimulus
   c. Excess or insufficiency of hormonal secretions
   d. (a) and (b)
   e. (b) and (c)
   f. All the above

5. List three of the most common symptoms of diabetes mellitus.

   1. _____

   2. _____

   3. _____

6. What is the primary difference between the two hyperglycemic states: diabetic ketoacidosis and hyperglycemic, hyperosmolar, nonketotic coma (HHNC)?

7. Is it safe to administer a source of sugar to a lethargic or unconscious person with diabetes?

8. Clients with diabetes insipidus would most likely come to the physical therapist with which of the following clinical symptoms?
   a. Severe dehydration, polydipsia
   b. Headache, confusion, lethargy
   c. Weight gain
   d. Decreased urine output

9. Clients who are taking corticosteroid medications should be monitored for the onset of Cushing's syndrome. You will need to monitor your client for which of the following problems?
   a. Low blood pressure, hypoglycemia
   b. Decreased bone density, muscle wasting
   c. Slow wound healing
   d. (b) and (c)

10. Parathyroid hormone secretion is particularly important in the metabolism of bone. The client with an oversecreting parathyroid gland would most likely have:
    a. Increased blood pressure
    b. Pathologic fractures
    c. Decreased blood pressure
    d. Increased thirst and urination

References

Atcheson SG, Ward JR, Lowe W: Concurrent medical disease in work-related carpal tunnel syndrome, *Arch Intern Med* 158(14):1506-1512, 1998.

Cody JD, Singer FR, Roodman GD et al: Genetic linkage of Paget disease of the bone to chromosome 18q, *Am J Hum Genet* 61(5):1117-1122, 1997.

Gagel RF, Goepfert H, Callender DL: Changing concepts in the pathogenesis and management of thyroid carcinoma, *CA Cancer J Clin* 46(5):261-283, 1996.

Gilliland BC, Gardner GC: Rheumatic disorders. In Ramsey PG, Larson EB, editors: *Medical therapeutics,* ed 2, Philadelphia, 1993, WB Saunders, pp 488-521.

Goodman TA, Simon LS: Osteoporosis: current issues in diagnosis and management, *J Musculoskel Med* 14(3):10-22, 1997.

Grokoest AW, Demartini FE: Systemic disease and carpal tunnel syndrome, *JAMA* 155:635-637, 1954.

Grossman LA, Kaplan HJ, Ownby FD, Grossman M: Carpal tunnel syndrome: initial manifestation of systematic disease, *JAMA* 176:259-261, 1961.

Leon A: Diabetes. In Skinner J, editor: *Exercise testing and exercise prescription for special cases: theoretical basis and clinical application,* ed 2, Philadelphia, 1993, Lea & Febiger, pp 153-183.

Lowe JC, Cullum ME, Graf LH et al: Mutations in the c-erbA beta 1 gene: do they underlie euthyroid fibromyalgia, *Med Hypotheses* 48(2):125-135, 1997.

Lowe JC, Lowe G: Facilitating the decrease in fibromyalgia pain during metabolic rehabilitation: an essential role for soft tissue therapies, *J Bodywork Movement Ther* 2(4):208-217, 1998.

Lowe JC, Reichman AJ, Honeyman GS et al: Thyroid status of fibromyalgia patients, *Clin Bull Myofascial Ther* 3(1):47-53, 1998a.

Lowe JC, Reichman AJ, Yellin BA: A case-control study of metabolic therapy for fibromyalgia: long term follow-up comparison of treated and untreated patients, *Clin Bull Myofascial Ther* 3(1):65-79, 1998b.

National Osteoporosis Foundation: *Osteoporosis and women: a major public health problem,* Washington, DC, 1991, The Foundation.

Orwoll ES, Bauer DC, Vogt TM et al: Axial bone mass in older women, *Ann Intern Med* 124:187-196, 1996.

Papapoulos SE: Paget's disease of bone: clinical, pathogenetic, and therapeutic aspects, *Baillieres Clin Endocrinol Metab* 11(1):117-143, 1997.

Phalen GS: The carpal tunnel syndrome: seventeen years' experience in diagnosis and treatment of six hundred and fifty-four hands, *J Bone Joint Surg* 48A(2):211-228, 1966.

Simmons G: *Far Eastern osteoporosis study,* Hong Kong, 1996, The Gordon Simmons Research Group Ltd.

Sinnett P: National Conference of the Australian Physiotherapy Association, Sydney, Australia, 1993.

Trivalle C, Doucet J, Chassagne P et al: Differences in the signs and symptoms of hypothyroidism in older and younger patients, *JAGS* 1(44):50-53, 1996.

Wallach S: Identifying and controlling Paget's disease, *J Musculoskel Med* 14(6):66-82, 1997.

Appendix

Osteoporosis Screening Evaluation

Name _____ Date _____

	YES	NO
1. Do you have a small, thin body?	☐	☐
2. Are you Caucasian or Asian?	☐	☐
3. Have any of your blood-related family members had osteoporosis?	☐	☐
4. Are you a postmenopausal woman?	☐	☐
5. Do you drink 2 or more ounces of alcohol each day? (1 beer, 1 glass of wine, or 1 cocktail = 1 ounce of alcohol)	☐	☐
6. Do you smoke more than 10 cigarettes each day?	☐	☐
7. Are you physically inactive? (Walking or similar exercise at least three times per week is average.)	☐	☐
8. Have you had both ovaries (with or without a hysterectomy) removed before age 40 years without treatment (hormone replacement)?	☐	☐
9. Have you been taking thyroid medication, antiinflammatories, or seizure medication for more than 6 months?	☐	☐
10. Have you ever broken your hip, spine, or wrist?	☐	☐
11. Do you drink or eat four or more servings of caffeine (carbonated beverages, tea, coffee, chocolate) per day?	☐	☐
12. Is your diet low in dairy products and other sources of calcium? (Three servings of dairy products or two doses of a calcium supplement per day are average.)	☐	☐

If you answer "yes" to three or more of these questions, you may be at greater risk for developing osteoporosis, or "brittle bone disease," and you should contact your physician for further information.

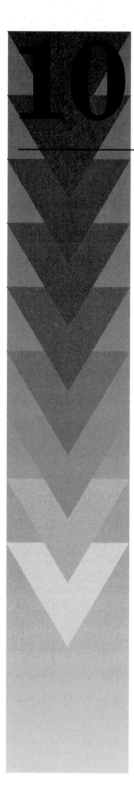

Overview of Oncologic Signs and Symptoms

A 56-year-old man has come to you for an evaluation without a referral. He has not seen any type of physician for at least 3 years. He is seeking an evaluation on the insistence of his wife, who has noticed that his collar size has increased two sizes in the last year and that his neck looks "puffy." He has no complaints of any kind (including pain or discomfort), and he denies any known trauma; however, his wife insists that he has limited ability in turning his head when backing the car out of the driveway. What questions would be appropriate for your first physical therapy interview with this client? What test procedures will you carry out during the first session? If you suggest to this man that he should see his physician, how would you make that recommendation? (See the Case Study at the end of the chapter.)

Cancer in its early stages is often asymptomatic, yet it is the second leading cause of death in the United States. Only heart disease claims more lives. There are more than 1 million new cases of cancer in the United States each year, with one in four Americans developing at least one cancer in his or her lifetime. In the past cancer was invariably fatal. Today, however, survival rates continue to improve for most cancers (except lung and bronchus), and there continues to be a reported reduced mortality from cancer (Rosenthal, 1998).

Fig. 10-1 summarizes current United States figures for cancer incidence and deaths by site and sex. Although prostate and breast cancers are the most common malignancies in men and women, respectively, the cancer most commonly causing death is still lung cancer (Landis et al, 1999).

Neoplasms are divided into three categories: benign, invasive, and metastatic. Within the categories of invasive and metastatic tumors, four large subcategories of malignancy have been identified and classified according to the cell type of origin (Table 10-1).

For the physical therapist, primary cancers arising from specific body structures are not as likely to present with musculoskeletal signs and symptoms. It is more likely that recurrence of a previously treated cancer will have metastasized from another part of the body (secondary neoplasm) with subsequent bone, joint, or muscular

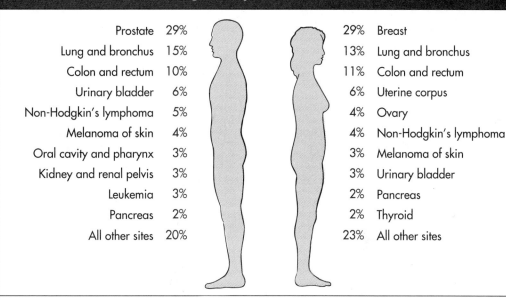

Estimated New Cancer Cases*
10 Leading Sites by Sex, United States, 1999

Prostate	29%			29%	Breast
Lung and bronchus	15%			13%	Lung and bronchus
Colon and rectum	10%			11%	Colon and rectum
Urinary bladder	6%			6%	Uterine corpus
Non-Hodgkin's lymphoma	5%			4%	Ovary
Melanoma of skin	4%			4%	Non-Hodgkin's lymphoma
Oral cavity and pharynx	3%			3%	Melanoma of skin
Kidney and renal pelvis	3%			3%	Urinary bladder
Leukemia	3%			2%	Pancreas
Pancreas	2%			2%	Thyroid
All other sites	20%			23%	All other sites

*Excludes basal and squamous cell skin cancers and in situ carcinomas except urinary bladder.

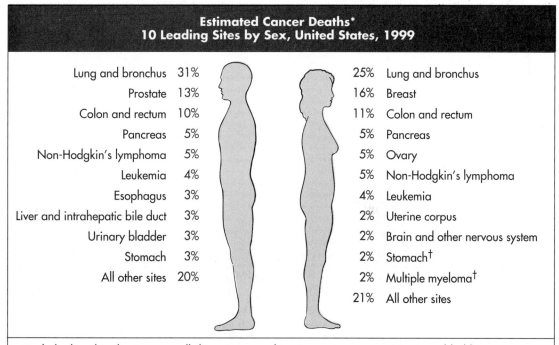

Estimated Cancer Deaths*
10 Leading Sites by Sex, United States, 1999

Lung and bronchus	31%			25%	Lung and bronchus
Prostate	13%			16%	Breast
Colon and rectum	10%			11%	Colon and rectum
Pancreas	5%			5%	Pancreas
Non-Hodgkin's lymphoma	5%			5%	Ovary
Leukemia	4%			5%	Non-Hodgkin's lymphoma
Esophagus	3%			4%	Leukemia
Liver and intrahepatic bile duct	3%			2%	Uterine corpus
Urinary bladder	3%			2%	Brain and other nervous system
Stomach	3%			2%	Stomach†
All other sites	20%			2%	Multiple myeloma†
				21%	All other sites

*Excludes basal and squamous cell skin cancers and in situ carcinomas except urinary bladder.
†These two cancers both received a ranking of 10; they have the same number of deaths and contribute the same percentage.

FIGURE 10-1 • Estimated new cases of cancer and cancer deaths by site for men and women. (From Landis SH, Murray T, Bolden S et al: Cancer statistics, 1999, *CA Cancer J Clin* 49(1):8-31, 1999.)

TABLE 10-1 ▼ Subcategories of Malignancy By Cell Type of Origin

Carcinomas	Sarcomas	Lymphomas	Leukemias
Arise from epithelial cells: Breast Colon Pancreas Skin Large intestine Lungs Stomach	Develop from connective tissues: Fat Muscle Bone Cartilage Synovium Fibrous tissue	Originate in lymphoid tissues: Lymph nodes Spleen Intestinal lining	Cancers of the hematologic system: Bone marrow
Metastasize via lymphatics	Metastasize hematogenously Local invasion	Spread by infiltration	Invasion and infiltration

presentation. Metastatic spread can occur as late as 15 to 20 years after initial diagnosis and medical treatment. For this reason the physical therapist must take care to conduct a thorough Subjective Examination including past medical history (see Chapter 2).

Other predisposing factors, such as age, sex, geographic location, heredity, lifestyle (e.g., consumption of alcohol, smoking cigarettes, poor diet),* or exposure to environmental and occupational toxins (e.g., asbestos, agricultural chemicals, chemical dyes) must also be considered during the interviewing process (see Chapter 2).

In particular, the physical therapist must pay close attention to the client's age in correlation with a personal or family history of cancer. Many cancers, such as prostate, colon, ovarian, and some chronic leukemias, have increased incidence in older adults. The incidence of cancer doubles after 25 years of age and increases with every 5-year increase in age until the mid-80s, when cancer incidence and mortality reach a plateau and even decline slightly.

Other cancers occur within very narrow age ranges. Testicular cancer is found in men from about 20 to 40 years of age. Breast cancer shows a sharp increase after age 45. Ovar-

ian cancer is more common in women older than 55. A number of cancers occur mainly in childhood, such as Ewing's sarcoma, acute leukemia, Wilms' tumor, and retinoblastoma.

▼ METASTASES

The spread of cancer cells from their primary site to secondary sites is called *metastases*. Cancer cells can spread throughout the body through the bloodstream, through the lymphatic system, or by local invasion and infiltration into surrounding tissues (Fig. 10-2). At secondary sites the malignant cells continue to reproduce, and new tumors or lesions develop.

Approximately 30% of clients with newly diagnosed cancers have clinically detectable metastases. At least 30% to 40% of the remaining clients who are clinically free of metastases harbor occult metastases. Only a third of newly diagnosed clients might potentially be cured by local therapeutic modalities alone, and that number may be optimistic.

Many individuals develop multiple sites of metastatic disease because of the potential of cancers to spread. A metastatic colony is the end result of a complicated series of tumor-host interactions called the *metastatic cascade*. Once a primary tumor is initiated and starts to move by local invasion,

---

*Experts at the National Cancer Institute now estimate that 35% of cancer deaths are attributable to diet alone (American Institute for Cancer Research, 1997).

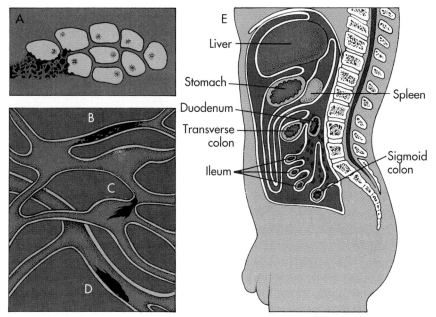

FIGURE 10-2 • Some modes of dissemination of cancer. **A,** Direct extension into neighboring tissue. **B,** Permeation along lymphatic vessels. **C,** Embolism via lymphatic vessels to the lymph nodes. **D,** Embolism via blood vessels (hematogenous spread). **E,** Invasion of a body cavity by diffusion. (Modified from Phipps JS et al, editors: *Medical-surgical nursing: concepts and clinical practice,* ed 4, St Louis, 1991, Mosby.)

tumor angiogenesis occurs (blood vessels from surrounding tissue grow into the solid tumor). Tumor cells then invade host blood vessels and are discharged into the venous drainage.

The usual mode of spread and eventual location of metastases varies with the type of cancer and the tissue from which the cancer arises. Patterns of blood flow, regional venous drainage, and lymphatic channels determine the distribution pattern of metastases. For example, prostatic carcinomas typically spread via the lymphatics to the bones of the pelvis and vertebrae, sometimes appearing as low back and/or pelvic pain radiating down the leg.

Primary tumors of the bone, such as osteogenic sarcoma, initially metastasize to the lungs. The high proportion of bone metastases in breast, prostate, and lung cancers is an example of selective homing of tumor cells to a specific organ (Woodhouse et al, 1997). For some cancers, such as malig-

nant melanoma, no typical pattern exists, and metastases may occur anywhere.

The five most common sites of metastasis are bone, lymph nodes, lung, liver, and brain. However, the physical therapist is most likely to observe symptoms affecting one of four systems (listed in order of prevalence in a physical therapy setting): (1) skeletal system, (2) central nervous system (CNS), (3) pulmonary system, and (4) hepatic system.

▼ CLINICAL MANIFESTATIONS OF MALIGNANCY

Neoplastic disease can cause backache, particularly in older adults, or shoulder pain in the presence of breast cancer. Although primary neoplasms of the spine are rare, myeloma and metastatic disease are more common.

In anyone with a known cancer, the onset of back pain suggests spinal metastases. An insidious onset of waist-level or midback pain that becomes progressively more severe and more persistent often occurs. The pain is usually unrelieved by lying down and frequently becomes worse at night. Unexplained weight loss with severe back pain aggravated by rest suggests metastatic carcinoma of the spine. Multiple myeloma can cause severe, unremitting backaches that are present at rest and become worse with recumbency (Seller, 1996).

Early Warning Signs

For many years, the American Cancer Society has publicized seven warning signs of cancer, the appearance of which could indicate the presence of cancer and the need for a medical evaluation. The following mnemonic is often used as a helpful reminder of these warning signs:

> **C**hanges in bowel or bladder habits
>
> **A** sore that does not heal in 6 weeks
>
> **U**nusual bleeding or discharge
>
> **T**hickening or lump in breast or elsewhere
>
> **I**ndigestion or difficulty in swallowing
>
> **O**bvious change in a wart or mole
>
> **N**agging cough or hoarseness
>
> *For the physical therapist:*
>
> Proximal muscle weakness
>
> Change in deep tendon reflexes

Awareness of these signals is useful, but it is generally agreed that these symptoms do not always reflect early curable cancer; nor does this list include all the possible signs for the different types of cancer.

For the physical therapist, idiopathic proximal muscle weakness may be an early sign of cancer. This syndrome of proximal muscle weakness is referred to as *carcinomatous neuromyopathy*. It is accompanied by changes in two or more deep tendon reflexes (ankle jerk usually remains intact). Muscle weakness may occur secondary to hypercalcemia, which is typically found in persons with multiple myeloma, a form of plasma cell cancer that affects bone marrow.

Pain is rarely an early warning sign of cancer, even in the presence of unexplained bleeding. Bleeding is an important sign of cancer, but a cancer is generally well established by the time bleeding occurs. Bleeding develops secondary to ulcerations in the central areas of the tumor or by pressure on or rupture of local blood vessels. As the tumor continues to grow, it may enlarge beyond its capacity to obtain necessary nutrients, resulting in revitalization of portions of the tumor.

This process of invading and compressing local tissue, shutting off blood supply to normal cells, is called *necrosis*. Tissue necrosis leads ultimately to secondary infection, severe hemorrhage, and the development of pain when regional sensory nerves become involved. Other symptoms can include pathologic fractures, anemia, and thrombus formation.

Skeletal Manifestations
(Coleman, 1997)

The skeleton is the most common organ affected by metastatic cancer, and tumors arising from the breast, prostate, thyroid, lung, and kidney possess a special propensity to spread to bone. Bone pain is the most common complication of metastatic bone disease, resulting from structural damage, rate of bone resorption, periosteal irritation, and nerve entrapment. Once tumor cells become housed in the skeleton, cure is no longer possible and only palliative therapy is administered.

Bone Pain

Tumor cells commonly metastasize to the most heavily vascularized parts of the skeleton, particularly the red bone marrow of the axial skeleton and the proximal ends of the long bones (humerus and femur), the vertebral column, pelvis, and ribs. Pain is usually deep, intractable, and poorly localized, sometimes described as burning or aching and accompanied by episodes of stabbing discomfort.

The pain is made worse by activity, especially weight bearing. It is often worse at night; neither sleep nor lying down provides relief. Pain may occur around joints because of mechanical, chemical, or bony change; pain and the rate of bone resorption appear to be linked. There is often disturbance of the highly innervated periosteum, giving bone pain its neurogenic-like qualities, especially its unrelenting, intractable quality.

Hypercalcemia

Hypercalcemia (excess calcium in the blood) occurs frequently in clients with metastatic bone disease who have osteolytic lesions. It is very common in cases of breast cancer and myeloma primarily because of an increase in bone resorption, which is caused, in turn, by the production of bone-active agents by the tumor cells that stimulate osteoclastic bone resorption. Hypercalcemia is characterized by CNS, musculoskeletal, cardiovascular, and gastrointestinal (GI) symptoms (see box, p. 342).

Neurologic Manifestations

Nerve and cord compression

Metastatic involvement of the vertebrae may result in epidural spinal cord compression with resultant quadriplegia or paraplegia and possible death. Symptoms caused by metastatic epidural disease and resultant compression may be only transient with proper medical treatment.

Symptoms of nerve and/or cord compression may occur when tumors invade and impinge directly on the spinal cord or more frequently because severe destructive osteolytic lesions lead to pathologic fracture (developing spontaneously or following trivial injury), fragility, and subsequent deformity of one or more vertebral bodies. Lung and breast cancer are the leading causes of epidural spinal cord compression, but lymphoma, multiple myeloma, and carcinomas of the prostate or kidney can also result in spinal cord and nerve root compression. This complication is becoming increasingly common, as individuals affected by cancer survive longer with medical treatment.

Other neurologic problems occur frequently in individuals with cancer. They are usually caused by one of three phenomena: (1) tumor metastases to the brain; (2) endocrine, fluid, and electrolyte abnormalities; or (3) remote effects of tumors on the CNS. When tumors produce signs and symptoms at a distance from the tumor or its metastasized sites, these "remote effects" of malignancy are collectively referred to as *paraneoplastic syndromes*.

The causes of these syndromes are not well understood. In contrast to the hormone syndromes in which the cancer directly produces a substance that circulates in blood to produce symptoms, the neurologic syndromes are generally produced by cancer stimulation of antibody production (Odell, 1993).

Brain tumors

Lung and breast cancer account for more than half of all metastatic brain lesions. Metastatic brain tumors can increase intracranial pressure, obstruct the normal flow of cerebrospinal fluid, change mentation, and reduce sensory and motor function [see later discussion of primary CNS tumors].

Paraneoplastic Syndromes

The most common cancer associated with paraneoplastic syndromes is small cell cancer of the lung. Clinical findings of paraneoplastic syndromes may resemble those of primary endocrine, metabolic, hematologic, or neuromuscular disorders. For example, the Lambert-Eaton myasthenic syndrome (LEMS) results in muscle weakness when autoantibodies directed against the presynaptic calcium channels at the neuromuscular junction cause impaired release of acetylcholine from presynaptic nerve terminals (Henson and Posner, 1993).

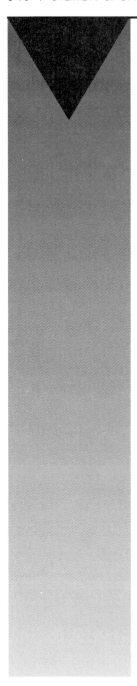

Case Example. A 72-year-old woman was referred to physical therapy by her neurologist with a diagnosis of "nerve entrapment" for a postural exercise program and home traction. She was experiencing symptoms of left shoulder pain with numbness and tingling in the ulnar nerve distribution. She had a moderate forward head posture with slumped shoulders and loss of height from known osteoporosis.

The woman's past medical history was significant for right breast cancer treated with a radical mastectomy and chemotherapy 20 years ago. She had a second cancer (uterine) 10 years ago that was considered separate from her previous breast cancer.

Further questioning about the presence of associated signs and symptoms revealed a significant disturbance in sleep pattern over the last 6 months with unrelenting shoulder and neck pain. There were no other reported constitutional symptoms, skin changes, or noted lumps anywhere. Vital signs were remarkable at the time of the physical therapy evaluation.

The physical therapy examination was consistent with the physician's diagnosis of nerve entrapment in a classic presentation. There were significant postural components to account for the development of symptoms. However, the therapist palpated several large masses in the axillary and supraclavicular fossa on both the right and left sides. There was no local warmth, redness, or tenderness associated with these lesions. The therapist requested permission to palpate the client's groin and popliteal spaces for any other suspicious lymph nodes. The rest of the examination findings were within normal limits.

Result. Returning this client to her referring physician was a difficult decision to make since the therapist did not have the benefit of the medical records or results of neurologic examination and testing. Given the significant past medical history for cancer, the woman's age, presence of progressive night pain, and palpable masses, no other reasonable choice remained. When asked if the physician had seen or felt the masses, the client responded with a definite "no."

There are several ways to approach handling a situation like this one, depending on the physical therapist's relationship with the physician. In this case the therapist had never communicated with this physician before. A telephone call was made to ask the clerical staff to check the physician's office notes. It is possible that the physician was aware of the masses, knew from medical testing that there was extensive cancer, and chose to treat the client palliatively. Since there was no indication of such, the therapist notified the physician's staff of the decision to return the client to the MD. A brief (one-page) written report summarizing the findings was given to the client to hand-carry to the physician's office.

Further medical testing was performed, and a medical diagnosis of lymphoma was made.

The paraneoplastic syndromes are of considerable importance because they may accompany relatively limited neoplastic growth and provide an early clue to the presence of certain types of cancer (e.g., osteoarthropathy caused by bronchogenic carcinoma or hypercalcemia from osteolytic skeletal metastases).

TABLE 10-2 ▼ Paraneoplastic Syndromes Having Musculoskeletal Manifestations

Malignancy	Rheumatic Disease	Clinical Features
Lymphoproliferative disease (leukemia)	Vasculitis	Necrotizing vasculitis
Plasma cell dyscrasia	Cryoglobulinemia	Vasculitis; Raynaud's phenomenon; arthralgia; neurologic symptoms
Hodgkin's disease	Immune complex disease	Nephrotic syndrome
Ovarian cancer	Reflex sympathetic dystrophy	Palmar fascitis and polyarthritis
Carcinoid syndrome	Scleroderma	Scleroderma-like changes; anterior tibia
Colon cancer	Pyogenic arthritis	Enteric bacteria cultured from joint
Mesenchymal tumors	Osteogenic osteomalacia	Bone pain, stress fractures
Renal cell cancer (and other tumors)	Severe Raynaud's phenomenon	Digital necrosis
Pancreatic cancer	Panniculitis	Subcutaneous nodules, especially in males

Modified from Gilkeson GS, Caldwell DS: Rheumatologic associations with malignancy, *J Musculoskel Med* 7(1):72, 1990.

The course of the paraneoplastic syndrome usually parallels that of the tumor. Therefore effective medical treatment (rather than physical therapy) should result in resolution of the syndrome. A paraneoplastic syndrome may be the first sign of a malignancy or recurrence of cancer that may be cured if detected early. Paraneoplastic syndromes with musculoskeletal manifestations are listed in Table 10-2.

Even such nonspecific symptoms as anorexia, malaise, weight loss, and fever are truly neoplastic and are probably due to the production of specific factors by the tumor itself. For example, anorexia is a common symptom in clients with cancer that is attributed to tumor production of the protein tumor necrosis factor (TNF), also called cachectin. Fever may be seen in clients with cancer in the absence of infection when it is produced by tumor induction of pyrogen formation by host white cells or by direct tumor production of a pyrogen.

Gradual, progressive muscle weakness during a period of weeks to months (especially of the pelvic girdle muscles) may occur. Proximal muscles are most likely to be involved. The weakness does stabilize. Reflexes of the involved extremities are present but diminished.

Paraneoplastic syndromes may be related to rheumatologic complaints with sudden onset. Clinical features of carcinoma poly-

TABLE 10-3 ▼ Muscular Disorders Associated With Malignancy

Dermatomyositis and polymyositis
Type II muscle atrophy
Myasthenia gravis
Lambert-Eaton myasthenic syndrome (LEMS)
Metabolic myopathies
Primary neuropathic diseases
  Amyotrophic lateral sclerosis
  Amyloidosis

From Gilkeson GS, Caldwell DS: Rheumatologic associations with malignancy, *J Musculoskel Med* 7(1):70, 1990.

arthritis primarily affect asymmetric joints of the lower extremities. Other rheumatologic conditions and muscular disorders can be associated with malignancy (Table 10-3). In clients who develop myopathies such as dermatomyositis (DM) or polymyositis (PM), the myositis may precede, follow, or arise concurrently with the malignancy. No particular type of cancer has been found to predominate in such cases, but the clients affected are generally older and respond poorly to medical treatment for the myositis.

Pulmonary Manifestations

Pulmonary metastases are the most common of all metastatic tumors because venous drainage of most areas of the body is through

▼ *Clinical Signs and Symptoms of*
Paraneoplastic Syndromes

- Fever
- Skin rash
- Clubbing of the fingers
- Pigmentation disorders
- Arthralgias
- Paresthesias
- Thrombophlebitis
- Proximal muscle weakness
- Anorexia, malaise, weight loss
- See Tables 10-2 and 10-3

▼ *Clinical Signs and Symptoms of*
Metastases*

- **Skeletal**
  Neurogenic bone pain
  Pain on weight bearing
  Hypercalcemia
    CNS (drowsiness, lethargy, headaches, depression or apathy, irritability, confusion)
    Musculoskeletal (weakness, muscle flaccidity, bone pain, pathologic fractures)
    Cardiovascular (cardiac arrest, hypertension)
    GI (anorexia, nausea, vomiting, abdominal pain, constipation, dehydration, polydipsia)
- **Neurologic**
  Nerve and cord compression
  Brain tumors (headache, altered mentation, sensory and motor disturbances)
  Paraneoplastic syndrome
- **Pulmonary**
  Pleural pain
  Dyspnea
- **Hepatic**
  Bilateral carpal/tarsal tunnel syndrome
  Abdominal pain and tenderness
  General malaise and fatigue

*Seen most often in a physical therapy practice.

the superior and inferior venae cavae into the heart, making the lungs the first organ to filter malignant cells. Parenchymal metastases are asymptomatic until tumor cells have expanded and reached the parietal pleura, where pain fibers are stimulated.

Pleural pain and dyspnea may be the first two symptoms experienced by the person. Tumor cells from the lung embolizing via the pulmonary veins and carotid artery can result in metastases to the CNS. Lung cancer is the most common primary tumor to metastasize to the brain. In any individual, any neurologic sign may be the presentation of a silent lung tumor (Gudas, 1987).

Hepatic Manifestations

Liver metastases are among the most ominous signs of advanced cancer. The liver filters blood coming in from the GI tract, making it a primary metastatic site for tumors of the stomach, colorectum, and pancreas.

Symptoms observed in a physical therapy practice include bilateral carpal/tarsal tunnel syndrome, possibly accompanied by abdominal pain and tenderness with general malaise and fatigue. Right upper quadrant pain with possible referral to the right shoulder may also occur with or without carpal tunnel syndrome.

▼ ONCOLOGIC PAIN

As mentioned earlier, pain is rarely an early warning sign of cancer and is uncommon in some cancers such as leukemia. However, pain occurs in 60% to 80% of clients with solid tumors.

This pain syndrome has multiple causes, and the therapist must always keep in mind common patterns of referred pain (Table 10-4). Some pain is caused by pressure on or displacement of nerves. Pain may

CLUES TO SCREENING FOR CANCER

- Age older than 50 years
- Previous personal history of any cancer, especially in the presence of carpal tunnel symptoms, back pain, shoulder pain, or joint pain of unknown or rheumatic cause at presentation
- Any woman with chest, breast, axillary, or shoulder pain of unknown cause
- Anyone with back, pelvic, groin, or hip pain accompanied by vague abdominal complaints, palpable mass

  For women: Prolonged or excessive menstrual bleeding (or in the case of the postmenopausal woman who is not taking hormone replacement, breakthrough bleeding)

  For men: Additional presence of sciatica and past history of prostate cancer
- When a back "injury" is not improving as expected or if symptoms are increasing
- Early warning signs, including proximal muscle weakness and changes in deep tendon reflexes
- Recent weight loss of 10 pounds or more within 1 month (weight gain is more typical with true musculoskeletal dysfunction because pain has limited physical activities)
- Constant pain (unrelieved by rest or change in position)
- Pain present at night
- Signs of nerve root compression must be screened for cancer as a possible cause
- Development of new neurologic deficits (e.g., weakness, sensory loss, reflex change, bowel or bladder dysfunction)
- Changes in size, shape, tenderness, and consistency of lymph nodes, especially painless, hard, rubbery lymph nodes present in more than one location and occurring for more than 4 weeks

TABLE 10-4 ▼ Common Patterns of Pain Referral

Pain Mechanism	Lesion Site	Referral Site
Visceral	Diaphragmatic irritation	Shoulder, lumbar spine
	Urothelial tract	Inguinal region and genitalia
Somatic	C7, T1 vertebrae	Interscapular area
	L1, L2 vertebrae	Sacroiliac joint and hip
	Hip joint	Knee
	Pharynx	Ipsilateral ear
Neuropathic	Nerve or plexus	Anywhere in distribution of a peripheral nerve
	Nerve root	Anywhere in corresponding dermatome
	Central nervous system	Anywhere in region of body innervated by damaged structure

Modified from Cherny NI, Portenoy RK: The management of cancer pain, *CA Cancer J Clin* 44:271, 1994.

also result from interference with blood supply or from blockage within hollow organs.

A common cause of cancer pain is metastasis of cancer to the bone. This type of pain can occur as a result of pathologic fracture with resultant muscle spasms; if the spine is involved, nerves may be affected. Pain may also result from iatrogenic causes such as surgery, radiation therapy, and chemotherapy. Immobility and inflammation also can lead to pain.

Signs and Symptoms Associated with Levels of Pain

The severity of pain varies from one client to another, but certain signs and symptoms are characteristic of particular levels of pain. For example, in *mild-to-moderate superficial pain,* a sympathetic nervous system response is usually elicited with hypertension, tachycardia, and tachypnea (rapid, shallow breathing).

In *severe or visceral pain,* a parasympathetic nervous system response is more characteristic, with hypotension, bradycardia, nausea, vomiting, tachypnea, weakness, or fainting. Depression and anxiety may increase the client's perception of pain, requiring additional psychologic and emotional support.

Biologic Mechanisms

Five biologic mechanisms have been implicated in the development of chronic cancer pain. The characteristics of the pain depend on tissue structure as well as on the mechanisms involved.

Bone Destruction

Bone destruction secondary to infiltration by malignant cells or resulting from metastatic lesions is the first and most common of the biologic mechanisms causing chronic cancer pain. Bone metastases cause increased release of prostaglandins and subsequent bone breakdown and resorption. The client's pain threshold is reduced through sensitization of free nerve endings. Bone pain may be mild to intense. Maladaptive outcomes of bone destruction may include sharp continuous pain that increases on movement or ambulation. The rich supply of nerves and tension or pressure on the sensitive periosteum or endosteum may cause bone pain.

Other factors contributing to the intense discomfort reported by clients include limited space for relief of pressure, altered local metabolism, weakening of the bone structure, and pathologic fractures ranging in size from microscopic to large.

Visceral Obstruction

Obstruction of a hollow visceral organ and ducts such as the bowel, stomach, or ureters is a second physiologic factor in the development of chronic cancer pain.

Viscus obstruction is most often due to the obstruction of an organ lumen by tumor growth. In the GI or genitourinary tracts, obstruction results in either a severe, colicky, crampy pain or true visceral pain that is dull, diffuse, boring, and poorly localized.

If a vein, artery, or lymphatic channel is obstructed, venous engorgement, arterial ischemia, or edema, respectively, will result. In these cases pain is described as being dull, diffuse, burning, and aching. Obstruction of the ducts leading from the gallbladder and pancreas is common in cancer of these organs, although jaundice is more frequently an earlier symptom than pain. Cancer of the throat or esophagus can obstruct these organs, leading to difficulties in eating or speaking.

Nerve Compression

Infiltration or compression of peripheral nerves is the third physiologic factor that produces chronic cancer pain and discomfort. Pressure on nerves from adjacent tumor masses and microscopic infiltration of nerves by tumor cells result in continuous, sharp, stabbing pain generally following the pattern of nerve distribution. The invading cells affect the conduction of impulses by the nervous system and sometimes result in constant, dull, poorly localized pain and altered sensation.

Blockage of the blood in arteries and veins, again both by pressure from tumor masses nearby and by infiltration, can decrease oxygen and nutrient supply to tissues. This deficiency can be perceived as pain similar in origin and character to cardiac pain, or angina pectoris, which is chest pain from insufficient supply of oxygen to the heart. Hyperesthesia or paresthesia may result.

Skin or Tissue Distension

Infiltration or distension of integument (skin) or tissue is the fourth physiologic phenomenon resulting in chronic, severe cancer pain. This type of pain is secondary to the painful stretching of skin or tissue because of underlying tumor growth. This stretching produces severe, dull, aching, and localized pain, with the severity of the pain increasing concurrently with increase of tumor size. Pain associated with headaches secondary to brain tumors is thought to be due to traction on pain-sensitive intracranial structures.

Tissue Inflammation, Infection, and Necrosis

Inflammation, infection, and necrosis of tissue may be the fifth and final cause of cancer pain. Inflammation, with its accompanying symptoms of redness, edema, pain, heat, and loss of function, may progress to infection, necrosis, and sloughing of tissue. If the inflammatory process alone is present, the pain is characterized by a sensitive tenderness. If, however, necrosis and tissue sloughing have occurred, pain may be excruciating.

▼ SIDE EFFECTS OF CANCER TREATMENT

For many years three basic modalities of cancer treatment have been used, either alone or in combination: surgery, radiation therapy, and chemotherapy. In recent years immunotherapies involving the use of cells of the immune system to prompt a tumor-killing response have been developed. Immunotherapy may be most effective when combined with conventional treatments, such as chemotherapy and radiation, to improve the success of treatment and decrease the side effects of conventional modalities.

Conventional cancer treatment has many side effects because the goal of treatment is to remove or to kill certain tissues. In any situation healthy tissue also is usually sacrificed.

The pharmaceuticals used in chemotherapy are cytotoxic (destructive), designed to kill dividing cells selectively by blocking the ability of DNA and RNA to reproduce and by lysing cell membranes. All types of dividing cells, not just the cancer cells, are affected.

In addition, a combination of drugs (each causing cell death through different pharmacologic mechanisms) is traditionally used for greater efficacy in the systemic treatment of some cancers (e.g., breast cancer). Hence an overlap of toxicities may result in greater side effects.

The effects of treatment for cancer can be debilitating physiologically, physically, and psychologically. Common physical side effects include severe mucositis, mouth sores, nausea and vomiting, fluid retention, pulmonary edema, cough, headache, CNS effects, malaise, fatigue, dyspnea, and loss of hair. Emotional and psychologic side effects are present but less evident (Table 10-5).

Aggressive chemotherapeutic agents and chest irradiation can cause cardiopulmonary dysfunction, especially in the treatment of Hodgkin's disease and breast and lung cancers. High-dose radiation can result in pericardial fibrosis (scarring of the pericardium) and constrictive pericarditis (inflammation of the pericardium). These conditions are usually asymptomatic until the client starts to exercise, and then exertional dyspnea is the first symptom.

Other causes of dyspnea include deconditioning, anemia, peripheral arterial disease, and increased physiologic demand for oxygen because of fever or infection. During radiation therapy the client may be more tired than usual. Resting throughout exercise is important, as are adequate nutrition and hydration.

The skin in the irradiated area may become red or dry and should be exposed to the air but protected from the sun and from tight clothing. Gels, lotions, oils, or other topical agents should not be used over the irradiated skin without a physician's approval. Clients may have other side effects, depending on the areas treated. For example, radiation to the lower back may cause nausea, vomiting, or diarrhea because the lower digestive tract is exposed to the radiation.

Because bone marrow suppression is a common and serious side effect of many chemotherapeutic agents and can be a side effect of radiation therapy in some instances, it is extremely important to monitor

TABLE 10-5 ▼ Side Effects of Cancer Treatment*

Surgery	Radiation	Chemotherapy	Biotherapy	Hormonal Therapy
Disfigurement	Radiation sickness	GI effects	Fever	Nausea
Loss of function	Immunosuppression	Anorexia	Chills	Vomiting
Infection	Decreased platelets	Nausea	Nausea	Hypertension
Increased pain	Decreased WBCs	Vomiting	Vomiting	Steroid-induced diabetes
Deformity	Infection	Diarrhea	Anorexia	Myopathy (steroid-
	Fatigue	Ulcers	Fatigue	induced)
	Fibrosis	Hemorrhage	Fluid reten-	Weight gain
	Burns	Bone marrow suppression	tion	Altered mental status
	Mucositis	Anemia	CNS effects	Hot flashes
	Diarrhea	Leukopenia		Sweating
	Edema	Thrombocytopenia		Impotence
	Hair loss	Skin rashes		Decreased libido
	Delayed wound	Neuropathies		
	healing	Hair loss		
	CNS effects	Sterilization		
	Malignancy	Phlebitis		

From Goodman CC, Boissonnault WG: *Pathology: implications for the physical therapist,* Philadelphia, 1998, WB Saunders, p 165.
  *The health care professional must remember that some of the delayed effects of radiation, such as cerebral injury, pericarditis, pulmonary fibrosis, hepatitis, intestinal stenosis, other GI disturbances, and nephritis, may be signs of recurring cancer. The physician must be notified by the affected individual of any new symptoms, change in symptoms, or increase in symptoms.

the hematologic values in clients receiving these treatment modalities. It is very important to review these values before any type of vigorous physical therapy is initiated. A guideline used by some physical therapy exercise programs is the Winningham Contraindications for Aerobic Exercise. According to these guidelines, aerobic exercise is contraindicated in chemotherapy clients when laboratory values are as follows (Winningham et al, 1986):

Platelet count	<50,000/mm³
Hemoglobin	<10 g/dl
White blood cell count	<3000/mm³
Absolute granulocytes	<2500/mm³

▼ SKIN AND BREAST CANCERS

Skin cancer and breast cancer are two of the more common cancers about which clients will ask physical therapists for advice. During the observation/inspection portion of any examination, the physical therapist may observe skin lesions that may need further medical investigation. Mortality is reduced when lesions are found early and promptly treated. For these reasons this special section on skin and breast cancer is included.*

Additionally, the woman with chest, breast, axillary, or shoulder pain of unknown origin at presentation must be questioned regarding breast self-examinations. Any recently discovered lumps or nodules must be examined by a physician. The client may need education regarding breast self-examination, and the physical therapist can provide this valuable information. Techniques of breast self-examination are commonly available in written form for the physical therapist or the client who is unfamiliar with these methods.

Skin Cancer

Skin cancer is the most common cancer diagnosed in the United States; the incidence of melanoma continues to rise faster than any other cancer (Rigel et al, 1996). It affects

---

*Other specific types of cancer affecting organ systems are discussed individually in each related chapter.

TABLE 10-6 ▼ Risk Factors for the Development of Skin Cancer

Nonmelanoma Skin Cancer	Malignant Melanoma
• Fair skin, blond or red hair • Male gender • Advancing age • Cumulative sun exposure*	• Fair skin, blond or red hair • Male gender • Marked freckling on the upper back • Short, intense episodes of sun exposure* • History of three or more blistering sunburns before age 20 years • History of 3 or more years in outdoor summer job or recreation during adolescence • Presence of actinic keratosis (sharply outlined horny growth, e.g., wart or callous)

From Hill LH, Ferrini RL: Skin cancer prevention and screening: summary of the American College of Preventive Medicine's Practice Policy Statements, *CA Cancer J Clin* 48(4):232-235, 1998.

*Recent studies have brought this belief into question (see text discussion).

men and women equally but seldom occurs in children before puberty.

The several different kinds of skin cancer are distinguished by the types of cells involved. Basal cell carcinoma, squamous cell carcinoma, and malignant melanoma are the three most common types of skin cancer. More than 90% of all skin cancers fall into the first two classifications, referred to as nonmelanoma skin cancer (NMSC). Although less prevalent, malignant melanoma is a more common cause of cancer death.

The cause of skin cancer is well known. Prolonged or intermittent exposure to ultraviolet (UV) radiation from the sun, especially when it results in sunburn and blistering damages DNA. The majority of all NMSCs occur on parts of the body unprotected by clothing (face, neck, forearms, and backs of hands) and in persons who have received considerable exposure to sunlight.

All adults are at risk for skin cancer, regardless of skin tone and hair color; however, some people are at much greater risk than others (Table 10-6). In general, individ-

uals with red, blond, or light-brown hair with light complexions and maybe freckles, many of Celtic or Scandinavian origin, are most susceptible; persons of African or Asian origin are least susceptible. The most severely affected people usually have a history of long-term occupational or recreational sun exposure.

Individuals with a history of skin cancer are at much greater risk for other, more serious forms of the disease. Anyone with a history of NMSC is at increased risk of cancer mortality. Although the biologic mechanisms are unknown, a history of NMSC should increase the clinician's alertness for certain noncutaneous cancer and melanoma (Kahn, 1998).

CLINICAL SIGNS AND SYMPTOMS
BASAL CELL CARCINOMA

Basal cell carcinoma involves the bottom layer of the epidermis and occurs mainly on any hair-bearing area exposed to the sun (e.g., face, neck, head, ears, or hands). Occasionally, basal cell carcinoma may appear on the trunk, especially the upper back and chest. These lesions grow slowly, attaining a size of 1 to 2 cm in diameter, often after years of growth. Metastases almost never occur, but neglected lesions may ulcerate and produce great destruction, ultimately invading vital structures.

There are a number of common forms of basal cell carcinoma: (1) pearly papule 2 to 3 mm in diameter and covered by tightly stretched epidermis laced with small delicate, branching vessels (telangiectasia); (2) pearly papule with a small crater in the center; (3) scaly, red, sharply outlined plaque; and (4) ill-defined pale, tough, scarlike tumor.

SQUAMOUS CELL CARCINOMA

Squamous cell carcinoma arises from the top of the epidermis and is found on areas often exposed to the sun, typically the rim of the ear, the face, the lips and mouth, and the dorsa of the hands. These lesions appear as small, red, hard nodules with a smooth or warty surface. The central portion may be scaly, ulcerated, or crusted. Premalignant lesions include sun-damaged skin or dysplasias (whitish discolored areas), scars, radiation-induced keratosis, actinic keratosis (rough, scaly spots), and chronic ulcers.

Metastases are uncommon but are much more likely to occur in lesions arising in chronic leg ulcers, burn scars, and areas of prior x-ray exposure. Although these tumors do not usually metastasize, they are potentially dangerous. They may infiltrate surrounding structures and metastasize to lymph nodes and eventually to distant sites, including bone, brain, and lungs, to become fatal. Invasive tumors are firm and increase in elevation and diameter. The surface may be granular and bleed easily.

MALIGNANT MELANOMA

Malignant melanoma (MM) is the most serious form of skin cancer. It arises from pigmented cells in the skin called melanocytes. The majority of MMs appear to be associated with the intensity rather than the duration of sunlight exposure, in contrast to basal and squamous cell carcinomas.* However, melanoma can appear anywhere on the body, not just on sun-exposed areas.

The clinical characteristics of early malignant melanoma are similar, regardless of anatomic site. Unlike benign pigmented lesions, which are generally round and symmetric, the shape of an early MM is often asymmetric. Whereas benign pigmented lesions tend to have regular margins, the borders of early MM are often irregular.

Compared with benign pigmented lesions, which are more uniform in color, MMs are usually variegated, ranging from various hues of tan and brown to black, sometimes intermingled with red and white. The diameters of MM are often 6 mm or larger when first identified.

---

*Recent studies have brought this belief into question, suggesting that nonmelanoma skin cancer is caused by the same kind of sporadic exposure that can lead to melanoma (Kricker et al, 1995; Gallagher et al, 1995). Further investigation to validate these studies is pending.

▼ **Clinical Signs and Symptoms of**
Early Melanoma

A Asymmetry: Uneven edges, lopsided in shape, one half unlike the other half
B Border: Irregularity, irregular edges, scalloped or poorly defined edges
C Color: Black, shades of brown, red, white, occasionally blue
D Diameter: Larger than a pencil eraser

During observation and inspection, the physical therapist should be alert to any potential signs of skin cancer. The major warning sign of melanoma is some change in a mole or "beauty mark." The Skin Cancer Foundation advocates the use of the ABCD method of early detection of melanoma and dysplastic (abnormal in size or shape) moles.

When a suspicious skin lesion is noted, the physical therapist must pose three questions:

- How long have you had this area of skin discoloration/mole/spot [use whatever brief description seems most appropriate]?
- Has it changed in the last 6 weeks to 6 months?
- Has your physician examined this area?

The most common sites of distant metastases associated with MM are the skin and subcutaneous tissue, lungs, and surrounding visceral pleura, although any anatomic site may be involved. In-transit metastases (unique malignancies that have spread from the primary tumor but may not have reached the regional lymph nodes) typically develop multiple bulky tumors on an arm or leg. Often these tumors cause pain, swelling, bleeding, ulceration, and decreased mobility (Ross, 1997).

Other signs that may be important include irritation and itching; tenderness, soreness, or new moles developing around the mole in question; or a sore that keeps crusting and does not heal within 6 weeks.

Benign moles tend to have smooth symmetric borders. Benign moles tend to be flat, hairless, round or oval, and <6 mm in diameter. Pigmentation is generally even, although there may be color variations, especially in shades of brown. Adolescents frequently have nevi with irregular borders, multiple shades of pigment, or both. Most are normal variations of the benign nevi, but any lesion that arouses clinical suspicion or is of concern to the client should be examined by a physician.

If any of these signs and symptoms are present in a client whose skin lesion(s) has not been examined by a physician, a medical referral is recommended. If the client is planning a follow-up visit with the physician within the next 2 to 4 weeks, the client is advised to point out the mole or skin changes at that time. If no appointment is pending, the client is encouraged to make a specific visit either to the family/personal physician or to a dermatologist.

Breast Cancer

The breast is the second most common site of cancer in women (skin cancer is first), and cancer of the breast is second only to lung cancer as a cause of death from cancer among women. The incidence of breast cancer began to rise steadily around 1940 and increased sharply around 1980. The steep rise since 1980 has been largely attributed to earlier, better detection with mammography. At the present rate of incidence, 1 of every 8 American women will develop breast cancer during her lifetime (Feuer, 1993).

Although the frequency of breast cancer in men is strikingly less than that in women, the disease in both sexes is remarkably similar in epidemiology, natural history, and response to treatment. Men with breast cancer are 5 to 10 years older than women at the time of diagnosis, with mean or median ages between 60 and 66 years. This apparent difference may occur because symptoms in men are ignored for a longer period and the disease is diagnosed at a more advanced state.

TABLE 10-7 ▼ Factors Associated with Breast Cancer

Gender	Women > men
Race	White
Age	Advancing age
	Peak incidence: 45-70
	Mean and median age: 60-61 (women)
	60-66 (men)
Family history	First-degree relative with breast cancer
	Premenopausal
	Bilateral
	Mother, daughter, or sister
Previous medical history	Previous personal history of cancer
	Breast
	Uterine
	Ovarian
	Colon
	Benign breast disease
Exposure to estrogen	Age at menarche <12
	Age at menopause >55
	Nulliparous (never pregnant)
	First live birth after age 35
	Environmental estrogens (esters)

Risk Factors

Despite the recent discovery of a "breast cancer gene,* researchers estimate that only 5% of breast cancers are a result of inherited genetic susceptibility. A large proportion are attributed to other factors, such as age, race, smoking, physical activity, alcohol intake, exposure to ionizing radiation,† and exposure to estrogens (Table 10-7).

As a general principle, the risk of breast cancer is linked to a woman's total lifelong exposure to estrogen. The increased inci-

---

*A predisposing gene for breast and ovarian cancer (BRCA-1) has been mapped to the long arm of chromosome 17. The disease is linked to this gene in almost all families having members with breast and ovarian cancer and in half of those families whose members have only breast cancer. All cases of bilateral breast cancer and ovarian cancer appear to be linked to this gene (Black and Solomon, 1993; Porter et al, 1993).

†Women who received multiple fluoroscopies for tuberculosis or radiation treatment for mastitis during their adolescent or childbearing years are at increased risk for breast cancer as a result of exposure to ionizing radiation. Irradiation was used for a variety of other medical conditions, including gynecomastia, thymic enlargement, eczema of the chest, chest burns, pulmonary tuberculosis, mediastinal lymphoma, and other cancers.

dence of estrogen-responsive tumors (tumors that are rich in estrogen receptors proliferate when exposed to estrogen) has been postulated to occur as a result of a variety of factors, such as prenatal and lifelong exposure to synthetic chemicals and environmental toxins, earlier age of menarche (first menstruation), improved nutrition in the United States, delayed and decreased childbearing, and longer average lifespan.

At the same time it should be remembered that many women diagnosed with breast cancer have no identified risk factors. More than 70% of breast cancer cases are not explained by established risk factors (Garfinkel, 1993). There is no history of breast cancer among female relatives in more than 90% of clients with breast cancer. However, first-degree relatives (mother, daughters, or sisters) of women with breast cancer have two to three times the risk of developing breast cancer than the general female population, and relatives of women with bilateral breast cancer have five times the normal risk.

Risk factors for men are similar to those for women, but at least half of all cases do not have an identifiable risk factor. Risk factors for men include heredity*, obesity, infertility, late onset of puberty, frequent chest x-ray examinations, history of testicular disorders (e.g., infection, injury, or undescended testes), and increasing age.

The presence of any of these factors may become evident during the interview with the client and should alert the physical therapist to potential neuromusculoskeletal complaints of a systemic origin that would require a medical referral.

Metastases

Metastases have been known to occur up to 25 years after the initial diagnosis of breast cancer. On the other hand, breast cancer can

---

*Men who have several female relatives with breast cancer and those in families in which the BRCA-2 mutation on chromosome 13q have a greater risk potential.

> ▼ **Clinical Signs and Symptoms of**
> ## Metastasized Breast Cancer
>
> - Palpable mass in supraclavicular, chest, or axillary regions
> - Unilateral upper extremity numbness and tingling
> - Back or shoulder pain
> - Pain on weight bearing
> - Leg weakness or paresis
> - Bowel/bladder symptoms

be a rapidly progressing, terminal disease. All distant visceral sites are potential sites of metastases. Bone is the most frequent site of metastases from breast cancer in men and women. Other primary sites of involvement are lymph nodes, remaining breast tissue, lung, brain, CNS, and liver, but this widely metastasizing disease has been found in almost every remote site. Women with metastases to the liver or CNS have a poorer prognosis.

Knowledge of the usual metastatic patterns of breast cancer and the common complications can aid early recognition and effective treatment. Spinal cord compression, usually from extradural metastases, may appear as back pain, leg weakness, and bowel/bladder symptoms.

CLINICAL SIGNS AND SYMPTOMS

Breast cancer usually consists of a nontender, firm, or hard lump with poorly delineated margins that is caused by local infiltration. Breast cancer in women has a predilection for the outer upper quadrant of the breast and the areola (nipple) area. Slight skin or nipple retraction is an important sign. Watery, serous, or bloody discharge from the nipple is an occasional early sign but is more often associated with benign disease.

The presenting complaint in about 70% of persons with breast cancer is a lump (usually painless) in the breast. About 90% of

Case Example. A 53-year-old woman with severe adhesive capsulitis was referred to a physical therapist by an orthopedic surgeon. A physical therapy program was initiated. When the client's shoulder flexion and abduction allowed for sufficient movement to place the client's hand under her head in the supine position, ultrasound to the area of capsular redundancy before joint mobilization was added to the treatment protocol.

During the treatment procedure the client was dressed in a hospital gown wrapped under the axilla on the involved side. With the client in the supine position, the upper outer quadrant of breast tissue was visible and the physical therapist observed skin puckering (peau d'orange) accompanied by a reddened area.

Result. It is always necessary to approach situations like this one carefully to avoid embarrassing or alarming the client. In this case the therapist casually observed, "I noticed when we raised your arm up for the ultrasound that there is an area of your skin here that puckers a little. Have you noticed any changes in your armpit, chest, or breast areas?"

Depending on the client's response, follow-up questions should include asking about distended veins, discharge from the nipple, itching of the skin or nipple, and the approximate time of the client's last breast examination (self-examination and physician examination). Although breast examination is not within the scope of a physical therapist's practice, palpation of lymph nodes and muscles such as the pectoral muscle groups can be performed.

There was no previous history of cancer, and further palpation did not elicit any other suspicious findings. The physical therapist recommended a physician evaluation, and a diagnosis of breast cancer was made.

breast masses are discovered by the individual. Less common symptoms are breast pain, nipple discharge, erosion/retraction/enlargement/itching of the nipple, redness, generalized hardness, or enlargement or shrinking of the breast.

Rarely, an axillary mass, swelling of the arm, or bone pain from metastases may be the first symptom. Back or bone pain, jaundice, or weight loss may be the result of systemic metastases, but these symptoms are rarely seen on initial presentation.

A tumor of any size in male breast tissue is associated with skin fixation and ulceration and deep pectoral fixation more often than a tumor of similar size in female breast tissue is because of the small size of male breasts. Lump masses that occur in the upper outer quadrant of the breast (usually women) involve the breast

▼ *Clinical Signs and Symptoms of*

Breast Cancer

- Nontender, firm or hard lump
- Skin or nipple retraction
- Discharge from nipple
- Erosion, retraction, enlargement, itching of nipple
- Redness or skin rash
- Generalized hardness, enlargement, or shrinking of breast
- Axillary mass
- Swelling of arm
- Bone or back pain
- Weight loss
- Jaundice

Case Example. A 67-year-old woman had loss of functional left shoulder motion (e.g., she could no longer reach the top shelf in her kitchen) as her only presenting complaint. During the Past Medical History portion of the interview, she mentioned that she had had a stroke 10 years ago. Her referring physician was unaware of this information.

Examination revealed mild loss of strength in the left upper extremity accompanied by mild sensory and proprioceptive losses. Palpation of the shoulder and pectoral muscles produced breast pain. The client had been aware of this pain, but she had attributed it to a separate medical problem. She was reluctant to report her breast pain to her physician. Objectively, there were positive trigger points of the left pectoral muscles and loss of accessory motions of the left shoulder.

Physical therapy treatment to eliminate trigger points and restore shoulder motion resolved the breast pain during the first week. Despite this woman's positive response to physical therapy treatment, given the age of this client, her significant past medical history for cerebrovascular injury, and the residual paresis, medical referral was still indicated.

At the first follow-up visit, a letter was sent with the client that briefly summarized the initial objective findings, her progress to date, and the current concerns. She returned for an additional week of physical therapy to complete the home program for her shoulder. A medical evaluation ruled out breast disease, but medical treatment (medication) was indicated related to her cardiovascular system.

tissue overlying the pectoral muscle. During palpation, breast tissue lumps move easily over the pectoral muscle, compared with a lump within the muscle tissue itself. Later signs of malignancy include fixation of the tumor to the skin or underlying muscle fascia.

A suspicious finding should be checked by a physician, especially in the case of the woman with identified risk factors. For this reason it is always important to ask the client about the risk factors identified in the text and previous medical history and to correlate this information with objective findings.

▼ GYNECOLOGIC CANCERS

Cancers of the female genital tract account for about 15% of all new cancers diagnosed in women. Although gynecologic cancers are the fourth leading cause of deaths from cancer in women in the United States, most of these cancers are highly curable when detected early. The most common cancers of the female genital tract are uterine endometrial cancer, ovarian cancer, and cervical cancer (Repetto et al, 1998).

Endometrial (Uterine) Cancer

Cancer of the uterine endometrium, or lining, is the most common gynecologic cancer, usually occurring in postmenopausal women between the ages of 55 and 70 years. Its occurrence is associated with endometrial hyperplasia, prolonged unopposed estrogen therapy (without progesterone), and, more recently, tamoxifen used in the treatment of breast cancer (Ball and Elkadry, 1998).

Clinical Signs and Symptoms of
Endometrial (Uterine) Cancer

- Vaginal bleeding or vaginal discharge after menopause (extremely significant sign)
- Persistent, irregular premenopausal bleeding, especially in obese women
- Abdominal or pelvic pain
- Weight loss, fatigue

CLINICAL SIGNS AND SYMPTOMS

Seventy-five percent of all cases of endometrial cancer occur in postmenopausal women who usually have abnormal vaginal bleeding or discharge at presentation. However, 25% of these cancers occur in premenopausal women, and 5% occur in women younger than 40 years. In a physical therapy practice the most common presenting complaint is pelvic pain without abnormal vaginal bleeding. Abdominal pain, weight loss, and fatigue may be present but unreported (Barakat, 1998).

Case Example. A 44-year-old slender, athletic woman with isolated left-knee pain of unknown cause was referred to physical therapy by her physician for a "strengthening program." She was actively involved in a variety of physical activities, including a co-ed baseball team, hiking club, and church basketball intramurals, but could not recall any specific injury, fall, or other impact to her leg. She had a pair of shoe orthotics prescribed by a podiatrist 5 years ago "to compensate for my excessive Q-angle."

The physical therapy examination was unremarkable for any joint swelling, redness, or palpable warmth. There was point tenderness along the medial joint line and a palpable though asymptomatic plica. The joint integrity was intact, and all special tests were negative. A neurologic screening examination was also considered within normal limits, although muscle strength for the quadriceps and hamstrings was diminished by pain. Pain was present on weight-bearing activities but did not prevent the woman from participating in all activities. There was no reported night pain, fever, or other associated signs and symptoms.

Without a definitive physical therapy diagnosis, a treatment plan was outlined to include modalities for pain and a stretching and strengthening program. Within a week's time this client's pain level escalated from 3 to 10 (on a scale from 1 to 10) with constant pain that kept her awake at night for hours. When she returned to the physical therapy clinic, she was using crutches and not bearing weight on the left leg.

Result. Therapists should be careful about assuming that physical therapy treatment has exacerbated a client's symptoms and instituting a change in program. If the treating therapist decided to continue physical therapy, trying some other approach, the physician should have been notified of the change in status.

Given the insidious onset of this joint pain and the rapidly progressive nature of the symptoms, this client was immediately sent back to her physician. A diagnosis of osseous metastasis was made, with early-stage endometrial carcinoma appearing as an unusual, isolated skeletal lesion. She was treated with aggressive multidisciplinary therapy, including limb salvage and physical therapy as part of her rehabilitation program. The early referral most likely contributed to her favorable prognosis and cancer-free status 2 years later.

Ovarian Cancer*

Ovarian cancer is the second most common reproductive cancer in women and the leading cause of death from gynecologic malignancies, accounting for more than half of all gynecologic-related cancer deaths.

The average American woman ovulates approximately 450 times during her lifetime. This "incessant ovulation" raises a woman's risk of developing ovarian cancer. The key to this connection may lie with the mechanics of ovulation. Each time an egg is released, it disrupts the surface of the ovary, stimulating ovarian cells to divide and repair the surface.

Risk increases with advancing age, and the incidence of ovarian cancer peaks between the ages of 40 and 70 years. Other factors that may influence the development of ovarian cancer include nulliparity (never being pregnant); history of breast, endometrial, or colorectal cancer; family history of ovarian cancer†; infertility; and early menopause.

Other possible, but not yet proven, factors include hormone replacement therapy (HRT), fertility drugs, use of talc-containing powders on the genital area, lactose intolerance, a high-fat diet, and excessive consumption of coffee and alcohol.

There is no reliable screening test to detect ovarian cancer in its early, most curable

---

▼ **Clinical Signs and Symptoms of**

Ovarian or Primary Peritoneal Cancer

- Persistent vague GI complaints
- Abdominal discomfort, bloating
- Indigestion, belching
- Early satiety
- Mild anorexia in a woman age 40 or older
- Urinary frequency
- Pelvic discomfort or pressure
- Ascites, pain, and pelvic mass (advanced disease)

---

stages. The CA-125 (carcinoembryonic antigen, a biologic marker) blood test and transvaginal ultrasonography help to determine whether an existing ovarian growth is benign or cancerous. Because the early-stage symptoms are quite nonspecific, most women do not seek medical attention until the disease is advanced.

The ovaries begin in utero, where the kidneys are located in the fully developed human and then migrate following the pathways of the ureters. Kidney stones moving down the pathway of the ureters cause flank pain radiating to the labia in the female.

Conversely, following the viscerosomatic referral patterns discussed in Chapter 2, ovarian cancer can cause back pain at the level of the kidneys. A Murphy's percussion text (see Chapter 7) would be negative; other symptoms of ovarian cancer might be present but unreported if the woman does not recognize their significance.

Cervical Cancer

Cancer of the cervix is the third most common gynecologic malignancy. Since the widespread introduction of the Pap smear as a standard screening tool, the diagnosis of cervical cancer at the invasive stage has decreased significantly, whereas the highly curable preinvasive carcinoma in situ (CIS) has increased.

---

*Extraovarian primary peritoneal carcinoma (EOPPC), a relatively newly defined disease that develops only in women, accounts for approximately 10% of cases with a presumed diagnosis of ovarian cancer. Characterized by abdominal carcinomatosis, uninvolved or minimally involved ovaries, and no identifiable primary form of cancer, EOPPC has been reported following bilateral oophorectomy performed for benign disease or prophylaxis (Eltabbakh and Piver, 1998). The occurrence of EOPPC may be explained by the common origin of the peritoneum and the ovaries from the coelomic epithelium. The various histologic differences of ovarian and peritoneal lesions are under extensive investigation at this time (Kunz and Rondez, 1998).

†The identification of the BRCA-1 gene on chromosome 17 and the subsequent evidence for a family of genes that may play a role in both the breast-ovarian syndrome and familial ovarian cancer offer the possibility of identifying women truly at risk for this disease (Young, 1995).

CIS is more common in women 30 to 40 years of age, and invasive carcinoma is more frequent in women over age 40 years.

Risk factors associated with the development of cervical cancer include early age at first sexual intercourse; early age at first pregnancy; low socioeconomic status; history of any sexually transmitted disease; history of multiple sex partners; and women whose mothers used the drug diethylstilbestrol (DES) during their pregnancy.

Viral infection also may be involved in the development of this cancer, and this factor is currently under investigation.

The American Cancer Society recommends that all women age 18 years and older and those younger than 18 years who are sexually active have an annual Pap smear and pelvic examination. After three negative annual examinations, the Pap smear may be performed less frequently at the advice of the physician. Women with risk factors for cervical cancer should be advised to have an annual Pap smear.

Women with abnormal Pap smears undergo a procedure that visualizes the cervical canal (colposcopy) and identifies abnormal areas to be biopsied. In some cases conization, or removal of a cone-shaped section of cervical tissue, may be necessary to obtain adequate tissue for diagnosis.

CLINICAL SIGNS AND SYMPTOMS

Early cervical cancer has no symptoms. Clinical symptoms related to advanced disease include painful intercourse; postcoital, coital, or intermenstrual bleeding; and a watery, foul-smelling vaginal discharge.

▼ CANCERS OF THE BLOOD AND LYMPH SYSTEM

Cancers arising from the bone marrow include acute leukemias, chronic leukemias, multiple myelomas, and some lymphomas. These cancers are characterized by the uncontrolled growth of blood cells.

The major lymphoid organs of the body are the lymph nodes and the spleen (Fig. 10-3). Cancers arising from these organs are called malignant lymphomas and are categorized as either Hodgkin's disease or non-Hodgkin's lymphoma.

Leukemia

Leukemia, a malignant disease of the blood-forming organs, is the most common malignancy in children and young adults. One half of all leukemias are classified as *acute,* with rapid onset and progression of disease resulting in 100% mortality within days to months without appropriate therapy. Acute leukemias are most common in children from 2 to 4 years of age, with a peak incidence again at age 65 years and older. The remaining leukemias are classified as *chronic,* which have a slower course and occur in persons between the ages of 25 and 60 years.

From these two broad categories, leukemias are further classified according to the specific malignant cell line (Table 10-8).

Leukemia develops in the bone marrow and is characterized by abnormal multiplication and release of white blood cell (WBC) precursors. The disease process originates during WBC development in the bone marrow or lymphoid tissue. In effect, leukemic cells become arrested in "infancy," with most of the clinical manifestations of the disease being related to the absence of functional "adult" cells, which are the product of normal differentiation.

With rapid proliferation of leukemic cells, the bone marrow becomes overcrowded with immature WBCs, which then spill over into the peripheral circulation. Crowding of the bone marrow by leukemic cells inhibits normal blood cell production. Decreased red blood cell (RBC) (erythrocyte) production results in anemia and reduced tissue oxygenation. Decreased platelet production results in thrombocytopenia and risk of hemorrhage. Decreased production of normal WBCs results in increased vulnerability to infection, especially because leukemic cells

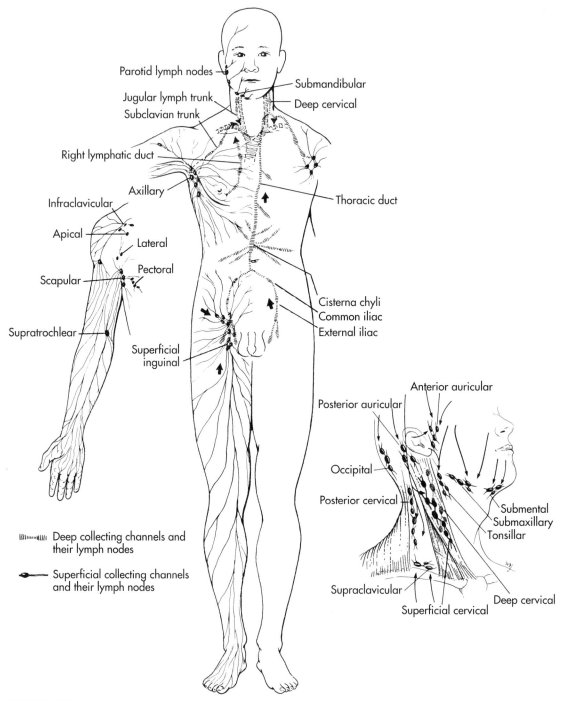

FIGURE 10-3 • **A,** Major lymphoid organs of the body: lymph nodes and spleen. (From Jacob SW, Francone CA: *Elements of anatomy and physiology*, ed 2, Philadelphia, 1989, WB Saunders.) **B,** Lymph nodes of the neck and their drainage. (From Swartz M: *Textbook of physical diagnosis*, Philadelphia, 1989, WB Saunders.)

TABLE 10-8 ▼ Overview of Leukemia

	ALL	ANLL (AML)	CLL	CML
Incidence				
Percentage of all leukemias	20%	20%	25%-40%	15%-20%
Adults	20%	85%	100%	95-100%
Children	80%-85%	10%-20%	—	3%
Age	Peak: 3-7 years 65+ (older adults)	15-40 years Incidence increases with age from 40-80+	50+	25-60 years
Etiology	Unknown Chromosomal abnormality Environmental factors Down's syndrome (high incidence)	Benzene Alkylating agents Radiation Myeloproliferative disorders Aplastic anemia	Chromosomal abnormalities Slow accumulation of CLL lymphocytes	Philadelphia chromosome Radiation exposure
Prognosis	Adult: Poor Child: 60% with aggressive treatment	Poor even with treatment 10%-15% survival	2-10 years survival Median survival: 6 years	Poor; 2-8 years Median survival: 3-4 years

From Goodman CC, Boissonnault WG: *Pathology: implications for the physical therapist,* Philadelphia, 1998, WB Saunders, p 368.
ALL, Acute lymphoblastic leukemia; *ANLL,* acute nonlymphocytic leukemia; *CLL,* chronic lymphocytic leukemia; *CML,* chronic myelogenous leukemia.

are functionally unable to defend the body against pathogens. Leukemic cells may invade and infiltrate vital organs such as the liver, kidneys, lung, heart, or brain.

CLINICAL SIGNS AND SYMPTOMS

Most of the clinical findings in acute leukemia are due to bone marrow failure (fatigue, bleeding, infection), which results from replacement of normal bone marrow elements by the malignant cells. The abnormal bleeding is caused by a lack of blood platelets required for clotting. Infections are due to a depletion of competent WBCs needed to fight infection.

For women, the abnormal bleeding may be prolonged menstruation leading to anemia. The Special Questions for Women (see Chapter 2) may elicit this kind of valuable information, which would then require medical referral. Less common manifestations include direct organ infiltration; clients may

experience easy bruising of the skin or abnormal bleeding from the nose, urinary tract, or rectum.

Lymphoproliferative malignancies such as leukemia and lymphoma may also involve the synovium and may lead to symptoms suggestive of a rheumatic disease. The most common presentation is a child with acute lymphoblastic leukemia who has joint pain and swelling that mimics juvenile rheumatoid arthritis (JRA) (Gilkeson and Caldwell, 1990).

The arthritic symptoms in such a child may be a consequence of leukemic synovial infiltration, hemorrhage into the joint, synovial reaction to an adjacent tumor mass, or crystal-induced synovitis.

Asymmetric involvement of the large joints is most commonly observed. Pain that is disproportionate to the physical findings may occur, and joint symptoms are often fleeting. Less frequent rheumatic manifestations of leukemia in children are back pain

▼ *Clinical Signs and Symptoms of*
Acute and Chronic Leukemias

- Abnormal bleeding
- Easy bruising of the skin
- Petechiae
- Epistaxis (nosebleeds) and/or bleeding gums
- Hematuria (blood in the urine)
- Rectal bleeding
- Infections, fever
- Weakness
- Easy fatigability
- Enlarged lymph nodes
- Bone and joint pain
- Weight loss
- Loss of appetite
- Pain or enlargement in the left upper abdomen (enlarged spleen)

▼ *Clinical Signs and Symptoms of*
Multiple Myeloma

- Recurrent bacterial infections (especially pneumococcal pneumonias)
- Anemia with weakness and fatigue
- Bleeding tendencies
- **Bone destruction**
  Skeletal/bone pain (especially pelvis, spine, and ribs)
  Spontaneous fracture
  Osteoporosis
  Hypercalcemia (confusion, increased urination, loss of appetite, abdominal pain, vomiting, and constipation)
- **Renal involvement**
  Kidney stones
  Renal insufficiency
- **Neurologic abnormalities**
  Carpal tunnel syndrome
  Back pain with radicular symptoms
  Spinal cord compression (motor or sensory loss, bowel/bladder dysfunction, paraplegia)

secondary to infiltration of the meninges by leukemic cells and long bone pain (Gilkeson and Caldwell, 1990).

Multiple Myeloma

Multiple myeloma, also known as plasma cell myeloma, is a primary malignant bone tumor associated with widespread osteolytic lesions (decreased areas of bone density), appearing radiographically as punched-out defects of bone. Excessive growth of plasma cells originating in the bone marrow destroys bone tissue.

Bone lesions and hypercalcemia are rare events in most hematologic malignancies, except in the case of multiple myeloma and adult T-cell leukemia/lymphoma (ATL) associated with human T-cell leukemia/lymphoma virus-1 (HTLV-1) infection. Morbidity and mortality associated with the extensive bone disease seen in clients with multiple myeloma is substantial (Roodman, 1997).

This disease can develop at any age from young adulthood to advanced age but peaks among persons between the ages of 50 and 70 years. It is more common in men and African-Americans. Molecular genetic abnormalities have been identified in the etiologic complex of this disease (Ozaki and Kosaka, 1998). Recent data suggest that a virus (Kaposi-associated herpes virus, HHV-8) may be implicated in AIDS-related cases (Pico et al, 1998).

CLINICAL SIGNS AND SYMPTOMS

The most common complications of multiple myeloma include bone destruction, renal failure, anemia, and neurologic abnormalities. The onset of multiple myeloma is usually gradual and insidious. Most clients pass through a long presymptomatic period

Case Example. At presentation, a 57-year-old man has rib pain that began 1 month ago. He could not think of any possible cause and denied any repetitive motions, recent trauma, forceful coughing, or history of tobacco use. Past medical history was significant for hepatitis A (10 years ago) and benign prostatic hypertrophy (BPH). The BPH is reportedly well controlled with medication, but he has noticed a decreased need to urinate and noted that he has been meaning to have a recheck of this problem.

On examination there was bilateral point tenderness over the posterior seventh and eighth ribs. Symptoms were not increased by respiratory movements, trunk movements, position, or palpation of the intercostal spaces. Trunk and extremity movements were considered within normal limits, and a neurologic screening examination was unremarkable.

The physical therapist could not account for the client's symptoms, given the history and clinical presentation. Further screening revealed that the client had noticed progressive fatigue and generalized aching over the last 2 weeks that he attributed to the flu. He had lost about 10 pounds during the week of vomiting and diarrhea. Vital signs were taken and were within normal limits. There were no other red-flag symptoms to suggest a systemic origin or symptoms.

Result. Without a proper physical therapy diagnosis on which to base treatment, the therapist did not have a clear treatment plan. There was not a well-defined musculoskeletal problem, but a variety of systemic variables were present (e.g., sudden weight loss and constitutional symptoms accounted for by the flu, oliguria, attributed to BPH, insidious onset of rib pain).

The therapist decided to treat the client for 7 to 10 days and reassess at that time. Treatment consisted of stretching, manual therapy, postural exercises, and Feldenkrais techniques. At the end of the prescribed time, there was no change in clinical presentation. The therapist asked a colleague in the same clinic for a second opinion at no charge to the client. An ultrasound test for possible rib fracture was performed and considered negative. No new findings were uncovered, and it was agreed collaboratively (including the client) to request a medical evaluation of the problem from the client's family physician. The client was subsequently diagnosed with multiple myeloma and treated medically.

that lasts 5 to 20 years. Early symptoms involve the skeletal system, particularly the pelvis, spine, and ribs. Some clients have backache or bone pain that worsens with movement.

BONE DESTRUCTION

Bone pain is the most common symptom of myeloma. It is caused by infiltration of the plasma cells into the marrow with subsequent destruction of bone. Initially, the skeletal pain may be mild and intermittent, or it may develop suddenly as a severe pain in the back, rib, leg, or arm, often the result of an abrupt movement or effort that has caused a spontaneous (pathologic) bone fracture. The pain is often radicular and sharply cutting to one or both sides and is aggravated by movement.

As the disease progresses, more and more areas of bone destruction and hypercalcemia develop. Symptoms associated with bone pain usually subside within days to weeks after initiation of antiresorptive agents. If left untreated, this disease will result in skeletal deformities, particularly of the ribs, sternum, and spine. Diffuse osteoporosis develops, accompanied by a negative calcium balance.

HYPERCALCEMIA

To rid the body of the excess calcium (hypercalcemia), the kidneys increase the output of urine, which can led to serious dehydration if there is an inadequate intake of fluids. This dehydration may be compounded by vomiting. Clients who have symptoms of hypercalcemia (confusion, increased urination, loss of appetite, abdominal pain, constipation, and vomiting) should seek immediate medical care because this condition can be life-threatening.

RENAL EFFECTS

Drainage of calcium and phosphorus from damaged bones eventually leads to the development of renal stones, particularly in immobilized clients. Renal insufficiency is the second most common cause of death, after infection, in clients with multiple myeloma.

In addition to bone destruction, multiple myeloma is characterized by disruption of RBC, leukocyte, and platelet production, which results from plasma cells crowding the bone marrow. Impaired production of these cell forms causes anemia, increased vulnerability to infection, and bleeding tendencies.

NEUROLOGIC COMPLICATIONS

Approximately 10% of persons with myeloma have amyloidosis, deposits of insoluble fragments of a monoclonal protein resembling starch. These deposits cause tissues to become waxy and immobile and may affect nerves, muscles, tendons, and ligaments, especially the carpal tunnel area of the wrist. Carpal tunnel syndrome with pain, numb-ness, or tingling of the hands and fingers may develop.

More serious neurologic complications may occur in 10% to 15% of clients with multiple myeloma. Spinal cord compression is usually observed early or in the late relapse phase of disease. Back pain is usually present as the initial symptom, with radicular pain that is aggravated by coughing or sneezing. Motor or sensory loss and bowel/bladder dysfunction are signs of more extensive compression. Paraplegia is a later, irreversible event.

Hodgkin's Disease

Hodgkin's disease is a chronic, progressive, neoplastic disorder of lymphatic tissue characterized by the painless enlargement of lymph nodes with progression to extralymphatic sites such as the spleen and liver.

In Caucasians, Hodgkin's disease demonstrates constant incidence rates, with a first peak occurring in adolescents and young adults and a second peak occurring in older adults (Greil, 1998). Men are affected more often than women, and boys are affected five times more often than girls.

Epidemiologic and clinical-pathologic features of Hodgkin's disease suggest that an infectious agent may be involved in this disorder. Recently, accumulated data provide direct evidence supporting a causal role of Epstein-Barr virus in a significant portion of cases (Dolcetti and Boiocchi, 1998).

Although Hodgkin's disease is not usually associated with acquired immunodeficiency disorders, there is a statistically significant increase in Hodgkin's disease among individuals infected with human immunodeficiency virus (HIV) (Levine, 1998).

Metastases

The exact mechanism of growth and spread of Hodgkin's disease remains unknown. The disease may progress by extension to adjacent structures or via the lymphatics because lymphoreticular cells inhabit all tissues of the body except the CNS. Hema-

▼ *Clinical Signs and Symptoms of*
Hodgkin's Disease

- Painless, progressive enlargement of unilateral lymph nodes, often in the neck
- Pruritus (itching) over entire body
- Unexplained fevers, night sweats
- Anorexia and weight loss
- Anemia, fatigue, malaise
- Jaundice
- Edema
- Nonproductive cough, dyspnea, chest pain, cyanosis
- Nerve root pain
- Paraplegia

tologic spread may also occur, possibly by means of direct infiltration of blood vessels.

CLINICAL SIGNS AND SYMPTOMS

Hodgkin's disease usually appears as a painless, enlarged lymph node, often in the neck, underarm, or groin. The physical therapist may palpate these nodes during a cervical spine, shoulder, or hip examination (see Fig. 10-3). Lymph nodes are evaluated on the basis of size, consistency, mobility, and tenderness. Lymph nodes up to 1 cm in diameter of soft to firm consistency that move freely and easily without tenderness are considered within normal limits. Lymph nodes >1 cm in diameter that are firm and rubbery in consistency or tender are considered suspicious. Enlarged lymph nodes associated with infection are more likely to be tender than slow-growing nodes associated with cancer.

Because lymph nodes enlarge in response to infections throughout the body, referral to a physician is not necessary on finding enlarged lymph nodes unless these nodes persist for more than 4 weeks or involve more than one area. However, the physician should be notified of these findings, and the client should be advised to have the lymph nodes checked at the next follow-up visit with the physician.

As always, *changes* in size, shape, tenderness, and consistency raise a red flag. Supraclavicular nodes are common metastatic sites for occult lung and breast cancers, whereas inguinal nodes implicate tumors arising in the legs, perineum, prostate, or gonads.

Other early symptoms may include unexplained fevers, night sweats, weight loss, and pruritus (itching). The itching occurs more intensely at night and may result in severe scratches because the client is unaware of scratching during the sleep state. The fever typically peaks in the late afternoon, and night sweats occur when the fever breaks during sleep. Fatigue, malaise, and anorexia may accompany progressive anemia. Some clients with Hodgkin's disease experience pain over the involved nodes after ingesting alcohol.

Symptoms may arise when enlarged lymph nodes obstruct or compress adjacent structures, causing edema of the face, neck, or right arm secondary to superior vena cava compression or causing renal failure secondary to urethral obstruction. Obstruction of bile ducts as a result of liver damage causes bilirubin to accumulate in the blood and discolor the skin. Mediastinal lymph node enlargement with involvement of lung parenchyma and invasion of the pulmonary pleura progressing to the parietal pleura may result in pulmonary symptoms, including nonproductive cough, dyspnea, chest pain, and cyanosis.

Dissemination of disease from lymph nodes to bones may cause compression of the spinal cord, leading to paraplegia. Compression of nerve roots of the brachial, lumbar, or sacral plexus can cause nerve root pain.

Non-Hodgkin's Lymphoma

Non-Hodgkin's lymphoma (NHL) is a group of lymphomas affecting lymphoid tissue and occurring in persons of all ages. It is more common in adults in their middle and older years (40 to 60 years). Although men are affected more often than women, the incidence of NHL in women is up by 36% since the early 1970s.

▼ *Clinical Signs and Symptoms of*

Non-Hodgkin's Lymphoma

- Enlarged lymph nodes
- Fever
- Night sweats
- Weight loss
- Bleeding
- Infection
- Red skin and generalized itching of un-known origin

Several possible etiologic mechanisms are hypothesized for NHL. Immunosuppression, possibly in combination with viruses or exposure to certain infectious agents could be the primary cause. Chemicals, UV light, blood transfusion, acquired and congenital immune deficiency, and autoimmune disorders increase the risk for NHL (Hardell and Axelson, 1998). Other studies link the disease to widespread environmental contaminants, such as benzene found in cigarette smoke, gasoline, automobile emissions, and industrial pollution.

CLINICAL SIGNS AND SYMPTOMS

NHLs present a clinical picture broadly similar to that of Hodgkin's disease, except that the disease is usually initially more widespread. The disease starts in the lymph node, although involvement of extranodal sites is more commonly seen in the NHLs than in Hodgkin's disease.

The most common manifestation is painless enlargement of one or more peripheral lymph nodes. Systemic symptoms are not as commonly associated with the NHLs as with Hodgkin's disease. Clients with non-Hodgkin's lymphomas often have remarkably few symptoms, even though many node areas or extranodal sites are involved.

Acquired Immunodeficiency Syndrome–Non-Hodgkin's Lymphoma (AIDS-NHL)

Only recently has AIDS-NHL emerged as a major sequela of HIV infection. It now occurs frequently in clients who survive other consequences of AIDS.

The etiologic basis of AIDS-NHL is still under investigation; profound cellular immunodeficiency plays a central role in lymphomagenesis. The molecular pathogenesis is a complex process involving both host factors and genetic alterations (Gaidano et al, 1998). Epstein-Barr virus (EBV) often accompanies NHLs. It is generally accepted that EBV acts in the pathogenesis of lymphoma owing to the alteration in balance between host and the latent EBV infection in immunodeficiency states, with an increased activity of the virus.

Other predisposing factors include age and sex. The median age at diagnosis of HIV-related NHL is 38 years, compared with 56 years for HIV-negative clients with NHL. Women are at relatively less risk of developing lymphoma than are men. The percentage of AIDS cases with NHL is shown not to vary between risk groups (homosexuals versus intravenous drug abusers) (Beral et al, 1991).

NHL is more likely to develop among clients who have Kaposi's sarcoma, a history of herpes simplex infection, and a lower neutrophil count.

CLINICAL SIGNS AND SYMPTOMS

The most common presentations of HIV-related NHL are systemic B symptoms (which may suggest an infectious process), a rapidly enlarging mass lesion, or both. At the time of diagnosis, approximately 75% of clients will have advanced disease. Extranodal disease frequently involves any part of the body, with the most common locations being the CNS, bone marrow, GI tract, and liver.

Although musculoskeletal lesions are not reported as commonly as pulmonary or CNS abnormalities in HIV-positive individuals, a wide variety of osseous and soft tissue changes are seen in this group. Diffuse adenopathy, lower extremity pain and swelling, subcutaneous nodules, and lytic lesions of the extremities are common (Aboulafia et al, 1998).

▼ SARCOMA

By definition, sarcoma is a fleshy growth and refers to a large variety of tumors arising in the connective tissues that are grouped together because of similarities in pathologic appearance and clinical presentation. Tissues affected include connective tissue, such as bone and cartilage (discussed subsequently under Bone Tumors); muscle; fibrous tissue; fat; and synovium.

The different types of sarcomas are named for the specific tissues affected (e.g., fibrosarcomas are tumors of the fibrous connective tissue; osteosarcomas are tumors of the bone; and chondrosarcomas are tumors arising in cartilage [Table 10-9]).

As a general category, sarcoma differs from carcinoma in the origin of cells comprising the tumor (see Table 10-1). As mentioned, sarcomas arise in connective tissue (embryologic mesoderm), whereas carcinomas arise in epithelial tissue (embryologic ectoderm) (i.e., cellular structures covering or lining surfaces of body cavities, small vessels, or visceral organs). Carcinomas affect structures such as the skin, large intestine, stomach, breast, and lungs. Generally, carcinomas tend to metastasize via the lymphatics, whereas sarcomas are more likely to metastasize hematogenously.

Malignant neoplasms or new growths that develop as *primary* lesions in the musculoskeletal tissues are relatively rare, representing less than 1% of malignant disease of all age groups and 6.5% of all cancers in children under the age of 15 years (American Cancer Society, 1993).

Secondary neoplasms that develop in the connective tissues as metastases from a primary neoplasm elsewhere (especially metastatic carcinoma) are common. Fibrosarcomas occurring after radiotherapy can occur usually after a significant latent period (4 years or more) (Borman et al, 1998).

A high grade (grade represents the likelihood of metastasis based on measures of cell differentiation and growth) and evidence of metastasis are associated with a poor prognosis for all neoplasms of bone or soft tissue (Peabody et al, 1998).

Soft Tissue Tumors

Soft tissue sarcomas comprise a group of relatively rare malignancies. Little is known about important epidemiologic or etiologic factors in clients with soft tissue sarcomas. There is no proven genetic predisposition to the development of soft tissue sarcomas.

Although researchers continue to explore the role of specific tumor suppressor genes and abnormalities in gene expression as these relate to sarcomas (Milas et al, 1998), there are two peaks of incidence in human sarcoma development: early adolescence and the middle decades. Soft tissue sarcomas can arise anywhere in the body. In adults, most soft tissue sarcomas arise in the extremities (usually the lower extremity, at or below the knee), followed by the trunk and retroperitoneum.

In contrast, the overwhelming majority of childhood soft tissue sarcomas are rhabdomyosarcomas, and the anatomic distribution of these lesions is entirely different (20% in the extremities, 40% in the head and neck region, and 25% in genitourinary

TABLE 10-9 ▼ Classification of Soft Tissue and Bone Tumors

Tissue of Origin	Benign Tumor	Malignant Tumor
Connective Tissue		
Fibrous	Fibroma	Fibrosarcoma
Cartilage	Chondroma:	Chondrosarcoma
	Enchondroma	
	Chondroblastoma	
Bone	Osteoma	Osteosarcoma
Bone marrow		Leukemia
		Multiple myeloma
		Ewing's sarcoma
Adipose (fat)	Lipoma	Liposarcoma
Synovial	Ganglion, giant cell of tendon sheath	Synovial sarcoma
Muscle		
Smooth muscle	Leiomyoma	Leiomyosarcoma
Striated muscle	Rhabdomyoma	Rhabdomyosarcoma
Endothelium (Vascular/Lymphatic)		
Lymph vessels	Lymphangioma	Lymphangiosarcoma
		Kaposi's sarcoma
Lymphoid tissue		Lymphosarcoma (lymphoma)
		Lymphatic leukemia
Blood vessels	Hemangioma	Hemangiosarcoma
Neural Tissue		
Nerve fibers and sheaths	Neurofibroma	Neurofibrosarcoma
	Neuroma	Neurogenic sarcoma
	Neurinoma (neurilemmoma)	
Glial tissue	Gliosis	Glioma
Epithelium		
Skin and mucous membrane	Papilloma	Squamous cell carcinoma
	Polyp	Basal cell carcinoma
Glandular epithelium	Adenoma	Adenocarcinoma

Data from Purtilo DT, Purtilo RB: *A survey of human disease,* ed 2, Boston, 1989, Little, Brown; Phipps W et al: *Medical-surgical nursing: concepts and clinical practice,* ed 4, St Louis, 1990, Mosby.

sites) (Lawrence, 1994). Many of the primary sites in children (e.g., orbit of the eye, paratesticular region, and prostate) are never primary sites for soft tissue sarcomas in adults.

Metastases

In children, tumors of the extremities tend to behave relatively aggressively, with a high incidence of nodal spread and distant metastases. In adults, soft tissue sarcomas rarely spread to regional lymph nodes, instead invading aggressively into surrounding tissues with early hematogenous dissemination, usually to the lungs.

Even with pulmonary metastases, the survival rate has greatly improved in the last decade with a multidisciplinary approach that includes multiagent chemotherapy and limb-sparing surgery (La Quaglia, 1998). However, as more people survive for increasingly longer periods, serious and potentially life-threatening complications of such therapy can develop months to years later.

CLINICAL SIGNS AND SYMPTOMS

Soft tissue sarcomas most often appear as asymptomatic soft tissue masses. Because these lesions arise in compressible tissues

▼ *Clinical Signs and Symptoms of*
Soft Tissue Sarcoma

- Persistent swelling or lump in a muscle (most common finding)
- Pain
- Pathologic fracture
- Local swelling
- Warmth of overlying skin

and are often far from vital organs, symptoms are few unless they are located close to a major nerve or in a confined anatomic space.

The most common manifestations of these neoplasms are swelling and pain. Pelvic sarcomas may appear with swelling of the leg or pain in the distribution of the femoral or sciatic nerve. Some people attribute swelling to a minor injury, reporting a misleading cause of onset to the therapist. The therapist must always keep this in mind when evaluating a client of any age.

More often, the neoplasm goes unnoticed until some trauma or injury requires medical attention and an x-ray study reveals the lesion. When pain is the most significant symptom, it is usually mild and intermittent, progressively becoming more severe and more constant with rapidly growing neoplasms.

No reliable physical signs are present to distinguish between benign and malignant soft tissue lesions. Consequently, all soft tissue lumps that persist or grow should be reported immediately to the physician.

Bone Tumors

Benign and malignant (primary) bone tumors are relatively rare, accounting for 1% of total deaths from cancer. Excluding multiple myeloma, the ratio of benign to malignant bone tumors is approximately 7:1.

Primary bone cancer affects children and young adults most commonly, whereas secondary bone tumors or metastatic neoplasms occur in adults with primary cancer (e.g., cancer of the prostate, breast, lungs, kidneys, thyroid).

The two most common childhood sarcomas of the bone are osteosarcoma (osteogenic sarcoma) and Ewing's sarcoma; both have a poor prognosis. This text is limited to the most common forms of bone tumors.

A history of sudden onset of severe pain usually indicates the complication of a pathologic fracture (a break in an already weakened bone). Local swelling can be detected when the lesion protrudes beyond the normal confines of the bone. The swelling of a benign lesion is usually firm and nontender. In the presence of a rapidly growing malignant neoplasm, however, the swelling is more diffuse and frequently tender (Fig. 10-4). The overlying skin may be warm because of the highly vascularized nature of neoplasms. If the lesion is close to a joint, function in that joint may be disturbed, with painful and restricted range of motion.

Bone pain (especially pain on weight bearing) that persists for more than 1 week and grows worse at night, often awakening the person, is usually the most common symptom of bone cancer. The pain is often associated with trauma during a game or exercise and may be dismissed in children as "growing pains."

Occasionally, a growing bone mass is the first sign of disease. Diagnosis is made by x-ray study and surgical biopsy, requiring immediate attention to suspicious symptoms by referral to the client's physician.

Osteosarcoma

Osteosarcoma (also known as osteogenic sarcoma) is the most common type of bone cancer, occurring between the ages of 10 and 25 years. It is more common in boys.

Although it can involve any bones in the body, because it arises from osteoblasts,

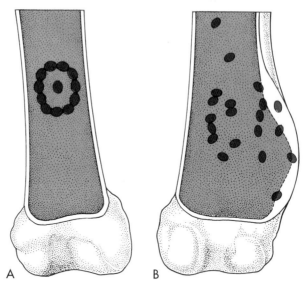

FIGURE 10-4 • **A,** Benign bone tumors have a characteristic sclerotic rim around the periphery of the lesion. The lesion is usually well defined, and there is no evidence of erosion of the cortex or a soft tissue mass. **B,** Malignant bone tumors can have lytic or slcerotic components. It is frequently difficult to know the extent of the lesion within the bone because there is no well-defined sclerotic rim around the tumor. The destructive process is diffuse within the medullary cavity of the bone, and the tumor may break through the cortex of the bone, producing Codman's triangle. Frequently an associated soft tissue mass is present. Medical differential diagnosis of this lesion is between an osteogenic sarcoma and a chondrosarcoma. (Modified from de Vita VT Jr, Hellman S, editors: *Cancer: principles and practice of oncology,* Philadelphia, 1982, JB Lippincott.)

the usual site is the epiphyses of the long bones, where active growth takes place (e.g., lower end of the femur, upper end of the tibia or fibula, and upper end of the humerus).

In general, 80% to 90% of osteosarcomas occur in the long bones; the axial skeleton is rarely affected. The growth spurt of adolescence is a peak time for the development of osteosarcoma. Half of all osteosarcomas are located in the upper leg above the knee, where the most active epiphyseal growth occurs.

Metastases. Bone tumors, unlike carcinomas, disseminate almost exclusively through the blood; bones lack a lymphatic system. Metastases to the lungs, pleurae, lymph nodes, kidneys, and brain and to other bones are common and occur early in the disease process. Hematogenous spread is to the lungs first and to other bones second.

With the use of adjuvant chemotherapy, the skeletal system has become a more common site of initial relapse. Local recurrence of either a benign or a malignant lesion is due to inadequate removal of the primary tumor. Most local recurrences develop within 24 months of attempted removal.

CLINICAL SIGNS AND SYMPTOMS

Osteosarcoma usually appears with pain in a lesional area, usually around the knee in clients with femur or tibia involvement. The pain is initially mild and intermittent but becomes progressive, more severe, and constant over time.

Most lesions produce pain as the tumor starts to expand the bony cortex and stretch the periosteum. A tender lump may develop, and a bone weakened by erosion of the metaphyseal cortex may break with little or no

▼ *Clinical Signs and Symptoms of*
Osteosarcoma

- Pain and swelling of the involved body part
- Loss of motion and functional movement of adjacent joints
- Tender lump
- Pathologic fracture
- Occasional weight loss
- Malaise
- Fatigue

▼ *Clinical Signs and Symptoms of*
Ewing's Sarcoma

- Increasing and persistent pain
- Increasing and persistent swelling over a bone (localized over the area of tumor)
- Decrease in movement if a limb bone is involved
- Fever
- Fatigue
- Weight loss

stress. This pathologic fracture often brings the person into the medical system, at which time a diagnosis is established by x-ray study and surgical biopsy. This neoplasm is highly vascularized, so that the overlying skin is usually warm.

Ewing's Sarcoma

Ewing's sarcoma is the second most common primary malignant bone tumor of children and the fourth most common malignant bone tumor overall (Vlasak and Sim, 1996).

It is most common between the ages of 5 and 16 years, with a slightly greater incidence in boys than in girls. Ewing's sarcoma rarely occurs in people of African origin. Almost any bone can be involved, but typically the pelvis, femur, tibia, ulna, and metatarsal are the most common sites for Ewing's sarcoma.

Metastases. Metastasis is predominantly hematogenous (to lungs and bone), although lymph node involvement may occur. Metastasis usually occurs late in the disease process, but aggressive chemotherapy has increased 5-year survival rats from 10% to 70% (Vlasak and Sim, 1996).

CLINICAL SIGNS AND SYMPTOMS

Ewing's sarcoma is a rapidly growing tumor that often outgrows its blood sup-

ply and quickly erodes the bone cortex, producing a painful, soft, tender, palpable mass.

The pain may be intermittent and may not be accompanied by swelling, resulting in a physical therapy referral. Systemic symptoms such as fatigue, weight loss, and intermittent fever may be present, especially in clients with metastatic disease. Fever may occur when products of bone degeneration enter the bloodstream. In addition, the blood supply to local areas of bone may be compromised, with resultant avascular necrosis of bone.

Ewing's sarcoma occurs most frequently in the long bones and the pelvis, the most common site being the distal metaphysis and the diaphysis of the femur. The next most common sites are the pelvis, tibia, fibula, and humerus.

Less common presentations of Ewing's sarcoma include primary rib tumor associated with a pleural effusion and respiratory symptoms, mandibular lesions presenting with chin and lip paresthesias, primary vertebral (cervical, lumbar) tumor with symptoms of nerve root or spinal cord compression, and primary sacral tumor with neurogenic bladder. Neurologic symptoms may occur secondary to nerve entrapment by the tumor, and misdiagnosis as lumbar disk disease can occur (Grubb et al, 1994).

Case Example. A 17-year-old male high school athlete noted low back pain 6 weeks ago. He was unable to identify a specific traumatic event or injury but noted that he had been "training pretty hard" the last 2 weeks. Spinal motions were all within normal limits with no apparent step suggestive of spondylolisthesis. There were no obvious postural changes, such as a scoliotic shift or unusual kyphosis/lordosis of the spinal curves.

The only positive evaluation findings included a mild left foot drop and an absent left ankle jerk. Pain was intensified on weight bearing and movement of any kind. Pain was not relieved by rest or aspirin. There was no fever or recent history of sore throat, upper respiratory or ear infection, and so on. After 1 week in physical therapy, the pain began radiating into the posterior aspect of the left thigh. The client had also noted for the first time paresthesias along the lateral side of the left leg. The pain had increased rather markedly over the past 2 weeks.

The therapist might assume that the physical therapy treatment aggravated this client's condition, causing increased symptoms. However, given the unknown cause of pain, symptoms inconsistent with musculoskeletal conditions (e.g., unrelieved by rest), combined with the recent change in symptoms and the presence of positive neurologic symptoms, this client was returned to the physician before continuing further therapy.

A blood test performed at that time indicated that the WBC count was 10,000 mm^3 (normal range = 4300 to 10,800 mm^3). Further testing, including a radiograph, resulted in a diagnosis of Ewing's sarcoma.

Chondrosarcoma

Chondrosarcoma, the most common malignant cartilage tumor, occurs most often in adults older than 40. However, when it does occur in the younger age group, it tends to be a higher grade of malignancy and capable of metastases.

It occurs most commonly in some part of the pelvic or shoulder girdles or long bones, such as the femurs. Chondrosarcomas are the most common malignant tumors of the sternum and scapula.

Chondrosarcoma is usually a relatively slow-growing malignant neoplasm that arises either spontaneously in previously normal bone or as a result of malignant change in a preexisting benign bone tumor (osteochondromas and enchondromas or chondromas).

Metastases. Although slow-growing chondrosarcoma has a high tendency for thrombus formation in the tumor blood vessels, with an increased risk for pulmonary embolism and metastatic spread to the lungs. Metastases develop late, so that the prognosis of chondrosarcoma is considerably better than that of osteosarcoma.

▼ *Clinical Signs and Symptoms of*
Chondrosarcoma

- Back or thigh pain
- Sciatica
- Bladder symptoms
- Unilateral edema

CLINICAL SIGNS AND SYMPTOMS

Clinical presentation of chondrosarcoma varies. *Peripheral chondrosarcomas* (arising from bone surface) grow slowly and may be undetected and quite large. Local symptoms develop only because of mechanical irritation; otherwise, pain is not a prominent symptom. Pelvic chondrosarcomas are often large and appear with pain referred to the back or thigh, sciatica caused by sacral plexus irritation, urinary symptoms from bladder neck involvement, or unilateral edema caused by iliac vein obstruction.

Conversely, *central chondrosarcomas* (arising within bone) appear with dull pain, and a mass is rare. Pain, which indicates active growth, is an ominous sign of a central cartilage lesion.

PRIMARY CENTRAL NERVOUS SYSTEM TUMORS
(Prados et al, 1998)

Primary tumors of the CNS arise within the CNS and include tumors that lie within the spinal cord (intramedullary), within the dura mater (extramedullary), or outside the dura mater (extradurally). About 80% of CNS tumors occur intracranially, and 20% affect the spinal cord and peripheral nerves. Of the intracranial lesions, about 60% are primary, and the remaining 40% are metastatic lesions, often multiple and most commonly from the lung, breast, kidney, and GI tract.

Although neurons are the most common cells in the brain, they have no significant capability for reproducing and have little potential for neoplastic changes that could result in a tumor. Glial cells, the supporting cells of the brain, are numerous and carry out many structural and metabolic functions. These cells give rise to a variety of intraaxial tumors that infiltrate and invade brain tissue. Extraaxial tumors have their origin in the skull, meninges, cranial nerves, or pituitary gland. These tumors have a compressive effect on the brain.

The CNS is surrounded by meninges that protect the brain and are responsible for maintaining the cerebrospinal-fluid pathways around the brain and the spinal cord. Meningiomas are common tumors, almost always benign, that arise from these structures. These tumors indent the brain and cause symptoms by pressure or by producing a reaction (e.g., irritation or edema) in adjacent brain.

Schwannomas are benign tumors of the nerve sheath surrounding the cranial nerves. They cause symptoms related to compression of the affected nerve. For example, schwannomas of the vestibular portion of the eighth cranial nerve (formerly called acoustic neuroma) cause hearing loss.

Any CNS tumor, even if well differentiated and histologically benign, is potentially dangerous because of the lethal effects of increased intracranial pressure and tumor location near critical structures. For example, a small, well-differentiated lesion in the pons or medulla may be more rapidly fatal than a massive liver cancer.

Primary CNS tumors rarely metastasize outside the CNS; there is no lymphatic drainage available, and hematogenous spread is also unlikely. In most cases CNS spread is contained in the cerebrospinal axis, involving local invasion or CNS seeding through the subarachnoid space and the ventricles.

Brain Tumors

The incidence of primary brain tumors is increasing in all ages; in children, it is second only to leukemia as a cause of death. Although the causes for this overall increase remain unknown, it is clear that it is not simply a matter of better diagnostic techniques. Adding the number of people who survive other primary cancers but later develop metastatic brain tumors increases the overall incidence dramatically.

Primary Malignant Brain Tumors

The most common primary malignant brain tumors are glioblastomas and astrocytomas. Low-grade gliomas, although usually thought of as benign, progress to more malignant forms in nearly 75% of all cases. Both glioblastomas and astrocytomas are usually fatal lesions, with median survivals

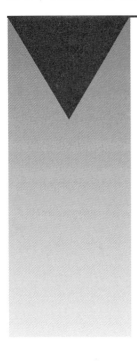

Case Example. A 75-year-old woman fell and sprained her right wrist. She visited her family physician, who prescribed an antiinflammatory agent and provided her with a soft wrist support. The woman continued to have painful swelling and could not use her hand to write, lift even small objects at home, or accomplish daily activities. Her physician referred her to a physical therapist for evaluation and treatment.

Although the clinical examination revealed a straightforward wrist sprain, the therapist observed that the client seemed confused and disoriented. Past medical history included breast cancer, diverticulosis, gallbladder removal, and hysterectomy. There were no current health concerns expressed by the client or her family.

Given the client's past history of cancer, knowing that confusion is not a "normal" sign of aging and that any neurologic sign can be an indicator of cancer, the physical therapist suggested that the family talk with the referring physician about these observations.

Result. The client progressed well with the wrist rehabilitation program. The family reported that the physician did not seem concerned about the developing confusion. No further medical testing was recommended. Six weeks later the client fell and broke her hip. At that time she was diagnosed with metastases to the bone and brain (CNS).

of about 1 year and 2 to 3 years, respectively, with conventional treatment (Young, 1998).

Metastatic Brain Tumors

Cancer can spread through bloodborne metastasis or via the cerebrospinal fluid pathways. Therefore the brain is a common site of metastasis. In fact, metastatic brain tumors are probably the most common form of malignant brain tumors. Up to 50% of individuals affected with cancers develop neurologic symptoms resulting from brain metastases. As mentioned previously, any neurologic sign can be the silent presentation of cancer metastasized to the CNS. The most common sources of brain metastases are cancers of the lung and breast, followed by metastases from melanomas and cancers of the colon and kidney (Young, 1998).

CLINICAL SIGNS AND SYMPTOMS

Symptoms of brain tumor are usually general or focal symptoms, depending on the size and location of the lesion. Two of the most common clinical manifestations of brain tumor are headache and personality change, but personality change is often attributed to depression, delaying the diagnosis of brain tumor. Headaches occur in 30% to 50% of persons with brain tumors and are usually bioccipital or bifrontal. They are usually intermittent and of increasing duration and may be intensified by a change in posture or by straining.

The headache is characteristically worse on awakening because of differences in CNS drainage in the supine and prone positions and usually disappears soon after the person arises. It may be intensified or precipitated by any activity that increases intracranial pressure, such as straining during a bowel movement, stooping, lifting heavy objects, or coughing.

Often, the pain can be relieved by taking aspirin, acetaminophen, or other moderate painkillers. Vomiting with or without nausea (unrelated to food) occurs in about 25% to 30% of people with brain tumors and of-

Clinical Signs and Symptoms of
Brain Tumors

- Increased intracranial pressure
  Headache, especially retroorbital
  Nausea and vomiting
  Visual changes (blurring, blind spots, diplopia)
- Changes in mentation
  Difficulty concentrating (e.g., reading)
  Memory loss
  Personality change, irritability
  Increased sleeping
- Seizures (without previous history)
- Sensory changes
- Muscle weakness or hemiparesis
- Bladder dysfunction
- Increased lower extremity reflexes compared with upper extremity reflexes
- Decreased coordination, ataxia
- Positive Babinski reflex
- Clonus (ankle or wrist)

ten accompanies headaches when there is an increase in intracranial pressure. If the tumor invades the meninges, the headaches will be more severe.

Focal manifestations of a space-occupying brain lesion are caused by the local compression or destruction of the brain tissue as well as by compression secondary to edema. Papilledema (edema and hyperemia of the optic disc) may be the first sign of intracranial tumors. Visual changes do not occur until prolonged papilledema causes optic atrophy.

Specific symptoms depend on where the tumor is located. For example, if a tumor is growing in the motor cortex, the client may develop isolated extremity weakness or hemiparesis. If the tumor is developing in the cerebellum, coordination may be affected. Tumors affecting the frontal lobes may produce personality changes. Seizures

occur in approximately one third of persons with metastatic brain tumors.

Spinal Cord Tumors

Spinal tumors are similar in nature and origin to intracranial tumors but occur much less often. They are most common in young and middle-aged adults, and they occur most often in the thoracic spine because of its length, proximity to the mediastinum, and proximity to direct metastatic extension from lymph nodes involved with lymphoma, breast cancer, or lung cancer.

Metastases

Most metastasis is disseminated by local invasion. Spinal cord tumors account for <15% of brain tumors. As mentioned, 10% of spinal tumors are themselves metastasized neoplasms from the brain.

One other means of dissemination is through the intervertebral foramina. The extradural space communicates through the intervertebral foramina with adjacent extraspinal compartments, such as the mediastinum and retroperitoneal space.

In most cases extradural tumors are metastatic, reaching the extradural space and then adjacent extraspinal spaces through this foraminal connection.

Tumors within the spinal cord (intramedullary) or outside the spinal cord (extramedullary) may metastasize to the dural tube to become intradural tumors.

CLINICAL SIGNS AND SYMPTOMS

Back pain at the level of the spinal cord lesion occurs in more than 80% of cases and may be aggravated by lying down, weight bearing, sneezing, or coughing.

Discomfort may be thoracolumbar back pain in a beltlike distribution; the pain may extend to the groin or the legs. The pain may be constant or intermittent, a dull ache or a sharp, knifelike sensation. Pain occurs most often at rest; pain occurring at night can awaken an individual from sleep; the person reports that it is impossible to go back to sleep.

Clinical manifestations of spinal tumors vary according to their location. Spinal cord compression is the most common pathologic feature of all tumors within the spinal column; symptoms occur in the body below the level of the tumor. Early characteristics of spinal cord compression include pain, sensory loss, muscle weakness, and muscle atrophy. Less commonly, chest or abdominal pain may occur, caused by nerve root compression from epidural tumor(s). Bowel and bladder dysfunction are late findings.

Pain associated with *extramedullary tumors* can be located primarily at the site of the lesion or may refer down the ipsilateral extremity, with radicular involvement from nerve root compression, irritation, or occlusion of blood vessels supplying the cord. Progressive cord compression is manifested by spastic weakness below the level of the lesion, decreased sensation, and increased weakness.

Intramedullary tumors produce more variable signs and symptoms. High cervical cord involvement causes spastic quadriplegia and sensory changes. Tumors in descending areas of the spinal cord produce motor and sensory changes appropriate to functions of that level.

Text Continued on page 379.

▼ **Clinical Signs and Symptoms of**
Spinal Cord Tumors

- Pain
- Decreased sensation
- Spastic muscle weakness
- Progressive muscle weakness
- Muscle atrophy
- Paraplegia or quadriplegia
- Thoracolumbar pain
- Unilateral groin or leg pain
- Pain at rest and/or night pain
- Bowel/bladder dysfunction (late finding)

OVERVIEW | **CANCER PRESENCE AND PAIN**

▼ ONCOLOGIC (CANCER) PAIN

Location:	See Table 10-4; localized bone pain
Referral:	May follow nerve distribution
Description:	Bone pain: Sharp, continuous
	Viscera: Colicky, cramping, dull, diffuse, boring, poorly localized
	Vein, artery, lymphatic channel: Dull, diffuse, burning, aching
	Nerve compression: Sharp, stabbing; follows nerve distribution or dull, poorly localized
	Inflammation: Sensitive tenderness
Intensity:	Varies from mild to severe or excruciating
	Bone pain: Increases on movement or weight bearing
Duration:	Usually constant; may be worse at night
Associated signs and symptoms:	With mild to moderate superficial pain: Sympathetic nervous system response (e.g., hypertension, tachycardia, tachypnea)

With severe or visceral pain: Parasympathetic nervous system response (e.g., hypotension, tachypnea, weakness, fainting)

Organ dependent (e.g., esophagus: difficulty eating or speaking; gallbladder: jaundice, nausea; nerve involvement: altered sensation, paresthesia; see individual visceral cancers)

▼ PARANEOPLASTIC SYNDROMES

Location:	Remote sites from primary neoplasm
Referral	Organ dependent
Description:	Asymmetric joint involvement
	Lower extremities primarily
	Concurrent arthritis and malignancy
	Explosive onset at late age
	See Tables 10-2 and 10-3
Intensity:	Symptom dependent
Duration:	Symptom dependent
Associated signs and symptoms:	Fever
	Skin rash
	Clubbing of the fingers
	Pigmentation disorders
	Arthralgias
	Paresthesias
	Thrombophlebitis
	Proximal muscle weakness
	Anorexia, malaise, weight loss
	Rheumatologic complaints

▼ SKIN (MELANOMA ONLY)

Location:	Anywhere on the body
	Women: Arms, legs, back, face
	Men: Head, trunk
	African-Americans: Palms, soles, under the nails
Referral:	None
Description:	Usually painless; see ABCD method of detection (text)
	Sore that does not heal

	Irritation and itching
	Cluster mole formation
	Tenderness and soreness around a mole
Intensity:	Mild
Duration:	Constant
Associated signs and symptoms:	None

▼ BREAST (Fig. 10-5)

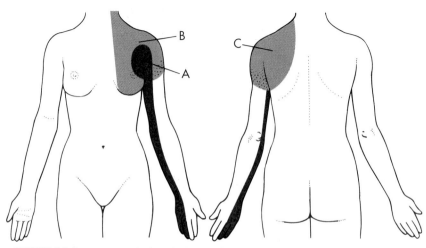

FIGURE 10-5 • Pain arising from the breast. **A,** Mammary pain referred into the axilla along the medial aspect of the arm. **B,** Referred pain to the supraclavicular level and into the neck. **C,** Diffusion around the thorax through the intercostal nerves. Pain may be referred to the back and the posterior shoulder.

Location:	Changes or pain occur anywhere on the breast or nipple
Referral:	May be painless
	Around the chest into the axilla, to the back at the level of the breast, occasionally into the neck and posterior aspect of the shoulder girdle
	Along the ulnar nerve distribution (medial aspect of the ipsilateral arm to the 4th and 5th digits)
Description:	Usually painless
	Involvement of breast tissue may result in sharp cutting or sharp aching
Intensity:	Mild to severe
Duration:	Intermittent to constant

Associated signs and symptoms:	May have no other symptoms
	May report discharge or bleeding from the breasts or nipples
	Distorted shape of the breast or nipple
	Enlarged rubbery lymph nodes
	Dimpling of the skin surface over the breast
	Unusual rash on the breast or nipple
	Unusual prominence of the veins over the breast

▼ GYNECOLOGIC

Location:	Usually asymptomatic; pelvis, sacroiliac, or low back
Referral:	Usually none; hip, groin
Description:	Discomfort
Intensity:	Mild
Duration:	Constant when present
Associated signs and symptoms:	Vaginal bleeding or discharge after menopause
	Persistent, irregular premenopausal bleeding, especially in obese women
	GI symptoms (abdominal bloating, belching, indigestion, early satiety, anorexia)

▼ LEUKEMIA

Location:	Usually painless; may have pain in the left abdomen; bone and joint pain possible
Referral:	None
Description:	Dull pain in the abdomen; may occur only on palpation
Intensity:	Mild to moderate
Duration:	Intermittent (with applied pressure)
Associated signs and symptoms	Enlarged lymph nodes
	Unusual bleeding from the nose or rectum, or blood in urine
	Prolonged menstruation
	Easy bruising of the skin
	Fatigue
	Dyspnea
	Weight loss, loss of appetite
	Fevers and sweats

▼ MULTIPLE MYELOMA

Location:	Skeletal pain, especially in the spine, sternum, rib, leg, or arm
Referral:	According to the location of the tumor
Description:	Sharp, knifelike
Intensity:	Moderate to severe
Duration:	Intermittent, progressing to constant
Associated signs and symptoms:	

Hypercalcemia: Dehydration (vomiting), polyuria, confusion, loss of appetite, constipation

Bone destruction with spontaneous bone fracture

Neurologic: Carpal tunnel syndrome; back pain with radicular symptoms; spinal cord compression (motor or sensory loss, bowel/bladder dysfunction, paraplegia)

▼ HODGKIN'S DISEASE

Location:	Lymph glands, usually unilateral neck or groin
Referral:	According to the location of the metastases
Description:	Usually painless, progressive enlargement of lymph nodes
Intensity:	Not applicable
Duration:	Not applicable
Associated signs and symptoms:	

Fever peaks in the late afternoon, night sweats

Anorexia and weight loss

Severe itching over the entire body

Anemia, fatigue, malaise

Jaundice

Edema

Nonproductive cough, dyspnea, chest pain, cyanosis

▼ NON-HODGKIN'S LYMPHOMA (including AIDS-NHL)

Location:	Peripheral lymph nodes
Referral:	Not applicable
Description:	Usually painless enlargement

Intensity:	Not applicable
Duration:	Not applicable
Associated signs and symptoms:	
	Constitutional symptoms (fever, night sweats, weight loss)
	Bleeding
	Generalized itching and reddened skin
	AIDS-NHL: Musculoskeletal lesions, subcutaneous nodules

▼ SOFT TISSUE TUMORS

Location:	Any connective tissue (e.g., tendon muscle, cartilage, fat, synovium, fibrous tissue)
Referral:	According to the tissue involved
Description:	Persistent swelling or lump, especially in the muscle
Intensity:	Mild, increases progressively to severe
Duration:	Intermittent, increases progressively to constant
Associated signs and symptoms:	
	Local swelling with tenderness and skin warmth
	Pathologic fracture

▼ BONE TUMORS

Location:	Can affect any bone in the body, depending on the specific type of bone cancer
Referral:	According to pattern and location of metastases
Description:	Sharp, knifelike, aching bone pain
	Occurs on movement and weight bearing, with pathologic fractures
	Pain at night preventing sleep
Intensity:	Initially mild, progressing to severe
Duration:	Usually intermittent, progressing to constant
Associated signs and symptoms:	
	Fatigue and malaise
	Weight loss
	Swelling and warmth over localized areas of tumor
	Soft, tender palpable mass over bone
	Loss of range of motion and joint function if limb bone is involved
	Fever
	Sciatica
	Unilateral edema

▼ PRIMARY CENTRAL NERVOUS SYSTEM: BRAIN TUMORS

Location: Intracranial

Referral: Specific symptoms depend on tumor location

Headaches*

Description: Bioccipital or bifrontal headache

Intensity: Mild to severe

Duration: Worse in morning on awakening

Diminishes or disappears soon after rising

Aggravating factors: Activity that increases intracranial pressure (e.g., straining during bowel movements, stooping, lifting heavy objects, coughing, bending over)

Prone/supine position at night during sleep

Relieving factors: Pain medications, including aspirin, acetaminophen

Associated signs and symptoms:

Papilledema

Altered mentation:

Increased sleeping

Difficulty in concentrating

Memory loss

Increased irritability

Poor judgment

Vomiting unrelated to food accompanies headaches

Seizures

Neurologic findings:

Positive Babinski reflex

Clonus (ankle or wrist)

Sensory changes

Decreased coordination

Ataxia

Muscle weakness

Increased lower extremity deep tendon reflexes

Transient paralysis

---

*Although the report of headache is common in a physical therapy practice, there is little agreement to the cause or how such headaches should be treated. Past medical history and associated signs and symptoms must be reviewed in all cases of headache to screen for the possibility of systemic origin.

▼ PRIMARY CENTRAL NERVOUS SYSTEM: SPINAL CORD TUMORS

Location:	Intramedullary (within the spinal cord)
	Extramedullary (within the dura mater)
	Extradural (outside the dura mater)
Referral:	Back pain at the level of the spinal cord lesion
	Pain may extend to the groin or legs
Description:	Dull ache; sharp, knifelike sensation
Intensity:	Mild to severe, progressive; night pain
Duration:	Intermittent, progressing to constant, or constant
Aggravating factors:	(Back pain) Lying down/rest
	Weight bearing
	Sneezing or coughing
Associated signs and symptoms:	Muscle weakness
	Muscle atrophy
	Sensory loss
	Paraplegia/quadriplegia
	Chest or abdominal pain
	Bowel/bladder dysfunction (late findings)

▼ PHYSICIAN REFERRAL

Early detection of cancer can save a person's life. Any suspicious sign or symptom discussed in this chapter should be investigated immediately by a physician. This is true especially in the presence of a positive family history of cancer, a previous personal history of cancer, the presence of environmental risk factors, and/or in the absence of medical or dental (oral) evaluation during the previous year.

Any recently discovered lumps or nodules must be examined by a physician. Any suspicious finding by report, on observation, or by palpation should be checked by a physician. Finding enlarged, tender lymph nodes does not require a referral to a physician unless these lymph nodes persist and involve more than one area because lymph nodes enlarge in response to infections throughout the body.

However, the physician should be notified of such findings, and the client should be advised to have the lymph nodes checked at the next follow-up visit with the physician. If the nodes remain enlarged over a long period (4 weeks or more), the client should be encouraged to contact the physician to discuss the need for follow-up. The exception is with individuals who have enlarged, *painless* lymph nodes. These people should notify their physician of these findings and make an appointment for follow-up at the physician's discretion.

If any signs of skin lesions are described by the client or if they are observed by the physical therapist, and the client has not been examined by a physician, a medical

GUIDELINES FOR PHYSICIAN REFERRAL

- Presence of recently discovered lumps or nodules or changes in previously present lumps, nodules, or moles, especially in the presence of a previous history of cancer or when accompanied by carpal tunnel or other neurologic symptoms.
- Palpable lump or nodule within the pectoral muscle tissue in the presence of previous history of breast cancer or identified risk factors for breast cancer (men and women).
- Notify physician of enlarged, painless, rubbery lymph nodes, especially if present in more than one area and for longer than 4 weeks.
- Presence of any of the early warning signs of cancer, including idiopathic muscle weakness accompanied by decreased deep tendon reflexes.
- Any unexplained bleeding from any area (e.g., rectum, blood in urine or stool, unusual or unexpected vaginal bleeding, breast, penis, nose, ears, mouth, mole, skin, or scar).
- Any sign or symptom of metastasis in someone with a previous history of cancer (see individual cancer types for specific clinical signs and symptoms; see also Clues to Screening for Cancer).
- Any man with pelvic, groin, sacroiliac, or low back pain accompanied by sciatica and a past history of prostate cancer.
- Bone pain, especially on weight bearing, that persists more than 1 week and is worse at night.

referral is recommended. If the client is planning a follow-up visit with the physician within the next 2 to 4 weeks, that client is advised to indicate the mole or skin changes at that time. If no appointment is pending, the client is encouraged to make a specific visit either to the family/personal physician or to a dermatologist.

Systemic Signs and Symptoms Requiring Physician Referral

The physical therapist is advised to ask the client further questions whenever any of the following signs and symptoms are reported or observed because they may indicate cancer or some other systemic disease. The client should therefore be referred to a physician for further evaluation.

Arthralgias
Bleeding mole
Bone pain
Change in bowel habits
Change in urinary habits
Change in voice
Chronic cough
Clubbing of the fingers
Drowsiness/confusion
Dysphagia
Dyspnea
Epistaxis
Fatigue, general malaise
Fevers and sweats
Headache
Hemoptysis (spitting blood)
Hoarseness
Itching/scratching
Jaundice
Loss of appetite
Lump or thickening
Pain at night disturbing sleep
Pain on weight bearing
Persistent nausea, vomiting, and neurologic findings
Prolonged menstruation
(Proximal) muscle weakness
Restlessness
Sore that does not heal
Unusual bleeding
Unusual discharge
Unusual skin lesions or rash
Wheezing

KEY POINTS TO REMEMBER

▶ Spinal malignancy involves the lumbar spine more often than the cervical spine and is usually metastatic rather than primary.

▶ Spinal cord compression from metastases may appear as back pain, leg weakness, and bowel/bladder symptoms.

▶ Fifty percent of clients with back pain from a malignancy have an identifiable preceding trauma or injury to account for the pain or symptoms. Always remember that clients may erroneously attribute symptoms to an event.

▶ Back pain may precede the development of neurologic signs and symptoms in any person with cancer.

▶ Signs of nerve root compression may be the first indication of cancer, in particular lymphoma, multiple myeloma, or cancer in the lung, breast, prostate, or kidney.

▶ The five most common sites of metastasis are the lymph nodes, liver, lung, bone, and brain.

▶ The presence of jaundice in association of any atypical presentation of back pain may indicate liver metastasis.

▶ Lung, breast, prostate, thyroid, and the lymphatics are the primary sites responsible for most metastatic bone disease.

▶ Monitoring physiologic responses (vital signs) to exercise is important in the immunosuppressed population. Watch closely for early signs (dyspnea, pallor, sweating, and fatigue) of cardiopulmonary complications of cancer treatment.

▶ To determine appropriate exercise levels for clients who are immunosuppressed, review blood test results (WBCs, RBCs, hematocrit, platelets).

▶ Besides the seven early warning signs of cancer, the physical therapist should watch for idiopathic muscle weakness accompanied by decreased deep tendon reflexes.

▶ Any woman with chest, breast, axillary, or shoulder pain of unknown origin at presentation must be screened for breast cancer.

▶ Changes in size, shape, tenderness, and consistency of lymph nodes raise a red flag. Supraclavicular nodes and inguinal nodes are common metastatic sites for cancer.

▶ No reliable physical signs distinguish between benign and malignant soft tissue lesions. All soft tissue lumps that persist or grow should be reported immediately to the physician.

SUBJECTIVE EXAMINATION

• SPECIAL QUESTIONS TO ASK

Special questions to ask will vary with each client and the clinical signs and symptoms presented at the time of the evaluation. The physical therapist should refer to the specific chapter representing the client's current complaints. The case study provided here is one example of how to follow up with necessary questions to rule out a systemic origin of musculoskeletal findings.

A previous history of drug therapy and current drug use may be important information to obtain because prolonged use of drugs such as phenytoin (Dilantin) or immunosuppressive drugs such as azathioprine (Imuran) and cyclosporine may lead to cancer. Postmenopausal use of estrogens has been linked with endometrial cancer.

Past Medical History

A previous personal/family history of cancer may be significant, especially any history of breast, colorectal, or lung cancer that demonstrates genetic susceptibility.

- Have you ever been exposed to chemical agents or irritants, such as asbestos, asphalt, aniline dyes, benzene, herbicides, fertilizers, wood dust, or others? **(Environmental causes of cancer)**

Early Warning Signs

With the seven early warning signs of cancer used as a basis for follow-up, one or all of these questions may be appropriate:

- Have you noticed any changes in your bowel movement or in the flow of urination?
  - *If yes,* ask pertinent follow-up questions as suggested in Chapter 7.
  - *If the client answers no,* it may be necessary to provide prompts or examples of what changes you are referring to (e.g., difficulty in starting or continuing the flow of urine, numbness or tingling in the groin or pelvis).
- Have you noticed any sores that have not healed properly?
  - *If yes,* where are they located? How long has the sore been present? Has your physician examined this area?
- Have you noticed any unusual bleeding (*for women:* including prolonged menstruation or *any* bleeding for the postmenopausal woman who is not taking hormone replacement) or prolonged discharge from any part of your body?
  - *If yes,* where? How long has this been present? Has your physician examined this area?
- Have you noticed any thickening or lump of any muscle, tendon, bone, breast, or anywhere else?
  - *If yes,* where? How long has this been present? Has your physician examined this area?*

---

*An asymptomatic mass that has been present for years and causes only cosmetic concern is usually benign, whereas a painful mass of short duration that has caused a decrease in function may be malignant.

- *If no (for women):* Do you examine your own breasts? How often do you examine them, and when was the last time you did a breast self-examination?

- Do you have any pain, swelling, or unusual tenderness in the breasts? **(Pain can be a symptom of cancer; cyclic pain is common with normal breasts, use of oral contraceptives, and fibrocystic disease)**

   - *If yes,* is this pain brought on by strenuous activity? **(Spontaneous/systemic or related to specific musculoskeletal cause** [e.g., use of one arm]**)**

- Have you noticed any rash on the breast or discharge from the nipple? **(Medications such as oral contraceptives, phenothiazines, diuretics, digitalis, tricyclic tranquilizers, reserpine, methyldopa, and steroids can cause clear discharge from the nipple; blood-tinged discharge is always significant)**

- Have you noticed any difficulty in eating or swallowing? Have you had a chronic cough, recurrent laryngitis, hoarseness, or any difficulty with speaking?

   - *If yes,* how long has this been happening? Have you discussed this with your physician?

- Have you had any change in digestive patterns? Have you had increasing indigestion or unusual constipation?

   - *If yes,* how long has this been happening? Have you discussed this with your physician?

- Have you had a recent, sudden weight loss, such as 10 to 15 pounds in 2 weeks, without dieting?

- Have you noticed any obvious change in color, shape, or size of a wart or mole?

   - *If yes,* what have you noticed? How long has this wart or mole been present? Have you discussed this problem with your physician?

- Have you had any unusual headaches or changes in your vision?

   - *If yes,* please describe. **(Brain tumors: bioccipital or bifrontal)**

   - Can you attribute these to anything in particular?

   - Do you vomit (unrelated to food) when your headaches occur? **(Brain tumors)**

- Have you been more tired than usual or experienced persistent fatigue during the last month?

- Can you think of any time during the past week when you may have bumped yourself, fallen, or injured yourself in any way? (Ask when in the presence of local swelling and tenderness.) **(Bone tumors)**

- Have you noticed any bone pain or problems with any of your bones? Is the pain affected by movement? **(Fractures cause sharp pain that increases with movement. Bone pain from systemic causes usually feels dull and deep and is unrelated to movement)**

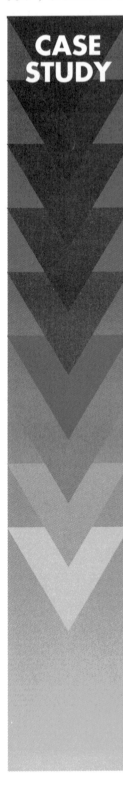

CASE STUDY

REFERRAL

A 56-year-old man has come to you for an evaluation without referral. He has not been examined by a physician of any kind for at least 3 years. He is seeking an evaluation on the insistence of his wife, who has noticed that his collar size has increased two sizes in the last year and that his neck looks "puffy." He has no complaints of any kind (including pain or discomfort), and he denies any known trauma, but his wife insists that he has limited ability in turning his head when backing the car out of the driveway.

PHYSICAL THERAPY INTERVIEW

First read the client's Family/Personal History form with particular interest in his personal or family history of cancer, presence of allergies or asthma, use of medications or over-the-counter drugs, previous surgeries, available x-ray studies of the neck or spine, and/or history of cigarette smoking (or other tobacco use). An appropriate lead-in to the following series of questions may be: "Because you have not seen a physician before your appointment with me, I will ask you a series of questions to find out if your symptoms require examination by a physician rather than treatment in this office."

Current Symptoms

What have you noticed different about your neck that brings you here today?

When did you first notice that your neck was changing (in size or shape)?

Can you remember having any accidents, falls, twists, or any other kind of potential trauma at that time?

Do you ever notice any pain, stiffness, soreness, or discomfort in your neck or shoulders?

> If *yes*, please describe (as per the outline in the Core Interview, Chapter 2).

Does this or any pain ever awaken you at night or keep you awake? (**Night pain associated with cancer**)

> If *yes*, follow up with appropriate questions. (See the Physical Therapy Interview.)

Associated Symptoms

Have you noticed any numbness or tingling in your arms or hands?

Have you noticed any swollen glands, lumps, or thickened areas of skin or muscle in your neck, armpits, or groin? (**Cancer screen**)

Do you have any difficulty in swallowing? Do you have recurrent hoarseness, influenza-like symptoms, or a persistent cough or cold that never seems to go away? (**Cancer screen**)

Have you noticed any low-grade fevers or night sweats? (**Systemic disease**)

Have you had any recent unexplained weight gain or loss? (You may need to explain that you mean a gain or loss of 10 to 15 pounds in as many days without dieting.) Have you had a loss of appetite? (**Cancer screen or other systemic disease**)

Do you ever have any difficulty with breathing or find yourself short of breath at rest or after minimal exercise? (**Dyspnea**)

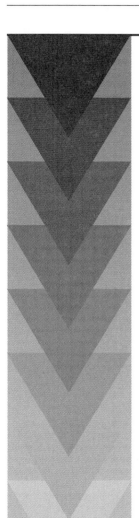

Do you have frequent headaches, or do you experience any dizziness, nausea, or vomiting? (**Systemic disease, carotid artery affected**)

FUNCTIONAL CAPACITY

What kind of work do you do?

Do you have any limitations caused by this condition that affect you in any way at work or at home? (**Occupational disease, limitations of activities of daily living [ADL] skills**)

Final Questions

How would you describe your general health?

Have you ever been diagnosed with cancer of any kind?

Is there anything that you would like to tell me that you think is important about your neck or your health in general?

TEST PROCEDURES DURING THE FIRST SESSION TO ASSESS THE MUSCULOSKELETAL SYSTEM

Observation/Inspection

Observe for the presence of swelling anywhere, tender or swollen lymph nodes (cervical, supraclavicular, and axillary), changes in skin temperature, unusual moles or warts. Perform a brief posture screen (general postural observations may be made while you are interviewing the client). Palpate for carotid artery and upper extremity pulses. Check vital signs and **TAKE THE CLIENT'S ORAL TEMPERATURE!**

Cervical AROM/PROM

Assess for muscle tightness, loss of joint motion (including accessory movements if indicated by a loss of passive motion). Assess for compromise of the vertebral artery, and, if negative, clear the cervical spine by using a quadrant test with overpressure (e.g., Spurling's test) and assess accessory movements of the cervical spine. Perform tests for thoracic outlet syndrome. Palpate the anterior cervical spine for pathologic protrusion while the client swallows.

Temporomandibular Joint (TMJ) Screen

Clear the joint above (i.e., TMJ) using AROM, observation, and palpation specific to the TMJ.

Shoulder Screen

Clear the joint below (i.e., shoulder) by using a screening examination (e.g., AROM/PROM and quadrant testing).

Neurologic Screen

Deep tendon reflexes, sensory screen (e.g., gross sensory testing for light touch), manual muscle test (MMT) screening using break testing of the upper quadrant, grip strength. If test(s) is abnormal, consider further neurologic testing (e.g., balance, coordination, stereognosia, in-depth sensory examination, dysmetria). Ask about the presence of recent visual changes, headaches, numbness, or tingling into the jaw or down the arm(s).

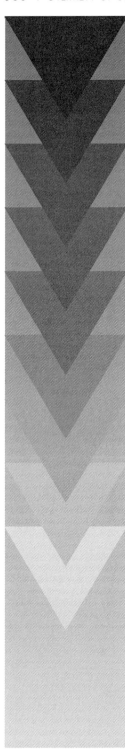

It is always recommended that the physical therapist give the client ongoing verbal feedback during the examination regarding evaluation results, such as: "I notice you can't turn your head to the right as much as you can to the left—from checking your muscles and joints, it looks like muscle tightness, not any loss of joint movement." . . . or . . . "I notice your reflexes on each side aren't the same (your right arm reacts more strongly than the left)—let's see if we can find out why."

RECOMMENDATION FOR PHYSICIAN VISIT

- I noticed on your intake form that you haven't listed the name of a personal or family physician. Do you have a physician?

- If *yes*, when was the last time you saw your physician? Have you seen your physician for this current problem?

Give the client a brief summary of your findings while making your recommendations; for example: "Mr. X., I notice today that although you don't have any ongoing neck pain, the lymph nodes in your neck and armpit are enlarged but not particularly tender. Otherwise, all of my findings are negative. Your loss of motion on turning your head is not unusual for a person your age and certainly would not cause your neck to increase in size or shape.

"Given the fact that you have not seen a physician for almost 3 years, I strongly recommend that you see a physician of your choice, or I can give you the names of several to choose from. In either case, I think some medical tests are necessary to rule out any underlying medical problem. For instance, a neck x-ray exam would be recommended before physical therapy treatment is started."

If the client has indicated a positive family history of cancer, it might be appropriate to suggest: "Given your positive family history of previous medical illnesses, the 3 years since you have seen a physician, and the lack of musculoskeletal findings, I strongly recommend . . ." It is important to provide the client with all the information available to you, but without causing undue alarm and emotional stress, which could actually prevent the client from seeking further testing.

If the client does give the name of a physician, you may ask for written permission (disclosure release) to send a copy of your results to the physician. If the client does not have a physician and requests recommendations from you, you may offer to send a copy of your results to the physician with whom the client makes an appointment. If you think that a problem may be potentially serious and you want this person to receive adequate follow-up without causing alarm, you may offer to let him make the appointment from your office, suggest that your secretary or receptionist make the appointment for him, or even offer to make the initial telephone contact yourself.

RESULT

This client did comply with the physical therapist's suggestion to see a physician and was diagnosed as having Hodgkin's disease (a cancer of the lymph system) without constitutional symptoms (i.e., without evidence of weight loss, fever, or night sweats). Medical treatment was initiated, and physical therapy treatment was not warranted.

PRACTICE QUESTIONS

1. Name three predisposing factors to cancer that the physical therapist must watch for during the interview process as red flags.

2. Complete the following chart in relation to physical therapy practice:

Type of Cancer	Metastasizes to	Results in
Prostate	Bones of pelvis and vertebrae	Low back and/or pelvic pain radiating down the leg
Osteogenic sarcoma		
Breast		
Malignant melanoma		
Lung		
Stomach or colon		

3. Which are the most common sites of metastasis?

   a. Skeletal system, lymphatic system, hepatic system, pulmonary system, central nervous system

   b. Bones, lungs, brain

   c. Hematologic and lymphatic systems

   d. Lymph nodes, lungs, liver

4. What is the significance of nerve root compression?

5. Complete the following mnemonic:

   C _____

   A _____

   U _____

   T _____

   I _____

   O _____

   N _____

6. Whenever a physical therapist observes, palpates, or receives a client report of a lump or nodule, what three questions must be asked?

7. How can the physical therapist determine whether a client's symptoms are caused by the delayed effects of radiation as opposed to being signs of recurring cancer?

8. Give a general *description* and *explanation* of the changes seen in deep tendon reflexes associated with cancer.

9. Why is weight loss a significant red-flag sign in a physical therapy practice?

10. What is a neoplastic syndrome?

Bonus Question

A client who has recently completed chemotherapy requires immediate medical referral if he has which of the following symptoms?

a. Decreased appetite

b. Increased urinary output

c. Mild fatigue but moderate dyspnea with exercise

d. Fever, chills, sweating

References

Aboulafia AJ, Khan F, Pankowsky D et al: AIDS-associated secondary lymphoma of bone: a case report with review of the literature, *Am J Orthop* 27(2):128-134, 1998.

American Cancer Society: *1993 cancer facts and figures,* Atlanta, 1993, The Society.

American Institute for Cancer Research: *Food, nutrition, and the prevention of cancer: a global perspective,* Washington, DC, 1997, The Institute.

Ball HG, Elkadry EA: Endometrial cancer: current concepts and management, *Surg Oncol Clin North Am* 7(2):271-284, 1998.

Barakat RR: Contemporary issues in the management of endometrial cancer, *CA Cancer J Clin* 48(5):299-314, 1998.

Beral V, Peterman T, Berkelman R et al: AIDS-associated non-Hodgkin lymphoma, *Lancet* 1:805-809, 1991.

Black DM, Solomon E: The search for the familial breast/ovarian cancer gene, *Trends Genet* 9(1):22-26, 1993.

Borman H, Safak T, Ertoy D: Fibrosarcoma following radiotherapy for breast cancer: a case report and review of the literature, *Ann Plast Surg* 41(2):201-204, 1998.

Coleman RE: Skeletal complications of malignancy, *CANCER Suppl* 80(8):1588-1594, 1997.

Dolcetti R, Boiocchi M: Epstein-Barr virus in the pathogenesis of Hodgkin's disease, *Biomed Pharmacother* 52(1):13-25, 1998.

Eltabbakh GH, Piver MS: Extraovarian primary peritoneal carcinoma, *Oncology* 12(6):813-819, 1998.

Feuer EJ: The lifetime risk of developing breast cancer, *J Natl Cancer Inst* 85:892-896, 1993.

Gaidano G, Carbone A, Dalla-Favera R: Genetic basis of acquired immunodeficiency syndrome-related lymphomagenesis, *J Natl Cancer Inst Monogr* 23:95-100, 1998.

Gallagher RP, Hill GB, Bajdik CD et al: Sunlight exposure, pigmentary factors, and risk of nonmelanocytic skin cancer. I. Basal carcinoma, *Arch Dermatol* 131:157-163, 1995.

Garfinkel L: Current trends in breast cancer, *CA Cancer J Clin* 43(1):5-6, 1993.

Gilkeson GS, Caldwell DS: Rheumatic associations with malignancy, *J Musculoskel Med* 7(1):64-79, 1990.

Greil R: Prognosis and management strategies of lymphatic neoplasias in the elderly. II. Hodgkin's disease, *Oncology* 55(4):265-275, 1998.

Grubb MR, Currier BL, Pritchard DJ et al: Primary Ewing's sarcoma of the spine, *Spine* 19:309-313, 1994.

Gudas S: The physical therapy challenge in disseminated cancer, *Oncol Sect News APTA* 5:3, 1987.

Hardell L, Axelson O: Environmental and occupational aspects on the etiology of non-Hodgkin's lymphoma. *Oncol Res* 10(1):1-5, 1998.

Henson JW, Posner JB: Neurological complications. In Holland JF et al, editors: *Cancer medicine,* ed 3, vols 1 and 2, Philadelphia, 1993, Lea & Febiger, pp 2268-2286.

Kahn HS: Increased cancer mortality following a history of nonmelanoma skin cancer, *JAMA* 280(10):910-912, 1998.

Kricker A, Armstrong BK, English DR et al: Does intermittent sun exposure cause basal cell carcinoma? A case-controlled study in Western Australia, *Int J Cancer* 60:489-494, 1995.

Kunz J, Rondez R: Correlation between serious ovarian tumors and extra-ovarian peritoneal tumors of the same histology, *Schweiz Rundsch Med Prax* 87(6):191-198, 1998.

Landis SH, Murray T, Bolden S et al: Cancer statistics, 1999, *CA Cancer J Clin* 49(1):8-31, 1999.

La Quaglia MP: Osteosarcoma: specific tumor management and results, *Chest Surg Clin North Am* 8(1):77-95, 1998.

Lawrence W: Soft tissue sarcomas in adults and children: a comparison, *CA Cancer J Clin* 44(4):197-199, 1994.

Levine AM: Hodgkin's disease in the setting of human immunodeficiency virus infection, *J Natl Cancer Inst Monogr* 23:37-42, 1998.

Milas M, Yu D, Pollock RE: Advances in the understanding of human soft tissue sarcomas: molecular biology and therapeutic strategies, *Oncol Rep* 5(5):1275-1279, 1998.

Odell WD: Ectopic hormones and humoral syndromes of cancer. In Holland JF et al, editors: *Cancer medicine,* ed 3, vols 1 and 2, Philadelphia 1993, Lea & Febiger, pp 896-904.

Ozaki S, Kosaka M: Multiple myeloma: new aspects of biology and treatment, *J Med Invest* 44(3-4):127-136, 1998.

Peabody TD, Gibbs CP, Simon MA: Current concepts review: evaluation and staging of musculoskeletal neoplasms, *J Bone Joint Surg Am* 80A(8):1204-1218, 1998.

Pico JL, Castagna L, Bourhis JH: Recent progress in the biology of multiple myeloma and future directions in treatment, *Hematol Cell Ther* 40(2):45-61, 1998.

Porter DE, Cohen BB, Wallace MR et al: Linkage mapping in familial breast cancer: improved localisation of a susceptibility locus on chromosome 17q12-21, *Int J Cancer* 53(2):188-198, 1993.

Prados MD, Berger MS, Wilson CB: Primary central nervous system tumors: advances in knowledge and treatment, *CA Cancer J Clin* 48(6):331-360, 1998.

Repetto L, Granetto C, Aapro M: Gynaecologic cancers, *Crit Rev Oncol Hematol* 27:147-150, 1998.

Rigel DS, Friedman RJ, Kopf AW: The incidence of malignant melanoma in the United states: issues as we approach the 21st century, *J Am Acad Dermatol* 34:839-847, 1996.

Roodman GD: Mechanisms of bone lesions in multiple myeloma and lymphoma, *CANCER Suppl* 80(8):1557-1563, 1997.

Rosenthal DS: Cancer: changing trends, *CA Cancer J Clin* 48(1):3-4, 1998.

Ross MI: Aid for patients with limb metastases, *World Melanoma Update* 1:15, 1997.

Seller RH: *Differential diagnosis of common complaints,* ed 3, Philadelphia, 1996, WB Saunders.

Vlasak R, Sim FH: Ewing's sarcoma, *Orthop Clin North Am* 27(3):591-603, 1996.

Winningham ML, McVicar M, Burke C: Exercise for cancer patients: guidelines and precautions, *Physician Sportsmed* 14:121-134, 1986.

Woodhouse EC, Chuaqui RD, Liotta LA: General mechanisms of metastasis, *CANCER Suppl* 80(8):1529-1537, 1997.

Young RC: Ovarian cancer, *CA Cancer J Clin* 45(2):69-70, 1995.

Young RF: The role of the gamma knife in the treatment of malignant primary and metastatic brain tumors, *CA Cancer J Clin* 48(3):177-188, 1998.

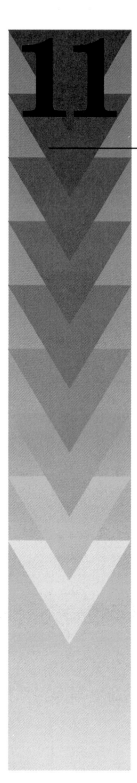

Overview of Immunologic Signs and Symptoms

Immunology, one of the few disciplines with a full range of involvement in all aspects of health and disease, is one of the most rapidly expanding fields in medicine today. Keeping current is difficult at best, considering the volume of new immunologic information generated by clinical researchers each year. The information presented here is a simplistic representation of the immune system and should be supplemented by the reader with any of the texts references.

Immunity denotes protection against infectious organisms. The immune system is a complex network of specialized organs and cells that has evolved to defend the body against attacks by "foreign" invaders. Immunity is provided by lymphoid cells residing in the immune system. This system consists of central and peripheral lymphoid organs (Fig. 11-1).

By circulating its component cells and substances, the immune system maintains an early warning system against both exogenous microorganisms (infections produced by bacteria, viruses, parasites, and fungi) and endogenous cells that have become neoplastic.

Immunologic responses in humans can be divided into two broad categories: humoral immunity, which takes place in the body fluids (humors) and is concerned with antibody and complement activities, and cell-mediated or cellular immunity, primarily intracellular, which involves a variety of activities designed to destroy or at least contain cells that are recognized by the body as being alien and harmful. Both types of responses are initiated by lymphocytes and are discussed in the context of lymphocytic function.

▼ SIGNS AND SYMPTOMS OF IMMUNE SYSTEM DYSFUNCTION (Cash, 1997)

As always in the evaluation of any client, the medical history is the most important variable, followed by the assessment of associated signs and symptoms. Many immune system disorders have a unique

Central   **Peripheral**

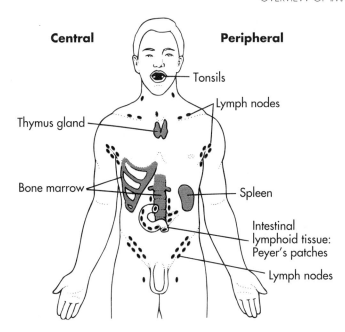

Tonsils

Lymph nodes

Thymus gland

Bone marrow

Spleen

Intestinal
lymphoid tissue:
Peyer's patches

Lymph nodes

FIGURE 11-1 • Organs of the immune system.

chronology or sequence of events that define them. When the immune system is involved, the most important questions will be:

- How long have you had this problem? (acute vs. chronic)

- Has the problem gone away and then recurred?

- Have additional symptoms developed or have other areas become symptomatic over time?

Family history is also important when assessing the role of the immune system in presenting signs and symptoms. Persons with fibromyalgia or chronic pain often have a family history of alcoholism, depression, migraine headaches, gastrointestinal (GI) disorders, or panic attacks. Clients with systemic inflammatory disorders may have a family history of an identical or related disorder such as rheumatoid arthritis, systemic lupus erythematosus, autoimmune thyroid disease, multiple sclerosis, or myasthenia gravis. Other rheumatic diseases that are often genetically linked include seronegative spondyloarthropathy.

For anyone with new onset of joint pain, a review of systems should include questions about symptoms or diagnoses involving other organ systems. In particular, the presence of dry, red, or irritated and itching eyes; chest pain with dyspnea; urethral or vaginal discharge; skin rash or photosensitivity; hair loss; diarrhea; or dysphagia should be assessed. A recent history of surgery may be indicative of bacterial or reactive arthritis, which requires immediate medical evaluation.

Symptoms of rheumatic disorders often include soft tissue and/or joint pain, stiffness, swelling, weakness, constitutional symptoms, Raynaud's phenomenon, and sleep disturbances. Inflammatory disorders such as RA and polymyalgia rheumatica are marked by prolonged *stiffness* in the morning lasting more than 1 hour. This stiffness is relieved with activity, but it recurs after the person sits down and subsequently attempts to resume activity. This is referred to as the gel phenomenon.

In anyone with *swelling,* especially single-joint swelling, it is necessary to distinguish whether this swelling is articular (as in

CLUES TO IMMUNE SYSTEM DYSFUNCTION

- Client with a history of rheumatoid arthritis taking disease-modifying antirheumatic drugs (DMARDs) de-velops symptoms of drug toxicity (e.g., rash, petechiae/ecchymosis, photosensitivity, dyspnea, nausea/vomiting, lymph node swelling, edema, oral ulcers, diarrhea)
- Long-term use of nonsteroidal antiinflammatory drugs (NSAIDs) or other antiinflammatory drugs, especially with new onset of GI symptoms, back or shoulder pain of unknown cause
- Long-term use of immunosuppressives or corticosteroids with onset of constitutional symptoms, especially fever
- Insidious onset of episodic back pain in a person younger than 40 who has a family history of spondyloarthropathy
- Joint pain preceded or accompanied by burning and urinary frequency (urethritis) and/or accompanied by eye irritation, crusting, redness, tearing, or burning usually lasting only a few days (**Conjunctivitis**) (**Reiter's syndrome**)
- Joint pain preceded or accompanied by skin rash or lesions (**Psoriatic arthritis; Lyme disease; rheumatic fever**)
- New onset of inflammatory joint pain (especially monoarticular joint involvement) postoperatively, especially accompanied by extraarticular signs or symptoms such as rash, diarrhea, urethritis) (**Reactive or bacterial arthritis);** mouth ulcers (**Reiter's syndrome, systemic lupus erythematosus;** raised skin patches (**psoriatic arthritis**)
- Development of neurologic symptoms 1 to 3 weeks after an infection (**Guillain-Barré syndrome**)

arthritis), periarticular (as in tenosynovitis), involves an entire limb (as with lymphedema), or occurs in another area (such as with lipoma or palpable tumors). The physical therapist will need to assess whether the swelling is intermittent, persistent, symmetric, or asymmetric and whether the swelling is minimal in the morning but worse during the day (as with dependent edema).

Generalized *weakness* is a common symptom of individuals with immune system disorders (especially fibromyalgia) in the absence of muscle disease. If the weakness involves one limb without evidence of weakness elsewhere, a neurologic disorder may be present. Anyone having trouble performing tasks with the arms raised above the head, difficulty climbing stairs, or arising from a low chair may have muscle disease.

Nail bed changes are especially indicative of underlying inflammatory disease. For example, small infarctions or splinter hemorrhages occur in endocarditis and systemic vasculitis. Characteristics of systemic sclerosis and limited scleroderma include atrophy of the fingertips, calcific nodules, digital cyanosis, and sclerodactyly (tightening of the skin). Dystrophic nail changes are characteristic of psoriasis. Spongy synovial thickening or bony hypertrophic changes (Bouchard's nodes) are present with rheumatoid arthritis and other hand deformities.

▼ IMMUNE SYSTEM PATHOPHYSIOLOGY

Immune disorders involve dysfunction of the immune response mechanism, causing over-responsiveness or blocked, misdirected, or limited responsiveness to antigens. These disorders may result from a developmental defect, infection, malignancy, trauma, metabolic disorder, or drug use.

Immunologic disorders may be classified as an immunodeficiency, hypersensitivity, autoimmunity, or immunoproliferative disorder.

When the immune system is underactive, or *hypoactive,* it is referred to as being immunodeficient or immunocompromised in the case of people undergoing chemotherapy for cancer or taking immunosuppressive drugs after organ transplantation.

When the immune system becomes overactive, or *hyperactive,* a state of hypersensitivity exists, leading to immunologic diseases such as allergies.

T cells act as modulators of immune reactions, so that along with clearance of antigen by macrophages, death of antibody-producing plasma cells, and certain humoral factors, the immune response ultimately ceases. Abnormalities in this control system lead to immunodeficiency, autoimmunity, and possibly hematologic diseases, such as aplastic anemia.

Autoimmune disorders occur when the immune system fails to distinguish self from nonself and misdirects the immune response against the body's own tissues. The resultant abnormal tissue reaction and tissue damage may cause systemic manifestations varying from minimal localized symptoms to systemic multiorgan involvement with severe impairment of function and life threatening organ failure.

Immunoproliferative disorders occur when abnormal reproduction or multiplication of the cells of the lymphoid system results in leukemia, lymphoma, and other related disorders. These have been covered in other parts of this text and are not discussed in this chapter.

Immunodeficiency Disorders

Acquired Immunodeficiency Syndrome

Human immunodeficiency virus (HIV) is a cytopathogenic virus that causes acquired immunodeficiency syndrome (AIDS). HIV has been identified as the causative agent, its genes have been mapped and analyzed, drugs that act against it have been found and tested, and vaccines against the HIV infection have been under development.

Acquired refers to the fact that the disease is not inherited or genetic but develops as a result of a virus. *Immuno* refers to the body's immunologic system, and *deficiency* indicates that the immune system is underfunctioning, resulting in a group of signs or symptoms that occur together called a *syndrome.*

People who are HIV-infected are vulnerable to serious illnesses called "opportunistic" infections or diseases, so named because they use the opportunity of lowered resistance to infect and destroy. These infections and diseases would not be a threat to most individuals whose immune systems functioned normally. *Pneumocystis carinii* pneumonia (PCP) continues to be a major cause of morbidity and mortality in the AIDS population.

Population groups at greatest risk include commercial sex workers (prostitutes) and their clients, homosexual men, injection drug users (IDUs), blood recipients, hemophiliacs, dialysis recipients, organ transplant recipients, fetuses of HIV-infected mothers, and people with sexually transmitted diseases (STDs). The latter group is estimated to have several times higher the risk for HIV infection compared with those having no STDs.

TRANSMISSION

Transmission of HIV occurs through horizontal transmission (from either sexual contact or parenteral exposure to blood and blood products) or through vertical transmission (from HIV-infected mother to infant). HIV is not transmitted through casual contact, such as the shared use of food, towels, cups, razors, or toothbrushes, or even by kissing.

Transmission always involves exposure to some body fluid from an infected client. The greatest concentrations of virus have been found in blood, semen, cerebrospinal fluid, and cervical/vaginal secretions. HIV has been found in low concentrations in tears, saliva, and urine, but no cases have been

AIDS AT A GLANCE

- **What it is:** AIDS, acquired immunodeficiency syndrome, is a contagious disease that destroys the T cells, a key component of the body's immune system.
- **What causes it:** AIDS is caused by the human immunodeficiency virus (HIV), spread through sexual contact, needles or syringes shared by injection drug users (IDUs), transfusion of infected blood or blood products, or perinatal transmission (from infected birthing mother to her infant).
- **Who gets it:** Primary persons infected with HIV have been homosexual men and IDUs. The Centers for Disease Control and Prevention (CDC) estimates that heterosexual contact is responsible for 3% of male cases and 34% of female cases. Although 1 million Americans are infected, the CDC reported a decline in the number of AIDS-related deaths for the first time since 1996.
- **Diagnosis:** Screening for AIDs is conducted by testing blood for the presence of antibodies to the AIDs virus or detection of pieces of proteins or genetic material from the virus. The test indicates only if a person has been exposed to the virus. There is a typical 6-month window of latency when those infected test negative. Other diagnostic tests may include the polymerase chain reaction (PCR), CD4+ T-lymphocyte count, and the p24 antigen test.
- **Prognosis:** According to the CDC, a person with a positive test has a 20% to 30% chance of developing AIDS over a 5-year period. At present, there is no cure, and death occurs as a result of "opportunistic" infections or cancers that the immunosuppressed body cannot resist.
- **Treatment:** Numerous types of drugs for AIDS are under investigation, including protease inhibitors and an effective AIDS vaccine.

transmitted by these routes. Several cases of HIV transmission through breast milk have been reported.

Any injectable drug, legal or illegal, can be associated with HIV transmission. It is not injection drug use that spreads HIV but the sharing of HIV-infected intravenous (IV) drug needles among individuals.

Despite the perception that only IV injection is dangerous, HIV also can be transmitted through subcutaneous and intramuscular injection. Use of infected needles for tattooing or body piercing are included in this category. Public health organizations have changed their terminology, substituting the acronym *IDU* (injection drug user) for the earlier term *IVDU* (intravenous drug user).

Injection drug users who sterilize their drug paraphernalia with a 1:10 solution of bleach to water before passing the needles are less likely to spread HIV.*

---

*For further information regarding this or other AIDS-related questions, contact the National AIDS Hotline (1-800-342-2437).

Blood and Blood Products. Parenteral transmission occurs when there is direct blood-to-blood contact with a client infected with HIV. This can occur through sharing of contaminated needles and drug paraphernalia ("works"), through transfusion of blood or blood products, by accidental needlestick injury to a health care worker, or from blood exposure to nonintact skin or mucous membranes.

Health care workers who have contact with clients with AIDS and who follow routine instructions for self-protection are a very low risk group.

Almost all persons with hemophilia born before 1985 have been infected with HIV. Heat-treated factor concentrates became available in 1985, involving a method of chemical and physical processes that completely inactivate HIV, eliminating the transmission of HIV to anyone with a clotting disorder who is receiving blood or blood products.

Additionally, HIV has been transmitted heterosexually from infected men with hemophilia to spouses or sexual partners in

▼ *Clinical Signs and Symptoms of*
Early Symptomatic HIV Infection

- Fever
- Night sweats
- Chronic diarrhea
- Fatigue
- Minor oral infections
- Headache
- (Women): Vaginal candidiasis
- Cough
- Shortness of breath
- Cutaneous changes (rash, nail bed changes, dry skin)

▼ *Clinical Signs and Symptoms of*
Advanced Symptomatic HIV Infection

- Kaposi's sarcoma
  - Multiple purple blotches and bumps on skin
- Opportunistic diseases (e.g., tuberculosis, *Pneumocystis carinii*, pneumonia, lymphoma, thrush; herpes I and II; toxoplasmosis)
  - Persistent dry cough
  - Fever, night sweats
  - Easy bruising
  - Thrush (thick, white coating on the tongue or throat, accompanied by a sore throat)
  - Muscle atrophy and weakness
  - Back pain
  - Side effects of medication

what is termed *the second wave* of infection and on to children born to infected couples.

CLINICAL SIGNS AND SYMPTOMS

Many individuals with HIV infection remain asymptomatic for years, with a mean time of approximately 10 years between exposure and development of AIDS. Systemic complaints such as weight loss, fevers, and night sweats are common. Cough or shortness of breath may occur with HIV-related pulmonary disease. GI complaints include changes in bowel function, especially diarrhea.

Cutaneous complaints are common and include dry skin, new rashes, and nail bed changes. Because virtually all these findings may be seen with other diseases, a combination of complaints is more suggestive of HIV infection than any one symptom.

Many persons with AIDS experience back pain, but the underlying causes may differ. Decrease in muscle mass with subsequent postural changes may occur as a result of the disease process or in response to medications. It is not uncommon for pain to develop in the back or another musculoskeletal location where there may have been a previous injury. This is more likely to occur when the T-cell count drops.

The therapist should review the potential side effects from medication used in the treatment of AIDS. The more commonly occurring symptoms include nausea, headaches, muscle pain, weakness, and fatigue.

Any woman at risk for AIDS should be aware of the possibility that recurrent or stubborn cases of vaginal candidiasis may be an early sign of infection with HIV. Pregnancy, diabetes, contraceptive pills, and antibiotics are also commonly linked to these fungal infections.

AIDS and Other Diseases

AIDS is a unique disease—no other known infectious disease causes its damage through a direct attack on the human immune system. Because the immune system is the final mediator of human host-infectious agent interactions, it was anticipated early that HIV infection would complicate the course of other serious human diseases.

This has proved to be the case, particularly for tuberculosis and certain sexually transmitted infections such as syphilis and the genital herpes virus. Cancer has been linked with AIDS since 1981; this link was discovered with the increased appearance of a highly unusual malignancy, Kaposi's sarcoma. Since then, HIV infection has been associated with a second malignancy, non-Hodgkin's lymphoma (NHL).

KAPOSI'S SARCOMA

This disease was first recognized as a malignant tumor of the inner walls of the heart, veins, and arteries in 1873 in Vienna, Austria. Before the AIDS epidemic, Kaposi's sarcoma (KS) was a rare tumor that primarily affected older people of Mediterranean and Jewish origin.

Clinically, KS in HIV-infected, immunodeficient persons occurs more often as purplish-red lesions of the trunk and head. The lesion is not painful or contagious. It can be flat or indurated and over time frequently progresses to a nodule. The mouth and many internal organs (especially those of the GI and respiratory tracts) may be involved either symptomatically or subclinically.

Prognosis depends on the status of the individual's immune system. People who die of AIDS usually succumb to opportunistic infections rather than to KS.

NON-HODGKIN'S LYMPHOMA*

Approximately 3% of AIDS diagnoses in all risk groups and in all areas originate through discovery of non-Hodgkin's lymphoma. The incidence of NHL increases with age and as the immune system weakens.

These malignancies are difficult to treat because clients often cannot tolerate the further immunosuppression that treatment causes. As with KS, prognosis depends largely on the initial level of immunity. Clients with adequate immune reserves may tolerate therapy and respond reasonably well. However, in people with severe immunodeficiency, survival is only 4 to 7 months on average. Clients diagnosed with HIV-related brain lymphomas have a very poor prognosis.

TUBERCULOSIS†

Tuberculosis (TB) was considered a stable, endemic health problem, but now, in association with the HIV/AIDS pandemic, TB is resurgent. The recent emergence of multiple drug-resistant TB, which has reached epidemic proportions in New York City, has created a serious and growing threat to the capacity of TB control programs (see discussion, Chapter 4).

In urban areas of the United States, the present upsurge in TB cases is occurring among young (aged 25 to 44 years) injection drug users, ethnic minorities, prisoners and prison staff because of poorly ventilated and overcrowded prison systems, homeless people, and immigrants from countries with a high prevalence of TB.

The first major interaction between HIV and TB occurs as a result of the weakening of the immune system in association with progressive HIV infection. The great majority of individuals exposed to TB are infected but not clinically ill. Their subclinical TB infection is kept in check by an active, healthy immune system. However, when a TB-infected person becomes infected with HIV, the immune system begins to decline, and at a certain level of immune damage from HIV, the TB bacteria become active, causing clinical pulmonary TB.

TB is the only opportunistic infection associated with AIDS/HIV that is directly transmissible to household and other contacts. Therefore each individual case of active TB is a threat to community health.

CLINICAL SIGNS AND SYMPTOMS

Pulmonary TB is the most common manifestation of TB disease in HIV-positive clients. When TB precedes the diagnosis of AIDS, disease is usually confined to the lung, whereas when TB is diagnosed after the onset of AIDS, the majority of clients also have extrapulmonary TB, most commonly involving the bone marrow or lymph nodes. Fever, night sweats, wasting, cough,

---

*See also NHL-AIDS, Chapter 10.

†See also Pulmonary Tuberculosis, Chapter 4.

and dyspnea occur in the majority of clients (see also Chapter 4).

The standard tuberculin test is not reliable in persons with HIV infection or AIDS because the weakened immune system may simply be unable to respond to the test. As a result, clinicians need to interpret the test differently for an HIV-infected person.

HIV NEUROLOGIC DISEASE

HIV neurologic disease may be the presenting symptom of HIV infection and can involve the central and peripheral nervous systems. Signs and symptoms range from mild sensory polyneuropathy to seizures, hemiparesis, paraplegia, and dementia.

Central Nervous System Disease. Central nervous system (CNS) disease in HIV-infected clients can be divided into intracerebral space-occupying lesions, encephalopathy, meningitis, and spinal cord processes. Toxoplasmosis is the most common space-occupying lesion in HIV-infected clients. Presenting symptoms may include headache, focal neurologic deficits, seizures, or altered mental status.

AIDS dementia complex (HIV encephalopathy) is the most common neurologic complication and the most common cause of mental status changes in HIV-infected clients. It is characterized by cognitive, motor, and behavioral dysfunction. This disorder is similar to Alzheimer's dementia but has less impact on memory loss and a greater effect on time-related skills (i.e., psychomotor skills learned over time, such as learning to read or playing piano).

Early symptoms of AIDS dementia involve difficulty with concentration and memory, personality changes, irritability, and apathy. Depression and withdrawal occur as the dementia progresses. Motor dysfunction may accompany cognitive changes and may result in poor balance, poor coordination, and frequent falls.

Progressive multifocal leukoencephalopathy (PML), localized lesions within the brain, causes demyelination in the brain and leads to death within a few months.

> **▼ *Clinical Signs and Symptoms of***
> **HIV Neurologic Disease**
>
> - Difficulty with concentration and memory
> - Personality changes (depressions, withdrawal, apathy)
> - Headaches
> - Seizures
> - Paralysis (hemiparesis, paraplegia)
> - Motor dysfunction (balance and coordination)
> - Gradual weakness of extremities
> - Numbness and tingling (peripheral neuropathy)
> - Radiculopathy

In addition to the brain, neurologic disorders related to AIDS and HIV may affect the spinal cord, appearing as myelopathies. A vacuolar myelopathy often appears in the thoracic spine and causes gradual weakness, painless gait disturbance characterized by spasticity, and ataxia in the lower extremities that progresses to include weakness of the upper extremities.

Peripheral Nervous System. Peripheral nervous system syndromes include inflammatory polyneuropathies, sensory neuropathies, and mononeuropathies. An inflammatory demyelinating polyneuropathy similar to Guillain-Barré syndrome occurs in HIV-infected clients.

Peripheral nerve disease is a common complication of the HIV infection. Cytomegalovirus (CMV), a highly host-specific herpes virus that infects the nerve roots, may result in an ascending polyradiculopathy characterized by lower extremity weakness progressing to flaccid paralysis.

The most common neuropathy develops into painful sensory neuropathy with numbness and burning or tingling in the feet, legs, or hands. Immobility caused by painful neuropathies can result in deconditioning and eventual cardiopulmonary decline.

Hypersensitivity Disorders

Although the immune system protects the body from harmful invaders, an overactive or overzealous response is detrimental. Overreaction to a substance, or hypersensitivity, is often referred to as an allergic response. Although the word *allergy* is widely used, the term *hypersensitivity* is more appropriate. Hypersensitivity designates an increased immune response to the presence of an antigen (referred to as an allergen) that results in tissue destruction.

The two general categories of hypersensitivity reaction are immediate and delayed. These designations are based on the rapidity of the immune response. In addition to these two categories, hypersensitivity reactions are divided into four main types (I to IV).

Type I Anaphylactic Hypersensitivity ("Allergies")

ALLERGY AND ATOPY

Allergy refers to the abnormal hypersensitivity that takes place when a foreign substance (allergen) is introduced into the body of a person likely to have allergies. The body fights these invaders by producing the special antibody immunoglobulin E (IgE). This antibody (now a vital diagnostic sign of many allergies), when released into the blood, breaks down mast cells, which contain chemical mediators, such as histamine, that cause dilation of blood vessels and the characteristic symptoms of allergy.

Atopy differs from allergy because it refers to a genetic predisposition to produce large quantities of IgE, causing this state of clinical hypersensitivity. The reaction between the allergen and the susceptible person (i.e., allergy-prone host) results in the development of a number of typical signs and symptoms usually involving the GI tract, respiratory tract, or skin.

CLINICAL SIGNS AND SYMPTOMS

Clinical signs and symptoms vary from one client to another according to the aller-gies present. With the Family/Personal History form used, each client should be asked what known allergies are present and what the specific reaction to the allergen would be for that particular person. The physical therapist can then be alert to any of these warning signs during treatment and can take necessary measures, whether that means grading exercise to the client's tolerance, controlling the room temperature, or appropriately using medications prescribed.

ANAPHYLAXIS

Anaphylaxis, the most dramatic and devastating form of type I hypersensitivity, is the systemic manifestation of immediate hypersensitivity. The implicated antigen is often introduced parenterally, such as by injection of penicillin or a bee sting. The activation and breakdown of mast cells systematically causes vasodilation and increased capillary permeability, which promotes fluid loss into the interstitial space, resulting in the clinical picture of bronchospasms, urticaria (wheals or hives), and anaphylactic shock.

Initial manifestations of anaphylaxis may include local itching, edema, and sneezing. These seemingly innocuous problems are followed in minutes by wheezing, dyspnea, cyanosis, and circulatory shock. Clinical signs and symptoms of anaphylaxis are listed by system in Table 11-1.

Clients with previous anaphylactic reactions (and the specific signs and symptoms of that individual's reaction) should be identified by using the Family/Personal History form. Identification information should be worn at all times by individuals who have had previous anaphylactic reactions.

For identified and unidentified clients, immediate action is required when the person has a severe reaction. In such situations the physical therapist is advised to call for emergency assistance.

Type II Hypersensitivity (Cytolytic or Cytotoxic)

These reactions usually occur during blood transfusion. Blood group incompatibility

TABLE 11-1 ▼ Clinical Aspects of Anaphylaxis by System

System	Signs and Symptoms
General	Malaise, weakness
	Sense of illness
Dermal	Hives, erythema
	Edema of the lips
Mucosal	Periorbital edema
	Nasal congestion and pruritus
	Flushing or pallor, cyanosis
Respiratory	Sneezing
	Rhinorrhea
	Dyspnea
Upper airway	Hoarseness, stridor
	Tongue and pharyngeal edema
Lower airway	Dyspnea
	Acute emphysema
	Air trapping: Asthma, bronchospasm
	Chest tightness; wheezing
Gastrointestinal	Increased peristalsis
	Vomiting
	Dysphagia
	Nausea
	Abdominal cramps
	Diarrhea (occasionally with blood)
Cardiovascular	Tachycardia
	Palpitations
	Hypotension
	Cardiac arrest
Central nervous system	Anxiety, seizures

Modified from Lawlor GJ, Rosenblatt HM: Anaphylaxis. In Lawlor GJ, Fischer TJ, editors: *Manual of allergy and immunology: diagnosis and therapy,* ed 2, Boston, 1988, Little, Brown, p 228.

▼ *Clinical Signs and Symptoms of*
Type II Hypersensitivity

- Headache
- Back (flank) pain
- Chest pain similar to angina
- Nausea and vomiting
- Tachycardia and hypotension
- Hematuria
- Urticaria (skin reaction)

causes cell lysis, which results in a transfusion reaction. The antigen responsible for initiating the reaction is a part of the donor red blood cell (RBC) membrane.

▼ *Clinical Signs and Symptoms of*
Type III Hypersensitivity

- Fever
- Arthralgias; synovitis
- Lymphadenopathy
- Urticaria
- Visceral inflammation (nephritis, pleuritis, pericarditis)

Manifestations of a transfusion reaction result from intravascular hemolysis of RBCs.

Type III Hypersensitivity (Immune Complex)

Immune complex disease results from formation or deposition of antigen-antibody complexes in tissues. For example, the antigen-antibody complexes may form in the joint space, with resultant synovitis, as in RA. Antigen-antibody complexes are formed in the bloodstream and become trapped in capillaries or are deposited in vessel walls, affecting the skin (urticaria), the kidneys (nephritis), the pleura (pleuritis), and the pericardium (pericarditis).

Serum sickness is another type III hypersensitivity response that develops 6 to 14 days after injection with foreign serum (e.g., penicillin, sulfonamides, streptomycin, thiouracils, hydantoin compounds). Deposition of complexes on vessel walls causes complement activation with resultant edema, fever, inflammation of blood vessels and joints, and urticaria.

Type IV Hypersensitivity (Cell-Mediated or Delayed)

In cell-mediated hypersensitivity a reaction occurs 24 to 72 hours after exposure to an allergen.

For example, type IV reactions occur after the intradermal injections of TB antigen. Graft-versus-host disease (GVHD) and

▼ *Clinical Signs and Symptoms of*
Type IV Hypersensitivity

- Itching
- Erythema
- Vesicular skin lesions
- Graft-versus-host disease (GVHD): skin, GI, hepatic dysfunction

transplant rejection are also type IV reactions. In GVHD, immunocompetent donor bone marrow cells (the graft) react against various antigens in the bone marrow recipient (the host), which results in a variety of clinical manifestations, including skin, GI and hepatic lesions.

Contact dermatitis is another type IV reaction that occurs after sensitization to an allergen, commonly a cosmetic, adhesive, topical medication, drug additive (e.g., lanolin added to lotions, ultrasound gels, or other preparations used in massage or soft tissue mobilization), or plant toxin (e.g., poison ivy). With the first exposure, no reaction occurs; however, antigens are formed. On subsequent exposures, hypersensitivity reactions are triggered, which leads to itching, erythema, and vesicular lesions. Anyone with known hypersensitivity (identified through the Family/Personal History form) should have a small area of skin tested before use of large amounts of topical agents in the physical therapy clinic. Careful observation throughout treatment is required.

Neurologic Disorders

Some neurologic disorders encountered by the physical therapist display features that suggest an immunologic basis for the disorder. Such diseases include myasthenia gravis, Guillain-Barré syndrome, and multiple sclerosis. Other dysfunctions, such as amyotrophic lateral sclerosis (ALS) and acute disseminated encephalomyelitis, also associated with immunologic dysfunction but seen less often by the physical therapist, are not discussed.

Myasthenia Gravis

Myasthenia gravis (MG) develops when, for unknown reasons, antibodies produced by the immune system block receptors in muscles that receive signals of acetylcholine (a chemical messenger generated by nerve impulses), thus impairing muscle function.

MG may begin at any time in life, including in the newborn infant, but there are two major peaks of onset. In early-onset MG, at age 20 to 30 years, women are more often affected than men. In late-onset MG, after age 50 years, men are more often affected.

CLINICAL SIGNS AND SYMPTOMS

Clinically, the disease is characterized by muscle weakness and fatigability, most commonly in muscles controlling eye movement, chewing, swallowing, and facial expressions. Symptoms show fluctuations in intensity and are more severe late in the day or after prolonged activity. Fluctuations also occur with superimposed illness,

▼ *Clinical Signs and Symptoms of*
Myasthenia Gravis

- Muscle fatigability and proximal muscle weakness aggravated by exertion
- Respiratory failure from progressive involvement of respiratory muscles
- Ptosis (extraocular muscle weakness resulting in drooping of the upper eyelid)
- Diplopia (double vision)
- Dysarthria (speech disturbance)
- Bulbar involvement
  - Alteration in voice quality
  - Dysphagia (speech impairment)
  - Nasal regurgitation
  - Choking, difficulty in chewing

menses, and air temperature (worsening with warming).

Proximal muscles are affected more than distal muscles, and difficulty in climbing stairs, rising from chairs, combing the hair, or even holding up the head occurs. Cranial muscles, neck muscles, respiratory muscles, and muscles of the proximal limbs are the primary areas of muscular involvement. Neurologic findings are normal except for muscle weakness. There is no muscular atrophy or loss of sensation. Muscular weakness ranges from mild to life-threatening (when involving respiratory muscles).

Guillain-Barré Syndrome (Acute Idiopathic Polyneuritis)

Guillain-Barré syndrome is a demyelinative disease that affects the peripheral nervous system (especially spinal nerves) and is characterized by an abrupt onset of paralysis. The disease affects all age groups, and incidence is not related to race or sex.

The exact cause of the disease is unknown, but it frequently occurs after an infectious illness. Upper respiratory infections, vaccinations, or viral infections such as measles, hepatitis, or mononucleosis commonly precede acute idiopathic polyneuritis by 1 to 3 weeks.

Like MG, acute idiopathic polyneuritis may be an autoimmune disease that occurs after surgery, a viral infection, or immunization. The immune system attacks its own myelin cells because they look similar to the molecules of the infecting virus. The immune system shifts into an accidental self-destructive overdrive.

CLINICAL SIGNS AND SYMPTOMS

The onset of acute idiopathic polyneuritis is generally characterized by a rapidly progressive weakness for a period of 3 to 7 days. It is usually symmetric, involving first the lower extremities, then the upper extremities, and then the respiratory musculature. Weakness and paralysis are frequently pre-

ceded by paresthesias and numbness of the limbs, but actual objective sensory loss is usually mild and transient.

Although muscular weakness is usually described as bilateral, progressing from the legs upward toward the arms, this syndrome may be missed when the client has unilateral symptoms that do not progress proximally.

Muscular weakness of the chest may appear early in this disease process as respiratory compromise. Respiratory involvement as such may be unnoticed until the person develops more severe symptoms associated with the Guillain-Barré syndrome.

The progression of paralysis varies from one client to another, often with full recovery from the paralysis. Usually symptoms develop over a period of 1 to 3 weeks, and the progression of paralysis may stop at any point. Once the weakness reaches a maximum (usually during the second week), the client's condition plateaus for days or even weeks before spontaneous improvement and eventual recovery begin, extending over a period of 6 to 9 months.

Cranial nerves, most commonly the facial nerve, can be involved. The tendon reflexes are decreased or lost early in the course of the illness. The incidence of residual neurologic deficits is higher than was previously recognized, and deficits may occur in as many as 50% of all cases.

There is no immediate cure for this disease, but medical support is vital during

▼ *Clinical Signs and Symptoms of*

Guillain-Barré Syndrome (Acute Idiopathic Polyneuritis)

- Muscular weakness (bilateral, progressing from the legs to the arms to the chest and neck)
- Diminished deep tendon reflexes
- Paresthesias (without loss of sensation)
- Fever, malaise
- Nausea

Case Example. A 67-year-old retired aeronautics engineer was referred to physical therapy by his physician for electrotherapy and therapeutic exercise. The physician's diagnosis was right-sided Bell's palsy. Past medical history was significant for an upper respiratory infection 2 weeks before the onset of his first symptoms.

The client reported difficulty in closing his eyes, chewing, and drinking, and he was unable to smile. There were no changes in sensation or hearing. During the neurologic examination the client was unable to raise his eyebrows or close his eyes, and there was obvious facial drooping on both sides. A gross manual muscle test revealed full (5/5) muscle strength in all four extremities, but muscle stretch reflexes were absent in all four extremities.

Result. The therapist recognized three red-flag symptoms in this case: (1) recent upper respiratory infection followed by the development of neurologic symptoms, (2) progressive development of symptoms from right-sided to bilateral between the time the client was evaluated by the physician and went to the physical therapist, and (3) absent deep tendon reflexes, an inconsistent finding for Bell's palsy.

The physical therapist contacted the physician by telephone to relay this information and confirm the treatment plan given this new information. The physician requested that the client return for further medical testing, and a revised diagnosis of Guillain-Barré syndrome was made.

The client's clinical status stabilized, and he returned to the physical therapist. The treatment plan was modified accordingly. This case again demonstrates the importance of performing a careful diagnostic examination, including screening for systemic disease and recognizing red-flag symptoms.

the progression of symptoms, particularly in the acute phase when respiratory function may be compromised. Physical therapy is initiated at an early stage to maintain joint range of motion within the client's pain tolerance and to monitor muscle strength until active exercises can be initiated.

The usual precautions for clients immobilized in bed are required to prevent complications during the acute phase. A major precaution is to provide active exercise at a level consistent with the client's muscle strength. Overstretching and overuse of painful muscles may result in a prolonged recovery period or a lack of recovery.

Multiple Sclerosis

Multiple sclerosis (MS) is the most common inflammatory demyelinating disease of the CNS, affecting areas of the brain and spinal cord but sparing the peripheral nerves. Symptoms appear usually between 20 and 40 years of age, with a peak onset of age 30 years. Onset is rare in children and in adults older than 50. Women are affected twice as often as men, and a family history of MS increases the risk tenfold. It would appear that MS susceptibility and age at onset are to some extent under genetic control (Sadovnick et al, 1998). Environmental factors may affect onset; MS is five times more prevalent in the temperate (colder) climates of North America and Europe than in tropical areas. Risk associated with geographic location appears to be correlated with the area where a person lived during the first decade of life.

The most widely accepted theory is that MS is an immune-mediated process with a viral trigger (Frozema, 1997). HHV-6, a strain of herpesvirus that is responsible for the childhood roseola and that remains dormant in nerve trunks, has been implicated, but this has not yet been proved.

According to this hypothesis, T cells that have been called up against the virus turn their focus to the myelin and continue to make intermittent attacks on it long after the virus has receded (Kimberlin and Whitley, 1998; Mayne et al, 1998).*

The disease is characterized by inflammatory demyelinating (destructive removal or loss) lesions that later form scars known as plaques, which are scattered throughout the CNS white matter, especially the optic nerves, cerebrum, and cervical spinal cord. When edema and inflammation subside, some remyelination occurs, but it is often incomplete. Axonal injury may cause permanent neurologic dysfunction (Trapp et al, 1998).

The progression of MS is difficult to predict and depends on several factors, including the person's age and the intensity of onset, the neurologic status at 5 years after the onset, and the course of exacerbations-remissions. The survival rate after the onset of symptoms is usually good, and death typically results from either respiratory or urinary infection.

CLINICAL SIGNS AND SYMPTOMS

Clinically, MS is characterized by multiple and varying signs and symptoms and by unpredictable and fluctuating periods of remissions and exacerbations.

Symptoms may vary considerably in character, intensity, and duration. Symptoms can develop rapidly over a course of minutes or hours; less frequently, the onset may be insidious, occurring during a period of weeks or months.

Symptoms depend on the location of the lesions, and early symptoms demonstrate involvement of the sensory, pyramidal, cerebellar, and visual pathways or disruption of cranial nerves and their linkage to the brainstem.

Motor symptoms. Many persons with MS experience weakness in the extremities, leading to difficulty with ambulation, coordination, and balance, with ataxia or tremor present if lesions are in the cerebellum. Spasticity and hyperreflexia are common

---

▼ **Clinical Signs and Symptoms of Multiple Sclerosis**

(Listed in declining order of frequency)

Symptoms
- Unilateral visual impairment
- Paresthesias
- Ataxia or unsteadiness
- Vertigo (sensation of rotation of self or surroundings)
- Fatigue
- Muscle weakness
- Bowel/bladder dysfunctions:
  - Frequency
  - Urgency
  - Incontinence
  - Retention
  - Hesitancy
- Speech impairment (slow, slurred speech)

Signs
- Optic neuritis
- Nystagmus
- Spasticity or hyperreflexia
- Babinski's sign
- Absent abdominal reflexes
- Dysmetria or intention tremor
- Labile or changed mood
- Lhermitte's sign

---

*If MS is a virus-induced autoimmune disease, it could be categorized under Autoimmune Disorders (see next section).

causes of disability with severe, uncontrollable spasms of the extremities. Profound fatigue or dysmetria (intention tremor) contribute to motor impairment (Rudick and Cohen, 1997).

Difficulties with speech (slow, slurred) or chewing and swallowing can occur if the brainstem or cranial nerves are affected. Urinary frequency, urinary urgency, incontinence, urinary retention, or urinary hesitancy commonly characterizes motor and/or sensory bowel/bladder dysfunctions.

Sensory symptoms. Unilateral visual impairment (e.g., double vision, visual loss, red-green color blindness) that comes and goes as a result of optic neuritis is often the first indication of a problem.

Extreme sensitivity to temperature changes is evident in more than 60% of the people diagnosed with MS. Elevated temperatures shorten the duration of the nerve impulse and worsen symptoms, whereas cooler temperatures actually restore conduction in blocked nerves and improve symptoms.

Paresthesias (numbness and tingling) accompanied by burning in the extremities can result in injury to the hands or feet. Lhermitte's sign (electric shocklike sensation down the spine and radiating to the extremities, initiated by neck flexion) is very suggestive of MS but can also occur with disk protrusion.

Autoimmune Disorders

Autoimmunity results from an inability to distinguish self from nonself, causing the immune system to direct immune responses against normal ("self") tissue. The body begins to manufacture antibodies directed against the body's own cellular components or specific organs. These antibodies are known as autoantibodies, and the diseases that they produce are called autoimmune diseases.

The exact cause of autoimmune diseases is not understood, but factors implicated in the development of autoimmune immunologic abnormalities may include genetics (familial tendency), sex hormones (women are affected more often than men by autoimmune diseases), viruses, stress, cross-reactive antibodies, altered antigens, or environment.

Autoimmune disorders may be classified as organ-specific diseases or generalized (systemic) diseases. Organ-specific diseases involve autoimmune reactions limited to one organ.

Organ-specific autoimmune diseases include thyroiditis, Addison's disease, Graves' disease, chronic active hepatitis, pernicious anemia, ulcerative colitis, and insulin-dependent diabetes. These diseases have been discussed in the text appropriate to the organ involved and are not covered further in this chapter.

Generalized autoimmune diseases involve reactions in various body organs and tissues (e.g., fibromyalgia, rheumatoid arthritis, systemic lupus erythematosus, and scleroderma). Systemic autoimmune diseases lead to a sequence of abnormal tissue reaction and damage to tissue that may result in diffuse systemic manifestations.

Fibromyalgia Syndrome

Fibromyalgia syndrome (FMS) is a noninflammatory condition appearing with generalized musculoskeletal pain in conjunction with tenderness to touch in a large number of specific areas of the body and a wide array of associated symptoms. FMS is much more common in women than in men. It occurs in age groups from preadolescents to early postmenopausal women. The condition is rare in older adults.

There is still much controversy over the exact nature of FMS and even debate over whether fibromyalgia is an organic disease with abnormal biochemical or immunologic pathologic aspects. Current theories suggest that it is a genetically predisposed condition with dysregulation of the neurohormonal and autonomic nervous systems. It may be triggered by viral infection, a traumatic event, or stress.

Fibromyalgia has been differentiated from myofascial pain in that FMS is considered

TABLE 11-2 ▼ Differentiating Myofascial Pain Syndrome from Fibromyalgia Syndrome

Myofascial Pain Syndrome	Fibromyalgia Syndrome
Trigger points	Tender points
Localized musculoskeletal condition	Systemic condition
No associated signs and symptoms	Wide array of associated signs and symptoms
Etiology: Overuse, repetitive motions; reduced muscle activity (e.g., casting or prolonged splinting)	Etiology: Neurohormonal imbalance; autonomic nervous system dysfunction

▼ *Clinical Signs and Symptoms of*
Fibromyalgia Syndrome

- Fatigue (mental and physical)
- Sleep disturbances, nocturnal myoclonus, nocturnal bruxism
- Tender points of palpation
- Myalgia (generalized aching)
- Chest wall pain mimicking angina pectoris
- Tendinitis, bursitis
- Temperature dysregulation
  - Raynaud's phenomenon; cold-induced vasospasm (hypersensitivity to cold)
  - Hypothermia (mild decrease in core body temperature)
- Dyspnea, dizziness, syncope
- Headache (throbbing occipital pain)
- Morning stiffness (more than 15 minutes)
- Paresthesia (numbness and tingling)
- Mechanical low back pain with sciatica-like radiation of pain
- Subjective swelling
- Irritable bowel symptoms
- Urinary urgency; irritable bladder syndrome
- Dry eyes/mouth (Sicca syndrome)
- Depression/anxiety
- Cognitive difficulties (e.g., short-term memory loss, decreased attention span)
- Premenstrual syndrome (PMS)

a systemic problem with multiple tender points as one of the key symptoms. Myofascial pain is a localized condition specific to a muscle and may involve as few as one or several areas.

The hallmark of myofascial pain syndrome is a trigger point, as opposed to tender points in FMS. Both disorders cause myalgia with aching pain and tenderness and exhibit similar local histologic changes in the muscle. Painful symptoms in both conditions are increased with activity, although fibromyalgia involves more generalized aching, whereas myofascial pain is more direct and localized (Table 11-2).

FMS has striking similarities to chronic fatigue syndrome (CFS), with a mix of overlapping symptoms that have some common biologic denominator. Diagnostic criteria for CFS focuses on fatigue, whereas the criteria for FMS focuses on pain, the two most prominent symptoms of these syndromes.

▼ *Differential Diagnosis of*
Fibromyalgia

Frequently misdiagnosed, fibromyalgia syndrome is often confused with any of the following:
- Hypothyroidism
- Polymyalgia rheumatica/giant cell arteritis
- Rheumatoid arthritis
- Polymyositis/dermatomyositis
- Systemic lupus erythematosus
- Myofascial pain syndrome
- Metabolic myopathy (e.g., alcohol)
- Neurosis (depression/anxiety)
- Metastatic cancer
- Chronic fatigue syndrome
- Temporomandibular joint dysfunction
- Disk disease

Modified from Harvey CK et al: Fibromyalgia. I. Review of the literature, *J Am Podiatr Med Assoc* 83(7):413, 1993.

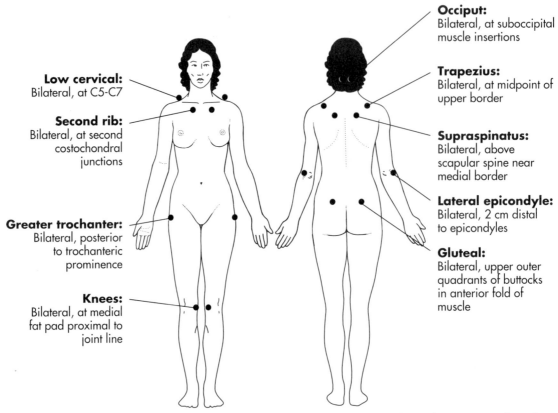

Occiput:
Bilateral, at suboccipital muscle insertions

Trapezius:
Bilateral, at midpoint of upper border

Supraspinatus:
Bilateral, above scapular spine near medial border

Lateral epicondyle:
Bilateral, 2 cm distal to epicondyles

Gluteal:
Bilateral, upper outer quadrants of buttocks in anterior fold of muscle

Low cervical:
Bilateral, at C5-C7

Second rib:
Bilateral, at second costochondral junctions

Greater trochanter:
Bilateral, posterior to trochanteric prominence

Knees:
Bilateral, at medial fat pad proximal to joint line

FIGURE 11-2 • Anatomic locations of tender points associated with fibromyalgia, according to the American College of Rheumatology. Digital palpation should be performed with an approximate force of 4 kg (enough pressure to indent a tennis ball). For a tender point to be considered positive, the subject must state that the palpation was "painful." A reply of "tender" is not considered a positive response. (From Goodman CC, Boissonnault WG: *Pathology: implications for the physical therapist,* Philadelphia, 1998, WB Saunders.

For a detailed description of the Manual Tender Point Survey, the reader is referred to Starz et al. (1997). A videotape reviewing the examination techniques is also available from Dennis C. Turk, Ph.D., Pain Evaluation and Treatment Institute, University of Pittsburgh School of Medicine, 4601 Baum Boulevard, Pittsburgh, PA 15123. Cost $10.00

CLINICAL SIGNS AND SYMPTOMS

The core features of FMS include widespread pain lasting more than 3 months and widespread local tenderness in all clients (Fig. 11-2). Primary musculoskeletal symptoms most frequently reported are (1) aches and pains, (2) stiffness, (3) swelling in soft tissue, (4) tender points, and (5) muscle spasms or nodules (Krsnich-Shriwise, 1997). Fatigue, morning stiffness, and sleep disturbance with nonrefreshed awakening may be present but are not necessary for the diagnosis.

Nontender control points (such as midforehead and anterior thigh) have been included in the examination by some clinicians, although they are not included in the American College of Rheumatology criteria. These control points may be useful in distinguishing FMS from a conversion reaction, referred to as psychogenic rheumatism, in which tenderness may be present everywhere. However, evidence suggests that individuals with FMS may have a generalized lowered threshold for pain on palpation and the control points may also be tender on occasion (Freundlich and Leventhal, 1997; Mountz et al, 1995).

AMERICAN COLLEGE OF RHEUMATOLOGY CRITERIA FOR THE CLASSIFICATION OF FIBROMYALGIA*

HISTORY OF WIDESPREAD PAIN

DEFINITION: Pain is considered widespread when all the following are present:

- Pain in the left side of the body
- Pain in the right side of the body
- Pain above the waist
- Pain below the waist
- Axial skeletal pain (cervical spine, anterior chest, thoracic spine, or low back)

In this definition shoulder and buttock pain is considered as pain for each involved side. "Low back" pain is considered lower segment pain.

PAIN IN 11 OF 18 TENDER POINTS ON DIGITAL PALPATION†

DEFINITION: Pain on digital palpation must be present in at least 11 of the following 18 tender point sites:

- Occiput: Bilateral, at the suboccipital muscle insertions
- Low cervical: Bilateral, at the anterior aspects of the intertransverse spaces at C5-C7
- Trapezius: Bilateral, at the midpoint of the upper border
- Supraspinatus: Bilateral, at origins, above the scapular spine near the medial border
- Second rib: Bilateral, at the second costochondral junctions, just lateral to the junctions on upper surfaces
- Lateral epicondyle: Bilateral, 2 cm distal to the epicondyles
- Gluteal: Bilateral, in upper outer quadrants of buttocks in anterior fold of muscle
- Greater trochanter: Bilateral, posterior to the trochanteric prominence
- Knees: Bilateral, at the medial fat pad proximal to the joint line

From Wolfe F et al: The American College of Rheumatology 1990 criteria for the classification of fibromyalgia, *Arthritis Rheum* 33:160-172, 1990.

*For classification purposes, clients are said to have fibromyalgia if both criteria are satisfied. Widespread pain must be present for at least 3 months. The presence of a second clinical disorder does not exclude the diagnosis of fibromyalgia.

†Digital palpation should be performed with an approximate force of 4 kg (approximately the pressure to indent a tennis ball.) For a tender point to be considered positive, the subject must state that the palpation was "painful"; a reply of "tender" is not to be considered painful.

Symptoms are aggravated by cold, stress, excessive or no exercise, and physical activity ("overdoing it"), including overstretching, and may be improved by warmth or heat, rest, and exercise, including gentle stretching.

Sleep disturbances in stage 4 of nonrapid eye movement sleep (needed for healing of muscle tissues), sleep apnea, difficulty getting to sleep or staying asleep, nocturnal myoclonus (involuntary arm and leg jerks), and bruxism (teeth grinding) cause clients with FMS to wake up feeling unrested and unrefreshed as if they had never gone to sleep (Millott and Berlin, 1997).

The American College of Rheumatology is the standard diagnostic tool currently used. The presence of generalized body pain, prescribed number of tender points, and presence of associated symptoms are essential in the diagnostic process because numerous other diseases and conditions may appear with pain, tenderness, and some of the symptoms commonly associated with FMS (Russell, 1998).

Rheumatoid Arthritis

Rheumatoid arthritis (RA) is a chronic, systemic, inflammatory disorder of unknown cause that can affect various organs but predominantly involves the synovial tissues of the diarthrodial joints. There are more than 100 rheumatic diseases affecting joints, muscles, and extraarticular systems of the body.

Women are affected with RA two to three times more often than men; however, women who are taking or have taken oral contraceptives are less likely to develop RA. Although it may occur at any age, RA is most common in persons between the ages of 20 and 40 years.

The etiologic factor or trigger for this process is as yet unknown. Support for a genetic predisposition comes from studies that RA clusters in families. One gene in particular (HLA-DRB1 on chromosome 6) has been identified in determining susceptibility.

Researchers hypothesize that an infection could trigger an immune reaction that is mediated through multiple complex genetic mechanisms and continues clinically even if the organism is eradicated from the body (Hunder et al, 1998).

Other nongenetic factors may also contribute to the development of RA. Because arthritis (and many related diseases) is more common in women, hormones have been implicated, but the relationship remains unclear. Environmental causes, such as chemicals (e.g., hair dyes, industrial pollutants), medications, food allergies, cigarette smoking, and stress remain under investigation as possible triggers for those individuals who are genetically susceptible to RA.

CLINICAL SIGNS AND SYMPTOMS

Clinical features of RA vary not only from person to person but also in an individual over the disease course. In most people the symptoms begin gradually during a period of weeks or months. Frequently malaise and fatigue prevail during this period, sometimes accompanied by diffuse musculoskeletal pain. Subsequently, specific joints exhibit pain, tenderness, swelling, and redness.

Inactivity, such as sleep or prolonged sitting, is commonly followed by stiffness. "Morning stiffness" usually lasting more than 1 hour occurs when the person arises in the morning or after prolonged inactivity. The duration of this stiffness is an accepted measure of the severity of the condition.

Clients should be asked: "After you get up in the morning, how long does it take until you are feeling the best you will feel for the day?" Pain and stiffness increase gradually as RA progresses and may limit a person's ability to walk, climb stairs, open doors, or perform other activities of daily living (ADLs). Weight loss, depression, and low-grade fever can accompany this process.

The inflammatory process may be under way for some time before swelling, tissue reaction, and joint destruction are seen. Structural damage usually begins between the first and second year of the disease (Anderson, 1997). When symptoms do occur, a symmetric pattern is characteristic, commonly involving the joints of the hands, wrists, elbows, and shoulders, usually sparing the distal interphalangeal (DIP) joints.

Chronic synovitis of the elbows, shoulders, hips, knees, and/or ankles creates special secondary disorders. When the shoulder is involved, limitation of shoulder mobility, dislocation, and spontaneous tears of the rotator cuff result in chronic pain and adhesive capsulitis. Destruction of the elbow articulations can lead to flexion contracture, loss of supination and pronation, and subluxation. Compressive ulnar nerve neuropathies may develop related to elbow synovitis. Symptoms include paresthesias of the fourth and fifth fingers and weakness in the flexor muscle of the little finger.

The joints of the wrist are frequently affected in RA, with variable tenosynovitis of

TABLE 11-3 ▼ Extraarticular Manifestations of Rheumatoid Arthritis

Organ System	Extraarticular Manifestations
Skin	Cutaneous vasculitis Rheumatoid nodules Ecchymoses/petechiae (drug-induced)
Eye	Episcleritis Scleritis Scleromalacia perforans Corneal ulcers/perforation Uveitis Retinitis Glaucoma Cataract
Lung	Pleuritis Diffuse interstitial fibrosis Vasculitis Rheumatoid nodules Caplan's syndrome Pulmonary hypertension
Heart and blood vessels	Pericarditis Myocarditis Coronary arteritis Valvular insufficiency Conduction defects Vasculitis Felty's syndrome
Nervous system	Mononeuritis multiplex Distal sensory neuropathy Cervical spine instability (spinal cord compression)

Modified from Andreoli TE et al: *Cecil essentials of medicine,* ed 3, Philadelphia, 1993, WB Saunders, p 566.

the dorsa of the wrists and, ultimately, interosseous muscle atrophy and diminished movement owing to articular destruction or bony ankylosis. Volar synovitis can lead to carpal tunnel syndrome.

In the feet, subluxation of the heads of the metatarsophalangeal joints and foreshortening of the extensor tendons give rise to "hammer toe" or "cock up" deformities. A similar process in the hands results in volar subluxation of the metacarpophalangeal joints and ulnar deviation of the fingers. An exaggerated inflammatory response of an extensor tendon can result in a spontaneous, often asymptomatic, rupture. Hyperextension of a proximal interphalangeal (PIP) joint and flexion of the DIP joint produce a swan neck deformity. The boutonniere deformity is a fixed flexion contracture of a PIP joint and extension of a DIP joint.

Involvement of the cervical spine by RA tends to occur late in more advanced disease. Clinical manifestations of early disease consist primarily of neck stiffness that is perceived through the entire arc of motion. Inflammation of the supporting ligaments of C1-C2 eventually produces laxity, sometimes giving rise to atlantoaxial subluxation. Spinal cord compression can result from anterior dislocation of C1 or from vertical subluxation of the odontoid process of C2 into the foramen magnum.

Extraarticular features, such as rheumatoid nodules, arteritis, neuropathy, scleritis, pericarditis, lymphadenopathy, and splenomegaly, occur with considerable frequency (Table 11-3). Once thought to be complications of RA, they are now recognized as being integral parts of the disease and serve to emphasize its systemic nature.

The subcutaneous nodules, present in approximately 25% to 35% of clients with RA, occur most commonly in subcutaneous or deeper connective tissues in areas subjected to repeated mechanical pressure, such as the olecranon bursae, the extensor surfaces of the forearms, the elbow, and the Achilles tendons.

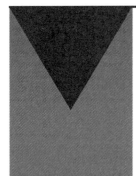

Case Example. A 67-year-old woman with a 13-year history of rheumatoid arthritis requiring gold and methotrexate fell and fractured her right acetabulum, requiring a total hip replacement. She was referred to physical therapy through a home health agency for "aggressive rehabilitation."

After 10 weeks she was walking unassisted after having progressed from a walker to a cane and participating in a swimming program sponsored by the local arthritis organization. She was discharged with a home program to continue working on strength and balance activities.

Six weeks later the therapist received a telephone call from the client's husband, who reported that there had been a gradual decline in her walking and asked the therapist for a reevaluation. The woman came into the outpatient clinic and was examined with the following findings.

The client had resumed the use of a cane, and her gait was characterized by wide-based stance, shortened steps, and trunk instability. She frequently took a few steps forward before tottering backward without falling. The client was unable to stand from a sitting position without assistance. When moving from a standing to a sitting position, she consistently fell backward. When asked about the new onset of any other symptoms, the client noted urinary urge incontinence, and the husband commented that she had just started having difficulty remembering the dates of their children's birthdays and the names of their grandchildren.

The physical therapist performed both an orthopedic and a neurologic screening examination and measured vital signs. The client's blood pressure was 135/78, pulse was 78, and temperature was considered normal. The orthopedic examination was consistent with a total hip replacement 6 months ago, with mild hip flexor weakness and mild loss of hip motion on the left (compared with the right). However, the neurologic examination raised some red flags.

Muscle tone was increased in the lower extremities, with proprioception and deep tendon reflexes decreased in both feet (right more than left). Pinprick, light-touch, and two-point discrimination were normal. Romberg's sign was absent, but a test for dysmetria of the upper extremities revealed mild cogwheeling. There was an observable tremor when the client's arms were stretched out in front of her trunk.

Result. Given the history of a progressive gait disturbance, new onset of urge incontinence, and positive findings on a neurologic screening examination, this client was referred to her family physician for a medical evaluation. The physical therapist explained to the client and her husband that these findings were not typical of someone who has had a total hip replacement or someone with rheumatoid arthritis (RA).

The client was examined by her family physician and referred to a neurologist. A magnetic resonance imaging (MRI) study was ordered, and a diagnosis of "basilar impression" was made. *Basilar impression* is the term used when the odontoid peg of C2 pushes up into the foramen magnum.

RA is a classic cause of this via atlantoaxial dislocation. The destructive inflammatory process of RA weakens ligaments that attach the odontoid to the atlas into the skull. The subsequent dislocation of the atlas on the axis can remain mobile, producing intermittent problems, or it can become fixed, giving persistent symptoms.

Modified from Williams ME, Richman J, Scatliff J: A 67-year-old woman with a progressive gait disturbance, *JAGS* 44(7):843-846, 1996.

TABLE 11-4 ▼ American Rheumatism Association Criteria for Classification of Rheumatoid Arthritis*

Criteria	Definition
Morning stiffness	Morning stiffness in and around the joints lasting at least 1 hour
Arthritis of three or more joint areas	Simultaneous soft tissue swelling or fluid (not bony overgrowth alone) observed by a physician; the 14 possible joint areas are (right or left) PIP, MCP, wrist, elbow, knee, ankle, and MTP joints
Arthritis of hand joints	At least one joint area swollen as above in wrist, MCP, or PIP joint
Symmetric arthritis	Simultaneous bilateral involvement of the same joint areas as above (PIP, MCP, or MTP joints without absolute symmetry is acceptable)
Rheumatoid nodules	Subcutaneous nodules, over bony prominences or extensor surfaces
Serum rheumatoid factor	Abnormal amounts of serum rheumatoid factor
Radiographic changes	Radiographic changes typical of rheumatoid arthritis on posteroanterior hand and wrist radiographs, which must include erosions or bony decalcification localized to involved joints (osteoarthritis changes alone do not qualify)

Modified from Harris ED, Jr: Clinical features of rheumatoid arthritis. In Kelley WN et al: *Textbook of rheumatology,* ed 4, Philadelphia, 1993, WB Saunders, p 874.

*For classification purposes, a client is said to have rheumatoid arthritis if he or she has satisfied at least four of the above seven criteria. Criteria 1 through 4 must be present for at least 6 weeks. Clients with two clinical diagnoses are not excluded. Designation as classic, definite, or probable rheumatoid arthritis is no longer made.

MCP, Metacarpophalangeal; *MTP,* metatarsophalangeal; *PIP,* proximal interphalangeal.

DIAGNOSIS

The clinical diagnosis of RA is based on careful consideration of three factors: the clinical presentation of the client, which is elucidated through history taking and physical examination; the corroborating evidence gathered through laboratory tests and radiography; and the exclusion of other possible diagnoses.

The physical presence of rheumatoid nodules and the presence of rheumatoid factor measured by laboratory studies are two indicators of RA, although some persons with actual rheumatoid factors are missed by commonly available methods.

Classification of RA (Table 11-4) is difficult in the early course of the disease, when articular symptoms are accompanied only by constitutional symptoms such as fatigue and loss of appetite, which are common to a number of chronic diseases. A full array of clinical signs and symptoms may not be manifest for 1 to 2 years.

A diagnosis of RA is established on the presentation of four of the seven listed criteria with a duration of joint signs and symptoms for at least 6 weeks.

Additional laboratory tests of significance in the diagnosis and management of RA include white blood cell (WBC) count, erythrocyte sedimentation rate, hemoglobin and hematocrit, urinalysis, and rheumatoid factor assay.

The number of WBCs will increase in the presence of joint inflammation, as will the erythrocyte sedimentation rate. Anemia may be present, and the rheumatoid factor will be elevated in clients with active RA. If the client's urinalysis reveals any protein, blood cells, or casts, SLE should be suspected. This type of abnormal urinalysis would necessitate further diagnostic evaluation and immediate physician referral.

Systemic Lupus Erythematosus

Systemic lupus erythematosus (SLE) belongs to the family of autoimmune rheumatic diseases. It is known to be a chronic, systemic, inflammatory disease characterized by injury to the skin, joints, kidneys, heart and blood-forming organs, nervous system, and mucous membranes.

Lupus comes from the Latin word for wolf, referring to the belief in the 1800s that the rash of this disease was caused by a wolf bite. The characteristic rash of lupus (especially a butterfly rash across the cheeks and nose) is red, leading to the term *erythematosus*.

There are two primary forms of lupus: discoid and systemic. *Discoid lupus* is a limited form of the disease confined to the skin. Discoid lupus rarely develops into systemic lupus. Individuals who develop the systemic form probably had systemic lupus at the outset, with the discoid rash as the main symptom. Treatment of discoid lupus will not prevent its progression to the systemic form.

Systemic lupus is usually more severe than discoid lupus and can affect almost any organ or system of the body. For some people, only the skin and joints will be involved. In others, the joints, lungs, kidneys, blood or other organs, or tissues may be affected.

The exact cause of SLE is unknown, although it appears to result from an immunoregulatory disturbance brought about by the interplay of genetic, hormonal, and environmental factors.

Some of the environmental factors that may trigger the disease are infections,* antibiotics (especially those in the sulfa and penicillin groups), exposure to ultraviolet (sun) light, and extreme physical and emotional stress, including pregnancy.

Although there is a known genetic predisposition, no known gene is associated with SLE. Lupus can occur at any age, but it is most common in persons between the ages of 15 and 40 years; it rarely occurs in older people. Women are affected 10 to 15 times more often than men, possibly because of hormones but the exact relationship remains unknown.

People of African, Native American, or Asian origin develop the disease more often than do whites. The effect of race on musculoskeletal morbidity is significant (Petri, 1998). There is no single characteristic clinical pattern of symptoms. Clients may differ dramatically in the relative severity and pattern of organ involvement. The distribution of damage in descending order includes musculoskeletal (25%); neuropsychiatric (15%); ocular (12%); renal, pulmonary, cardiovascular (10%) (see Lupus Carditis, Chapter 3); GI and skin (7%); peripheral vascular and diabetes (6%); and malignancy (2.5%) (Petri, 1996). Although these symptoms may not be

▼ **Clinical Signs and Symptoms of**
Systemic Lupus Erythematosus

Although lupus can affect any part of the body, most people experience symptoms in only a few organs. The most common symptoms associated with lupus are listed here.

Sign/Symptom
- Constitutional symptoms
- Achy joints (arthralgia)
- Arthritis (swollen joints)
- Arthralgia
- Skin rashes (malar)
- Pulmonary involvement
- Anemia
- Kidney involvement
- Sun or light sensitivity (photosensitivity)
- Hair loss
- Raynaud's phenomenon (fingers turning white or blue in the cold)
- CNS involvement:
  - Seizures
  - Headache
  - Peripheral neuropathy
  - Cranial neuropathy
  - Cerebral vascular accidents
  - Organic brain syndrome
  - Psychosis
- Mouth, nose, or vaginal ulcers

---

*New evidence supporting the long-suspected Epstein-Barr virus (EBV) has been found (James, 1997; Vaughan, 1997).

Case Example. A 33-year-old woman with a known diagnosis of systemic lupus erythematosus came to the physical therapy clinic with the following report: "Three weeks ago, I was carrying a heavy briefcase with a strap around my shoulder. I put weight on my right leg and felt my hip joint slip in the back with immediate pain, and I was unable to put any weight on that leg. I moved my hip around in the socket and was able to get immediate relief from the pain, but it felt like it could catch at any time." The client also reported that "it feels like my left hip is 2 inches higher than my right."

The client reported prolonged (over 7-year) use of prednisone and a past medical history of proteinuria and compromised kidney function. Muscle weakness 2 years ago resulted in a muscle biopsy and a diagnosis of "abnormal" muscle tissue of unknown cause. The client developed a staph infection from the biopsy, which resolved very slowly.

Other past medical history included a motor vehicle accident 2 years ago, at which time her knees went through the dashboard, which left both knees "numb" for a year after the accident.

Aggravating and relieving factors from this visit fit a musculoskeletal pattern of symptoms, and objective examination was consistent with lumbar/sacroiliac mechanical dysfunction with a multitude of other compounding factors, including bilateral posterior cruciate ligament laxity, poor posture, obesity, and emotional lability.

Physical therapy treatment was initiated, but a week later, when the client woke up at night to go to the bathroom, she swung her legs over the edge of her bed and experienced immediate hip and diffuse low back pain and lower extremity weakness.

She went to the emergency department by ambulance and later was admitted to the hospital. She was evaluated by a neurologist (results unknown), recovered from her symptoms within 24 hours, and was released after a 3-day hospitalization. She was directed by her primary care physician to continue outpatient physical therapy services.

This case example is included to point out the complexity of treating a musculoskeletal condition in a client with a long-term chronic inflammatory disease process requiring years of steroidal antiinflammatory medications. Before including any resistive exercises, muscle energy techniques, or joint or self-mobilization techniques, the therapist must be aware of any clinically significant changes in bone density and the presence of developing osteoporosis.

After consulting with this client's physician, conservative symptomatic treatment was planned. Within 2 weeks, she experienced another middle-of-the-night acute exacerbation of symptoms. A subsequent magnetic resonance image resulted in a diagnosis of disk extrusion (annulus fibrosus perforated with diskal material in the epidural space) at two levels (L4-L5 and L5-S1).

present at disease onset, most persons develop manifestations of multisystem disease.

Musculoskeletal changes. Arthralgias and arthritis are the most common presenting manifestations of SLE. Acute migratory or persistent nonerosive arthritis may involve any joint, but typically the small joints of the hands, wrists, and knees are symmetrically involved. Lupus does not directly affect the spine, but syndromes such as costochondritis and cervical myofascial syndrome associated with SLE are commonly treated in a physical therapist practice (Van Vollenhoven, 1996).

One fourth of all persons with lupus develop progressive musculoskeletal damage with deforming arthritis, osteoporosis with fracture and vertebral collapse, and osteomyelitis. Often these musculoskeletal complications occur as a result of the drugs necessary for treatment.

Approximately 30% of people with SLE have coexistent fibromyalgia, independent of race. Fibromyalgia is identified as a major contributor of pain and fatigue, but a medical differential diagnosis is required to rule out hypothyroidism, anemia, or pulmonary lupus (interstitial lung disease or pulmonary hypertension) (Petri, 1997).

Peripheral neuropathy. Peripheral neuropathy may be motor, sensory (stocking-glove distribution), or mixed motor and sensory polyneuropathy. These may develop subacutely in the lower extremities and progress to the upper extremities. Numbness on the tip of the tongue and inside the mouth is also a frequent complaint. Touch, vibration, and position sense are most prominently affected, and the distal limb reflexes are depressed.

Scleroderma (Progressive Systemic Sclerosis) (PSS)

Scleroderma, one of the lesser known chronic multisystem diseases in the family of rheumatic diseases, is characterized by inflammation and fibrosis of many parts of the body, including the skin, blood vessels, synovium, skeletal muscle, and certain internal organs such as kidneys, lungs, heart, and GI tract.

There are two major subsets, limited cutaneous (previously known as the CREST syndrome) and diffuse cutaneous scleroderma. The major differences between these two types are the degree of clinically involved skin and the pace of disease.

Limited scleroderma is often characterized by a long history of Raynaud's phe-

---

▼ Clinical Signs and Symptoms of Scleroderma

Limited Cutaneous Sclerosis (iSSc)
- CREST syndrome

  Calcinosis (abnormal deposition of calcium salts in tissues; usually on the fingertips and over bony prominences)

  Raynaud's phenomenon persisting for years

  Esophageal dysmotility, dysphagia, heartburn

  Sclerodactyly (chronic hardening and shrinking of fingers and toes)

  Telangiectasia (spiderlike hemangiomas formed by dilation of a group of small blood vessels; occurs most commonly on the face and hands)

Diffuse Cutaneous Sclerosis (dSSc)
- Raynaud's phenomenon (acute onset)
- Trunk and extremity skin changes (swelling, thickening, hardening)
- Ulcerations of the fingers secondary to constriction of small blood vessels
- Polyarthralgia (joint pain affecting large and small joints with inflammation, stiffness, swelling, warmth, and tenderness)
- Tendon friction rubs
- Flexion contractures of large and small joints
- Visceral involvement
  - Interstitial lung disease (dyspnea on exertion, chronic cough, pleurisy)
  - Esophageal involvement
  - Renal failure (headache, blurred vision, seizures, malaise)
  - GI disease (bloating, cramps, diarrhea or constipation)
  - Myocardial involvement (cardiomyopathy, pericarditis, pericardial effusions, arrhythmias)

---

nomenon before the development of other symptoms. Skin thickening is limited to the hands, frequently with digital ulcers. Esophageal dysmotility is common. Although limited scleroderma is generally a milder form than diffuse scleroderma, life-threatening complications can occur from small intestine involvement and pulmonary hypertension.

Diffuse scleroderma has a much more acute onset, with many constitutional symptoms, arthritis, carpal tunnel syndrome, and marked swelling of the hands and legs. Widespread skin thickening occurs, progressing from the fingers to the trunk. Internal organ problems, including GI effects and pulmonary fibrosis (see Systemic Sclerosing Lung Disease, Chapter 4), are common, and severe life-threatening involvement of the heart and kidneys occurs (Steen, 1998).

Although the cause of scleroderma is unknown, researchers suspect a complex interaction of genetic and environmental factors. Scleroderma can occur in individuals of any age, race, or sex, but it occurs most commonly in young or middle-age women (ages 25 through 55).

CLINICAL SIGNS AND SYMPTOMS

Skin. Raynaud's phenomenon and tight skin are the hallmarks of systemic sclerosis (SSc). Virtually all clients with SSc have Raynaud's phenomenon, which is defined as episodic pallor of the digits following exposure to cold or stress associated with cyanosis, followed by erythema, tingling, and pain. Raynaud's phenomenon primarily affects the hands and feet and less commonly the ears, nose, and tongue.

The appearance of the skin is the most distinctive feature of SSc. By definition, clients with diffuse SSc have taut skin in the more proximal parts of extremities, in addition to the thorax and abdomen. However, the skin tightening of SSc begins on the fingers and hands in nearly all cases. Therefore the distinction between limited and diffuse SSc may be difficult to make early in the illness.

Musculoskeletal. Articular complaints are very common in PSS and may begin at any time during the course of the disease. The arthralgias, stiffness, and frank arthritis seen may be difficult to distinguish from those of RA, particularly in the early stages of the disease.

Involved joints include the metacarpophalangeals, PIPs, wrists, elbows, knees, ankles, and small joints of the feet.

Muscle involvement is usually mild with weakness, tenderness, and pain of proximal muscles of the upper and lower extremities.

Late scleroderma is characterized by muscle atrophy, muscle weakness, deconditioning and flexion contractures.

Viscera. Involvement of the GI tract is the third most common manifestation of SSc, following only skin changes and Raynaud's phenomenon. Esophageal hypomotility occurs in more than 90% of clients with either diffuse or limited SSc. Similar changes occur in the small intestine, resulting in reduced motility and causing intermittent diarrhea, bloating, cramping, malabsorption, and weight loss.

The overall course of scleroderma is highly variable. Once remission occurs, relapse is uncommon. The diffuse form generally has a worse prognosis because of cardiac involvement, such as cardiomyopathy, pericarditis, pericardial effusions, or arrhythmias.

Spondyloarthropathy

Spondyloarthropathy represents a group of noninfectious, inflammatory, erosive rheumatic diseases that target the sacroiliac joints, the bony insertions of the annulus fibrosi of the intervertebral disks, and the facet or apophyseal joints. They are not seropositive for rheumatoid factor, and the progressive joint fibrosis present is associated

---

▼ **History Associated With**
Spondyloarthropathy

- Insidious onset of each episode of backache
- First episode of backache occurs before 30 years of age
- Each episode lasts for months
- Pain intensifies after rest
- Pain lessens with movement
- Family history of a spondyloarthropathy

with the genetic marker human leukocyte antigen (HLA-B27).

This group of diseases includes ankylosing spondylitis (AS; also known as Marie-Strümpell disease), Reiter's syndrome, psoriatic arthritis, and arthritis associated with chronic inflammatory bowel disease (see discussion, Chapter 6). Spondyloarthropathy is more common in men,* who by gender have a familial tendency toward the development of this type of disease.

ANKYLOSING SPONDYLITIS

Ankylosing spondylitis (AS) is a chronic, progressive inflammatory disorder of undetermined cause. It is actually more an inflammation of fibrous tissue affecting the entheses, or insertions of ligaments and capsules into bone, than of synovium, as is common in other rheumatic disorders. The sacroiliac joints, spine, and large peripheral joints are primarily affected, but this is a systemic disease with widespread effects. People with AS may experience arthritis in other joints, such as the hips, knees, and shoulders along with fever, fatigue, loss of appetite, and redness and pain of the eyes.

CLINICAL SIGNS AND SYMPTOMS

The classic presentation of AS is insidious onset of middle and low back pain and stiffness for more than 3 months in a person (usually male) under age 40 years. It is usually worse in the morning, lasting more than 1 hour, and is characterized as either achy or sharp ("jolting"), typically localized to the pelvis, buttocks, and hips; this pain can be confused with sciatica. A neurologic examination will be within normal limits.

Paravertebral muscle spasm, aching, and stiffness are common, but some clients may have slow progressive limitation of motion

with no pain at all. Most clients have sacroiliitis as the earliest feature seen on x-ray films before clinical involvement extends to the lumbar spine.

On physical examination, decreased mobility in the anteroposterior and lateral planes will be symmetric. The Wright-Schöber test is used to confirm reduction in spinal motion associated with AS (Magee, 1997). The sacroiliac joint is rarely tender by direct palpation. As the disease progresses, the inflamed ligaments and tendons around the vertebrae ossify (turn to bone), causing a rigid spine and the loss of lumbar lordosis.

In the most severe cases the spine becomes so completely fused that the person may be locked in a rigid upright position or in a stooped position, unable to move the neck or back in any direction.

Peripheral joint involvement usually (but not always) occurs after involvement of the spine. Typical extraspinal sites include the manubriosternal joint, symphysis pubis, shoulder, and hip joints.

If the ligaments that attach the ribs to the spine become ossified, diminished chest expansion (<2 cm) occurs, making it difficult to take a deep breath. Chest wall stiffness seldom leads to respiratory disability as long as diaphragmatic movement is intact. This process of vertebral and costovertebral fusion results in the formation of syndesmophytes (Fig. 11-3). This reparative process also forms linear bone ossification along the outer fibers of the annulus fibrosus of the disk.

This bridging of the vertebrae is most prominent along the anterior longitudinal ligament and occurs earliest in the thoracolumbar region. Destructive changes of the upper and lower corners of the vertebrae (at the insertion of the annulus fibrosus of the disk) are responsible for the vertebral squaring. Late in the disease the vertebral column takes on an appearance that is referred to as "bamboo spine."

Extraarticular Features. Uveitis, conjunctivitis, or iritis occurs in nearly 25% of clients and follows a course that is unrelated to the severity of the joint disease. Ocular symptoms may precede spinal symptoms by several weeks or even years. Pulmonary

---

*Some studies now suggest that the disease has a more uniform sex distribution, but it may be milder in women with more peripheral joint manifestations than spinal disease (Gomez et al, 1997; Ostensen and Ostensen, 1998). Diagnosis is delayed or inappropriate until disease progression can be identified radiographically.

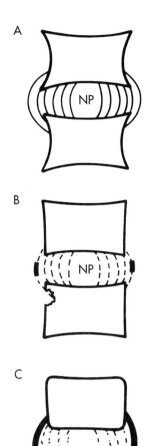

A

B

C

FIGURE 11-3 • Pathogenesis of the syndesmophyte. The syndesmophyte, along with destruction of the sacroiliac joint, is the hallmark of the inflammatory spondyloarthropathies, such as ankylosing spondylitis. It should be distinguished from the osteophyte, which is characteristic of degenerative spondylosis. **A,** Normal intervertebral disk. The inner fibers of the annulus fibrosus are next to the nucleus pulposus (*NP*). The outer fibers insert into the periosteum of the vertebral body at least one third the distance toward the next end-plate. **B,** With early inflammation, the corners of the bodies are reabsorbed and appear to be square or even eroded. Fine deposits of amorphous apatite (calcium phosphate, a mineral constituent of bone) first appear on radiographs as thin, delicate calcification in the outer fibers of the midannulus. **C,** The process progresses to bridging calcification, with the syndesmophyte extending from one midbody to the next. Thus the spine takes on its bamboo-like appearance on radiographs. (From Hadler NM: *Medical management of the regional musculoskeletal diseases,* Orlando, Fla, 1984, Grune & Stratton, p 5.)

▼ **Clinical Signs and Symptoms of**
Ankylosing Spondylitis

Early Stages
- Intermittent, low-grade fever
- Fatigue
- Anorexia, weight loss
- Anemia
- Painful limitation of cervical joint motion
- Sacroiliitis (inflammation, pain, and tenderness in the sacroiliac joints)
- Spasm of the paravertebral muscles
- Intermittent low back pain (nontraumatic, insidious onset)
- Loss of normal lumbar lordosis (positive Schöber's test)

Advanced Stages
- Constant low back pain
- Ankylosis (immobility and consolidation or fusion) of the sacroiliac joints and spine
- Muscle wasting in shoulder and pelvic girdles
- Marked dorsocervical kyphosis
- Decreased chest expansion
- Arthritis involving the peripheral joints (hips and knees)

Extraskeletal
- Cauda equina syndrome
- Iritis or iridocyclitis (inflammation of the iris; occurs in 25% of all cases)
- Carditis (10% occurrence)
- Pericarditis and pulmonary fibrosis (rare)
- Fatigue and weight loss
- Low-grade fever

changes (chronic infiltrative or fibrotic bullous changes of the upper lobes) occur in 1% to 3% of persons with AS and may be confused with TB.

Cardiomegaly, conduction defects, and pericarditis are well-recognized cardiovascular complications of AS. Occasionally, renal manifestations precede other symptoms of AS.

Complications. The very stiff osteoporotic spine of clients with AS is prone to *fracture* from even minor trauma. The most common site of fracture is the lower cervical spine. Risk of neurologic damage may be compounded by the development of epidural hematoma from lacerated vessels.

Severe neck or occipital pain possibly referring to the retroorbital or frontal area is the presenting symptom of *atlantoaxial subluxation*. This underappreciated entity may be either an early or a late manifestation, but it is frequently seen in clients with persistent peripheral arthritis.

Movement aggravates pain, and progressive myelopathy develops from cord compression, leading to motor/sensory disturbance in bladder and bowel control. The diagnosis of atlantoaxial subluxation is usually made from lateral x-ray views of the cervical spine in flexion and extension.

Spondylodiscitis (erosive and destructive lesions of vertebral bodies) is seen in clients with long-standing disease. Intervertebral disk lesions occur at multiple levels, especially in the thoracolumbar region.

Cauda equina syndrome is a late manifestation of the disease, with an average interval of 24 years between onset of AS and the syndrome (Tullous et al, 1990). The initial deficit is loss of sensation of the lower extremities, along with urinary and rectal sphincter disturbances and/or perineal pain and weakness. Neurologic abnormalities in AS are usually related to nerve impingement or spinal cord trauma.

Spinal stenosis occurs as a result of bony overgrowth of the spinal ligaments and facet joints. Symptoms are pain and numbness of the lower extremities brought on by walking and relieved by rest.

REITER'S SYNDROME

Reiter's syndrome, or reactive arthritis, is characterized by a triad of arthritis, conjunctivitis, and nonspecific urethritis, although some clients develop only two of these three problems. Reiter's syndrome occurs mainly in young adult men between the ages of 20 and 40 years, although women and children can be affected.

Reactive arthritis typically begins acutely 2 to 4 weeks after venereal infections or bouts of gastroenteritis. Most cases occur in young men and are believed to result from venereally acquired infections. Food-borne enteric infections affect both men and women. The onset of Reiter's syndrome can be abrupt, occurring over several days or more gradually over several weeks.

HLA-B27, present in a high-frequency pattern supports a genetic predisposition for the development of this syndrome after a person is exposed to certain bacterial infections or after sexual contact. Having HLA-B27 does not necessarily mean that the person will develop this syndrome but indicates that the person will have a greater chance of developing Reiter's syndrome than do persons without this marker.

Reiter's syndrome can be differentiated from AS by the presence of urethritis and

▼ ***Clinical Signs and Symptoms of***
Reiter's Syndrome

Articular Manifestations
- Polyarthritis (occurs several days or weeks after symptoms of infection appear)
- Sacroiliac joint changes
- Low back and buttock pain
- Small joint involvement, especially the feet (heel pain)
- Plantar fasciitis
- Low-grade fever
- Urethritis (when present, precedes other symptoms by 1 to 2 weeks)
- Conjunctivitis and iritis, bilaterally

Extraarticular Manifestations
- Skin involvement: Inflammatory hyperkeratotic lesions of the toes, nails, and soles resembling psoriasis
- May be preceded by bowel infection: diarrhea, nausea, vomiting
- Anorexia and weight loss

Case Example. At presentation, a 22-year-old man had left heel pain that had developed 3 weeks before his appointment in physical therapy. He could not attribute any trauma to the foot and was not involved in any sports or athletic activities. Previous medical history was minimal except for an appendectomy when he was 18 years old.

The client reported that his pain was the worst when he first got out of bed in the morning but improved with stretching and taking aspirin. He did not wear any orthotics or special shoes. The physical therapist did not ask about the presence of associated signs or symptoms.

No obvious gait abnormalities were observed. On palpation of the foot, there was no warmth, bruising, or redness in the area of the plantar fascia or calcaneus. Tenderness was reported along the plantar fascia, with a painful response to palpation of the tendinous attachment to the calcaneus. Ankle range of motion and muscle strength of the left lower leg were within normal limits. There was no tenderness of the surrounding bones, tendons, or muscles. A neurologic screen was also considered normal.

The physical therapist treated this client by using a treatment protocol for plantar fasciitis, including ultrasound, deep friction massage, and stretching exercises. Symptoms subsided and the client was discharged. Six weeks later he returned with recurrence of the original symptoms and new onset of low back pain.

The therapist reevaluated the client, including an in-depth evaluation of postural components and performing a back screening examination, but again did not ask any questions related to associated signs and symptoms. Before his next appointment, the client called and canceled further physical therapy treatment.

Result. A follow-up call determined that this young man had developed other symptoms, such as fever, red and itching eyes, and urinary frequency. He went to a walk-in clinic and was referred to an internist and received a diagnosis of Reiter's syndrome.

Whenever a client has musculoskeletal pain or symptoms of unknown cause, a series of questions must be posed to screen for medical disease. This is especially important when symptoms do not respond to treatment, when symptoms recur, or when new musculoskeletal symptoms develop.

Although joint pain, heel pain, or back pain usually occurs after the development of conjunctivitis, enteritis, or urethritis in Reiter's syndrome, this young man developed musculoskeletal symptoms first. At the time of the initial physical therapy evaluation, he was experiencing fatigue, low-grade fever, and malaise that he could not account for and that did not relate to his heel pain.

conjunctivitis, the prominent involvement of distal joints, and the presence of asymmetric radiologic changes in the sacroiliac joints and spine.

CLINICAL SIGNS AND SYMPTOMS

Arthritis associated with Reiter's syndrome often occurs precipitously and frequently affects the knees and ankles, lasting weeks to months. The distribution of the arthritis begins in the weight-bearing joints, especially of the lower extremities.

The arthritis may vary in severity from absence to extreme joint destruction. Involvement of the feet and spine is most common and is associated with HLA-B27 positivity. Affected joints are usually warm, tender, and edematous, with pain on active and passive movement. A dusky-blue discoloration or frank erythema accompanied by exquisite tenderness is a sign of a septic joint. Although the joints usually begin to improve after 2 or 3 weeks, many people continue to have pain, especially in the heels and back.

Low back and buttock pain are common in reactive arthritis; such pain is caused by sacroiliac or other spinal joint involvement. Sacroiliac changes seen on x-ray films are usually asymmetric and similar to those of AS. Small joint involvement, especially in the feet, is more common in Reiter's syndrome than in AS and is often asymmetric.

In addition to arthritis, inflammation typically occurs at bony sites where tendons, ligaments, or fascia have their attachments or insertions (entheses). Enthesitis most commonly occurs at the insertions of the plantar aponeurosis and Achilles tendon, on the calcaneus, leading to heel pain—one of the most frequent, distinctive, and disabling manifestations of the disease. Other common sites for enthesitis include ischial tuberosities, iliac crests, tibial tuberosities, and ribs, with associated musculoskeletal pain at sites other than joints (Arnett, 1997).

The *conjunctivitis* of Reiter's syndrome is mild and characterized by irritation with redness, tearing, and burning usually lasting a few days (or less commonly as long as several weeks). The process is ordinarily self-limiting.

Urethritis manifested by burning and urinary frequency is often the earliest symptom. A profuse and watery diarrhea can precede the onset of urethritis in Reiter's syndrome.

PSORIATIC ARTHRITIS

Psoriatic arthritis (PsA) is a chronic, recurrent, erosive, inflammatory arthritis associated with the skin disease psoriasis. It is not just a variant of RA but is a distinct disease that combines features of both rheumatoid arthritis and the spondyloarthropathies. Psoriasis is quite common, affecting 1% to 3% of the general population. This arthritis occurs in one third of clients with psoriasis.

In contrast to RA, there is no gender predilection in PsA. Both sexes are affected equally, although women tend to develop symmetric polyarthritis, and spinal involvement is more common in men. PsA can occur at any age although it usually occurs between the ages of 20 and 30 years. The onset of the arthritis may be acute or insidious and is usually preceded by the skin disease.

The cause of psoriasis and PsA is unknown. Genetic factors appear to play a role in the development of this disease. The presence of the histocompatibility complex marker HLA-B27 and other HLA antigens is not uncommon, and they occur in clients with peripheral arthritis and spondylitis.

The presence of these genetic markers may be associated with an increased susceptibility to unknown infectious or environmental agents or to primary abnormal autoimmune phenomena. As yet, no known immunologic pathogenic mechanism has been demonstrated.

CLINICAL SIGNS AND SYMPTOMS

Skin lesions that characterize psoriasis are readily recognized as piles of well-defined, dry, erythematous, often overlapping silver-scaled papules and plaques. These may appear in small, easily overlooked patches or may run together and cover wide areas. The scalp, extensor surfaces of the elbows and knees, back, and buttocks are common sites. The lesions, which do not usually itch, come and go and may be present for years before the onset of arthritis.

Nail lesions, including pitting, ridging (transverse grooves), cracking, onycholysis (loosening or separation of the nail) brown-yellow discoloration, and destruction of the nail, are the only clinical feature that may identify clients with psoriasis in whom arthritis is likely to develop. The nail changes may be mistaken for those produced by a fungal infection.

Arthritis appears as an early and severe sign in a symmetric distal distribution (DIP joints of fingers and toes before involvement of metacarpophalangeal/metatarsophalangeal (MCP/MTP) joints) in half of all clients with PsA, which distinguishes it from RA. Severe erosive disease may lead to marked deformity of the hands and feet, called arthritis mutilans. Wrists, ankles, knees, and elbows can also be involved.

Clients report pain and stiffness in the inflamed joints, with morning stiffness that lasts more than 30 minutes. Other evidence of inflammation includes pain on stressing the joint, tenderness at the joint line, and the presence of effusion. Painful symptoms are aggravated by prolonged immobility and are reduced by physical activity.

Marked vertebral involvement can result in *ankylosis of the spine.* This differs from AS in a number of respects, most notably in the tendency for many of the syndesmophytes to arise not at the margins of the vertebral bodies but from the lateral and anterior surfaces of the bodies. *Sacroiliac changes,* including erosions, sclerosis, and ankylosis similar to that in Reiter's syndrome, occur in 10% to 30% of clients with PsA.

Soft-tissue involvement, similar to clinical manifestations of spondyloarthropathy, occurs often in PsA. Enthesitis, or inflammation at the site of tendon insertion or muscle attachment to bone, is frequently observed at the Achilles tendon, plantar fascia, and pelvic bones. Also common are tenosynovitis of the flexor tendons of the hands, extensor carpi ulnaris, and other sites.

Dactylitis, which occurs in more than one third of PsA clients, is marked by diffuse

▼ **Clinical Signs and Symptoms of**
Psoriatic Arthritis

- Fever
- Fatigue
- Dystrophic nail bed changes
- Polyarthritis
- Psoriasis
- Sore fingers (sometimes sausagelike swelling)

swelling of the whole finger. Inflammation in this typical "sausage finger" extends to the tendon sheaths and adjacent joints.

Extraarticular features similar to those seen in clients with other seronegative spondyloarthropathies are frequently seen. These extraarticular lesions include iritis, mouth ulcers, urethritis, and, less commonly, colitis and aortic valve disease.

INFECTIOUS ARTHRITIS

Arthritis as a direct result of infection is one of the most common musculoskeletal system disorders encountered in general medicine. At presentation, the client has high fever, chills, an elevated WBC count, and general sepsis. There is usually a single painful, swollen joint, most often a knee, ankle, elbow, or shoulder. Aspirated synovial fluid is cloudy yellow or sometimes green or slightly bloody, and blood or synovial fluid culture is positive for staphylococci or pneumococci.

Septic arthritis is seen frequently in older or debilitated clients. Clients who have diabetes or another disorder associated with immune suppression, such as RA, or chronic renal failure or who have undergone joint surgery or renal transplantation are also at risk. Other potential risk factors include malignancy, hemophilia, injection drug abuse, SLE, chronic liver disease, and anemia.

LYME DISEASE

In the early 1970s, a mysterious clustering of juvenile arthritis occurred among children in Lyme, Connecticut, and in surrounding towns. Medical researchers soon recognized the illness as a distinct disease, which they called Lyme disease. They were able to identify the deer tick infected with a spiral bacterium or spirochete (later named *Borrelia burgdorferi*) as the key to its spread.

The number of reported cases of Lyme disease, as well as the number of geographic areas in which it is found, has been increasing. Most cases are concentrated in the coastal northeast, the mid-Atlantic states, Wisconsin, Minnesota, Oregon, and northern California. Children may be more susceptible than are adults simply because they spend more time outdoors and are more likely to be exposed to ticks.

CLINICAL SIGNS AND SYMPTOMS

In most individuals the first symptom of Lyme disease is a red rash, known as *erythema migrans,* that starts as a small red spot that expands over a period of days or weeks, forming a circular, triangular, or oval rash. Sometimes the rash resembles a bull's-eye because it appears as a red ring surrounding a central clear area. The rash can range in size from that of a dime to the entire width of a person's back, appearing within a few weeks of a tick bite and usually at the site of the bite, which is often the axilla or groin. As infection spreads, several rashes can appear at different sites on the body.

Erythema migrans is often accompanied by flulike symptoms such as fever, headache, stiff neck, body aches, and fatigue. Although these symptoms resemble those of common viral infections, Lyme disease symptoms tend to persist or may occur intermittently over a period of several weeks to months.

Arthritis appears several months after infection with *B. Burgdorferi.* Slightly more than half of the people who are not treated with antibiotics develop recurrent attacks of painful and swollen joints that last a few

▼ **Clinical Signs and Symptoms of Lyme Disease**

Early infection (one or more may be present at different times during infection)
- Red rash (erythema migrans)
- Flulike symptoms (fever, headache, stiff neck, fatigue)
- Migratory musculoskeletal pain (joints, bursae, tendons, muscle, or bone)
- Neurologic symptoms:
  - Severe headache (meningitis)
  - Numbness, pain, weakness of extremities
  - Poor motor coordination
  - Cognitive dysfunction: Memory loss, difficulty in concentrating, mood changes, sleep disturbances

Less Common Symptoms
- Eye problems such as conjunctivitis
- Heart abnormalities and myocarditis

Late Infection (months to years after infection)
- Arthritis, intermittent or chronic
- Encephalopathy (mood and sleep disturbances)
- Neurocognitive dysfunction
- Peripheral neuropathy

days to a few months. About 10% to 20% of untreated clients will go on to develop chronic arthritis.

In most clients Lyme arthritis is monoarticular or oligoarticular (few joints), most commonly affecting the knee, but the arthritis can shift from one joint to another. Other large joints, such as the shoulder and elbow, are also commonly affected. Involvement of the hands and feet is uncommon, and it is these features that help differentiate Lyme arthritis from RA (Steere, 1995).

Neurologic symptoms (including cognitive dysfunction referred to as neurocognitive symptoms) may appear because Lyme disease can affect the nervous system. Symptoms include stiff neck, severe headache

Case Example. A 54-year-old business executive developed searing neck and back pain and was diagnosed as having a cervical disk protrusion. He was sent to physical therapy but had a very busy travel schedule and was unable to make even half of his scheduled appointments.

He chose to discontinue physical therapy, but his symptoms worsened and the pain became so intense that he was unable to go to work some mornings. He also started experiencing numbness in his right arm along the ulnar nerve distribution. After a lengthy trial of physical therapy, there was no discernible improvement subjectively, by client report, or objectively, as measured by functional improvement.

Anterior cervical diskectomy was performed to remove the fifth cervical disk but with no change in symptoms postoperatively. There was significant right extremity paresis, with maximal functional loss of the right hand and continued neck and back pain.

This client was eventually discharged from further physical therapy services and underwent a second surgical procedure with no improvement in his condition. A year later he telephoned the therapist to report that he had been diagnosed with Lyme disease. This man spent his vacations in the woods of Connecticut and Long Island, but this important piece of information was never gleaned from his past medical history.

Despite the lengthy time before diagnosis, the client was almost entirely recovered and ready to return to work after completing a course of antibiotics.

associated with meningitis, Bell's palsy, numbness, pain or weakness in the limbs, or poor motor coordination. Memory loss, difficulty in concentrating, mood changes, and sleep disturbances have also been associated with Lyme disease.

Nervous system involvement can develop several weeks, months, or even years following an untreated infection. These symptoms last for weeks or months and may recur.

Cardiac involvement occurs in less than 1% of the people affected by Lyme disease. Symptoms of irregular heartbeat, dizziness, and dyspnea occur several weeks after the infection and rarely last more than a few days or weeks. Recovery is usually complete.

Finally, although Lyme disease can be divided into early and later stages, each with a different set of complications, these stages may vary in duration, may overlap, or may even be absent. Clinical manifestations may first appear from 3 to 30 days after the tick bite but usually occur within 1 week.

Lyme disease is still mistaken for other ailments, including Guillain-Barré syndrome, MS, and FMS, and can be difficult to diagnose. The only distinctive hallmark unique to Lyme disease, the erythema migrans rash, is absent in at least one fourth of those who become infected. Many people are unaware that they have been bitten by a tick.

In general, the sooner treatment is initiated, the quicker and more complete the recovery, with less chance for the development of subsequent symptoms of arthritis and neurologic problems.

Following treatment for Lyme disease, some persons still have persistent fatigue and achiness, which can take months to subside. Unfortunately, a bout with Lyme disease is no guarantee that the illness will be prevented in the future. The disease can strike more than once in the same individual if she or he is reinfected with the Lyme disease bacterium.

BACTERIAL ARTHRITIS

Bacterial arthritis can be caused by a wide variety of organisms, including gonococci, staphylococci, streptococci, enterobacteria, *Pseudomonas* species, and *Haemophilus influenzae*. In most clients bacterial arthritis begins with infection, such as sinusitis, bedsores, pneumonia, or septicemia, or an abdominal or genitourinary tract infection. The bacteria travel through the bloodstream and eventually invade and infect the synovium. Occasionally, bacterial arthritis results from a penetrating injury (including arthrocentesis) or from an infection in the periarticular tissues.

Many clients with bacterial arthritis have been immunocompromised by severe illness, particularly neoplasm, or by treatment with immunosuppressive drugs such as corticosteroids or cytotoxic agents.

Chronic arthritis in any form, especially RA, predisposes the joint to bacterial arthritis. Other predisposing factors include previous joint surgery, especially if a plastic or metal prosthesis has been implanted, and injection drug abuse.

CLINICAL SIGNS AND SYMPTOMS

Bacterial arthritis is typically monoarticular, begins abruptly, and is characterized by inflammatory symptoms of pain and swelling. Symptoms progressively worsen in 12 to 48 hours. In later stages the infected

▼ *Clinical Signs and Symptoms of*
Bacterial Arthritis

- Constitutional symptoms, especially fever and chills
- Rapid onset of monoarticular (single-joint) involvement (knee, shoulders, wrist, ankle, elbow, hand [decreasing order of prevalence])
- Inflammatory symptoms: Redness, warmth, pain, swelling
- Range of motion restricted
- Skin lesions near involved joint
- Local tenosynovitis

joint is usually tender, warm, swollen, and red. Both active and passive motions are painful and almost always limited.

Large joints, particularly the knee but also the shoulder, elbow, wrist, ankle, and hip, are affected more often than the small joints of the hands and feet. Infection can occur in the spine, with poorly localized back pain as the initial symptom. The sternoclavicular and sacroiliac joints often become infected in injection drug users.

Immediate referral is necessary whenever clinical manifestations similar to bacterial arthritis are observed. Left untreated, bacterial arthritis causes cartilage and bone damage that can proceed rapidly to total joint destruction within a few weeks.

▼ PHYSICIAN REFERRAL

In most immunologic disorders, physicians must rely on the client's history and clinical findings in association with supportive information from diagnostic tests to make a differential diagnosis. Often, there are no definitive diagnostic tests, such as in the case of MS. The physician instead relies on objectively measured central nervous system abnormalities, a history of episodic exacerbations, and remissions of symptoms with progressive worsening of symptoms over time.

In the early stages of treating disorders such as MS, Guillain-Barré syndrome, and myositis, factors such as the effect of fatigue on the client's progress and fragile muscle fibers necessitate that the physical therapist keep close contact with the physician, who will use a physical examination and laboratory tests to determine the most opportune time for an exercise program. While the physician is monitoring serum enzyme levels and the overall medical status of the client, the physical therapist will continue to provide the physician with essential feedback regarding objective findings, such as muscle tenderness, muscle strength, and overall physical endurance.

A careful history and close clinical observations may elicit indications that the client

GUIDE TO PHYSICIAN REFERRAL

- See also Clues to Immune System Dysfunction on p. 392
- New onset of joint pain within 6 weeks of surgery, especially when accompanied by constitutional symptoms, rash, or skin lesions
- Development of progressive neurologic symptoms within 1 to 3 weeks of a previous infection or recent vaccination
- Evidence of spinal cord compression in anyone with cervical rheumatoid arthritis who has progressed from generalized stiffness to new onset of cervical laxity (C1-C2 subluxation or dislocation)

GUIDELINES FOR IMMEDIATE MEDICAL ATTENTION

- Anyone exhibiting signs and symptoms of anaphylactic shock (see Table 11-1)

is demonstrating signs and symptoms unrelated to a musculoskeletal disorder. Because the immune system can implicate many of the body systems, the physical therapist should not hesitate to relay to the physician any unusual findings reported or observed.

Clinical Signs and Symptoms Requiring Physician Referral

Anaphylactic reaction
Ataxia
Bowel/bladder dysfunction
Calcinosis
Change in voice
Choking, difficulty in chewing
Chronic diarrhea
Dry eyes/mouth
Dysarthria
Dysphagia
Dyspnea on exertion
Easy bruising
Enlarged lymph nodes
Fatigue
Fever, malaise
Finger ulceration
Headache
Heartburn
Hoarseness
Incoordination
Increased deep tendon reflexes
Joint inflammation
Loss of appetite
Morning stiffness
Muscle fatigue with exertion
Myalgia
Myositis (inflamed muscle)
Nausea, vomiting
Night sweats
Paresthesias
Persistent, dry cough
Polyarthralgia
Positive Babinski/clonus
Progressive dyspnea
Proximal muscle weakness
Ptosis
Raynaud's phenomenon
Recurrent influenza-like symptoms
Recurrent vaginal candidiasis
Skin rash or thickening
Sleep disturbances
Spasticity
Speech impairment
Subcutaneous nodules
Tender points
Thrush in the mouth/tongue
Vertigo
Visual disturbances (diplopia, nystagmus, scotomas)
Weight loss
Wheals

KEY POINTS TO REMEMBER

▶ Pain in the knees, hands, wrists, or elbows may indicate an autoimmune disorder; aching in the bones can be caused by expanding bone marrow.

▶ Any change in cough, pain, or fever and any change or new presentation of symptoms should be reported to the physician.

▶ Be alert to any warning signs of hypersensitivity response (allergic reaction) during therapy and be prepared to take necessary measures (e.g., graded exercise to client tolerance, control of room temperature, client use of medications).

▶ Immediate emergency procedures are required when a client has a severe allergic reaction (anaphylactic shock).

▶ For the client with Guillain-Barré syndrome, active exercise must be at a level consistent with the client's muscle strength. Overstretching and overuse of painful muscles may result in prolonged or lack of recovery.

▶ For the client with multiple sclerosis, treatment should take place in the coolest (temperature) setting possible.

▶ For the client with rheumatoid arthritis or ankylosing spondylitis, the risk of fracture from the development of atlantoaxial subluxation necessitates the use of extreme caution in treatment procedures. The most common site of fracture is the lower cervical spine.

SUBJECTIVE EXAMINATION

• SPECIAL QUESTIONS TO ASK

Signs and symptoms of immune disorders can appear in any body system. A thorough review of the Family/Personal History form, subjective interview, and appropriate follow-up questions will help the physical therapist identify signs and symptoms that are not part of a musculoskeletal pattern. Special attention should be given to the question on the Family/Personal History form concerning general health. Clients with immune disorders or immunocompromised clients often have poor general health or recurrent infections.

Past Medical History

- Have you ever been told that you had/have an immune disorder, autoimmune disease, or cancer? (Predisposes the person to other diseases)

- Have you ever received radiation treatment? (Diminishes blood cell production, predisposes to infection)

- Have you ever had an organ transplant (especially kidney) or removal of your thymus? **(Myasthenia gravis)**

Associated Signs and Symptoms

- Do you have difficulty with combing your hair; raising your arms; getting out of a bathtub, bed, or chair; or climbing stairs? **(Myasthenia gravis)**

- Do you have difficulty when raising your head from the pillow when you are lying down on your back? **(Myasthenia gravis)**

- Do you have difficulty with swallowing, or have you noticed any changes in your voice? **(Myasthenia gravis)**

- Have you noticed any changes in your skin texture or pigmentation? Do you have any skin rashes? **(Scleroderma, allergic reactions, systemic lupus erythematosus, rheumatoid arthritis, dermatomyositis, psoriatic arthritis, AIDS, Lyme disease)**

  - Have you noticed any association between the development of the skin rash and pain or swelling in any of your joints (or other symptoms)?

  - Do these other symptoms go away when the skin rash clears up?

  - Have you been exposed to ticks? For example, have you been out walking in the woods or in tall grass or in contact with pets? **(Lyme disease)**

- Have you had any recent vision problems? **(Multiple sclerosis, systemic lupus erythematosus)**

- Have you had any body tattooing or ear/body piercing done in the last 6 weeks to 6 months? **(AIDs, hepatitis)**

- Have you had any difficulties with urination, for example, a change in appearance of urine, accidents, increased frequency? **(Multiple sclerosis, myasthenia gravis, Reiter's syndrome)**

For the person with known allergies (check the Family/Personal History form):

- What are the usual symptoms that you experience in association with your allergies?

- Describe a typical allergic reaction for you.

- Do the symptoms relate to physical changes (e.g., cold, heat, or dampness)?

- Do the symptoms occur in association with activities (e.g., exercise)?

- Do you take medication for your allergies?

For the client reporting fatigue and weakness:

- Do you feel tired all the time or only after exertion?

- Do you get short of breath after mild exercise or at rest?

- How much sleep do you get at night?

- Do you take naps during the day?

- Have you ever been told by a physician that you are anemic?

- How long have you had this weakness?

- Does it come and go, or is it persistent (there all the time)?

- Are you able to perform your usual daily activities without stopping to rest or nap?

For the client with sudden onset of joint pain (Reiter's syndrome):

- Have you recently noticed any crusting, redness, or burning of your eyes?
- Have you noticed any burning when you urinate?
- Have you noticed an increase in the number of times you urinate?
- Have you had any bouts of diarrhea over the last 1 to 3 weeks (before the onset of joint pain)?

For the client with fever (fevers recurring every few days, fevers that rise and fall within 24 hours, and fevers that recur frequently should be documented and reported to the physician):

- When did you first notice this fever?
- Is it constant or does it come and go?
- Does your temperature fluctuate?

  If yes, over what period of time does this occur?

FIBROMYALGIA SYNDROME (FMS) SCREEN

1. Do you have trouble sleeping through the night?	YES	NO
2. Do you feel rested in the morning?	YES	NO
3. Are you stiff and sore in the morning?	YES	NO
4. Do you have daytime fatigue/exhaustion?	YES	NO
5. Do your muscle pain and soreness travel?	YES	NO
6. Do you have tension/migraine headaches?	YES	NO
7. Do you have irritable bowel symptoms (e.g., nausea, diarrhea, stomach cramping)?	YES	NO
8. Do you have swelling, numbness, or tingling in your arms or legs?	YES	NO
9. Are you sensitive to temperature and humidity or changes in the weather?	YES	NO

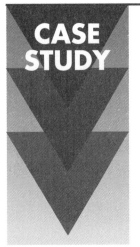

CASE STUDY

REFERRAL

A 28-year-old Hispanic man has come to you for an evaluation without a medical referral. He has seen no medical practitioner for his current symptoms, consisting of an unusual gait pattern and weakness of the lower extremities, which he noticed during the last 2 days. He speaks English with a heavy accent, making it difficult to obtain a clear medical history, but the Personal/Family History form indicates no previous or current health or medical problems of any kind. He does note that he has had influenza in the last 3 weeks but that he is fully recovered now.

PHYSICAL THERAPY INTERVIEW

Using the format outlined in the chapter on The Physical Therapy Interview (Chapter 2), begin with an open-ended question and follow up with additional appropriate questions incorporating the following:

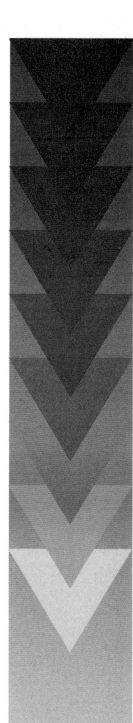

Current Symptoms

Tell me why you are here (open-ended question) . . . Or you may prefer to say, "I notice from your intake form that you have had some weakness in your legs and a change in the way you walk. What can you tell me about this?"

When did you first notice these changes?

What did you notice that made you think that something was happening?

Just before the development of these symptoms, did you injure yourself in any way that you can remember?

Did you have a car accident, fall down, or twist your trunk or hips in any unusual way?

Do you have any pain in your back, hips, or legs? If yes, follow the outline in The Physical Therapy Interview to elicit a further description.

Associated Symptoms

Have you had any numbness or tingling in your back, buttocks, or hips or down your legs?

Have you had any other changes in sensation in these areas, such as a burning or prickling feeling?

Have you had the "flu," a cold, an upper respiratory infection, or other infection recently?

Have you had a fever or elevated temperature in the last 48 hours?

Do you think that you have a temperature right now?

Have you noticed any other symptoms that I should know about?

Give the client time to answer the question. Prompt him or her if you need to with various suggestions (include any others that seem appropriate to the information and responses already given by the client), such as:

> Nausea or dizziness
>
> Diarrhea or constipation
>
> Unusual fatigue
>
> Recent headaches
>
> Choking, difficulty with chewing
>
> Shortness of breath with mild exertion (e.g., walking to the car or even at rest)
>
> Vomiting
>
> Cold sweats during the day or night
>
> Changes in vision or speech
>
> Skin rashes
>
> Joint pains

Have you noticed any other respiratory, lung, or breathing problems?

Final Question

Is there anything else you think that I should know about your current condition or general health that I have not asked yet?

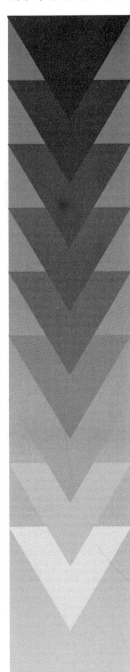

PROCEDURES TO CARRY OUT DURING THE FIRST SESSION

Given the client's report of lower extremity weakness and antalgic gait of sudden onset without precipitating cause, the following possible problems should be ruled out during the objective assessment:

Neurologic disease or disorder (immunologically based or otherwise), such as:

> Discogenic lesion
>
> Tumor
>
> Myasthenia gravis (unlikely because of the man's age)
>
> Guillain-Barré syndrome
>
> Multiple sclerosis

Other possible immunologic disorders

> AIDS dementia (unlikely from the way the history was presented)

Psychogenic disorder (e.g., hysteria, anxiety, alcoholism, or drug addiction)

Observation/Inspection

- Take the client's vital signs.
- Note any obvious changes, such as muscle atrophy, difficulty with breathing or swallowing, facial paralysis, intention tremor.
- Describe the gait pattern: Observe for ataxia, incoordination, positive Trendelenburg position, balance, patterns of muscular weakness or imbalance, other gait deviations.

Neurologic Screen

- All deep tendon reflexes
- Manual muscle testing of proximal-to-distal large muscle groups looking for a pattern of weakness
- Babinski sign and clonus
- Gross sensory screen looking for any differences in perceived sensation, proprioception, or vibration from one side to the other
- Test for dysmetria, balance, and coordination

Orthopedic Assessment

- Lower extremity range of motion (ROM): Active and passive
- Back, lower quadrant evaluation protocol (Magee, 1997)

TESTING RESULTS

In the case of this client, the interview revealed very little additional information because he denied any other associated (systemic) signs or symptoms and denied bowel/bladder dysfunction, precipitating injury or trauma, and neurologic indications such as numbness, tingling, or paresthesias. Although he was difficult to understand, the physical therapist thought that the client had understood the questions and had answered them truthfully. Subjectively, he did not appear to be a malingerer or a hysterical/anxious individual.

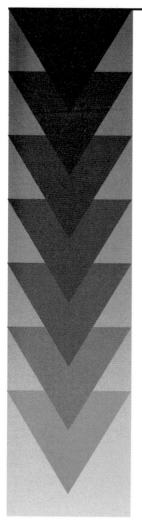

The client's gait pattern could best be described as ataxic. His lower extremities would not support him fully, and he frequently lost his balance and fell down, although he denied any pain or warning that he was about to fall.

Objective findings revealed inconsistent results of muscle testing: The proximal muscles were more involved than the distal muscles (difference of one grade: proximal muscles = fair grade; distal muscles = good grade), but repeated tests elicited alternately strong, weak, or cogwheel responses, as if the muscles were moving in a ratching motion against resistance through the ROM.

The only other positive findings were slightly diminished deep tendon reflexes of the lower extremities compared with the upper extremities, but, again, these findings were inconsistent when tested over time.

FINAL RESULTS

Because the subjective and objective examinations were so inconsistent and puzzling, the therapist asked another therapist to briefly examine this client. In turn, they decided to ask the client to return either at the end of the day or for the first appointment of the next day to reexamine him for any changes in the pattern of his symptoms. It was more convenient for him to return the next day and he did.

At that time it became clear that the therapist's difficulty in understanding the client had less to do with his use of English as a second language and more to do with an increasingly slurred speech pattern. His gait remained unchanged, but the muscle strength of the proximal pelvic muscles was consistently weak over several trials spread out during the therapy session, which lasted for 1 hour. This time the therapist checked the muscles of his upper extremities and found that the scapular muscles were also unable to move against any manual resistance. Deep tendon reflexes of the upper extremities were inconsistently diminished, and reflexes of the lower extremities were now consistently diminished.

The client was referred to a physician for further follow-up and was not treated at the physical therapy clinic that day. He was examined by his family physician, who referred him to a neurologist. A diagnosis of Guillain-Barré syndrome was confirmed when the client's symptoms progressed dramatically, requiring hospitalization.

PRACTICE QUESTIONS

1. Fibromyalgia syndrome is a:
   a. Musculoskeletal disorder
   b. Psychosomatic disorder
   c. Neurosomatic disorder
   d. Noninflammatory rheumatic disorder

2. Which of the following best describes the pattern of rheumatic joint disease?
   a. Pain and stiffness in the morning gradually improves with gentle activity and movement during the day.
   b. Pain and stiffness accelerate during the day and are worse in the evening.

c. Night pain is frequently associated with advanced structural damage associated with rheumatoid arthritis.

d. Pain is brought on by activity and resolves predictably with rest.

3. Match the following skin lesions with the associated underlying disorder (not all letter choices will be used):

a. Raised, scaly patches

b. Flat or slightly raised malar on the face

c. Petechiae

d. Tightening of the skin

e. Kaposi's sarcoma

f. Erythema migrans

g. Hives

h. Subcutaneous nodules

___ Psoriatic arthritis

___ Systemic lupus erythematosus

___ HIV infection

___ Scleroderma

4. A new client has come to you with a primary report of new onset of knee pain and swelling. Name three clues that this client might give from his medical history that should alert you to the possibility of immunologic disease.

5. A positive Schöber's test, inability to touch the occiput to the wall while standing erect, and a flattened lumbar curve in the upright position are all signs of:

a. Reiter's syndrome

b. Infectious arthritis

c. Ankylosing spondylitis

d. (a) or (b)

e. (a) or (c)

6. What is Lhermitte's sign, and what does it signify?

7. Proximal muscle weakness may be a sign of:

a. Paraneoplastic syndrome

b. Neurologic disorder

c. Myasthenia gravis

d. Scleroderma

e. (b), (c), and (d)

f. All the above

8. Which of the following skin assessment findings in the HIV-infected client would require physician referral (and possible medical diagnosis of AIDS)?

a. Darkening of the nail beds

b. Purple-red blotches or bumps on the trunk and head

c. Cyanosis of the lips and mucous membranes

d. Painful blistered lesions of the face and neck

9. The most common cause of change in mental status of the HIV-infected client is related to:

a. Meningitis

b. Alzheimer's disease

c. Space-occupying lesions

d. AIDS dementia complex

10. Symptoms of anaphylaxis that would necessitate immediate medical treatment or referral are:

a. Hives and itching

b. Vocal hoarseness, sneezing, and chest tightness

c. Periorbital edema

d. Nausea and abdominal cramping

References

Anderson RJ: Rheumatoid arthritis. B. Clinical and laboratory features. In Klippel JH, editor: *Primer on the rheumatic diseases,* ed 11, Atlanta, 1997, Arthritis Foundation, pp 161-167.

Arnett FC: Reactive arthritis (Reiter's syndrome) and enteropathic arthritis. In Klippel JH, editor: *Primer on the rheumatic diseases,* ed 11, Atlanta, 1997, Arthritis Foundation, pp 184-188.

Cash JM: Evaluation of the patient. A History and physical examination. In Klippel JH, editor: *Primer on the rheumatic diseases,* ed 11, Atlanta, 1997, Arthritis Foundation, pp 89-94.

Freundlich B, Leventhal L: Diffuse pain syndromes. In Klippel JH, editor: *Primer on the rheumatic diseases,* ed 11, Atlanta, 1997, Arthritis Foundation, pp 123-127.

Frozema C: Multiple sclerosis, *AJN* 97(11):48-49, 1997.

Gomez KS, Raza K, Jones SD et al: Juvenile onset ankylosing spondylitis: more girls than we thought? *J Rheumatol* 24(4):735-737, 1997.

Hunder GG, Kaye RL, Lane NE: Rheumatoid arthritis: progress in research and clinical management, *J Musculoskel Med* 15(11):22-35, 1998.

James JA: An increased prevalence of Epstein-Barr virus infection in young patients suggests a possible etiology for SLE, *J Clin Invest* 100(12):3019-3026, 1997.

Kimberlin DW, Whitley RJ: Human herpesvirus-6: neurologic implications of a newly-described viral pathogen, *J Neurovirol* 4(5):474-485, 1998.

Krsnich-Shriwise S: Fibromyalgia syndrome: an overview, *Phys Ther* 77(1):68-75, 1997.

Magee DJ: *Orthopedic physical assessment,* ed 3, Philadelphia, 1997, WB Saunders.

Mayne M. Krishan J, Metz L et al: Infrequent detection of human herpesvirus 6 DNA in peripheral blood mononuclear cells from multiple sclerosis patients, *Ann Neurol* 44(3):391-394, 1998.

Millott MK, Berlin RM: Treating sleep disorders in patients with fibromyalgia, *J Musculoskel Med* 14(6):25-34, 1997.

Mountz JM, Bradley LA, Modell JG et al: Fibromyalgia in women: abnormalities of regional cerebral blood flow in the thalamus and the caudate nucleus are associated with low pain threshold levels, *Arthritis Rheum* 38:926-928, 1995.

Ostensen M, Ostensen H: Ankylosing spondylitis: the female aspect, *J Rheumatol* 25(1):120-124, 1998.

Petri MA: Women and arthritis. Conference sponsored by the National Institute of Arthritis and Musculoskeletal and Skin Diseases, Washington DC, May 10, 1996.

Petri MA: Clinical challenges in SLE: moving beyond corticosteroids, *J Musculoskel Med* 14(8):64-75, 1997.

Petri MA: The effect of race on incidence and clinical course in systemic erythematosus: the Hopkins Lupus Cohort, *J Am Med Wom Assoc* 53(1):9-12, 1998.

Rudick RA, Cohen JA: Management of multiple sclerosis, *N Engl J Med* 337(22):1604-1611, 1997.

Russell LJ: Fibromyalgia syndrome: formulating a strategy for relief, *J Musculoskel Med* 15(11):4-21, 1998.

Sadovnick AD, Yee IML, Ebers GC et al: Effect of age at onset and parental disease status on sibling risks for MS, *Neurology* 50(3):719-723, 1998.

Shapiro LS: Effective intervention in scleroderma renal crisis, *J Musculoskel Med* 14(3):25-36, 1997.

Starz TW, Sinclair JD, Okifuji A et al: Putting the finger on fibromyalgia: the Manual Tender Point Survey, *J Musculoskel Med* 14(1):61-67, 1997.

Steen VD: Clinical manifestations of systemic sclerosis, *Semin Cutan Med Surg* 17(1):48-54, 1998.

Steere AC: Musculoskeletal manifestations of Lyme disease, *Am J Med* 98(suppl 4A):4A-44S, 1995.

Trapp BD, Peterson BS, Ransohoff RM et al: Axonal transection in the lesions of multiple sclerosis, *N Engl J Med* 338(5):278-285, 1998.

Tullous MW, Skerhut HEI, Story JL et al: Cauda equina syndrome of long-standing ankylosing spondylitis: case report and review of the literature, *J Neurosurg* 73:441-447, 1990.

Van Vollenhoven RF: Systemic lupus erythematosus: managing early, mild disease, *J Musculoskel Med* 13(8):24-39, 1996.

Vaughan JH: The Epstein-Barr virus and systemic lupus erythematosus, *J Clin Invest* 100(12):2939-2940, 1997.

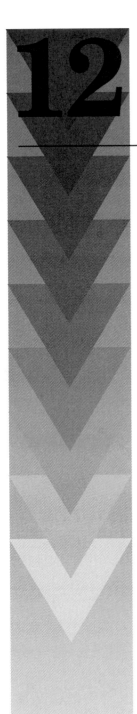

Systemic Origins of Musculoskeletal Pain

The potential for referral of pain from systemic diseases to specific muscles and joints is well documented in the medical literature. These referral patterns most often affect the back and shoulder but may also appear in the chest, thorax, hip, groin, or sacroiliac joint.

Up to this point the text has focused on each organ system and the pain or other signs and symptoms referred from organs to musculoskeletal sites. In this chapter the focus is turned around so that the reader can quickly refer to the site of presenting pain or other symptoms and determine possible systemic involvement. The physical therapist may then question the client, as suggested, and determine the possible need for a medical referral. For an in-depth discussion of the specific systemic causes of musculoskeletal signs or symptoms, the reader is referred to the individual chapters within this text.

▼ DECISION-MAKING PROCESS

As discussed in Chapter 1, four guiding parameters are used throughout this text to help physical therapists with the decision-making process. These parameters are:

- Client history
- Pain patterns/pain types
- Associated signs and symptoms of systemic diseases
- Systems review

It is essential that the physical therapist conduct a thorough interview and correlate the subjective findings with the objective findings to recognize presenting conditions that require medical follow-up.

Accordingly, the physical therapist will want to obtain the client's history, conduct a systems review, and remain familiar with types of pain, pain patterns, and signs and symptoms that may suggest systemic origins of problems appearing in the musculoskeletal system.

These guidelines for collecting and correlating subjective and objective information are suggested for any client who demonstrates one or more of the characteristics outlined in Chapter 1 (see box, When to Screen for Disease, Chapter 1, and Table 2-5).

Client History

A carefully taken, detailed medical history is the most important single element in the evaluation of a client who has musculoskeletal pain of unknown origin or cause. It is essential for the recognition of systemic disease that may be causing muscle or joint symptoms.

Symptoms are likely to appear some time before striking physical signs of disease are evident and before laboratory tests are useful to the physician in detecting disordered physiology. Thus an accurate and sufficiently detailed history provides historical clues that can be significant in determining when the client should be referred to a physician.

Pain Patterns/Pain Types

An in-depth discussion of pain patterns and pain types is presented in Chapter 1, with a corresponding Assessment of Pain and Symptoms in Chapter 2. In this chapter pain associated with each anatomic part (e.g., back, chest, shoulder, pelvis, sacrum/sacroiliac, hip, and groin) is discussed and differentiated as systemic from musculoskeletal whenever possible.

Characteristics of pain, such as onset, description, duration, pattern, aggravating and relieving factors, and associated signs and symptoms, are presented in Chapter 2 (see especially Table 2-4). Reviewing this comparison will assist the therapist in recognizing a systemic in contrast to a musculoskeletal presentation of signs and symptoms.

Associated Signs and Symptoms

After reviewing the client history and identifying pain types or pain patterns, the phys-

ical therapist must ask the client about the presence of additional signs and symptoms. Signs and symptoms associated with systemic disease are often present but go unidentified either because the client does not volunteer the information or the therapist does not ask.

Systems Review

Clusters of these associated signs and symptoms usually accompany the pathologic state of each organ system. As part of the physical therapy assessment, the therapist must conduct a review of systems. General questions about fevers, excessive weight gain or loss, and appetite loss should be followed by questions related to specific organ systems (see Systems Review chart, Chapter 1).

▼ BACK PAIN

Back pain is a symptom, not a diagnosis, but many times a specific diagnosis is impossible or unavailable. Back pain may arise in the spine from mechanical, inflammatory, metabolic, or neoplastic disorders, or it can be referred from abdominal or pelvic disease.

The therapist must be aware that many different diseases can appear as low back pain. The clues about the quality of pain, the age of the client, and the presence of systemic complaints or associated signs and symptoms indicate the need to investigate further. The history and physical therapy examination provide essential clues in determining the need for referral to a physician.

Effect of Position

Systemic back pain is not relieved by recumbency. The bone pain of metastasis or myeloma tends to be more continuous, progressive, and prominent when the client is recumbent. A history of fever and chills with or without previous infection anywhere in the body may indicate a low-grade infection. Fever in anyone taking immunosuppressants is a red-flag symptom indicating a possible underlying infection.

Beware of the client with acute backache who is unable to lie still because almost all clients with regional or nonspecific backache seek the most comfortable position (usually recumbency) and stay in that position. In contrast, persons with systemic backache move. In particular, visceral diseases, such as pancreatic neoplasm, pancreatitis, and posterior penetrating ulcers, often have a systemic backache that causes the client to curl up, sleep in a chair, or pace the floor at night.

Back pain that is unrelieved by rest or change in position, or pain that does not fit the expected mechanical or neuromusculoskeletal pattern, should serve as a red flag. When the symptoms cannot be reproduced, aggravated, or altered in any way during the examination, additional questions to screen for medical disease are indicated.

Night Pain

Long-standing night pain unaltered by positional change suggests a space-occupying lesion, such as a tumor. Systemic back pain may get worse at night, especially when caused by vertebral osteomylelitis, septic diskitis, cushing's disease, osteomalacia, primary and metastatic cancer, Paget's disease, ankylosing spondylitis, or tuberculosis (of the spine).

Age

The risk of certain diseases associated with back pain increases with advancing age; these include systemic diseases and neoplastic disorders. If a client has had a low backache for years, progressive serious disease is unlikely. However, 6 weeks to 6 months of increasing backache, often in an older client, may be a signal of lumbar metastases, especially in a person with a past history of cancer.

Associated Signs and Symptoms

When back pain is accompanied by severe or chronic pain and fever, referral to a physician is necessary. Other possible associated symptoms may include fatigue, dyspnea, sweating after only minor exertion, and GI symptoms. See Clues Suggesting Systemic Back Pain on p. 454.

Back pain accompanied by sustained morning stiffness may be caused by a spondyloarthropathy (disease of the joints of the spine). Extraarticular involvement of the eyes, skin, and GI system often accompanies spondyloarthropathy. Such symptoms present a red flag identifying clients who should be referred to a physician.

Referred pain originates in organs outside the spine that share pain innervation with areas of the lumbosacral spine. Collicky pain is associated with spasm in a hollow viscus. Severe, tearing pain with sweating and dizziness may originate from an expanding abdominal aortic aneurysm. Burning pain may originate from a duodenal ulcer (see Clues Suggesting Systemic Back Pain).

The therapist should look for clusters of signs and symptoms that may suggest involvement of a particular system. Using the Systems Review chart in chapter 1 can be very helpful in identifying systemic disease.

Classification: Sources of Back Pain

There are many ways to examine and classify back pain. In this discussion back pain is divided, first by the source of symptoms: visceral, neurogenic, vasculogenic, spondylogenic, psychogenic, and primary or secondary cancer.

Second, back pain is divided into anatomic location of symptoms: cervical, thoracic, scapular, lumbar, and sacroiliac joint/sacral.

Visceral Back Pain

Visceral back pain is not very often confused with pain originating in the spine because sufficient specific symptoms and signs are usually present to localize the problem correctly. It is the unusual presentation of systemic disease in the physical therapist's practice that will make it more difficult to recognize.

Visceral back pain is more likely to result from disease in the abdomen and pelvis than from intrathoracic disease, which usually refers pain to the neck and shoulder. Disorders of the GI, pulmonary, urologic, and gynecologic systems can cause stimulation of sensory nerves supplied by the same segments of the spinal cord, resulting in referred back pain.

Back pain associated with perforation of organs, gynecologic conditions, or gastroenterologic disease seldom mimics "typical back pain." Most often, past medical history, clinical presentation, and associated signs and symptoms will alert the physical therapist to an underlying systemic origin of musculoskeletal symptoms. Any client older than 45 with back pain, especially with insidious onset or unknown cause, must have vital signs taken, including body temperature.

Careful questioning can elicit important information that the client withheld, thinking it was irrelevant to the problem, such as low back pain alternating with abdominal pain at the same level or back pain alternating with bouts of bloody diarrhea.

Neurogenic Back Pain

Neurogenic back pain is not easily differentiated. Sciatica alone or sciatica accompanying back pain is an important but unreliable symptom. For example, diabetic neuropathy can cause nerve root irritation or prostatic metastases to the lumbar and pelvic regions, or other neoplasms of the spine can create a clinical picture that is indistinguishable from sciatica of musculoskeletal origin (Table 12-1). This similarity may lead to long and serious delays in diagnosis. Such a situation may require persistence on the part of the therapist and client in requesting further medical follow-up.

Spinal stenosis caused by a narrowing of the spinal canal, nerve root canals, or inter-vertebral foramina may produce neurogenic claudication. The canal tends to be narrow at the lumbosacral junction, and the nerve roots in the cauda equina are tightly packed. The emerging nerve root exits through a shallow lateral recess and may be compressed easily. Any combination of degenerative changes, such as disk protrusion, osteophyte formation, and ligamentous thickening, reduces the space needed for the spinal cord and its nerve roots.

Confusion with spinal stenosis syndromes may occur when atheromatous change in the internal iliac artery results in ischemia to the sciatic nerve. The subsequent sciatic pain with vascular claudication-like symptoms may go unrecognized as a vascular problem. Knowing vascular and neurogenic pain patterns, combined with careful subjective and objective examination (Table 12-2), the physical therapist may be able to recognize the need for medical intervention. This is especially true in the treatment of unusual cases of sciatica or back pain with leg pain.

The client with neurogenic back pain may develop a characteristic pattern of symptoms, with back pain, numbness, and paresthesia in the leg developing after the person walks a few hundred yards (neurogenic claudication). The person may be forced to stop walking and obtains relief after resting. The patterns of symptoms is similar to that of intermittent claudication associated with vascular insufficiency, the major differences being response to rest and position of the spine (Fig. 12-1; see Table 12-2).

The vertebral canal is wider when the spine is flexed, so relief from neurogenic pain may be obtained when the spine is flexed forward. Some individuals will squat as if to tie their shoe laces to assume a flexed spine position in public situations.

Vasculogenic Back Pain

Back pain of a vascular origin may be mistaken for those of a wide variety of musculoskeletal, neurologic, and arthritic disorders. Conversely, in a client with known vascular disease, a primary disorder that

TABLE 12-1 ▼ Causes of Sciatica

Neuromuscular Causes			Systemic/Extraspinal Causes*
Disorder	Symptoms	Physical Signs	Disorders
Diskogenic			Vascular ischemia of sciatic nerve
Disk herniation	Low back pain with radiculopathy and paravertebral muscle spasm; pain aggravated by sitting, Valsalva's maneuver, and sciatic stretch	Restricted spinal movement; restricted spinal segment; positive Lasègue's sign or straight-leg raise (SLR)	Neoplasm (primary or metastases) Diabetes (diabetic neuropathy)
Lateral entrapment syndrome (spinal stenosis)	Buttock and leg pain with radiculopathy; pain often relieved by sitting, aggravated by extension of spine	Similar to disk herniation	Megacolon Pregnancy Staphylococcal infection (e.g., bacterial endocarditis)
Nondiskogenic			Intrapelvic aneurysm (internal iliac artery)
Sacroilitis	Low back and buttock pain	Tender sacroiliac joint; positive lateral compression test; positive Patrick's test (often associated with peripheral arthritis)	Abscess
Piriformis syndrome	Low back and buttock pain with referred pain down the leg	Pain and weakness on resisted abduction/external rotation of the thigh	
Iliolumbar syndrome	Pain in iliolumbar ligament area (posterior iliac crest); referred leg pain	Tender iliac crest and increased pain with lateral or side bending	
Trochanteric bursitis	Buttock and lateral thigh pain; worse at night and with activity	Tender greater trochanter; rule out associated leg-length discrepancy	
Ischiogluteal bursitis	Buttock and posterior thigh pain; worse with sitting	Tender ischial tuberosity; positive SLR and Patrick's tests; rule out associated leg-length discrepancy	
Posterior facet syndrome	Low back pain	Lateral bending in spinal extension increases pain; side bending and rotation to the opposite side are restricted at the involved level(s)	
Fibromyalgia	Back pain, difficulty sleeping, anxiety and depression	Multiple tender points (see Fig. 11-2)	

Modified from Namey TC, An HC: Sorting out the causes of sciatica, *Mod Med* 52:132, 1984.
    *Clinical symptoms of systemic/extraspinal sciatica can be very similar to sciatica associated with disk protrusion. See also Table 12-2.

originates elsewhere may go undiagnosed (e.g., low back pain of a musculoskeletal origin, spinal cord tumor, peripheral neuritis, arthritis of the hip) because all symptoms are attributed to cardiovascular insufficiency.

Vascular back pain may be described as throbbing and almost always is increased with any activity that requires greater cardiac output and diminished or even relieved when the workload or activity is stopped. Atherosclerosis and the resulting peripheral arterial disease are the underlying causes of vascular back pain. Often the client history will reveal significant cardiovascular risk factors such a smoking, hypertension, diabetes, advancing age, or elevated serum cholesterol (see Table 3-3 and discussion of peripheral vascular disease in Chapter 3).

Peripheral arterial disease accompanied by intermittent claudication can be confused with neurogenic claudication. Intermittent claudication of a vascular origin is distinguished from other leg pain by its characteristic occurrence while walking or exercis-

TABLE 12-2 ▼ Symptoms and Differentiation of Leg Pain

	Vascular Claudication	Neurogenic Claudication	Peripheral Neuropathy	Restless Legs Syndrome
Description	Pain* is usually bilateral No burning or dysesthesia	Pain is usually bilateral but may be unilateral Burning and dysesthesia in the back, buttocks, and/or legs	Pain, aching, and numbness of feet (and hands) Motor, sensory, and autonomic changes: burning, prickling, or tingling may be present; extreme sensitivity to touch (or numbness); weakness, falling (foot drop), muscle atrophy; infection, ulcers, gangrene	Crawling, creeping sensation in legs; involuntary Involuntary contractions of calf muscles, occurring especially at night Pain† can be mild to severe, lasting seconds, minutes, or hours
Associated signs and symptoms	Decreased or absent pulses Color and skin changes in feet Normal deep tendon reflexes; may be absent in people older than 60 Sciatica possible (ischemia)	Normal pulses Good skin nutrition Depressed or absent ankle jerks Positive straight-leg raise Sciatica	Pulses may be affected, depending on underlying pathologic condition (e.g., diabetes) Deep tendon reflexes diminished or absent May have positive straight-leg raise May have sciatica	Sleep disturbance, paresthesias
Location	Usually calf first but may occur in the buttock, hip, thigh, or foot	Low back, buttock, thighs, calves, feet	Feet and hands in stocking-glove pattern	Feet, calves, legs
Aggravating factors	Pain is consistent in all spinal positions; brought on by physical exertion (e.g., walking); increased by climbing stairs or walking uphill	Increased in spinal extension Increased with walking; less painful when walking uphill	Depends on underlying cause (e.g., uncontrolled glucose levels with diabetes; progressive alcoholism)	Caffeine, pregnancy, iron deficiency
Relieving factors	Relieved promptly by standing still, sitting down, or resting (1-5 minutes)	Pain decreased by sitting, lying down, bending forward, or flexion exercises (may persist for hours)	Relieved by pain medications and relaxation techniques; treatment of underlying cause	Eliminate caffeine; increase iron intake, movement, walking, moderate exercise; medications; stretching; maintain hydration; heat or cold
Ages affected	40-60+	40-60+	Varies depending on underlying cause	Variable
Cause	Atherosclerosis in peripheral arteries	Neoplasm or abscess Disk protrusion Osteophyte formation Ligamentous thickening	More than 100 causes: diabetes; medications; accidents; nerve compression; metal toxicity; nutritional deficiency; diseases such as rheumatoid arthritis, systemic lupus erythematosus, AIDS; cancer, hypothyroidism, alcoholism	Cause unknown; may be a sleep disorder, arterial disorder, or dysautonomic disorder of the autonomic nervous system; may occur with dehydration or as a side effect of

*"Pain" associated with vascular claudication may also be described as an "aching," "cramping," or "tired" feeling.
†"Pain" associated with restless legs syndrome may not be painful but may be described as a "frantic," "unbearable," or "compelling" need to move the legs.

ing, prompt relief on rest, and the fact that a change in the position of the spine does not alter the client's symptoms (see Fig. 12-1 and Table 12-2).

The medical diagnosis is often difficult to make because vascular and neurogenic claudication occur in approximately the same age group and can coexist in the same individual.

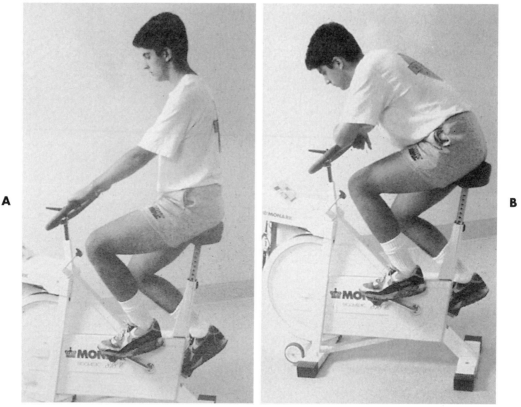

FIGURE 12-1 • Bicycle test. Assessing the underlying cause of intermittent claudication: Vascular or neurogenic? The effect of stooping over while pedaling on vascular claudication is negligible, whereas a change in spine position can aggravate or relieve claudication of a neurogenic origin. **A,** The client is seated on an exercise bicycle and asked to pedal against resistance without using the upper extremities except for support. If pain into the buttock and posterior thigh occurs, followed by tingling in the affected lower extremity, the first part of the test is positive, but whether it is vascular or neurogenic remains undetermined. **B,** While pedaling, the client leans forward. If the pain subsides over a short time, the second part of the test is positive for neurogenic claudication. The test is confirmed when the client sits upright again and the pain returns. (From Magee DJ: *Orthopedic physical assessment*, ed 2, Philadelphia, 1992, WB Saunders.)

Vascular studies and medical diagnostic testing may be required to help determine which problem dominates.

Back pain associated with abdominal aortic aneurysm is usually accompanied by a pulsating sensation or palpable abdominal pulse (see text discussion, Chapter 3). Although the underlying cause is most often atherosclerosis, the therapist should be aware that aging athletes involved in weight lifting are at risk for tears in the arterial wall, resulting in an aneurysm. There is often a history of intermittent claudi-cation and decreased or absent peripheral pulses.

The location of vasculogenic pain depends on the location of the vascular pathologic evidence (see Table 3-6). Gradual *obstruction of the aortic bifurcation* produces bilateral buttock and leg pain, weakness and fatigue of the lower extremities, atrophy of the leg musculature, absent femoral pulses, and color and temperature changes in the lower extremities.

When the pathology is in the *iliac artery*, symptoms may include pain in the low back,

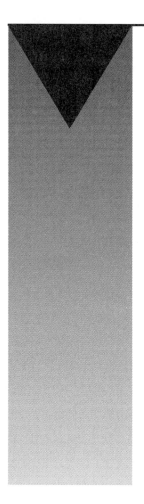

Case Example. A 73-year-old man was referred to a physical therapist by his family practitioner for evaluation of middle to low back pain that started when he stepped down from a curb. He was not experiencing radiating pain or sciatica and appeared to be in good general health. His medical history included bronchial asthma treated with oral corticosteroids and an abdominal hernia repaired surgically 10 years ago.

Vital signs were measured and appeared within normal limits for the client's age. There were no constitutional symptoms, no fever present, and no other associated signs or symptoms to suggest the presence of origin of back pain.

There was a marked decrease in thoracic and lumbar range of motion from T10 to L1 and tenderness throughout this same area. No other objective findings were noted despite a careful screening examination.

The client was treated conservatively over a 2-week period but without change in his painful symptoms and without improvement in spinal movement. A second therapist in the same clinic was consulted for a reevaluation without significant differences in findings. Several suggestions were made for alternative treatment techniques. After 2 more weeks without change in client symptoms, a medical referral was made.

Result. Radiographic testing demonstrated ischemic vertebral collapse secondary to chronic corticosteroid administration. Diffuse osteopenia and a compression fracture of the tenth thoracic vertebral body were also mentioned in the medical report. Long-term corticosteroid therapy and irradiation therapy for cancer are risk factors for ischemic or avascular necrosis. Hip or back pain in the presence of these factors should be examined carefully. In this case the client's age, lack of improvement with a variety of treatment techniques, and history of long-term corticosteroid use necessitated a return to the referring physician for further medical evaluation.

buttock, and leg of the affected side and numbness.

Involvement of the *femoral artery,* along its course or at the femoropopliteal junction, produces thigh and calf pain and pulses absent below femoral pulse.

Obstruction of the *popliteal artery* or its branches produces pain in the calf, ankle, or foot.

Spondylogenic Back Pain

Bone tenderness and pain on weight bearing usually characterize spondylogenic back pain (or the symptoms produced by bone lesions). Associated signs and symptoms may include weight loss, fever, deformity, and night pain. There are numerous conditions capable of producing bone pain, but only the most common systemic disorders that produce back pain of spondylogenic origin are included.

OSTEOPOROSIS (see also Chapter 9)

Osteoporosis has many different causes and predisposes a person to vertebral body fracture, back pain, and deformity. Senile osteoporosis is found in aging men, whereas postmenopausal osteoporosis occurs in women.

The acute pain of a compression fracture superimposed on chronic discomfort, often in the absence of a history of trauma, may be

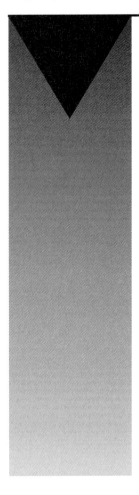

Case Example. A 68-year-old woman with a long history of degenerative arthritis of the spine was referred to physical therapy for conservative treatment toward a goal of improving function despite her painful symptoms. Her symptoms were diffuse bilateral lumbosacral back pain into the buttocks and thighs, which increased with walking or any activity and did not subside substantially with rest (except for prolonged rest and immobility).

On examination, this client moved slowly and with effort, complaining of the painful symptoms described. There was no tenderness of the sacroiliac joint or sciatic notch but a subjective report of tenderness over L4-L5 and L5-S1. There was no palpable step-off or dip of the spinous processes for spondylolisthesis and no paraspinal spasm, but a marked right lumbar scoliosis with a lateral shift to the left was noted. The client reported knowledge of scoliosis since she was a child.

A neurologic screening examination revealed normal straight-leg raise and normal sensation and reflexes in both lower extremities. Motor examination was unremarkable for an inactive 68-year-old woman. Dorsalis pedis and posterior tibialis pulses were palpable but weak bilaterally.

Despite physical therapy treatment and compliance on the part of the client with a home program, her symptoms persisted and progressively worsened. She returned to her physician with a report of these findings. Further testing showed that in addition to degenerative arthritis of the lumbrosacral spine, there was secondary stenosis and marked aortic calcification, indicting a vascular component to her symptoms.

Surgery was scheduled: an L4 to L5 laminectomy with fusion, iliac crest bone graft, and decompression foraminotomies. Postoperatively, the client subjectively reported 80% improvement in her symptoms with an improvement in function, although she was still unable to return to work.

the only presenting symptom. The client may recall a "snap" associated with mild pain, or there may have been no pain at all after the "snap." More intense pain may not develop for hours or until the next day.

Back pain over the thoracic or lumbar spine that is intensified by prolonged sitting, standing, and the Valsalva maneuver may resolve after 3 or 4 months as the fractures of the vertebral bodies heal. The pain may persist because of microfractures of biomechanical effects from deformity.

Other symptoms include pain on percussion over the fractured vertebral bodies, paraspinal muscle spasms, loss of height, and kyphoscoliosis.

OSTEOMALACIA (see also Chapter 9)

Osteomalacia is a metabolic bone disease in which the bone is weakened and vulnerable to fractures, which may produce back pain and progressive kyphoscoliosis. Osteomalacia may be caused by vitamin D deficiency, intestinal disorders, drugs, metabolic acidosis, phosphate deficiencies, renal disease, and primary and secondary mineralization defects.

Symptoms may include back pain, fractures, bone tenderness on palpation, muscle weakness, kyphoscoliosis, bowing of the lower extremities, and enlargement of the costochondral junctions.

VERTEBRAL OSTEOMYELITIS

Vertebral osteomyelitis is a bone infection most often affecting the first and second lumbar vertebrae, causing low back pain. There are many causative factors. Osteomyelitis may occur in diabetics, injection drug users (IDUs), alcoholics, clients taking corticosteroid drugs, clients with spinal cord injury and neurogenic bladder, and otherwise debilitated or immune-suppressed clients.

Osteomyelitis also can occur after surgery, open fractures, penetrating wounds, skin breakdown and ulcers, and systemic infections. *Staphylococcus aureus* is the most common causative organism. It may result from a hematogenous spread through arterial and venous routes secondary to surgically implanted hardware for internal fixation of the spine, pelvic inflammatory disease, or genitourinary tract infection.

Acute hematogenous osteomyelitis is seen most commonly in children, usually originating in the metaphysis of a long bone. Precipitating trauma is often present in the history, and well-localized, acute bone pain of 1 day to several days' duration is the primary symptom. The pain is most commonly severe enough to limit or restrict the use of the involved extremity, and fever and malaise consistent with sepsis are usual.

In the adult, usually two adjacent vertebrae and their intervening disk are involved, and the vertebral body(ies) may undergo destruction and collapse. Abscess formation may result, with possible neurologic involvement.

The most consistent clinical finding is marked local tenderness over the spinous process of the involved vertebrae with "nonspecific backache." Movement is painful, and there is marked muscular guarding of the paravertebral muscles and the hamstrings. The involved vertebrae are usually exquisitely sensitive to percussion, and pain is more severe at night. There may be no rise in temperature or abnormality in white blood cell count because generalized sepsis is not present, but an elevated erythrocyte sedimentation rate is likely.

DISK SPACE INFECTION

Disk space infection is a form of subacute osteomyelitis involving the vertebral endplates and the disk in both children and adults. Symptoms associated with postoperative disk space infection occur 2 to 8 weeks after diskectomy. Diskitis of an infectious type occurs following bacteremia secondary to urinary tract infection, with or without instrumentation (e.g., catheterization or cystoscopy).

Adults with disk space infection often complain of low back pain localized around the disk area. The pain can range from mild to "excruciating"; excruciating pain is accompanied by restricted movement and constant pain, present both day and night. The pain is usually made worse by activity, but unlike most other causes of back pain, it is *not* relieved by rest. If the condition becomes chronic, pain may radiate into the abdomen, pelvis, and lower extremities.

Physical examination may reveal localized tenderness over the involved disk space, paraspinal muscle spasm, and restricted lumbar motion. A straight-leg raise (SLR) may be positive, and fever is common.

RHEUMATIC DISEASES

Rheumatic diseases such as ankylosing spondylitis, Reiter's syndrome, psoriatic arthritis, and arthritis associated with chronic inflammatory bowel (enteropathic) disease may appear with back and sacroiliac joint pain. Clients with these diseases have a genetic predisposition to these arthropathies, which are triggered by a number of environmental factors such as trauma and infection. Each of these clinical entities has been discussed in detail in Chapter 11.

Spondyloarthropathy is characterized by morning pain that improves with activity. There is limitation of motion in all directions and tenderness over the spine and sacroiliac joints. The most significant finding in ankylosing spondylitis is that the client has night (back) pain and morning stiffness as the two major complaints, but asymmetric sacroiliac involvement with

Case Example. A 72-year-old man with leg myalgia and stabbing back pain of 2 weeks' duration was referred to physical therapy for evaluation by a rural nurse practitioner. When questioned about past medical history, the client reported a prostatectomy 22 years ago with no further problems. He was not aware of any other associated signs and symptoms but reported a recurring dermatitis that was being treated by his nurse practitioner. There were no skin lesions associated with the dermatitis present at the time of the physical therapist evaluation.

The examination revealed spasm of the thoracolumbosacral paraspinal muscles bilaterally. The client reported extreme sensitivity to palpation of the spinous processes at L3 and L4. Spinal accessory motions could not be tested because of the client's state of acute pain and immobility. Hip flexion and extension reproduced the symptoms and produced additional radiating flank pain. A straight-leg raise (SLR) caused severe back pain with each leg at 30 degrees on both sides. A neurologic examination was otherwise within normal limits. Vital signs were taken: blood pressure = 180/100 mm Hg; heart rate = 100 beats/min; temperature = 101° F.

Result. Although the client was treated locally to modulate the painful symptoms, the therapist contacted the nurse practitioner by telephone to report the findings, especially the vital signs and results of the SLR. It was determined that the client needed a medical evaluation, and he was referred to a physician's center in the nearest available city. A summary of findings from the physical therapist was sent with the client along with a request for a copy of the physician's report.

The client returned to the physical therapist's clinic with a copy of the physician's report with the following diagnosis: *Clostridium perfringens* septic diskitis (made on the basis of blood culture). The prescribed treatment was intravenous antibiotic therapy for 6 weeks, progressive mobilization, and a spinal brace to be provided and fitted by the physical therapist. The client's back pain subsided gradually over the next 2 weeks, and he was followed up at intervals until he was weaned from the brace and resumed normal activities.

Septic diskitis may occur following various invasive procedures, or it may be related to occult infections, urinary tract infections, septicemia, and dermatitis. Contact dermatitis was the most likely underlying cause in this case.

radiation into the buttock and thigh can occur.

In addition to back pain, these rheumatic diseases usually include a constellation of associated signs and symptoms, such as fever, skin lesions, anorexia, and weight loss, that alert the physical therapist to the presence of systemic disease.

Polymyalgia rheumatica and fibromyalgia syndrome are muscle syndromes associated with lumbosacral pain. Fibromyalgia syndrome refers to a syndrome of pain and stiffness that can occur in the back with localized tender areas. Both these disorders are also discussed in Chapter 11.

HYPERCORTISOLISM

Cushing's syndrome, or hypercortisolism, results from overactivity of the adrenal gland, with consequent hypersecretion of glucocorticoids. Iatrogenic Cushing's syndrome, another form of this disorder, results from exogenous administration of synthetic glucocorticoids in supraphysiologic amounts.

Although it is a relatively rare condition, it can cause demineralization of bone; in severe cases this may lead to pathologic fractures. More commonly, wedging of the vertebrae, kyphosis, bone pain, and back pain secondary to bone loss occur.

Psychogenic Back Pain*

Psychogenic back pain is observed in the hysterical client or in the client who has extreme anxiety that increases the person's perception of pain. The hysterical client has severe pain as a product of inadequate defense mechanisms or severe anxiety. The anxiety leads to muscle tension, more anxiety, and then to muscle spasm. In either situation, look for bizarre signs, such as:

- Paraplegia with only stocking-glove anesthesia
- Reflexes inconsistent with the presenting problem or other symptoms present
- Cogwheel motion of muscles for weakness
- SLR in the sitting versus the supine position (person is unable to complete SLR in supine but can easily perform an SLR in a sitting position)
- SLR supine with plantar flexion instead of dorsiflexion reproduces symptoms

Primary or Secondary Cancer

Spinal malignancy involves the lumbar spine more often than the cervical spine and is usually metastatic from breast, lung, prostate, or kidney neoplasm, rather than from primary spinal tumors. Multiple myeloma is the most common primary malignancy involving the spine, often resulting in diffuse osteoporosis.

Prompt identification of malignancy is important, starting with a knowledge of previous cancers. Early recognition and treatment does not always improve prognosis for survival from metastatic cancer, but it does reduce the risk of cord compression and paraplegia. It is important to remember that the history can be misleading. For example, almost 50% of clients with back pain from a malignancy have an identifiable (or attributable) antecedent injury or trauma (Mazanec et al,1993).

Key findings from the history are age older than 50, significant recent weight loss, previous malignancy, and constant pain that is not relieved by positional change or rest and is present at night, disturbing the person's sleep.

For example, in multiple myeloma pain is not relieved while the person is supine (this must be differentiated from vertebral compression fractures). Back pain associated with malignant retroperitoneal lymphadenopathy from lymphomas or testicular cancers is characterized as persistent, poorly localized low back pain present at night but relieved by forward flexion. Pain may be so excruciating while lying down that the person can sleep only while sitting in a chair hunched forward over a table.

Red flags requiring medical evaluation or reevaluation include back pain or symptoms that are not improving as expected, steady pain irrespective of activity, symptoms that are increasing, or the development of new or progressive neurologic deficits, such as weakness, sensory loss, reflex changes, bowel or bladder dysfunction, or myelopathy. The erythrocyte sedimentation rate, serum calcium level, and alkaline phosphatase level are usually elevated if cancer is present (Mazanec, 1996).

Neoplasm (whether primary or secondary) may interfere with the sympathetic nerves; if so, the foot on the affected side is warmer than the foot on the unaffected side. Paresis in the absence of nerve root pain suggests a tumor. Severe weakness without pain is very suggestive of spinal metastases. Gross muscle weakness with a full range of straight leg raise (SLR) and without a

---

*See also Psychologic Factors in Pain Assessment, Chapter 1.

history of recent acute sciatica at the upper two lumbar levels is also suggestive of spinal metastases.

A short period of increasing central backache in an older person is always a red-flag symptom. The pain spreads down both lower limbs in a distribution that does not correspond with any one nerve root level. Bilateral sciatica then develops, and the back pain becomes worse.

Classification: Location of Back Pain

After a view of back pain classified as to its source or origin and symptomatic presentation, back pain will be addressed as it presents itself anatomically.

Cervical Pain

Pain in the neck, shoulder, and arm may be caused by a local biomechanical dysfunction or a systemic disorder. Referred pain of a systemic origin may occur from infectious disease, such as vertebral osteomyelitis, or from cancer, cardiac, pulmonary, or abdominal disorders (Table 12-3).

CANCER

Cervical bone or spinal cord tumors may be primary (rare) or, more often, metastatic lesions. Persistent, local neck pain of unknown cause, with or without neurologic signs and symptoms, should be cause to screen for medical disease. Severe, constant pain, especially night pain that is not relieved by rest or change of position, is a red flag.

Occipital headache may accompany the neck pain, and there may be a palpable external mass anywhere in the neck or upper torso regions. Any time that urinary incontinence occurs with the onset of cervical pain, spinal cord compression must be considered and a medical referral is required (see Spinal Cord Tumors, Chapter 10).

Anterior and cervical pain should always be assessed for gastrointestinal (GI)-associated signs and symptoms (including eating disorders involving chronic vomiting), with palpation done during swallowing. Difficulty swallowing may be due to vertebral subluxation, osteophyte projection, disk protrusion into the esophagus or pharynx, or soft-tissue swelling in the throat (including neoplasm) (see Clues to screening for Cancer, Chapter 10).

CARDIAC CONDITIONS

Angina may cause chest pain radiating to the anterior neck and jaw, sometimes appearing only as neck and/or jaw pain and misdiagnosed as temporomandibular joint (TMJ) dysfunction. Postmenopausal women who are not taking hormonal replacement therapy are the most likely candidates for this type of presentation. Angina and/or myocardial infarction can appear as isolated midthoracic back pain in men or women (see Figs. 3-8 and 3-9) or as arm and shoulder pain that can be misdiagnosed as arthritis or other musculoskeletal pathologic conditions (see discussion of shoulder pain in this chapter).

PULMONARY CONDITIONS

Pancoast's tumors of the lung may invade the roots of the brachial plexus as they enlarge, appearing as pain in the C8 to T1 region. Other signs may include wasting of the muscles of the hand and/or Horner's syndrome with unilateral constricted pupil, ptosis, and loss of facial sweating (see Lung Cancer, Chapter 4).

Tracheobronchial irritation can cause pain to be referred to sites in the neck or anterior chest at the same levels as the points of irritation in the air passages (see Fig. 4-1). This irritation may be caused by inflammatory lesions, irritating foreign materials, or cancerous tumors.

Assessing for associated signs and symptoms will usually bring to light important red flags to assist the physical therapist in recognizing an underlying pulmonary problem. Neck pain that is reproduced or increased with inspiratory movements or accompanied by

TABLE 12-3 ▼ Viscerogenic Causes of Neck and Back Pain

	Cervical	Thoracic/Scapular	Lumbar	Sacroiliac/Sacral
Cancer	Metastatic lesions (leukemia, Hodgkin's disease) Cervical bone tumors Cervical cord tumors Lung cancer Esophageal cancer	Mediastinal tumors Metastatic extension Pancreatic cancer	Metastatic lesions Prostate cancer Testicular cancer Pancreatic cancer	Metastatic lesions Prostate cancer
Cardiac	Angina Myocardial infarction	Angina Myocardial infarction Aortic aneurysm	Abdominal aortic aneurysm Endocarditis	Endocarditis

Pulmonary	Pancoast's tumor
	Tracheobronchial irritation
		Pleuropulmonary disorders
		  Respiratory viral infection
		  Empyema
		  Pleurisy
		  Pneumothorax		

Renal		Acute pyelonephritis
		Kidney disease
			Kidney disorders
			  Acute pyelonephritis
			  Perinephritic abscess
			  Nephrolithiasis
			  Ureteral colic
			  Urinary tract infection	

Gastrointestinal*	Esophagitis
	Esophageal cancer
		Esophagitis (severe)
		Esophageal spasm
		Peptic ulcer
		Acute cholecystitis
		Biliary colic
		Pancreatic disease
			Small intestine
			  Obstruction (neoplasm)
			  Irritable bowel syndrome
			  Crohn's disease
			Pancreatic disease
				Ulcerative colitis
				Colon cancer
				Irritable bowel syndrome
				Crohn's disease

Gynecologic			Gynecologic disorders	Gynecologic disorders

Other	Vertebral osteomyelitis
	Retropharyngeal abscess
		Acromegaly	Spinal tuberculosis (rare)	Spondyloarthopathy
				  Ankylosing spondylitis
				  Reiter's syndrome
				  Psoriatic arthritis
				  Inflammatory bowel (IBD) arthritis
				Paget's disease

*Although these systems are anatomically separate, because of the interrelationship between gastrointestinal, hepatic, and biliary systems, disorders associated with any of these systems are consolidated under gastrointestinal.

dyspnea, persistent cough, hemoptysis, or constitutional symptoms requires further screening assessment. See Clues to Pulmonary Symptoms, Chapter 4.

GASTROINTESTINAL CONDITIONS

Esophageal pain may occur in the anterior neck, usually with a burning sensation ("heartburn") or other symptoms related to eating or swallowing (e.g., dysphagia, odynophagia). Clients with eating disorders who repeatedly binge and then purge by vomiting may report anterior neck pain without realizing the correlation between eating behaviors and symptoms. Esophageal varices associated with chronic alcoholism may appear as anterior neck pain but usually occur at the xiphoid process and are recognized as heartburn.

When assessing neck pain, the therapist should look for other associated signs and symptoms, such as sore throat; pain that is relieved with antacids, the upright position, fluids, or avoidance of eating; and pain that is aggravated by eating, bending, or recumbency. See Clues to Screening for Gastrointestinal Disease, Chapter 6.

Certain types of drugs (e.g., antidepressants, antihypertensives, asthma medications) can make swallowing difficult, requiring a careful evaluation during the client interview.

Thoracic Pain

Systemic origins of musculoskeletal pain in the thoracic spine (see Tables 12-3 and 12-4) are usually accompanied by constitutional symptoms and other associated symptoms. Often these additional symptoms develop after the initial onset of back pain, and the client may not relate them to the back pain and therefore may fail to mention them.

The close proximity of the thoracic spine to the chest and respiratory organs requires careful screening for pleuropulmonary symptoms in anyone with back pain of unknown cause or past medical history of cancer or chronic pulmonary problems. Thoracic pain can also be referred from the kidney, biliary duct, esophagus, stomach, gallbladder, pancreas, and heart.

CANCER

Tumors occur most often in the thoracic spine because of its length, the proximity to the mediastinum, and direct metastatic extension from lymph nodes with lymphoma, breast, or lung cancer. The client may report symptoms typical of cancer.

Tumor involvement in the thoracic spine may produce ischemic damage to the spinal cord or early cord compression since the ratio of canal diameter to cord size is small, resulting in rapid deterioration of neurologic status.

CARDIAC CONDITIONS

Thoracic aortic aneurysm, angina, or acute myocardial infarction are the most likely cardiac causes of thoracic back pain. Usually, there is a cardiac history and associated signs and symptoms, such as weak or thready pulse, extremely high or extremely low blood pressure, or unexplained perspiration and pallor.

TABLE 12-4 ▼ Location of Systemic Thoracic/Scapular Pain

Systemic Origin	Location
Cardiac	
Myocardial infarct	Midthoracic spine
Pulmonary	
Basilar pneumonia	Right upper back
Empyema	Scapula
Pleurisy	Scapula
Pneumothorax	Ipsilateral scapula
Renal	
Acute pyelonephritis	Costovertebral angle (posteriorly)
Gastrointestinal	
Esophagitis	Midback between scapulae
Peptic ulcer: stomach/duodenal	Sixth through tenth thoracic vertebrae
Gallbladder disease	Midback between scapulae; right upper scapula or subscapular area
Biliary colic	Right upper back; midback between scapulae; right interscapular or subscapular areas
Pancreatic carcinoma	Midthoracic or lumbar spine
Other	
Acromegaly	Midthoracic or lumbar spine

In the case of *abdominal aortic aneurysm* with low thoracic back pain, the client may describe a pulsating sensation in the abdomen. The therapist will detect a corresponding palpable abdominal pulse (see Aneurysm, Chapter 3).

PULMONARY CONDITIONS

Although reproducing pain or increased pain on respiratory movements is considered a hallmark sign of pulmonary involvement, symptoms of pleural, intercostal, muscular, costal, and dural origin all increase with coughing or deep inspiration. Only pain of a cardiac origin is ruled out when symptoms increase in association with respiratory movements. For this reason the therapist must always carefully correlate clinical presentation with client history and associated signs and symptoms when assessing for pulmonary disease (see Clues to Screening for Pulmonary Disease, Chapter 4).

RENAL CONDITIONS

Acute pyelonephritis (see Fig. 7-4) and other kidney conditions appear with aching pain at one or several costovertebral areas, posteriorly, just lateral to the muscles at T12 to L1, from acute distension of the capsule of the kidney. The pain is usually dull and constant, with possible radiation to the pelvic crest or groin. The client may describe febrile chills, frequent urination, hematuria, and shoulder pain (if the diaphragm is irritated). Percussion to the flank areas reveals tenderness; the therapist should perform Murphy's percussion test (see Fig. 7-5).

GASTROINTESTINAL CONDITIONS

Severe esophagitis (see Fig. 6-8) may refer pain to the thoracic spine. This pain is usually accompanied by epigastric pain and heartburn. As with cervical pain of GI origin, there may be a history of alcoholism with esophageal varices or an underlying eating disorder.

The pain of *peptic ulcer* (see Fig. 6-9) occasionally occurs only in the midthoracic back between T6 and T10, either at the midline or immediately to one side or the other of the spine. Posterior penetration of the retroperitoneum with blood loss and resultant referred thoracic pain is most often caused by long-term use of nonsteroidal antiinflammatory drugs (NSAIDs). The therapist should look for a correlation between symptoms and the timing of meals, as well as the presence of blood in the feces or relief of symptoms with antacids.

Acute cholecystitis (gallbladder infection), *biliary colic,* or *pancreatic disease* (see Fig. 8-2) may refer intense, sudden, paroxysmal pain to the right upper quadrant of the back. There may be pain in the right shoulder, right scapula, or interscapular or subscapular areas. The therapist should be observant for any report of fever and chills, nausea and indigestion, changes in urine or stool, or signs of jaundice.

Scapular Pain

Most causes of scapular pain occur along the vertebral border and result from various primary musculoskeletal lesions. However, cardiac, pulmonary, renal, and GI disorders can cause scapular pain.

Specific questions to rule out potential systemic origin of symptoms are listed in each individual chapter. For example, if the client reports any renal involvement, the therapist can use the questions at the end of Chapter 7 to assess further for medical disease. Renal and cardiac causes of scapular pain are not discussed further in this section (see previous section, Thoracic Pain).

PULMONARY CONDITIONS

Respiratory viral infections, empyema, pleurisy, or pneumothorax all can cause scapular pain. Clients with these respiratory origins of pain usually also show signs of general malaise and associated symptoms related to the pulmonary system (e.g., dyspnea, cough, hemoptysis, tachypnea, cyanosis). Respiratory movements usually aggravate painful symptoms. In the case of pneumothorax, sitting upright is the only comfortable position.

GASTROINTESTINAL CONDITIONS

Gallbladder disease and biliary colic from other causes may also refer pain to the interscapular or right subscapular area (see Fig. 8-2). The client may not associate GI symptoms with the scapular pain or discomfort. The therapist can use specific questions to rule out potential GI problems (see Special Questions to Ask, Chapter 6).

Lumbar Pain (Low Back Pain)
(see Tables 12-2 and 12-5)

CANCER

Metastatic lesions affecting the lumbar spine occur most commonly from breast, lung, prostate, kidney, or GI cancer and from myelomas and lymphomas. The high frequency of metastatic involvement of the spine may be due to tumor spread via the paravertebral venous plexus. This thin-walled and valveless venous system probably accounts for the higher incidence of metastases in the thoracic spine from breast carcinoma and in the lumbar region from prostatic carcinoma.

Prostate cancer is the second most common cancer among men and is often diagnosed when the man seeks medical assistance because of symptoms of urinary obstruction or sciatica. The sciatic pain affects the low back, hip, and leg and is caused by metastasis to the bones of the pelvis, lumbar spine, or femur. Associated symptoms may include melena, sudden moderate-to-high fever, chills, and changes in bowel or bladder function. Men who have reached the fifth decade or more are most commonly affected.

Testicular cancer represents the most common malignancy in men from ages 15 to 35. It is the second most common malignancy from ages 35 to 39. The usual presentation of testicular cancer is a painless swelling nodule in one gonad, noted incidentally by the client or his sexual partner. This is described as a lump or hardness of the testis, with occasional heaviness or a dull, aching sensation in the lower abdomen or scrotum. Acute pain is the presenting symptoms in about 10% of affected men.

Involvement of the epididymis or spermatic cord may lead to pelvic or inguinal lymph node metastases, although most tumors confined to the testis itself will spread

---

TABLE 12-5 ▼ Low Back Pain: Symptoms and Causes

Symptom	Possible Cause
Night pain unrelieved by rest or position change	Tumor
Fever, chills, sweats	Infection
Unremitting, throbbing lumbar pain	Aortic aneurysm
Abdominal pain radiating to midback	Pancreatitis, gastrointestinal disease, peptic ulcer
Morning stiffness that improves as day goes on	Inflammatory arthritis
Leg pain increased by walking and relieved by standing	Vascular claudication
Leg pain increased by walking, unaffected by standing, but relieved by sitting	Neurogenic claudication
"Stocking-glove" numbness	Referred pain, nonorganic pain
Global pain	Nonorganic pain
Long-standing back pain aggravated by activity	Deconditioning
Pain increased by sitting	Discogenic disease
Sharp, narrow band of pain radiating below the knee	Herniated disk
Chronic spinal pain (unsatisfying job/home life)	Stress
Back pain dating to specific injury	Strain or sprain
Back pain in athletic teenager	Epiphysitis, juvenile diskogenic disease, spondylolysis, or spondylolisthesis

Modified from Nelson BW: A rational approach to the treatment of low back pain, *J Musculoskel Med* 10(5):75, 1993.

primarily to the retroperitoneal lymph nodes. Subsequent cephalad drainage may be to the thoracic duct and supraclavicular nodes. Hematogenous spread to the lungs, bone, or liver may occur as a result of direct tumor invasion.

In about 10% of affected individuals, dissemination along these pathways results in thoracic, lumbar, supraclavicular, neck, or shoulder pain or mass as the first symptom. Other symptoms related to this pathway of dissemination may include respiratory symptoms or GI disturbance.

As discussed earlier, pain caused by neoplasm is typically progressive, is more pronounced at night, and may not have a clear association with activity level (as is more characteristic of mechanical back pain).

The usual progression of symptoms in clients with cord compression is back pain followed by radicular pain, lower extremity weakness, sensory loss, and, finally, loss of sphincter (bowel and bladder) control.

CARDIAC CONDITIONS

On occasion, an *abdominal aortic aneurysm* (see Fig. 3-10) can cause severe back pain. Prompt medical attention is imperative because rupture can result in death. The clients are usually men in the sixth or seventh decade of life who have a deep, boring pain in the midlumbar region.

Other historical clues of coronary disease or intermittent claudication of the lower extremities may be present. An objective examination may reveal a pulsing abdominal mass. Peripheral pulses may be diminished or absent.

Bacterial endocarditis frequently appears initially with musculoskeletal symptoms, including arthralgia, arthritis, low back pain, and myalgias. Half of these clients will have only musculoskeletal symptoms, without other signs of endocarditis. The early onset of joint pain and myalgia is more likely if the client is older and has had a previously diagnosed heart murmur or prosthetic valve.

Almost one third of clients with bacterial endocarditis have low back pain. In many persons it is the principal musculoskeletal symptom reported. Back pain is accompanied by decreased range of motion and spinal tenderness. Pain may affect only one side, and it may be limited to the paraspinal muscles.

Endocarditis-induced low back pain may be very similar to that associated with a herniated lumbar disk: it radiates to the leg and may be accentuated by raising the leg, coughing, or sneezing. The key difference is that neurologic deficits are usually absent in clients with bacterial endocarditis.

RENAL CONDITIONS

Kidney disorders such as acute pyelonephritis and perinephric abscess of the kidney may be confused with a back condition. Most renal and urologic conditions appear with a combination of systemic signs and symptoms accompanied by pelvic, flank, or low back pain. The client may have a history of recent trauma or a past medical history of urinary tract infections to alert the clinician to a possible renal origin of symptoms.

In *pyelonephritis,* an aching pain is noted in one or both costovertebral areas (see Fig. 7-4). The client usually has a fever and shaking chills, and the flank areas are tender to percussion.

Nephrolithiasis (kidney stones) may appear as back pain radiating to the flank or the iliac crest (see Fig. 7-4). Kidney stones may occur in the presence of diseases associated with hypercalcemia (excess calcium in the blood), such as hyperparathyroidism, metastatic carcinoma, multiple myeloma, senile osteoporosis, specific renal tubular disease, hyperthyroidism, and Cushing's disease. Other conditions associated with calculus formation are infection, urinary stasis, dehydration, and excessive ingestion or absorption of calcium.

Ureteral colic, caused by passage of a kidney stone (calculus), appears as excruciating pain that radiates down the course of the ureter into the urethra or groin area. These attacks are intermittent and may be accompanied by nausea, vomiting, sweating, and tachycardia. Localized abdominal muscle spasm may be present. The urine usually contains erythrocytes or is grossly bloody.

Urinary tract infection affecting the lower urinary tract is related directly to irritation of the bladder and urethra. The intensity of symptoms depends on the severity of the infection. Although low back pain may be the client's chief complaint, further questioning usually elicits additional urologic symptoms, such as urinary frequency, urinary urgency, dysuria, or hematuria. Clients can be asymptomatic with regard to urologic symptoms, making the physical therapy diagnosis more difficult.

GASTROINTESTINAL CONDITIONS

Actue pancreatitis may appear as epigastric pain radiating into the middle to low back in the region of L1 (see Fig. 6-12). Pain from the head of the pancreas is felt to the right of the spine, whereas pain from the body and tail is perceived to the left of the spine.

Associated symptoms, which are usually GI-related, may include diarrhea, anorexia, pain after a meal, and unexplained weight loss. The pain is relieved initially by heat, which decreases muscular tension, and may be relieved by leaning forward, sitting up, or lying motionless. The therapist should remain alert for the client with low back pain who seems to benefit from heat modalities but then suddenly gets worse and does not improve with physical therapy treatment.

Diseases of the small intestine (e.g., Crohn's disease, irritable bowel syndrome, obstruction from neoplasm) usually produce abdominal pain, but the pain may be referred to the back if the stimulus is sufficiently intense or if the individual's pain threshold is low (see Fig. 6-10). The abdominal pain may be alternating with episodes of back pain, but since both do not occur together, the client does not recognize the relationship. There will almost always be accompanying GI symptoms to alert the careful examiner.

GYNECOLOGIC CONDITIONS

Gynecologic disorders can cause midpelvic or low back pain and discomfort (see also Pelvic Pain in this chapter). The woman (most often between the ages 20 and 45) may have sharp, bilateral, and cramping pain in the lower quadrants. Menstrual pain can be referred to the rectum, lower sacrum, or coccyx. Tumors, masses, or even endometriosis may involve the sacral plexus or its branches, causing severe, burning pain.

Gynecologic conditions causing back pain can include retroversion (tipping back) of the uterus, ovarian cysts, uterine fibroids, endometriosis, pelvic inflammatory disease, cystocele (herniation of the bladder into the vagina), rectocele (herniation of part of the rectum into the vagina), or normal pregnancy.

Usually, there is a history of a chronic or long-standing gynecologic disorder, and the association between back pain and gynecologic disorder has been established. There may be a history of sexual assault, incest, sexually transmitted disease, ectopic preg-

▼ *Associated Signs and Symptoms of* **Gynecologic Disorders**

- Missed menses, irregular menses, history of menstrual disturbances
- Tender breasts
- Nausea, vomiting
- Chronic constipation (with laxative and enema dependency)
- Pain on defecation
- Fever, night sweats, chills
- History of vaginal discharge
- Abnormal uterine bleeding
  - Late menstrual periods with persistent bleeding
  - Irregular, longer, heavier menstrual periods, no specific pattern
  - Any postmenopausal bleeding

nancy, use of an intrauterine contraceptive device, dysuria, or a recent abortion. With a cystocele or rectocele, there may be a history of multiparity (two or more pregnancies resulting in live offspring), prolonged labor, instrument (e.g., forceps) delivery, chronic cough, or lifting heavy objects.

Gynecologic-related back pain can be confused with ruptured appendix, ectopic pregnancy, or perforation of GI abscesses. For this reason back pain accompanied by pelvic pain or correlated with menses requires a gynecologic/obstetric examination before physical therapy treatment begins.

Whenever there is an absence of objective musculoskeletal findings, a history of gynecologic involvement, or associated signs and symptoms of gynecologic disorders, the physical therapist is encouraged to ask appropriate questions to determine the need for a gynecologic evaluation (see Special Questions for Women, Chapter 2).

Sacroiliac Joint/Sacral Pain
(see Table 12-2)

The most common clinical presentation of sacroiliac pain is in a person who has had a memorable *physical event* that initiated the pain, such as a misstep off a curb, anal intercourse, lifting of a heavy object in a twisted position, or childbirth, possibly because of the relationship of birthing positions to pelvic/low back/sacral pain. The person usually experiences severe pain over the posterior sacroiliac joint and medial buttock, with some distal referral.

The most typical pain referral patterns of *systemic disease* to the sacrum and sacroiliac joint include endocarditis, prostate cancer, gynecologic disorders, rheumatic diseases that target the sacroiliac area (e.g., spondyloarthropathies), and Paget's disease.

Disorders of the large intestine and colon, such as ulcerative colitis, Crohn's disease (regional enteritis), carcinoma of the colon, and the irritable bowel syndrome, can refer pain to the sacrum when the rectum is stimulated. Similarly, the pain is reduced or relieved after the person passes gas or completes a bowel

movement. It may be appropriate to ask a client: "Is your pain relieved by passing gas or having a bowel movement?"

Most commonly, unless pain causes muscle spasm, splinting, and subsequent biomechanical changes, affected clients demonstrate a remarkable lack of objective findings to implicate the sacroiliac joint or sacrum as the causative factor in the symptoms presented.

Sacral pain in the absence of history of trauma or overuse is a clue to the presentation of systemic backache. Pain elicited by pressing on the sacrum with the client in a prone position suggests sacroiliitis (inflammation of the sacroiliac joint).

The principles guiding evaluation of sacroiliac joint and/or sacral pain are consistent with the information presented throughout this text and, in particular, in this section on back pain (see also Clues Suggesting Systemic Back Pain). Each of the disorders listed in Table 12-3 usually has its own unique systemic presentation, with clues available in the past medical history and presence of associated signs and symptoms.

▼ HIP PAIN

The physical therapist is well acquainted with hip pain as a result of regional neuromuscular or musculoskeletal disorders. Regional pain can be referred to the hip from the low back, sacroiliac joint, sacrum, or knee. Overlying soft tissue structures such as femoral hernia, bursitis, or fasciitis; muscle impairments such as weakness, loss of flexibility, hypertonus or hypotonus, strain, sprain, or tears; peripheral nerve injury or entrapment, including meralgia paresthetic, can also cause localized hip pain.

Hip pain from the upper lumbar vertebrae can refer pain into the anterior aspect of the thigh, whereas hip pain from the lower lumbar vertebrae and sacrum is usually felt in the gluteal region, with radiation down the back or outer aspect of the thigh.

CLUES SUGGESTING SYSTEMIC BACK PAIN

GENERAL

- Age younger than 20 and older than 45 with no history of a precipitating event
- Nocturnal back pain
- Pain that causes constant movement or makes the client curl up in the sitting position
- Back pain with constitutional symptoms: fatigue, nausea, vomiting, diarrhea, fever, sweats
- Back pain accompanied by unexplained weight loss
- Back pain accompanied by extreme weakness in the leg(s), numbness in the groin or rectum, or difficulty controlling bowel or bladder function (cauda equina syndrome)
- Back pain that is insidious in onset and progression (remember to assess for unreported sexual assault or physical abuse)
- Sacral pain in the absence of history of trauma (e.g., falls, assault, or anal intercourse) or overuse
- Back pain that is unrelieved by recumbency
- Back pain that does not vary with exertion or activity
- Back pain that is relieved by sitting up and leaning forward (pancreas)
- Back pain that is accompanied by multiple joint involvement (gastrointestinal, rheumatoid arthritis, fibromyalgia) or by sustained morning stiffness (spondyloarthropathy)
- Severe, persistent back pain with full and painless movement of the spine
- *(For women):* Sudden, localized back pain that does not diminish in 10 days to 2 weeks in postmenopausal women who are not taking hormone replacement therapy (osteoporosis with compression fracture)

PAST MEDICAL HISTORY

- Previous history of cancer, Crohn's disease, or bowel obstruction
- Long-term use of nonsteroidal antiinflammatory drugs (gastrointestinal bleeding), steroids, or immunosuppressants (infectious cause)
- Recent history or previous history of recurrent upper respiratory infection or pneumonia
- Recent history of surgery, especially back pain 2 to 8 weeks after diskectomy (disk space infection)
- History of osteoporosis and/or previous vertebral compression fracture(s)
- History of heart murmur or prosthetic valve in an older client who currently has low back pain of unknown cause (bacterial endocarditis)
- History of intermittent claudication and heart disease in a man with deep midlumbar back pain; assess for pulsing abdominal mass (abdominal aortic aneurysm)
- History of diseases associated with hypercalcemia, such as hyperparathyroidism, multiple myeloma, senile osteoporosis, hyperthyroidism, Cushing's disease, or specific renal tubular disease not appearing with back pain radiating to the flank or iliac crest (kidney stone)

GASTROINTESTINAL

- Back and abdominal pain at the same level (may occur simultaneously or alternately); check for gastrointestinal history or associated signs and symptoms
- Back pain with abdominal pain at a lower level than the back pain; look for its source in the back
- Back pain associated with meals (increase or decrease in symptoms)
- Back pain accompanied by heartburn or relieved by antacids

CLUES SUGGESTING SYSTEMIC BACK PAIN cont'd

- Associated signs and symptoms (dysphagia, odynophagia, melena, early satiety with weight loss, tenderness over McBurney's point, positive iliopsoas or obturator sign, bloody diarrhea)
- Sacral pain occurs when the rectum is stimulated, such as during a bowel movement or when passing gas and relieved after each of these events

PULMONARY

- Associated signs and symptoms (dyspnea, persistent cough, fever and chills)
- Back pain is aggravated by respiratory movements (deep breathing, laughing, coughing)
- Back pain is relieved by breath holding or Valsalva maneuver
- Autosplinting by lying on the involved side or holding firm pillow against the chest/abdomen decreases the pain
- Spinal/trunk movements (e.g., trunk rotation, trunk side bending) do not reproduce symptoms (exception; an intercostal tear caused by forceful coughing from underlying diaphragmatic pleurisy can result in painful movement but is also reproduced by local palpation)
- Weak and rapid pulse accompanied by fall in blood pressure (pneumothorax)

CARDIOVASCULAR

- Back pain that is described as "throbbing"
- Back pain accompanied by leg pain that is relieved by standing still or rest
- Back pain that is present in all spinal positions and increased by exertion
- Back pain accompanied by a pulsating sensation or palpable abdominal pulse
- Low back, pelvic, and/or leg pain with temperature changes from one leg to the other (involved side warmer: venous occlusion or tumor; involved side colder: arterial occlusion)
- Back injury occurred during weight lifting in someone with known heart disease or past history of aneurysm

RENAL/UROLOGIC

- Renal and urethral pain is felt throughout T9-L1 dermatomes
- Back pain at the level of the kidneys can be caused by ovarian or testicular cancer
- Back pain and shoulder pain, either simultaneously or alternately, may be renal/urologic in origin
- Associated signs and symptoms (blood in urine, fever, chills, increased urinary frequency, difficulty starting or continuing stream of urine, testicular pain in men)
- Assess for costovertebral angle tenderness; pain is affected by change of position (pseudorenal pain)
- History of traumatic fall, blow, lift (musculoskeletal)

GYNECOLOGIC

- History or current gynecologic disorder (e.g., uterine retroversion, ovarian cysts, uterine fibroids, endometriosis, pelvic inflammatory disease, sexual assault/incest, intrauterine contraceptive device, multiple births with prolonged labor or forceps use)
- Associated signs and symptoms (missed or irregular menses, tender breasts, cyclic nausea and vomiting, chronic constipation, vaginal discharge, abnormal uterine bleeding or bleeding in a postmenopausal woman)

CLUES SUGGESTING SYSTEMIC BACK PAIN cont'd

- Low back and/or pelvic pain developing soon after a missed menstrual cycle; blood pressure may be significantly low, and there may be concomitant shoulder pain when hemorrhaging occurs (ectopic pregnancy)

NONORGANIC (PSYCHOGENIC) (see discussion, Chapter 1)

- Widespread low back tenderness with overreaction to superficial palpation
- Assess for nonorganic signs such as axial loading (downward pressure on the top of the head) or shoulder-hip rotation (client rotates shoulder and hips with feet planted)
- Regional pain, numbness, weakness, sensory disturbances

ONCOLOGIC

- Back pain with severe lower extremity weakness without pain, with full range of motion but recent history of sciatica
- Temperature differences: involved side warmer when tumor interferes with sympathetic nerves
- Associated signs and symptoms: significant weight loss; night pain disturbing sleep; extreme fatigue; constitutional symptoms such as fever, sweats; other organ/system-dependent symptoms such as urinary changes (urologic), cough, and dyspnea (pulmonary); abdominal bloating or bloody diarrhea (gastrointestinal)

Additionally, pain from a pathologic condition of the hip can be referred to the low back, sacroiliac or sacral areas, groin, anterior thigh, knee, or ankle. Postoperatively, orthopedic pins may migrate, referring pain from the hip to the back, tibia, or ankle. Referred pain originating from a pathologic condition of the hip can be confused with pain referred from ligamentous structures of the lumbar spine or sacroiliac joints.

The therapist must be aware that disorders affecting the organs within the pelvic and abdominal cavities can also refer pain to the hip region (Table 12-6) mimicking a primary musculoskeletal lesion. A careful history and physical examination usually differentiate these entities from true hip disease.

Cancer

Spinal metastases to the femur or lower pelvis may appear as hip pain. With the exception of myeloma and a rare lymphoma, metastasis to the synovium is unusual. Therefore joint motion is not compromised by these bone lesions. Although any tumor of the bone may appear at the hip, some benign and malignant neoplasms have a propensity to occur in this location.

Osteoid osteoma, a small, benign but painful tumor, is relatively common, with 20% of lesions occurring in the proximal femur and 10% found in the pelvis. The client usually is in the second decade of life and complains of chronic dull hip, thigh, or knee pain that is worse at night and is alleviated by activity and aspirin. There is usually an antalgic gait and point tenderness over the lesion with restriction of hip motion.

A great many varieties of benign and malignant tumors may appear differently, depending on the age of the client, the site, and the duration of the lesion. Other bone tumors that cause hip pain, such as chondroblastoma, chondrosarcoma, giant cell tumors, and Ewing's sarcoma, are discussed in greater detail in Chapter 10.

TABLE 12-6 ▼ Causes of Hip Pain

Systemic	Neuromusculoskeletal*
Cancer	Low back, sacroiliac joint, sacral or knee dysfunction
Spinal metastasis	Osteoarthritis
Bone tumors	Femoral hernia
Osteoid osteoma	Bursitis (trochanteric, iliopectineal, iliopsoas, ischial)
Chondrosarcoma	Fasciitis
Giant cell tumor	Muscle impairment (weakness, loss of flexibility, hypertonus, or hypo-
Ewing's sarcoma	tonus, sprain/strain/tear)
	Stress reactions/fractures
Cardiovascular	Peripheral nerve injury or entrapment
Arterial insufficiency	Meralgia paresthetica
Urologic/renal	
Inflammatory diseases	
Abdominal or peritoneal inflammation	
(psoas abscess)	
Crohn's disease	
Appendicitis	
Pelvic inflammatory disease	
Ankylosing spondylitis	
Reiter's syndrome	
Other	
Osteoporosis	
Tuberculosis	
Sickle cell anemia	
Hemophilia	

*This is not an exhaustive list. It includes the most commonly encountered adult neuromusculoskeletal causes of hip pain.

Cardiovascular Conditions

As with low back and leg pain associated with arterial insufficiency, hip pain can also occur. All the same general principles for identifying back or leg pain from a cardiovascular origin apply to hip pain (see discussion, Sources of Back Pain, Table 12-2, and Clues Suggesting Systemic Back Pain).

Urologic Conditions

Referred symptoms from ureteral colic can be distinguished from musculoskeletal hip pain by the history, presence of urologic symptoms, and pattern of pain. The therapist needs to perform Murphy's percussion test to rule out kidney involvement (see discussion, Chapter 7).

Inflammatory and Infectious Diseases

Abdominal or peritoneal inflammation, which leads to irritation of the psoas muscle and psoas abscess, may present as hip pain. (See discussion of Psoas Abscess, Chapter 6.)

Psoas abscess, a localized collection of pus, most commonly affects the right hip and can be caused by any peritoneal inflammatory process such as diverticulitis, Crohn's disease, appendicitis, or pelvic inflammatory disease. Hip pain associated with such an abscess may also involve the medial aspect of the thigh and femoral triangle areas. Once the abscess is formed, muscular spasm may be provoked, producing hip flexion and even contracture. The leg also may be pulled into internal rotation.

Psoas abscess must be differentiated from trigger points of the psoas muscle, causing

Case Example. A 46-year-old male runner with a sudden onset of right hip pain and the diagnosis of trochanteric bursitis was referred to physical therapy for modalities and exercise.

The major criteria for a medical diagnosis of trochanteric bursitis are marked tenderness to deep palpation of the greater trochanter and relief of pain after peritrochanteric injection with a local anesthetic and corticosteroid. The absence of greater trochanter tenderness and the presence of a nonscapular pattern of restriction of the hip were not consistent with the given diagnosis. Local injection was not administered. If an injection had been given, tochanteric bursitis may have been eliminated from the list of possible diagnoses.

Result. The results of the physical therapy examination warranted further medical evaluation, and the client was returned to the physician. Magnetic resonance imaging (MRI) testing indicated a nondisplaced, complete stress fracture of the femoral neck.

An open reduction and internal fixation procedure was performed, and the client received six treatments of postoperative outpatient physical therapy for range-of-motion exercises and ambulation with touch-down weight bearing. The client was ambulatory without an assistive device or weight-bearing restrictions 5 weeks after surgery.

Because of changes in the health care delivery system, the combination of deemphasis on diagnostic testing and emphasis on the use of a nonspecialist will result in a greater number of clients being seen in physical therapy with potentially serious consequences. It is incumbent on physical therapists to make the first decision in the diagnostic process: Is the client a candidate for physical therapy?

From Jones DL, Erhard RE: Differential diagnosis with serious pathology: a case report, *Phys Ther* 76(5):S89-S90, 1996.

the psoas minor syndrome, which is easily mistaken for appendicitis. Hemorrhage within the psoas muscle, either spontaneous or associated with anticoagulation therapy for hemophilia, can cause a painful compression syndrome of the femoral nerve. Systemic causes of hip pain from psoas abscess are usually associated with loss of appetite or other GI symptoms, fever, and night sweats.

Symptoms from the ilopsoas trigger point are aggravated by weight-bearing activities and are relieved by recumbency or rest. Relief is greater when the hip is flexed (Travell and Simons, 1992). (See ilipsoas test, Chapter 6.)

Ankylosing spondylitis is primarily an arthritis of the spine. One fifth of the affected people notice the first symptoms in the peripheral joints, and approximately one third ultimately develop hip disease. Late in the disease, marked hip flexion contractures are present and bony ankylosis of the hip may occur.

Spinal tuberculosis that occurs as an opportunistic disease associated with autoimmunodeficiency syndrome (AIDS) can also cause hip pain as a result of a psoas abscess. Usually there is a known diagnosis of AIDS and tuberculosis as well as a positive iliopsoas test (see Chapter 6) to alert the therapist of the underlying systemic cause.

Case Example. A 78-year-old woman went to the emergency department over a weekend for knee pain. She reported a knee joint replacement 6 months ago because of arthritis. X-ray examination showed that the knee prosthetic was intact without any complications (e.g., no swelling, no fractures, no infection, nothing loose). She was told to contact her orthopedic surgeon the following Monday for a follow-up visit. The woman decided to see the physical therapist who was involved with her postoperative rehabilitation instead.

The physical therapist's interview and examination revealed the following information. There was no perceived or reported pain anywhere but in the knee. The pain pattern was constant (always present) but was made worse by weight-bearing activities. The knee was not warm, red, or swollen. There were no other associated signs and symptoms or constitutional symptoms present, and vital signs were within normal limits for her age range.

Range of motion was better than at the time of previous discharge, but painful symptoms were elicited with a gross manual muscle-screening examination. After a test of muscle strength, the woman was experiencing intense pain and was unable to put any weight on the painful leg.

The physical therapist was insistent that the woman visit her physician immediately and arranged by phone for an emergency appointment that same day.

Result. Orthopedic examination with pelvic and hip x-ray films showed a hip fracture necessitating an immediate total hip replacement the same day. The knee is an uncommon site for referred pain of systemic origin and especially monoarticular symptoms.

There was no history or accompanying signs and symptoms to suggest systemic origin of knee pain, but the pain on weight bearing made worse after muscle testing was a red-flag symptom for bone involvement. Hip fractures can masquerade as knee pain, although this is also uncommon.

Prompt diagnosis of hip fractures is important in preventing complications. This therapist chose to err on the side of conservatism with a medical evaluation rather than proceed with a physical therapy plan. Sometimes the "treat-and-see" approach to symptoms assessment works well, but if there are any red flags, a physician referral is required.

Other Conditions

Osteoporosis may result in hip fracture and accompanying hip pain, especially in postmenopausal women who are not taking hormone replacement. Osteoporosis accompanying the postmenopausal period—when combined with a circulatory impairment, postural hypotension, or some medications—can increase a person's risk of falling and incurring hip fracture.

Transient osteoporosis of the hip can occur during pregnancy, although the incidence is fairly low. Symptoms include progressive hip pain, sometimes referred to the lateral thigh. The pain develops shortly before or during the last trimester and is aggravated by weight bearing. The pain subsides and the x-ray appearance returns to normal within several months following delivery.

Any evaluation procedures that produce significant shear through the femoral head

CLUES SUGGESTING SYSTEMIC HIP AND GROIN PAIN

- See also Clues Suggesting Systemic Back Pain; general concepts from the back also apply to the hip and groin (see especially Cardiovascular discussion)
- History of AIDS-related tuberculosis, sickle cell anemia, or hemophilia
- Normal hip rotations are present when the client is tested in the supine position with the hips in neutral extension (zero degrees of hip flexion) but with reproduction of painful symptoms
- Presence of rebound tenderness, positive McBurney's iliopsoas, or obturator test (see Chapter 6)
- Hip or groin pain accompanied by or alternating with signs and symptoms associated with the gastrointestinal system, urologic/renal system, hematologic system, cardiovascular system, or constitutional symptoms, especially fever and night sweats
- Hip pain in a young adult that is worse at night and alleviated by activity and aspirin (osteoid osteoma)
- Hip or groin pain with any of the clues suggesting cancer (see Chapter 10), especially anyone with a previous history of cancer and men between the ages of 18 and 24 years experiencing hip or groin pain of an unknown cause (testicular cancer)
- Painless, progressive enlargement of lymph nodes that persist for more than 4 weeks or that involve more than one area (groin and popliteal areas)
- Signs and symptoms of a stress reaction or stress fracture (requires medical referral):

  Pain increases with activity and improves with rest

  Pain localizes to a specific area of bone

  Applying a translational, rotational, or impact stress (heel strike test or hopping on the involved side) to the bone reproduces the symptoms

  Local swelling at the fracture site develops if causative activity is not stopped

Clinical Signs and Symptoms of
Hip Avascular Necrosis

- Pain in the groin or thigh
- Tenderness to palpation over the hip joint
- Antalgic gait with a limp
- Hip motion decreased in flexion, internal rotation, and abduction

Clinical Signs and Symptoms of
Hip Hemarthrosis

- Pain in the groin and thigh
- Fullness in the hip joint, both anterior in the groin and over the greater trochanter
- Limited motion in hip flexion, abduction, and external rotation (allows most room for the blood in the joint capsule)

of a pregnant woman must be performed by the physical therapist with extreme caution. The transient osteoporosis of pregnancy is not limited to the hip, and vertebral compression may also occur.

Tubercular disease of the hip is rare in developed countries, but it may occur in the AIDS population when tuberculosis develops as an opportunistic disease. The client usu-

ally appears with a chronic limp and pain in the hip that persists at rest. Approximately 60% of affected individuals do not have constitutional symptoms, although the tuberculin skin test is usually positive, and radiographs are similar to those for septic arthritis.

Sickle cell anemia resulting in avascular necrosis (death of cells caused by lack of blood supply) of the hip and hemarthrosis (blood in the joint) associated with *hemophilia* are two of the most common hematologic diseases that cause pain in the hip.

Hemarthrosis associated with hemophilia may affect the hip, with hemorrhaging within the psoas muscle. The subsequent bleeding-spasm cycle produces increased hip pain and hip flexion spasm/contracture.

▼ PELVIC PAIN

Pelvic diseases can cause primary pelvic pain and also refer pain to the low back, thigh, groin, and rectum. Usually pelvic diseases appear as acute illnesses with sudden onset of severe pain accompanied by nausea and vomiting, fever, and abdominal pain. The physical therapist is more likely to see the atypical presentation of systemic-related central lumbar and sacral pain, which is easily mistaken for mechanical pain.

The anterior pelvic wall is part of the musculature of the abdominal cavity. The lateral walls are covered by the iliopsoas and obturator muscles, and inferiorly the outlet is guarded by the levator ani and pubococcygeus muscles, with which the corresponding muscles of the opposite side form the pelvic diaphragm.

Because the pelvic cavity is in direct communication with the abdominal cavity, any organ disease or systemic condition of either the pelvic cavity or the abdominal cavity can cause primary pelvic pain or referred musculoskeletal pain, as described in this section. Other causes of pelvic pain are listed in Table 12-7.*

_____
*A useful resource for the physical therapist and interested clients is the International Pelvic Pain Society: (205) 877-2950. The Section on Women's Health of the American Physical Therapy Association is also available.

Types of Pelvic Pain

Pelvic pain may be *visceral pain,* caused by stimulation of autonomic nerves (T11 to S3); *somatic pain,* caused by stimulation of sensory nerve endings in the pudendal nerves (S2, S3); or *peritoneal pain.*

Peritoneal pain may be caused by disruption of the autonomic nerve supply of the visceral pelvic peritoneum, which covers the upper third of the bladder, the body of the uterus, and the upper third of the rectum and the rectosigmoid junction. It is insensitive to touch but responds with pain on traction, distension, spasm, or ischemia of the viscus.

Peritoneal pain may also occur in relation to the parietal pelvic peritoneum, which covers the upper half of the lateral wall of the pelvis and the upper two thirds of the sacral hollow—all supplied by somatic nerves.

These somatic nerves also supply corresponding segmental areas of skin and muscles of the trunk and the anterior abdominal wall. Painful stimulation of the parietal pelvic peritoneum may cause referred segmental pain and spasm of the iliopsoas muscle and muscles of and the anterior abdominal wall (see discussion, Chapter 1, and Fig. 1-2).

Causes of Pelvic Pain

Musculoskeletal Conditions

Musculoskeletal causes of pelvic pain are normally easily recognized by the physical therapist. They are usually made worse by exercise and weight bearing and are relieved by rest, stretching, or trigger point release. There may be a history of fall or trauma, and trunk and lumbar rotation aggravates the symptoms.

Musculoskeletal dysfunction of the pelvic girdle and low back may be manifested as dyspareunia (painful intercourse). Hypertonus of the pelvic floor and pelvic floor trigger points can contribute to entrance dyspareunia. Deep thrust dyspareunia may

TABLE 12-7 ▼ Causes of Pelvic Pain

Systemic	Neuromusculoskeletal
Cancer	Hip, sacroiliac joint, low back or sacral dysfunction*
Vascular disorders	Muscle impairment (hamstring, abdominals, rectus femoris, adductor muscles, pelvic floor muscles, levator ani)†
Arterial occlusion	
Venous thrombosis	
Pelvic congestion	
Varicosities or pelvic congestion	
Renal/urologic	Psoas abscess
	Femoral hernia
Gastrointestinal disorders	Stress reactions/fractures
Inflammatory bowel disease (IBD)	Pubic sprain/separation
Crohn's disease	Sexual, birth, or activity-related trauma or injury
Ulcerative colitis	Levator ani syndrome
Diverticular disease	Tension myalgia
Irritable bowel syndrome (IBS)	Coccygodynia
	Neurologic disorders
Gynecologic	Nerve entrapment
Pregnancy (including ectopic)	Incomplete spinal cord lesion
Uterovaginal prolapse	Multiple sclerosis
Vulvodynia	Pudendal neuralgia
Dysmenorrhea	
Endometriosis	
Premenstrual tension	
Tumors/fibroids	
Ovarian cysts or varicosities	
Gynecalgia	
Other	
Psychogenic	
Trauma/sexual assault	
Sexually transmitted disease	
Surgery (abdominal/laparotomy, tubal, pelvic)	
Infection/inflammation	
Spontaneous or therapeutic abortion	
Septic arthritis	
Ankylosing spondylitis	
Ileal Crohn's disease	
Irritable bowel syndrome	
Acute or chronic appendicitis	
Osteomyelitis	
Vaginal infection	
Pelvic inflammatory disease (PID)	
Postpartum infection	
Fibromyalgia	
Autonomic nervous system dysfunction	
Paget's disease	

*The combined medical and physical therapy differential diagnosis includes many origins of pathologic conditions, including joint laxity; subluxations or displacements; thoracolumbar hypermobility; bursitis; osteoarthritis; spondyloarthropathy; fracture; postural, ligamentous, or osteoporosis/osteomalacia. (This list is not exhaustive.)

†As with joint dysfunction, the differential diagnosis of muscle pathologic conditions can include many origins (e.g., trigger points, tendinous avulsion, strain/sprain/tear, weakness, loss of flexibility, hypertonus or hypotonus, diastasis recti).

be related to sacroiliac or low back dysfunction. Dyspareunia symptoms that are reduced in alternate positions may indicate a musculoskeletal component, especially when other signs and symptoms characteristic of musculoskeletal dysfunction are also present (Baker, 1998).

The therapist must remember that pelvic pain or symptoms can be referred from systemic or neuromusculoskeletal origins from the hip, sacroiliac joint, sacrum, or low back. Likewise, pelvic diseases can refer pain and symptoms to the low back, groin, and thigh. When making a physical therapy diagnosis regarding low back or pelvic pain, the therapist must assess for pelvic floor laxity or tension,‡ psoas abscess, trigger points, history of birth or sexual trauma, and any associated signs and symptoms.

Anterior pelvic pain occurs most often as a result of any disorder affecting the hip joint, including inflammatory arthritis; upper lumbar vertebrae (disk pathology is rare at these segments); pregnancy with separation of the symphysis pubis; local injury to the insertion of the rectus abdominis, rectus femoris, or adductor muscles; femoral neuralgia; and psoas abscess.

Stress reactions of the pubis or ilium, sometimes called stress fractures, can occur during traumatic labor and delivery, but they are more common in osteomalacia and Paget's disease, producing anterior pelvic pain. Traumatic stress reactions can also occur in joggers, military personnel, athletes, and pregnant women during delivery. Symptoms may include pain in the involved areas that is aggravated by active motion of the limb or deep pressure and weight bearing during ambulation.

Femoral hernia accounts for 20% of hernias in women, causing lateral wall pelvic

‡The pelvic floor is a muscular floor that provides support for the abdominal contents and sphincter control for the perineal openings. When this muscular floor sags or sustains a muscle tear during childbirth or sexual trauma, weakness results in pelvic laxity and disrupts the positioning and functioning of the pelvic organs, also affecting the function of the lumbrosacral spine.

pain when the hernia strangulates. The referred pain pattern is located down the medial side of the thigh to the knee. Immediate surgical repair is indicated.

Posterior pelvic pain originating in the lumbosacral, sacroiliac, coccydynial, and sacrococcygeal regions usually appears as localized pain in the lower lumbar spine and over the sacrum, often radiating over the sacroiliac ligaments. Pain radiating from the sacroiliac joint can commonly be felt in both the buttock and the posterior thigh and is often aggravated by rotation of the lumbar spine on the pelvis. A proximal hamstring injury, including avulsion of the ischial epiphysis in the adolescent, can also cause posterior pelvic and buttock pain.

Coccydynial and sacrococcygeal pain is a common presentation in women, often associated with a fall on the buttocks or traumatic childbirth. It appears with the person having difficulty sitting on firm surfaces and having pain in the coccygeal region on defecation or straining.

Levator ani syndrome and tension myalgia may produce symptoms of pain, pressure, and discomfort in the rectum, vagina, perirectal area, or low back and can mimic a diskogenic problem. The spasm and tenderness in the levator ani may occur in both men and women. It can be caused by birthing trauma, neurologic abnormalities in the lumbrosacral spine, sexual assault or sexual trauma, or anal fissures from anal intercourse. There may be pain during sexual intercourse and throbbing pain during bowel movement with accompanying constipation and impaired bowel and bladder function.

Cancer

The female pelvis is a depository for malignant tissue after incomplete removal of a primary carcinoma within the pelvis, for recurrence of cancer after surgical resection or radiotherapy of a pelvic neoplasm, or for metastatic deposits from a primary lesion elsewhere in the abdominal cavity.

Ovarian cancer or extraovarian primary peritoneal carcinoma may cause pelvic discomfort but usually with accompanying GI, abdominal, or urinary signs and symptoms (see Ovarian Cancer, Chapter 10).

Primary colonic and rectal tumors spread locally—via the lymphatics or the blood stream. Extension through the bowel wall may fix the tumor to the musculoskeletal walls of the pelvic cavity or to surrounding organs. This may produce fistulas into the small intestine, bladder, or vagina. Advanced rectal tumors can become "fixed" to the sacral hollow. Deep pain within the pelvis may indicate spread of neoplasm into the sacral nerve plexuses.

Vascular Conditions

The iliac arteries may be gradually occluded by atherosclerosis or obstructed by an embolus. The resultant ischemia produces pain in the affected limb but may also give rise to pelvic pain. Whether the occlusion is thrombotic or embolic, the client will complain of pain in the affected limb and probably pain in the buttocks.

The pain is characteristically aggravated by exercise (claudication). The affected limb becomes colder and paler. In sudden occlusion, diminished sensation to pinprick may be observed on examination. Femoral and distal arteries should be palpated for pulsation.

Thrombosis of the large iliac veins may occur spontaneously, following injury to the lower limb and pelvis, or it may appear after pelvic surgical procedures. An estimated 30% of clients have asymptomatic deep vein thrombosis after major surgery. Thrombosis occluding the iliac vein produces an enlarged, warm, and painful leg; only occasionally is discomfort in the pelvis noted.

Varicose veins of the ovaries (varicosities) cause the blood in the veins to flow downward rather than toward the heart. This is a recently discovered source of chronic pelvic pain that sometimes results in a pelvic congestion syndrome (PCS) when there are extensive varices in the broad ligaments along with grossly dilated ovarian veins. Varicosity of the gonadal venous plexus can occur in men, but it is more readily diagnosed by the presentation of observable varicosities of the scrotum.

Symptoms of ovarian varicosities reflect the vascular incompetence associated with venous insufficiency. These symptoms include pelvic pain that worsens toward the end of the day or after standing for a long time, pain after intercourse, sensation of heaviness in the pelvis, and prominent varicose veins elsewhere on the body, especially the buttocks and thighs (Gasparini et al, 1998; Tarazov et al, 1997).

Renal/Urologic Conditions

Infection of the bladder or kidney, kidney stones, renal failure (chronic kidney disease), spasm of the urethral smooth muscle, and tumors in any of the renal urologic organs can refer pain to the lower lumbar and pelvic regions, mimicking musculoskeletal dysfunction. Pelvic floor tension myalgia can develop in response to these conditions and create pelvic pain. The primary pain pattern may radiate around the flanks to the lower abdominal region, the genitalia, and the anterior/medial thighs.

Usually, the most common diseases of this system appear as an obvious medical problem. In the physical therapy setting the past medical history and associated signs and symptoms provide important red-flag clues.

The therapist needs to review the past medical history and ask the client about the presence of painful urination or changes in urination and constitutional symptoms such as fever, chills, sweats, and nausea or vomiting.

Gastrointestinal Conditions

The small bowel, sigmoid, and rectum may be affected by gynecologic disease, and the response will occur in relation to the pressure or displacement of these organs by direct swelling or by reaction to an adjacent infection or to the spilling of blood, menstrual fluid, or infected material. Bowel function is usually altered, but sometimes normal bowel function may alternate with bowel symptoms, and the client does not see a pattern or relationship until asked about bowel function.

Crohn's disease, a chronic inflammation of all layers of the bowel wall (see Chapter 6) may affect the terminal ileum and cecum or the rectum and sigmoid colon in the pelvis. In addition to pelvic and low back pain, the systemic manifestations of Crohn's disease may include intermittent fever with sweats, malaise, anemia, arthralgias, and bowel symptoms.

Diverticular disease of the colon (diverticulosis), an acquired condition most common in the fifth to seventh decades, appears with intermittent symptoms. Moderate-to-severe pain in the left lower abdomen and the left side of the pelvis may be accompanied by a feeling of bowel distension and bowel symptoms such as hard stools, alternating diarrhea and constipation, mucus in the stools, and rectal bleeding.

Irritable bowel syndrome (IBS) produces persistent, colicky lower abdominal and pelvic pain associated with anorexia, belching, abdominal distension, and bowel changes. The symptoms are produced by excessive colonic motility and spasm of the bowel (spastic colon).

Gynecologic Conditions

Gynecologic causes of pelvic pain are related to the classic pathologic subdivision of congenital anomaly, inflammatory process (including infection), neoplasia, or trauma. In addition, there may be pelvic pain associated with pregnancy and endometriosis.

Children younger than 14 years rarely experience pelvic pain of gynecologic origin. Infection is the most likely cause and is limited to the vulva and vagina. Theoretically, infection can ascend to involve the peritoneal cavity, causing iliopsoas abscess and pelvic, hip, or groin pain, but this rarely happens in this age group.

Pelvic pain associated with normal *pregnancy* is similar to low back pain, as discussed earlier in this chapter. About 1% of all pregnancies are outside the endometrium (or ectopic), with the majority of ectopic implantations being in the fallopian tube. Risk factors include tubal ligation; sexually transmitted diseases; pelvic inflammatory disease; infertility or infertility treatments; a previous tubal, pelvic, or abdominal surgery; or the use of an intrauterine contraceptive device (IUCD).

Symptoms of an ectopic pregnancy are usually unexplained vaginal spotting to bursts of bleeding and sudden lower abdominal and pelvic cramping shortly after the first missed menstrual period. At first the pain may be a vague "twinge" or soreness on the affected side; later it can be sharp and severe.

Gradual hemorrhage causes pelvic (and sometimes low back) pain and pressure, but rapid hemorrhage results in hypotension or shock. Tubal rupture is common, bringing about medical attention and diagnosis.

Uterovaginal prolapse can cause low-grade and persistent pelvic pain. Prolapse can be caused by a combination of basic anatomic structure, the effects of pregnancy and labor, postmenopausal hormone deficiency, and poor general muscular fitness. The addition of obesity, chronic cough, and constipation makes permanent correction of this disorder difficult.

Secondary prolapse may occur with large intrapelvic tumors, with sacral nerve disorders, or following surgical resection. Pain is primarily due to stretching of the ligamentous supports and secondarily to the excoriation (scratch or abrasion) that can occur to the prolapsed cervical or vaginal tissue.

The pain of prolapse is central, suprapubic, and dragging in the groin, and there is a sensation of a lump at the vulva. Symptoms are relieved by rest and lying down and may be aggravated by sitting, walking, coughing, sexual intercourse, or straining. There are no significant associated signs and symptoms.

Dysmenorrhea, defined as painful cramping during menstruation, can be primary (of unknown cause) or secondary as a result of a pelvic pathologic condition related to endometriosis, intrauterine tumors or polyps (myomas), uterine prolapse, pelvic inflammatory disease, cervical stenosis, and adenomyosis (benign invasive growths of the endometrium into the muscular layers of the uterus).

Dysmenorrhea is characterized by spasmodic, cramplike pain that comes and goes in waves and radiates over the lower abdomen and pelvis, thighs, and low back, sometimes accompanied by headache, irritability, mental depression, fatigue, and GI symptoms.

Endometriosis is a pathologic condition in which tissue resembling the mucous membrane lining the uterus occurs outside the normal location in the uterus but within the pelvic cavity, including the ovaries, pelvic peritoneum, bowel, and diaphragm. It occurs most often in the reproductive years and in up to 50% of women with infertility (Giudice, 1998). Severity of pain is related more to the site than to the extent of disease. If untreated, endometriosis spreads progressively, and natural remission takes place only with menopause.

Pelvic pain associated with endometriosis can be referred to the rectum and lower sacral or coccygeal regions, starting before or after the onset of menstruation and improving after cessation of menstrual flow, with cyclic recurrence. As the condition extends, pain remains throughout the cycle, with exacerbation at menstruation and, finally, constant severity.

Other symptoms may include rectal discomfort during bowel movements, diarrhea, constipation, recurrent miscarriage, and infertility.

Although a pathologic cause can be identified for most cases of chronic pelvic pain, a small percentage remains for which no physical cause can be determined, and the term *gynecalgia* is used. Women with gynecalgia syndrome are usually 25 to 40 years of age and have at least one child. The symptoms are of at least 2 years' duration (and often many more), with acute exacerbation from time to time.

Pain associated with gynecalgia is vague and poorly localized, although it is usually confined to the lower abdomen and pelvis, radiating to the groin and upper and inner thighs. Other symptoms include dyspareunia, menstrual change, low back pain, urinary and bowel changes, fatigue, and obvious anxiety and depression.

CLUES SUGGESTING SYSTEMIC PELVIC PAIN*

GENERAL

- Pelvic pain described as "achy" or "comes and goes in waves" and is poorly localized (person cannot point to one spot)
- Pelvic pain that is aggravated by walking, sexual intercourse, coughing, or straining
- Pain that is not clearly affected by position changes or specific movements, especially when accompanied by night pain unrelieved by change in position
- Pelvic pain that is not reduced or eliminated by scar tissue mobilization, soft tissue mobilization, or release of trigger points of the myofascial structures in the pelvic cavity

ASSOCIATED SIGNS AND SYMPTOMS

- Pelvic pain in the presence of yellow, odorous vaginal discharge
- Positive McBurney's or iliopsoas/obturator tests (see Chapter 6)
- Pelvic pain with constitutional symptoms, especially nausea and vomiting, gastrointestinal symptoms (possible enteropathic origin)
- Presence of painful urination; urinary incontinence, urgency, frequency; nocturia; blood in the urine; or other urologic changes

PAST MEDICAL HISTORY

- History of dysmenorrhea, ovarian cysts, previous pelvic/bladder surgeries, pelvic inflammatory disease, sexually transmitted disease, fibromyalgia, sexual assault/incest/trauma, chronic yeast/vaginal infections, chronic bladder or urinary tract infections, chronic irritable bowel syndrome
- Recent therapeutic or spontaneous abortion
- Recent intrauterine contraceptive device (IUCD), especially the copper-T IUCD in the presence of pelvic inflammatory disease (PID) or in women with a history of PID

Other Conditions

Psychogenic pain is often ill defined, and its anatomic distribution depends more on the person's concepts than on clinical disease processes. Pelvic pain may coevolve with marital dysfunction (Mathias et al, 1996). Such pain does not usually radiate; commonly, the client has multiple unrelated symptoms, and the fluctuations in the course of symptoms are determined more by crises in the person's psychosocial life than by physical changes. (See also Psychologic Factors in Pain Assessment, Chapter 1).

Surgery, in particular hysterectomy, is associated with varying amounts of pain from problems such as scar formation or hematoma formation with infection, which causes backache and pelvic pain. Lower ab-

dominal discomfort, vaginal discharge, and fatigue may accompany pelvic pain or discomfort months after gynecologic surgery.

Other types of abdominal, pelvic, or tubal surgery, such as laparotomy, tubal ligation, or laminectomy, can also be followed by pelvic pain, usually associated with low back pain. The therapist must include questions about recent surgical procedures during the client interview.

Infection or inflammation within the pelvis from acute appendicitis, diverticulitis, Crohn's disease, osteomyelitis, septic arthritis of the sacroiliac joint, urologic disorders, sexually transmitted infections (e.g., *Chlamydia trachomatis*), and salpingitis (inflammation of the fallopian tube) can produce both visceral and somatic

CLUES SUGGESTING SYSTEMIC PELVIC PAIN cont'd

- History of previous gynecologic, colon, or breast cancer
- History of prolonged labor, use of forceps or vacuum extraction, and/or multiple births

GYNECOLOGIC

- Pelvic pain that is relieved by rest, placing a pillow or support under the hips and buttocks in the supine position, or "getting off your feet"
- Pelvic pain that is correlated with menses or sexual intercourse
- Pelvic pain that occurs after the first menstrual cycle is missed, especially if the woman is using an IUCD or has had a tubal ligation (see text for other risk factors), with shoulder pain also present (ruptured ectopic pregnancy); assess for low blood pressure
- Presence of pregnancy

VASCULAR

- History of heart disease with a clinical presentation of pelvic, buttock, and leg pain that is aggravated by activity or exercise (claudication)
- Pelvic pain accompanied by buttock and leg pain with changes in skin and temperature on the affected side (arterial occlusion or venous thrombosis), especially in the presence of known heart disease or recent pelvic surgery
- Pain that worsens toward the end of the day, accompanied by pain after intercourse and in the presence of varicose veins elsewhere in the body (ovarian varicosities)

---

*Frequently pelvic and low back pain occur together or alternately. Whenever pelvic pain is listed, the reader should consider this as "pelvic pain with or without low back or sacral pain."

---

pelvic pain because of the involvement of the parietal peritoneum. Secondary pelvic infection may follow surgery, septic abortion, or pregnancy as a result of the entry of endogenous bacteria into the damaged pelvic tissues.

All these disorders have similar signs and symptoms during the acute phase. The woman may not have any pain but will report low back and/or pelvic "discomfort," or she may experience acute, sharp, severe aching on both sides of the pelvis. Accompanying groin discomfort may radiate to the inner aspects of the thigh.

Right-sided abdominal or pelvic inflammatory pain is often associated with appendicitis, whereas left-sided pain is more likely associated with diverticulitis. Bilateral pain may indicate infection. The pain may be aggravated by increased abdominal pressure

(e.g., coughing, walking). The therapist must always test for iliopsoas or obturator abscesses (see discussion, Chapter 6).

Other red-flag symptoms may be reported in response to specific questions about disturbance in urination, odorous vaginal discharge, tachycardia, dyspareunia (painful or difficult intercourse), or constitutional symptoms such as fever, general malaise, and nausea and vomiting.

▼ GROIN PAIN (Table 12-8)

The physical therapist is not likely to be faced with a client complaining of just groin pain or symptoms. It is more typical to see a person who has low back, hip, or sacroiliac

TABLE 12-8 ▼ Causes of Groin Pain

Systemic Causes	Musculoskeletal Causes
Spinal cord tumors	Adductor muscle strain
	Internal oblique avulsion
Ureteral pain	Stress reaction or fracture
Ascites	Pubalgia
Hemophilia	Osteitis pubis
Gastrointestinal bleeding	Trauma (including sexual assault)
	Inguinal hernia
Abdominal Aortic aneurysm	Hip joint pathologic conditions
	Trigger points

problems with a secondary complaint of groin pain. However, on examination, the physical therapist may palpate enlarged lymph nodes in the groin area, or the client may indicate these nodes to the examiner.

Painless, progressive enlargements of lymph nodes that persist for more than 4 weeks or that involve more than one area are an indication of a need for a medical referral.

Hodgkin's disease arises in the lymph glands most commonly on one side of the neck or groin, but lymph nodes also enlarge in response to infections throughout the body. Lymph nodes in the groin area can become enlarged specifically related to sexually transmitted diseases.

The presence of painless, hard lymph nodes that are also similarly present at other sites (e.g., popliteal space) is always a red-flag symptom. As always, the physical therapist must question the client further regarding the onset of symptoms and the presence of any associated symptoms, such as fever, weight loss, bleeding, and skin lesions. The client must seek medical diagnosis to be certain of the cause of enlarged lymph nodes.

Musculoskeletal Causes

The most common musculoskeletal cause of groin pain is strain of the adductor muscles, most often involving the adductor longus.

The history includes a specific trauma or injury, which occurs primarily at the junction of the muscle fibers with the extended tendon of origin. Acutely, this injury causes pain with passive stretching or active contraction; eccentric activation may be even more painful. Acute injury may be followed in several days by ecchymosis.

Other musculoskeletal causes of groin pain may include avulsion of the internal oblique abdominal muscle, trauma (including sexual assault), inguinal hernia (fairly common in young athletes), pubalgia, osteitis pubis, and hip joint disease such as slipped capital femoral epiphysis, intraarticular disease, and avulsion of the rectus femoris from the anterior inferior iliac spine and the sartorius from the anterior superior iliac spine.

Stress reactions or stress fractures of the femur or pelvis can cause hip or groin pain. These type of injuries occur most often in women in the military who participate in long marches; they also occur in women athletes and are associated with abnormal eating patterns, secondary amenorrhea (cessation of menstruation), and low estrogen levels. The therapist may want to inquire concerning menstrual history and a possible eating disorder when interviewing a young female athlete presenting with lower groin, hip, or lower extremity pain.

Palpation over the injured bone may reproduce the painful symptoms, but when the stressed bone lies deep within the tissue, the therapist may be able to reproduce the pain by stressing the bone with translational or rotational force (e.g., hip rotation). Performing a heel strike test or having the client hop on the affected leg may also reproduce the pain. Swelling is not usually evident early in the course of a stress reaction or fracture but it will develop if the person continues athletic activity (Griffin, 1995).

Pubalgia is characterized by pain in the inguinal area, most often near the middle of the inguinal ligament. The pain results from an abdominal wall muscular injury. Active abdominal flexion (e.g., sit-ups) and passive stretching of abdominal muscles (e.g., prone extension) cause pain. This problem occurs most frequently in soccer players.

Osteitis pubis, which may be mistaken for adductor strain, is located at the symphysis pubis and is characterized by tenderness to direct pressure about the symphysis. This is also most likely to occur in participants of any active sport.

Underlying hip joint pathologic conditions can also mimic adductor strain. Pain associated with this entity is described as being directly in the inguinal area and limits hip rotation.

Active trigger points along the upper rim of the pubis and the lateral half of the inguinal ligament may lie in the lower internal oblique muscle and possibly in the lower rectus abdominis. These trigger points can cause increased irritability and spasm of the detrusor and urinary sphincter muscles, producing urinary frequency, retention of urine, and groin pain (Travell and Simons, 1983).

Systemic Causes

Primary and secondary *spinal cord tumors* may initially appear with discomfort in the thoracolumbar area in a beltlike distribution. The pain may extend to the groin or legs and may be constant or intermittent; a dull ache; or a sharp, knifelike sensation.

The pain can be primarily at the site of the lesion or may refer to the ipsilateral groin and down the ipsilateral extremity with radicular involvement (nerve root compression or irritation).

Ureteral pain is felt in the groin and genital area (see Fig. 7-6) with radiation forward around the flank into the lower abdominal quadrant. Abdominal muscle spasm with rebound tenderness can occur on the same side as the source of pain. Abdominal rebound tenderness results when the adjacent peritoneum becomes inflamed. The therapist should test for rebound tenderness (see McBurney's point, Chapter 6). The pain also can be generalized throughout the abdomen and associated with nausea, vomiting, and impaired intestinal motility.

Ascites, an abnormal accumulation of serous (edematous) fluid within the peritoneal cavity, also can cause low back pain or groin pain. This condition is associated with liver disease and alcoholism. The person has a distended abdomen, possible abdominal hernias, lumbar lordosis, and possible edema bilaterally in the ankles at presentation.

Hemophilia may involve GI bleeding accompanied by low abdominal and groin pain caused by bleeding into the wall of the large intestine or iliopsoas muscle. This retroperitoneal hemorrhage produces a muscle spasm of the iliopsoas muscle with a subsequent hip flexion contracture. Other symptoms may include melena, hematemesis, and fever.

Abdominal aortic aneurysm may be asymptomatic, and discovery occurs on physical or x-ray examination of the abdomen or lower spine for some other reason. The most common symptom is awareness of a pulsating mass in the abdomen, with or without pain, followed by abdominal and back pain. Groin pain and flank pain may be experienced because of increasing pressure on other structures. For detailed information, see Chapter 3.

▼ CHEST PAIN

The four types of pain discussed in Chapter 1 (cutaneous, deep somatic or parietal, visceral, and referred) also apply to the chest. A physical therapist must be able to evaluate whether or not chest pain is caused by a systemic problem.

Parietal chest pain* is the most common systemic chest discomfort encountered in a physical therapy practice. It is usually associated with infectious diseases but is also seen in pneumothorax, rib fractures, pulmonary embolism with infarction, and other systemic conditions.

---

*Parietal (somatic) pain refers to pain generating from the wall of any cavity, such as the chest or pelvic cavity (see Fig. 3-3). Although the visceral pleura are insensitive to pain, the parietal pleura are well supplied with pain nerve endings.

Parietal Pain

Pain fibers, originating in the parietal pleura, are conveyed through the chest wall as fine twigs of the intercostal nerves. Irritation of these nerve fibers results in pain in the chest wall that is usually described as knifelike and is sharply localized close to the chest wall, occurring cutaneously (in the skin).

Pain from the thoracic viscera and true chest wall pain are both felt in the chest wall, but visceral pain is referred to the area supplied by the upper four thoracic nerve roots. Report of pain in the lower chest usually indicates local disease, but upper chest pain may be caused by disease located deeper in the chest.

Parietal pain may appear as unilateral chest pain (rather than midline only) because at any given point the parietal peritoneum obtains innervation from only one side of the nervous system. It is usually not reproduced by palpation.

There are few nerve endings (if any) in the visceral pleurae (linings of the various organs), such as the heart or lungs.* Extensive disease may develop within the body cavities without the occurrence of pain until the process extends to the parietal pleura. Neuritis (constant irritation of nerve endings) in the parietal pleura then produces the pain described in this section.

Pleural pain may be aggravated by any respiratory movement involving the diaphragm, such as sighing, deep breathing, coughing, sneezing, laughing, or the hiccups. It may be referred along the costal margins or into the upper abdominal quadrants. Inflammation of the diaphragmatic pleura produces ipsilateral shoulder pain via the phrenic nerve.

Systemic Causes of Chest Pain

There are many causes of chest pain, both cardiac and noncardiac in origin (Table 12-9).

---

*The exception to this statement is in the area of the pericardium (sac enclosed around the entire heart), which is adjacent to the diaphragm (see Fig. 3-3).

TABLE 12-9 ▼ Causes of Chest Pain

Systemic Causes	Neuromusculoskeletal Causes
Cancer Mediastinal tumors	Tietze's syndrome Costochondritis Hypersensitive xiphoid, xiphodynia Slipping rib syndrome Trigger points Myalgia Rib fracture, costochondral dislocations Cervical spine disorders Neurologic Nerve root, intercostal neuritis Herpes zoster virus (shingles) Dorsal nerve root irritation Thoracic outlet syndrome Postoperative pain Breast Mastodynia Trigger points Trauma
Cardiac Myocardial ischemia (angina) Pericarditis Myocardial infarct Dissecting aortic aneurysm Aortic aneurysm Aortic stenosis or regurgitation Mitral valve prolapse†	
Pleuropulmonary Pulmonary embolism Pneumothorax Pulmonary hypertension† Cor pulmonale Pneumonia with pleurisy	
Epigastric/Upper Gastrointestinal Esophagitis† Esophageal spasm† Upper gastrointestinal ulcer Cholecystitis Pancreatitis	
Breast Fibrocystic changes Menstrual influences Breast tumor Abscess Mastitis Lactation problems	
Other Anemia Rheumatic diseases Anxiety† Cocaine use Anabolic steroids Fibromyalgia	

†Relieved by nitroglycerin because it relaxes smooth muscle.

Two conditions may be present at the same time, each contributing to chest pain. For example, someone with cervicodorsal arthritis could also experience reflux esophagitis or coronary disease.

Paying attention to past medical history, recognizing unusual clinical presentation for a neuromuscular or musculoskeletal condition, and keeping in mind the Clues to Differentiating Chest Pain will help the therapist evaluate difficult cases.

Cancer

Occasionally, the therapist may palpate a painless sternal or chest wall mass when evaluating the head and neck region. Most mediastinal tumors are the result of a metastatic focus from a distant primary tumor and remain asymptomatic unless they compress mediastinal structures or invade the chest wall.

The primary tumor is usually a lymphoma (Hodgkin's lymphoma in a young adult or non-Hodgkin's lymphoma in a child or older adult), multiple myeloma (primarily observed in people over 60 years of age), or carcinoma of the breast, kidney, or thyroid.

When involvement of the chest wall and nerve roots results in pain, the pattern is more diffuse, with radiation of pain to the affected nerve roots. Irritation of an intercostal nerve from rib metastasis produces burning pain that is unilateral and segmental in distribution. Sensory loss or hyperesthesia over the affected dermatomes may be noted.

Cardiovascular Conditions

Cardiac-related pain may arise secondary to angina, myocardial infarction, pericarditis, endocarditis, mitral valve prolapse, or aortic aneurysm. Cardiac-related chest pain also can occur when there is normal coronary circulation, as in the case of clients with pernicious anemia. Affected clients may have chest pain or angina on physical exertion because of the lack of nutrition to the myocardium.

The therapist should keep in mind that coronary disease may go unnoticed because the client has no anginal or infarct pain associated with ischemia. This situation occurs when collateral circulation is established to counteract the obstruction of the blood flow to the heart muscle. Anastomoses (connecting channels) between the branches of the right and left coronary arteries eliminate the person's perception of pain until challenged by physical exertion or exercise in the physical therapy setting.

These conditions and the accompanying signs and symptoms, including cardiac chest pain, are discussed in Chapter 3 and will not be discussed further in this chapter.

Pleuropulmonary Conditions

Pulmonary chest pain usually results from obstruction, restriction, dilation, or distension of the large airways or large pulmonary artery walls. Specific diagnoses include pulmonary artery hypertension, pulmonary embolism, mediastinal emphysema, pleurisy, pneumonia, and pneumothorax. Pleuropulmonary disorders are discussed in detail in Chapter 4.

Chest pain that tends to be sharply localized, that worsens with coughing, deep breathing, or other respiratory movements, or motion of the chest wall, and that is relived by maneuvers that limit the expansion of a particular part of the chest (e.g., autosplinting) is likely to be pleuritic in origin.

Epigastric/Upper Gastrointestinal Conditions

Epigastric pain is typically characterized by substernal or upper abdominal (just below the xiphoid process) discomfort (Fig. 12-2). This may occur with radiation posteriorly to the back secondary to long-standing duodenal ulcers. Lesions of the upper esophagus may cause pain in the (anterior) neck, whereas lesions of the lower esophagus are more likely to be characterized by pain originating from the xiphoid process, radiating around the thorax to the middle of the back.

Epigastric pain or discomfort may occur in association with disorders of the liver, gallbladder, common bile duct, and pancreas, with referral of pain to the interscapular, subscapular, or middle/low back regions. This type of pain pattern can be mistaken for angina pectoris or myocardial infarction (e.g., hypotension occurring with pancreatitis produces a reduction of coronary blood flow with the production of angina pectoris).

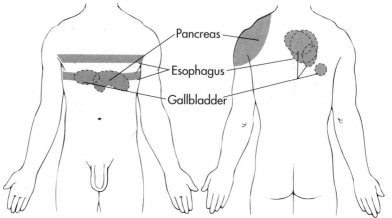

FIGURE 12-2 • Chest pain caused by gastrointestinal disease with referred pain to the shoulder and back.

Pain in the lower substernal area may arise as a result of reflux esophagitis (regurgitation of gastroduodenal secretions). It may be gripping, squeezing, or burning, described as "heartburn" or "indigestion." Like that of angina pectoris, the discomfort of reflux esophagitis may be precipitated by recumbency or by meals; however, unlike angina, it is not precipitated by exercise and is relieved by antacids.

Gastrointestinal disorders may cause chest pain with radiation of pain to the shoulders and back (see Fig. 12-2). Cholecystitis (gallbladder inflammation) appears as discrete attacks of epigastric or right upper quadrant pain, usually associated with nausea, vomiting, and fever and chills. The pain has an abrupt onset, is either steady or intermittent, and is associated with tenderness to palpation in the right upper quadrant. The pain may be referred to the back and right scapular areas. Rarely, the left upper quadrant and anterior chest pain can occur. Dark urine and jaundice indicate that the stone has obstructed the common duct.

Acute pancreatitis causes pain in the upper part of the abdomen that radiates to the back (usually anywhere from T10 to L2) and may spread out over the lower chest. Fever and abdominal tenderness may develop.

Gastric duodenal peptic ulcer may occasionally cause pain in the lower chest rather

▼ Symptoms Associated with Gastrointestinal Disorders

- Chest pain (may radiate to back)
- Nausea
- Vomiting
- Blood in stools
- Pain on swallowing or associated with meals
- Jaundice
- Heartburn or indigestion
- Dark urine

than in the upper abdomen. Antacid and food often immediately relieve pain caused by an ulcer. Ulcer pain is not produced by effort and lasts longer than angina pectoris.

Breast Conditions

Breast pain is most commonly caused by fibrocystic changes within a certain region of breast tissue or functional menstrual cycle influences. Other causes may include benign and malignant tumors, inflammatory breast disease such as mastitis (inflammation of the breast), lactation (breastfeeding problems), abscess, trigger points, breast implants, or mastodynia (mammary neuralgia).

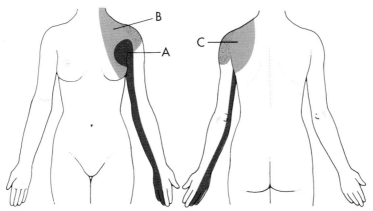

FIGURE 12-3 • Pain arising from the breast. **A,** Mammary pain referred into the axilla along the medial aspect of the arm. **B,** Referral pattern to the supraclavicular level and into the neck. **C,** Breast pain may be diffuse around the thorax through the intercostal nerves. Pain may be referred to the back and the posterior shoulder.

Although it is more typical in women, both men and women can have chest, back, scapular, and shoulder pain referred by a pathologic condition of the breast. Only those conditions most likely to be seen in a physical therapist's practice are included in this discussion.

The typical referral pattern for breast pain is around the chest into the axilla, to the back at the level of the breast, and occasionally into the neck and posterior aspect of the shoulder girdle (see Figs. 12-3 and 12-4). The pain may continue along the medial aspect of the ipsilateral arm to the fourth and fifth digits, mimicking pain of the ulnar nerve distribution.

Jarring or movement of the breasts and movement of the arms may aggravate this pain pattern. Pain in the upper inner arm may arise from outer quadrant breast tumors, but pain in the local chest wall may point to any pathologic condition of the breast. The physical therapist should examine lymph nodes in the axillae and supraclavicular space; any large, firm, hard, or fixed nodes should be reported to the physician (Cady et al, 1998).

Breast cancer and cysts develop more frequently in individuals who have a family history of breast disease. A previous history of cancer is always cause to question the client further regarding the onset and pattern of current symptoms. This is especially true when a woman with a previous history of breast cancer or cancer of the reproductive system appears with shoulder, chest, hip, or sacroiliac pain of unknown cause.

Any report of palpable breast nodules, lumps, or changes in the appearance of the breast requires medical follow-up, especially when there is a personal or family history of breast disease. The skin surface over a tumor may be red, warm, edematous, firm, and painful. There may be skin dimpling over the lesion, with attachment of the mass to surrounding tissues preventing normal mobilization of skin, fascia, and muscle.

Although breast examination is not within the scope of a physical therapist's practice, the client should be questioned about the presence of these signs. Palpation of the underlying muscle and lymph nodes in the supraclavicular and axillary regions should be part of the physical therapist's examination in anyone with chest pain (See further discussion, Breast Cancer, Chapter 10.)

Trigger points in the lateral margin of the pectoralis major, pectoralis minor, or anterior scalene muscle may appear as breast pain or tenderness. These hypersensitive spots in the musculature can refer pain to the chest in a manner that confusingly simulates the pain of coronary insufficiency in persons with no history or evidence of cardiac disease (see further discussion of trigger points in Musculoskeletal Disorders, this section).

Breast pain may be differentiated from the aching pain arising from the pectoral muscles by a history of upper extremity overuse usually associated with pectoral myalgia. Resistance to isometric movement of the upper extremities reproduces the symptoms of a pectoral myalgia but does not usually aggravate pain associated with breast tissue. Additionally, palpation of the underlying muscle reproduces the painful symptoms.

Breast implants, whether used for cosmetic reasons or after mastectomy, can develop capsular contraction (painful contraction of the scar tissue that forms around the implant), followed by implant rupture, hematomas, and infections. Any woman experiencing chest or breast pain should be asked about a personal history of previous breast surgeries, including mastectomy, breast reconstruction, or breast implantation or augmentation.

Mastodynia (irritation of the upper dorsal intercostal nerve) that causes chest pain is almost always associated with ovulatory cycles, especially premenstrually. The association between symptoms and menses may be discovered during the physical therapist's interview when the client responds to Special Questions for Women (see Chapter 2). The presentation is usually unilateral breast or chest pain and occurs initially at the premenstrual period and later more persistently throughout the menstrual cycle.

Other Conditions

An *anxiety state* called neurocirculatory asthenia that produces chest pain is the most common noncardiac cause of chest pain. Psychogenic chest pain may be manifested in the form of cardiac or respiratory symptoms mimicking myocardial infarction.

There are several types of chest discomfort caused by anxiety. The pain may be sharp, intermittent, or stabbing and located in the region of the left breast. The area of pain is usually no larger than the tip of the finger but may be as large as the client's hand. It is often associated with a local area of hyperesthesia of the chest wall.

Anxiety-related pain may be located precordially (region over the heart and lower part of the thorax) or retrosternally (behind the sternum). It may be of variable duration, lasting no longer than a second or for hours or days. This type of pain is unrelated to effort or exercise. Distinguishing this sensation from myocardial ischemia requires medical evaluation.

Discomfort in the upper portion of the chest, neck, and left arm, again unrelated to effort, may occur. There may be a sense of persistent weakness and unpleasant awareness of the heartbeat. Previously, radiation of chest discomfort to the neck or left arm was considered to be diagnostic of atherosclerotic coronary heart disease. More recently, stress testing and coronary arteriography have shown that chest discomfort of this type can occur in clients with normal coronary arteriograms.

Some individuals with anxiety-related chest pain may have a choking sensation in the throat caused by hysteria. There may be associated hyperventilation. Palpitation,

▼ **Clinical Signs and Symptoms of**
Breast Pathology

- Family history of breast disease
- Palpable beast nodules or lumps and previous history of chronic mastitis
- Breast pain with possible radiation to inner aspect of arm(s)
- Skin surface over a tumor may be red, warm, edematous, firm, and painful
- Firm, painful site under the skin surface
- Skin dimpling over the lesion with attachment of the mass to surrounding tissues, preventing normal mobilization of skin, fascia, and muscle
- Unusual nipple discharge
- Pain aggravated by jarring or movement of the breasts
- Pain that is not aggravated by resistance to isometric movement of the upper extremities

▼ *Clinical Signs and Symptoms of*
Chest Pain Caused by Anxiety

- Dull, aching discomfort in the substernal region and in the anterior chest
- Sinus tachycardia
- Fatigue
- Fear of closed-in places
- Diaphoresis
- Dyspnea
- Dizziness
- Choking sensation
- Hyperventilation: numbness and tingling of hands and lips

▼ *Clinical Signs and Symptoms of*
Anabolic Steroid Use

- Chest pain
- Elevated blood pressure
- Ventricular tachycardia
- Weight gain (10 to 15 pounds in 2 to 3 weeks)
- Peripheral edema
- Acne on the face, upper back, chest
- Altered body composition with marked development of the upper torso
- Stretch marks around the back and chest
- Needle marks in large muscle groups
- Development of male pattern baldness
- Gynecomastia (breast tissue development)
- Frequent hematoma or bruising
- Personality changes (rapid mood swings, sudden increased aggressive tendencies)
- Females: secondary male characteristics (deeper voice, breast atrophy, abnormal facial and body hair); menstrual irregularities

claustrophobia, and occurrence of symptoms in crowded places are common.

Hyperventilation occurs in persons with and without heart disease and may be misleading. Such clients have numbness and tingling of the hands and lips and feel as if they are going to "pass out." For a more detailed explanation of anxiety and its accompanying symptoms (e.g., hyperventilation), see Chapter 1.

Cocaine use can cause chest pain because it produces vasoconstriction and myocardial ischemia and enhances vasoconstriction at sites of atherosclerotic disease. Cocaine remains the most common of illicit drug-related causes of severe chest pain, bringing the person to the emergency department (Hoffman and Hollander, 1997; Jay 1998). The physical therapist is more likely to see the unusual presentation.

Many people with chest pain have used cocaine within the last week but deny its use. Careful questioning (see Chapter 2) may assist the physical therapist in identifying a possible correlation between chest pain and cocaine use.

*Anabolic steroid use** has increased in the last decade among young males (including

adolescents) and can also contribute to chest pain by accelerating atherosclerosis. Any young adult with chest pain of unknown cause, possibly accompanied by dyspnea and elevated blood pressure and without clinical evidence of neuromusculoskeletal involvement, may have a history of anabolic steroid use. The alert therapist may recognize the associated signs and symptoms accompanying chronic use of these steroids.

Musculoskeletal Causes

Musculoskeletal causes of chest (wall) pain must be differentiated from pain of cardiac, pulmonary, epigastric, and breast origin (see Table 12-9) before physical therapy treatment begins.

Chest pain can occur as a result of cervical spine disorders because nerves originating as high as C3 and C4 can extend as far

---

*Anabolic steroids are synthetic derivatives of testosterone and alter cardiac cellular and physiologic function. The effects persist long after their use has been discontinued (Sullivan et al, 1998).

as the nipple line. Pectoral, suprascapular, dorsal scapular, and long thoracic nerves originate in the lower cervical spine, and impingement of these nerves can cause chest pain.

Musculoskeletal disorders such as myalgia associated with muscle exertion, myofascial trigger points, costochondritis, or xiphoiditis can produce pain in the chest and arms. Compared with angina pectoris, the pain associated with these conditions may last for seconds or hours, and prompt relief does not occur with the ingestion of nitroglycerin.

Tietze's syndrome, costochondritis, a hypersensitive xiphoid, and the slipping rib syndrome must be differentiated from problems involving the thoracic viscera, particularly those of the heart, great vessels, and mediastinum, as well as from illness originating in the head, neck, or abdomen.

Tietze's Syndrome

Tietze's syndrome (inflammation of a rib and its cartilage; costal chrondritis) may be one possible cause of anterior chest wall pain, manifested by painful swelling of one or more costochondral articulations.* In most cases, the cause of Tietze's syndrome is unknown. Onset is usually before 40 years of age, with a predilection for the second and third decades. However, it also occurs in children.

Approximately 80% of clients have only single sites of involvement, most commonly the second or third costal cartilage (costochondral joint). Anterior chest pain may begin suddenly or gradually and may be associated with increased blood pressure, increased heart rate, and pain radiating down the left arm. Pain is aggravated by sneezing, coughing, deep inspirations, twisting motions of the trunk, horizontal shoulder

---

*Other causes of sternal swelling may include an infectious process from tuberculosis, aspergillosis, brucellosis, staphylococcal infection, or pseudomonal disease producing sternal osteomyelitis. Tuberculosis and fungal infections are commonly observed in the immunocompromised person.

▼ **Clinical Signs and Symptoms of**
Tietze's Syndrome or Costochondritis

- Sudden or gradual onset of upper anterior chest pain
- Pain/tenderness of costochondral joint(s)
- Bulbous swelling of the involved costal cartilage (Tietze's syndrome)
- Mild-to-severe chest pain that may radiate to the left shoulder and arm
- Pain is aggravated by sneezing, coughing, inspiration, bending, recumbency, or exertion

abduction and adduction, or the "crowing rooster" movement of the upper extremities.

These symptoms may seem similar to those of a heart attack, but the raised blood pressure, reproduction of painful symptoms with palpation or pressure, and aggravating factors differentiate Tietze's syndrome from myocardial infarction.

Costochondritis

Costochondritis, also known as anterior chest wall syndrome, costosternal syndrome, and parasternal chondrodynia (pain in a cartilage), is used interchangeably with Tietze's syndrome, although these two conditions are not the same. Costochondritis is more common than Tietze's syndrome.

Although both disorders are characterized by inflammation of one or more costal cartilages, costochondritis refers to pain in the costochondral articulations without swelling. This disorder is observed in people older than 40. It tends to affect the third, fourth, and fifth costochondral joints and occurs more often in women than in men.

Costochondritis is characterized by pain of the anterior chest wall that may radiate widely, stimulating intrathoracic (including cardiac) or intraabdominal disease. Costochondritis can be similar to muscular pain and is elicited by pressure over the costochondral junctions.

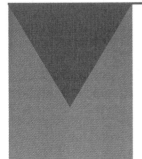

Case Example. A 53-year-old woman was referred by her physician with a diagnosis of left anterior chest pain. Her past medical history was significant for a hysterectomy 10 years ago for prolonged bleeding. She has been a 4- to 5-pack/day smoker for 30 years but has cut down to ½ pack/day for the last 2 months.

The woman described the onset of her pain as sudden, crushing chest pain radiating down the left arm, occurring for the first time 6 weeks ago. She was transported to the emergency department, but tests were negative for cardiac incident. Blood pressure at the time of the emergency admittance was 195/110 mm Hg. She was released from the hospital with a diagnosis of "stress-induced chest pain."

Ten days ago the client experienced the same type of episode of chest pain but described radiating pain around the chest and under the armpit to the upper back. Today her symptoms include extreme tenderness and pain in the left chest with deep pain described as penetrating straight through her chest to her back. There is no numbness or tingling and no pain down the arm but a residual soreness in the left arm.

The client believes that her symptoms may be "stress-induced" but expresses some doubts about this since her symptoms persist and no known cause has been found. She relates that because of divorce proceedings and child custody hearings, she is under extreme stress at this time.

The woman is employed at a sawmill and performs tasks that require repetitive shoulder flexion and extension in using a hydraulic apparatus on a sliding track. Lifting (including overhead lifting) is required occasionally but is limited to items less than 20 pounds.

Examination. The neurologic screen was negative. The deep tendon reflexes were within normal limits; strength testing was limited by pain but with a strong initial response elicited; and no changes in sensation, two-point discrimination, or proprioception were observed.

There was exquisite pain on palpation of the left pectoral muscle with tenderness and swelling noted at the second, third, and fourth costochondral joints. Painful and radiating symptoms were reproduced with resisted shoulder horizontal adduction. Active shoulder range of motion was full but with a positive painful arc on the left. There was also painful reproduction of the radiating symptoms down the arm with palpation of the left supraspinatus and biceps tendons.

The painful chest/arm/upper back symptoms were not altered by respiratory movements (deep breathing or coughing), but the client was unable to lie down without extreme pain.

Result. The physical therapy assessment resulted in a physical therapy diagnosis of Tietze's syndrome secondary to repetitive motion and exacerbated by emotional stress* with concomitant shoulder impingement syndrome. Physical therapy treatment resulted in initial rapid improvement of symptoms with full return to work 6 weeks later.

---

*It should be noted that although the physical therapist's assessment recognized emotional stress as a factor in the client's symptoms, it is not always in the client's best interests to include this information in the documentation. Although the medical community is increasingly aware of the research surrounding psychoneuroimmunology (see discussion, Chapter 1), workmen's compensation and other third-party payers may use this information to deny payment.

TABLE 12-10 ▼ Trigger Point Pain Guide

Location	Potential Muscles Involved	Location	Potential Muscles Involved
Front of chest pain	Pectoralis major Pectoralis minor Scaleni Sternocleidomastoid (sternal) Sternalis Iliocostalis cervicis Subclavius External abdominal oblique	Lumbar pain	Longissimus thoracis Iliocostalis lumborum Iliocostalis thoracis Multifidi Rectus abdominis
		Sacral and gluteal pain	Longissimus thoracis Iliocostalis lumborum Multifidi
Side of chest pain	Serratus anterior Lattissimus dorsi	Abdominal pain	Rectus abdominis Abdominal obliques
Low thoracic back pain	Iliocostalis thoracis Multifidi Serratus posterior inferior Rectus abdominis Lattissimus dorsi		Transversus abdominis Iliocostalis thoracis Multifidi Pyramidalis

Modified from Travell JG, Simons DG: *Myofascial pain and dysfunction: the trigger point manual,* Baltimore, 1983, Williams & Wilkins, p 574.

This condition may follow trauma or may be associated with systemic rheumatic disease. It can persist for months. Inflammation of upper costal cartilages may cause annoying chest pain, whereas inflammation of lower costal cartilages is more likely to cause abdominal or low back discomfort.

Hypersensitive Xiphoid

The hypersensitive xiphoid (xiphodynia) is tender to palpation, and local pressure may cause nausea and vomiting. This syndrome is manifested as epigastric pain, nausea, and vomiting.

Slipping Rib Syndrome

In the slipping rib syndrome (usually the tenth rib), the involved cartilage moves upward and overrides the cartilage above it, thus causing pain. The physical therapist is usually able to identify readily either of these causes of chest pain following a careful musculoskeletal examination.

Trigger Points

Trigger points (hypersensitive spots in the skeletal musculature) involving a variety of muscles (Table 12-10) may produce precordial pain (Fig. 12-4). Abdominal muscles have multiple referred pain patterns that may reach up into the chest or midback and produce heartburn or deep epigastric pain. Although these patterns strongly mimic cardiac pain, myofascial trigger point pain shows a much wider variation in its response to daily activity than does angina pectoris (Travell and Simons, 1983).

There may be a history of upper respiratory infection with repeated forceful coughing. The therapist should also ask about muscle strain from lifting weights overhead, from pushups, and from prolonged, vigorous activity that requires forceful abdominal breathing, such as severe coughing, running a marathon, or repetitive bending and lifting.

On examination, the physical therapist should palpate for tender points and taut bands of muscle tissue, squeeze the involved muscle, observe for increased pain with palpation, test for increased pain with resisted motion, and correlate symptoms with respiratory movements.

Chest pain from serratus anterior trigger points may occur at rest in severe cases. Clients with this myofascial syndrome may report that they are "short of breath" or that they are in pain when they take a deep

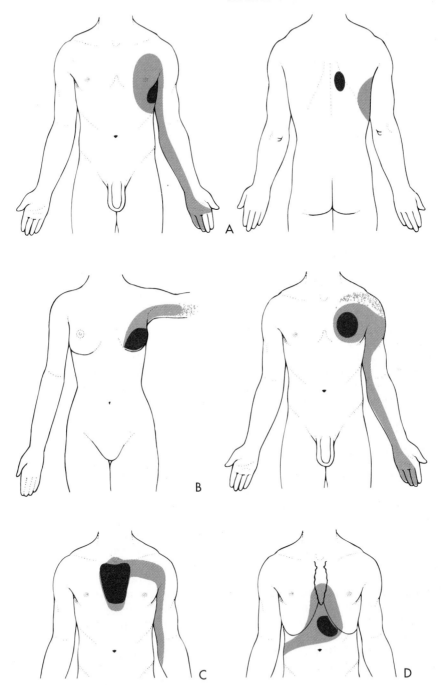

FIGURE 12-4 • **A,** Referred pain pattern from the left serratus anterior muscle. **B,** Left pectoralis major muscle: referred pain pattern in a woman and a man. **C,** Referred pain pattern from the left sternalis muscle. **D,** Referred pain from the external oblique abdominal muscle can cause "heartburn" in the anterior chest wall. (**A, C,** and **D** from Travell JG, Simons DG: *Myofascial pain and dysfunction: the trigger point manual,* vol 1, Baltimore, 1983, Williams & Wilkins. **B,** Modified from Travell JG, Simons DG: *Myofascial pain and dysfunction: the trigger point manual,* vol 1, Baltimore, 1983, Williams & Wilkins.)

breath. Serratus anterior trigger points on the left side of the chest can contribute to the pain associated with myocardial infarction. This pain is rarely aggravated by the usual tests for range of motion at the shoulder but may result from a strong effort to protract the scapula. Palpation reveals tender points that increase symptoms, and there is usually a palpable taut band present within the involved muscles.

One of the most extensive patterns of pain from irritable trigger points is the complex pattern from the anterior scalene muscle. This may produce ipsilateral sternal pain, anterior chest wall pain, breast pain, or pain along the vertebral border of the scapula, shoulder, and arm, radiating to the thumb and index finger.

When active trigger points occur in the left pectoralis muscle, the referred pain (anterior chest, to the precordium and down the inner aspect of the arm) is easily confused with that of coronary insufficiency. Pacemakers placed superficially can cause pectoral trigger points. In the case of pacemaker-induced trigger points, the physical therapist can teach the client trigger point self-treatment to carry out at home.

Chest pain that persists long after an acute myocardial infarction is often due to myofascial trigger points. Travell and Simons (1983) note that in acute myocardial infarction, pain is commonly referred from the heart to the midregion of the pectoralis major and minor muscles (see discussion of viscerosomatic sources of pain, Chapter 1).

The injury to the heart muscle initiates a viscerosomatic process that activates trigger points in the pectoral muscles. After recovery from the infarction, these self-perpetuating trigger points tend to persist in the chest wall. As with all myofascial syndromes, inactivation of the trigger points eliminates the client's symptoms of chest pain.

Myalgia

Myalgia or muscular pain can cause chest pain separate from trigger point pain but with a similar etiologic basis of prolonged or repeated movement. As mentioned earlier, the physical therapy interview must include questions about recent upper respiratory infection with repeated forceful coughing and recent activities of a repetitive nature that could cause sore muscles (e.g., painting or washing walls; calisthenics, including push-ups; or lifting heavy objects or weights).

Squeezing the muscle belly will reproduce painful chest symptoms. The discomfort of myalgia is almost always described as aching and may range from mild to intense. Diaphragmatic irritation may be referred to the ipsilateral neck and shoulder, lower thorax, lumbar region, or upper abdomen as a muscular aching pain. Myalgia in the respiratory muscles is well localized, reproducible by palpation, and exacerbated by movement of the chest wall.

Rib Fractures

Periosteal (bone) pain associated with fractured ribs can cause sharp, localized pain at the level of the fracture with an increase in symptoms associated with trunk motions and respiratory movements, such as deep inspiration, laughing, sneezing, or coughing. The pain may be accompanied by a grating sensation during breathing. This localized pain pattern differs from bone pain associated with chronic disease affecting bone marrow and endosteum, which may result in poorly localized pain of varying degrees of severity.

Occult (hidden) rib fractures may occur, especially in a client with a chronic cough or someone who has had an explosive sneeze. Fractures may occur as a result of trauma (e.g., motor vehicle accident, assault), but painful symptoms may not be perceived at first if other injuries are more significant.

A history of long-term steroid use in the presence of rib pain of unknown cause should raise a red flag. Rib fractures must be confirmed by x-ray diagnosis. Rib pain without fracture may indicate bone tumor or disease affecting bone, such as multiple myeloma.

Cervical Spine Disorders

Cervicodorsal arthritis may produce chest pain that is seldom similar to that of angina pectoris. It is usually sharp and piercing but may be described as a deep, boring, dull discomfort. There is usually unilateral or bilateral chest pain with flexion or hyperextension of the upper spine or neck. The chest pain may radiate to the shoulder girdle and down the arms and is not related to exertion or exercise. Rest may not alleviate the symptoms, and prolonged recumbency makes the pain worse.

Diskogenic disease can also cause referred pain to the chest, but there is usually evidence of disk involvement observed with diagnostic imaging and the presence of neurologic symptoms.

Neurologic Causes

Neurologic disorders such as intercostal neuritis and dorsal nerve root radiculitis or a neurovascular disorder such as thoracic outlet syndrome can cause chest pain. The most commonly recognized neuritis is herpes zoster (shingles).

Intercostal Neuritis

Intercostal neuritis, such as herpes zoster or shingles produced by a viral infection of a dorsal nerve root, can cause neuritic chest wall pain, which can be differentiated from coronary pain.

Neuritic pain occurs unrelated to effort and lasts longer (weeks, months, or years) than angina. The pain may be constant or intermittent and can vary from light burning to a deep visceral sensation. It may be associated with chills, fever, headache, malaise, and skin rash. Symptoms are confined to the somatic distribution of one of the involved spinal nerve(s).

There is an increased incidence of herpes zoster in clients with lymphoma, tuberculosis, leukemia, and AIDS, but it can be triggered by trauma or injection drugs or occur with no known cause.

Clusters of grouped vesicles appear unilaterally along cranial or spinal nerve dermatomes after 1 to 2 days of pain, itching, and hyperesthesia. The lesions follow nerve

Clinical Signs and Symptoms of
Herpes Zoster (Shingles)

- Fever, chills
- Headache and malaise
- 1 to 2 days of pain, itching, and hyperesthesia
- Skin eruptions (vesicles) appear along dermatomes 4 or 5 days after the other symptoms

pathways and do not cross the body midline, although nerves of both sides may be involved. The skin eruptions evolve into crusts on the skin and clear in about 2 weeks, unless the period between the pain and the eruption is longer than 2 days. Postherpetic neuralgia, with its burning and paroxysmal stabbing pain, may persist for long periods.

Herpes zoster is a communicable disease and requires some type of isolation. Specific precautions depend on whether the disease is localized or disseminated and the condition of the client. Persons susceptible to chickenpox should avoid contact with the affected client and stay out of the client's room.

Dorsal Nerve Root Irritation

Dorsal nerve root irritation of the thoracic spine is another neuritic condition that can refer pain to the chest wall. This condition can be caused by infectious processes (e.g., radiculitis or inflammation of the spinal nerve root dural sheath). However, the pain is more likely to be the result of mechanical irritation caused by spinal disease or deformity (e.g., bone spurs secondary to osteoarthritis or the presence of cervical ribs placing pressure on the brachial plexus).

The pain of dorsal nerve root irritation can appear as lateral or anterior chest wall pain with referral to one or both arms through the brachial plexus. Although it

> ### ▼ Clinical Signs and Symptoms of
> ### Dorsal Nerve Root Irritation
>
> - Lateral or anterior chest wall pain
> - History of back pain
> - Pain is aggravated by exertion of only the upper body
> - May be accompanied by neurologic signs
>   - Numbness
>   - Tingling
>   - Muscle atrophy

mimics the pain pattern of coronary heart disease, such pain is more superficial than cardiac pain. Like cardiac pain, dorsal nerve root irritation can be aggravated by exertion of only the upper extremities. However, unlike cardiac pain, exertion of the lower extremities has no exacerbating effect. It is usually accompanied by other neurologic signs, such as muscle atrophy and numbness or tingling.

Thoracic Outlet Syndrome

Thoracic outlet syndrome (TOS) refers to compression of the neural and vascular structures that leave or pass over the superior rim of the thoracic cage. Various names have been given to this condition, including first thoracic rib, cervical rib, scalenus anticus, costoclavicular, and hyperabduction syndromes, according to the presumed site of major neurovascular compression.

The compressive forces associated with this problem usually affect the upper extremities in the ulnar nerve distribution but can result in episodic chest pain mimicking coronary heart disease. There may be radiating pain to the neck, shoulder, scapula, or axilla, but usually associated changes in sensation and neurologic findings point to chest pain with an underlying neurologic cause (Table 12-11).

Paresthesias (burning, pricking sensation) and hypoesthesia (abnormal decrease in sensitivity to stimulation) are common. Anesthesia and motor weakness are reported in about 10% of the cases.

When a vascular compressive component is involved, there may be more diffuse pain in the limb, with associated fatigue and weakness. With more severe arterial compromise, the client may describe coolness, pallor, cyanosis, or symptoms of Raynaud's phenomenon. Although vascular in origin, these symptoms are differentiated from coronary artery disease by the local or regional presentation, affecting only a single extremity or only the upper extremities.

Symptoms may be related to occupational activities, poor posture, sleeping with arms elevated over the head, or acute injuries such as cervical flexion/extension (whiplash). Most people become symptomatic in the third or fourth decade, and women are affected three times more often than are men.

Palpation of the supraclavicular space may elicit tenderness or may define a prominence indicative of a cervical rib. The effect on pulse of Adson's maneuver (deep inspiration with the neck fully extended and the head rotated toward the side of symptoms), the hyperabduction test (arm extended overhead), and the costoclavicular test (exaggerated military attention posture) should be compared in both arms. Other tests are described in orthopedic assessment texts (Magee, 1997). There may be a difference of 10 mm Hg or more in blood pressure from one arm to the other when a unilateral vascular compressive force is present.

Postoperative Pain

Postoperative chest pain following cardiac transplantation or other open heart procedures is usually due to the sternal incision and musculoskeletal manipulation during surgery. Coronary insufficiency does not appear as chest pain because of cardiac denervation.

CLUES TO DIFFERENTIATING CHEST PAIN*

- Chest pain with sudden drop in blood pressure or symptoms such as dizziness, dyspnea, vomiting, or unexplained sweating while standing or ambulating for the first time after surgery, an invasive medical procedure, assault, or accident involving the chest or thorax (pneumothorax)
- Range of motion (e.g., trunk rotation of side bending, shoulder motions) does not reproduce symptoms (exception: intercostal tear caused by forceful coughing associated with diaphragmatic pleurisy)
- Lack of musculoskeletal objective findings; squeezing the underlying pectoral muscles does not reproduce symptoms; resisted motion (e.g., horizontal shoulder abduction or adduction) does not reproduce symptoms; heat and stretching do not reduce or eliminate the symptoms
- Review symptoms of anxiety (Table 1-3)
- Chest pain relieved by antacid (reflux esophagitis), rest from exertion (angina), recumbency (mitral valve prolapse), squatting (hypertrophic cardiomyopathy), passing gas (gas entrapment syndrome), or taking nitrolglycerin (see Table 12-9)

PAST MEDICAL HISTORY

- History of repetitive motion, overuse, prolonged activity (e.g., marathon), long-term use of steroids, assault, or other trauma
- History of flu, trauma, upper respiratory infection, shingles, recurrent pneumonia, chronic bronchitis, or emphysema
- History of breast cancer or other cancer, heart disease or previous myocardial infarction, recent upper respiratory infection (forceful coughing)
- Prolonged use of cocaine or anabolic steroids

CANCER (see also Clues to Screening for Cancer, Chapter 10)

- Nocturnal pain, pain without precise movement aggravation, or pain that fails to respond to treatment
- Weight loss in the presence of immobility when weight gain would otherwise be expected
- Presence of painless sternal or chest wall mass or painless, hard lymph nodes

CARDIOVASCULAR (see Table 3-4)

- Onset of chest pain occurs 5 to 10 minutes after initiating physical or sexual activity (lag time associated with angina)
- Assess the effect of exertion; reproduction of chest, shoulder, or neck symptoms with exertion of only the lower extremities may be cardiovascular
- Chest, neck, or shoulder pain that is aggravated by physical exertion, exposure to temperature changes, strong emotional reactions, or a large meal (coronary artery disease)
- Atypical chest pain associated with dyspnea, arrhythmias, and light-headedness or syncope

PLEUROPULMONARY (see also Clues to Pulmonary Symptoms, Chapter 4)

- Autosplinting (lying on the involved side) quiets chest wall movements and reduces or eliminates pain
- Pain is not reproduced by palpation
- Assess for the three ps (pleuritic pain exacerbated by respiratory movements, pain on palpation associated with musculoskeletal condition, pain with changes in neck, trunk, or shoulder position indicating musculoskeletal origin)
- Increased symptoms occur with recumbency (abdominal contents push up against diaphragm and in turn against the parietal pleura; see Fig. 12-6)
- Presence of associated signs and symptoms such as persistent cough, dyspnea (rest or exertional), or constitutional symptoms

CLUES TO DIFFERENTIATING CHEST PAIN cont'd

GASTROINTESTINAL (Upper GI/Epigastric) (see also Clues to Screening for Gastrointestinal Disease, Chapter 6)

- Food has an effect on symptoms; presence of GI symptoms, simultaneously or alternately
- Symptoms are relieved by antacids, food, passing gas, or assuming the upright position
- Symptoms radiate from the chest posteriorly to the upper back, interscapular, subscapular, or T10 to L2 areas
- Symptoms are not reproduced or aggravated by effort or exertion
- Presence of associated signs and symptoms such as nausea, vomiting, blood in stool, or pain on swallowing
- Presence of associated signs and symptoms such as nausea, vomiting, dark urine, jaundice, flatulence, indigestion, abdominal fullness or bloating, blood in stool, pain on swallowing

BREAST

- Appearance (or report) of lump, nodule, discharge, skin puckering, or distended veins
- Jarring or movement of the breast tissue increases or reproduces the pain in the presence of a breast pathologic condition
- Resisted isometric shoulder horizontal adduction or abduction usually does not reproduce breast pain
- Recent childbirth and/or breast feeding (pectoral myalgia, mastitis)
- Association between painful symptoms and menstrual cycle
- Presence of axillary or supraclavicular lymph nodes that are large, firm, hard, or fixed

NEUROMUSCULOSKELETAL

- Symptoms described using words typical of neuromusculoskeletal origin (e.g., aching, burning, hot, scalding, searing)
- History of associated back pain
- Positive hyperabduction test or other tests for thoracic outlet syndrome
- Presence of trigger points; elimination of trigger point(s) reduces or eliminates symptoms (see Table 12-10 and Fig. 12-4)
- Symptoms are elicited easily by palpation (e.g., squeezing the pectoral muscle belly, palpating the chest wall, intercostal spaces, or costochondral junction), reproducing the pain
- Symptoms are reproduced by resisted horizontal shoulder abduction, adduction, or other shoulder movements
- Symptoms are relieved by heat and stretching
- Costochondritis or Tietze's syndrome may be accompanied by an increase in blood pressure but is usually palpable and aggravated by trunk movements
- Presence of neurologic involvement (e.g., numbness, tingling, muscle atrophy)
- Pain referred along peripheral nerve pathway (dorsal nerve root irritation)
- Pain is unrelated to effort and lasts hours or weeks to months
- Associated signs and symptoms: numbness and tingling, muscle atrophy; rash, fever, chills, headache, malaise (neuritis or shingles)

---

*The reader should think "chest, neck, and/or shoulder" because these may occur simultaneously, alternately, or in various combinations. Most of these principles apply to all three anatomic sites.

TABLE 12-11 ▼ Assessing Symptoms of Thoracic Outlet Syndrome*

*With the use of special tests, patterns of positive objective findings may help characterize thoracic outlet syndrome.

| Vascular Component | Neural | |
	Upper Plexus	Lower Plexus
3-minute elevated test	Point tenderness over C5-C6	Pressure above clavicle elicits pain
Adson's test	Pressure over lateral neck elicits pain	Ulnar nerve tenderness when pal-
Swelling (arm/hand)	and/or numbness	pated under axilla or along inner
Discoloration of hand	Pain with head turned and/or tilted to	arm
Costoclavicular test	opposite side	Tinel's sign for ulnar nerve in axilla
Hyperabduction test	Weak biceps	Hypoesthesia in ulnar nerve distribu-
Upper extremity claudication	Weak triceps	tion
Differences in blood pressure	Weak wrist	Serratus anterior weakness
Skin temperature changes	Hypoesthesia in radial nerve distribution	Weak hand grip
Cold intolerance	3-minute abduction stress test	

▼ SHOULDER PAIN

Systemic disease affecting the breast and any organs in the chest or abdomen may present itself clinically as shoulder pain (Fig. 12-5; Table 12-12). Many neuromuscu-loskeletal conditions in the neck, cervical spine, axilla, thorax, thoracic spine, and chest wall can also refer pain to the shoulder. The physical therapist must always assess above and below the involved joint for referred musculoskeletal pain and screen for medical disease.

Differential diagnosis of shoulder pain is sometimes especially difficult because any pain that is felt in the shoulder often affects the joint as though the pain were originating in the joint (Mennell, 1964). Shoulder pain with any of the components listed in Clues to Differentiating Shoulder Pain should be approached as a manifestation of systemic visceral illness, even if shoulder movements exacerbate the pain or if there are objective findings at the shoulder.

Many visceral diseases are notorious for appearing as unilateral shoulder pain (Table 12-13). Esophageal, pericardial, or myocardial diseases, aortic dissection, and diaphragmatic irritation from thoracic or abdominal diseases (Fig. 12-6) all can appear as unilateral pain.

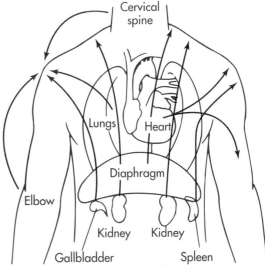

FIGURE 12-5 • Musculoskeletal and systemic structures referring pain to the shoulder. (Modified from Magee DJ: *Orthopedic physical assessment*, ed 2, Philadelphia, 1992, WB Saunders, p 125.)

"Frozen shoulder," or adhesive capsulitis a condition in which both active and passive glenohumeral motions are restricted, can be associated with diabetes mellitus, hyperthyroidism, ischemic heart disease, and lung diseases (tuberculosis, emphysema, chronic bronchitis) (Connolly, 1998). Shoulder pain (unilateral or bilateral) progressing to adhesive capsulitis can occur 6 to 9 months after

TABLE 12-12 ▼ Systemic Causes of Shoulder Pain

Shoulder pain may be referred from the neck, chest (thorax or thoracic spine), and abdomen and from systemic diseases. The following have been diagnosed as having the onset or origin of presenting symptoms in the shoulder.

Neck	Chest	Abdomen	Systemic Disease
Bone tumors	Angina/myocardial infarct	Liver disease	Collagen vascular disease
Metastases	Post-coronary artery bypass	Ruptured spleen	Gout
Tuberculosis	graft (CABG)	Spinal metastases	Syphilis/gonorrhea
Nodes in neck	Bacterial endocarditis	Dissecting aortic	Sickle cell anemia
(from metastases,	Pericarditis	aneurysm	Hemophilia
leukemia, and	Aortic aneurysm	Diaphragmatic irritation	Rheumatic disease
Hodgkin's disease)	Empyema and lung abscess	Peptic ulcer	Metastatic cancer
Cervical cord tumors	Pulmonary tuberculosis	Gallbladder disease	Breast
	Pancoast's tumor	Subphrenic abscess	Prostate
	Lung cancer (bronchogenic carci-	Hiatal hernia	Kidney
	noma)	Pyelonephritis	Lung
	Spontaneous pneumothorax	Diaphragmatic hernia	Thyroid
	Nodes in mediastinum/axilla	Ectopic pregnancy	Testicle
	Metastases in thoracic spine	(rupture)	Diabetes mellitus (adhe-
	Breast disease	Upper urinary tract	sive capsulitis)
	Primary or secondary cancer		
	Mastodynia		
	Hiatal hernia		

Modified from Zohn DA: *Musculoskeletal pain: diagnosis and physical treatment,* ed 2, Boston, 1988, Little, Brown, p 178.

a coronary artery bypass graft (CABG). Similarly, any intensive care unit (ICU) or coronary care unit (CCU) patient can experience shoulder impingement causing shoulder pain and loss of motion resulting in adhesive capsulitis.

Using the past medical history and assessing for the presence of associated signs and symptoms will alert the physical therapist to any red flags suggesting a systemic origin of shoulder symptoms. For example, a ruptured ectopic pregnancy with abdominal hemorrhage can produce left shoulder pain in a woman of childbearing age. Usually there is a history of missed menses.

Other examples include left shoulder pain lasting several days after laparoscopy* or distension of the renal cap from kidney disorders with pain to the ipsilateral shoulder (again, via pressure on the diaphragm). In the first case a recent surgery would be part

of the past medical history. In the case of a kidney disorder causing shoulder pain, accompanying urologic symptoms are usually present.

The client may not recognize the connection between gallbladder removal by laparoscopy and subsequent shoulder pain or painful urination and shoulder pain. It is the physical therapist's responsibility to assess musculoskeletal symptoms, making a physical therapy differential diagnosis that includes ruling out the possibility of systemic disease.

Pulmonary Diseases and Shoulder Pain

Extensive disease may occur in the periphery of the lung without pain until the process extends to the parietal pleura. Pleural irritation then results in sharp, localized pain that is aggravated by any respiratory movement.

Clients usually note that the pain is alleviated by lying on the affected side, which di-

---

*During the procedure air is introduced into the peritoneum to expand the area. This gas bubble can put pressure on the diaphragm and refer pain to the shoulder.

TABLE 12-13 ▼ Shoulder Pain

Right Shoulder		Left Shoulder	
Systemic Origin	**Location**	**Systemic Origin**	**Location**
Peptic ulcer	Lateral border, R scapula	Ruptured spleen	L shoulder (Kehr's sign)
Myocardial ischemia	R shoulder, down arm	Myocardial ischemia	L pectoral/L shoulder
Hepatic/biliary:		Pancreas	L shoulder
Acute cholecystitis	R shoulder; between scapulae; R subscapular area	Ectopic pregnancy (rupture)	L shoulder (Kehr's sign)
Liver abscess	R shoulder		
Gallbladder	R upper trapezius		
Liver disease (hepatitis, cirrhosis, metastatic tumors)	R shoulder, R subscapula		
Pulmonary:	Ipsilateral shoulder; upper trapezius	Pulmonary:	Ipsilateral shoulder; upper trapezius
Pleurisy		Pleurisy	
Pneumothorax		Pneumothorax	
Pancoast's tumor		Pancoast's tumor	
Kidney	Ipsilateral shoulder	Kidney	Ipsilateral shoulder
		Postoperative laparoscopy	L shoulder (Kehr's sign)

minishes the movement of that side of the chest ("autosplinting"). Shoulder pain of musculoskeletal origin is usually aggravated by lying on the symptomatic shoulder.

Pneumonia in the older adult may appear as shoulder pain when the affected lung presses on the diaphragm; usually there are accompanying pulmonary symptoms, but confusion may be the only other associated sign.

Cardiac Diseases and Shoulder Pain

Pain of cardiac and diaphragmatic origin is often experienced in the shoulder because the heart and diaphragm are supplied by the C5 to C6 spinal segment, and the visceral pain is referred to the corresponding somatic area (see Fig. 1-2).

Bacterial Endocarditis

The most common musculoskeletal symptom in clients with bacterial endocarditis is arthralgia, generally in the proximal joints. The shoulder is the most commonly affected site, followed (in declining incidence) by the knee, hip, wrist, ankle, metatarsophalan-

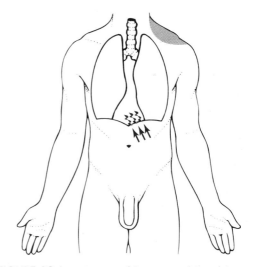

FIGURE 12-6 • Irritation of the peritoneal (outside) or pleural (inside) surface of the central area of the diaphragm refers sharp pain to the upper trapezius muscle, neck, and supraclavicular fossa. The pain pattern is ipsilateral to the area of irritation. Irritation to the peripheral portion of the diaphragm refers sharp pain to the costal margins and lumbar region (not shown).

geal, and metacarpophalangeal joints and by acromioclavicular involvement.

Most endocarditis clients with arthralgias have only one or two painful joints, although some may have pain in several joints. Painful symptoms begin suddenly in one or two joints, accompanied by warmth, tenderness, and redness. One helpful clue: As a rule, morning stiffness is not as prevalent in clients with endocarditis as in those with rheumatoid arthritis or polymyalgia rheumatica.

Pericarditis

The inflammatory process accompanying pericarditis may result in an accumulation of fluid in the pericardial sac, preventing the heart from expanding fully. The subsequent chest pain of pericarditis (see Fig. 3-9) closely mimics that of a myocardial infarction because it is substernal, is associated with cough, and may radiate to the shoulder. It can be differentiated from myocardial infarction by the pattern of relieving and aggravating factors.

For example, the pain of a myocardial infarction is unaffected by position, breathing, or movement, whereas the pain associated with pericarditis may be relieved by kneeling with hands on the floor, leaning forward, or sitting upright. Pericardial pain is often worse with breathing, swallowing, or belching.

Aortic Aneurysm

Aortic aneurysm appears as sudden, severe chest pain with a tearing sensation (see Fig. 3-10), and the pain may extend to the neck, shoulders, lower back, or abdomen but rarely to the joints and arms, which distinguishes it from a myocardial infarction. Isolated shoulder pain is not associated with aortic aneurysm.

Shoulder pain associated with *angina* and *myocardial infarct* is presented in Chapter 3. (See also Figs. 3-7 and 3-8.) Because of the well-known association between shoulder pain and angina, cardiac chest pain may be medically diagnosed without ruling out other causes, such as adhesive capsulitis or supraspinatus tendinitis.

Using a review of symptoms approach (see Systems Review, Chapter 1) and a specific musculoskeletal shoulder examination, the physical therapist can screen to differentiate between a medical pathologic condition and mechanical dysfunction (Smith, 1998).

Reflex Sympathetic Dystrophy

Reflex sympathetic dystrophy (RSD), also known as complex regional pain syndrome (CRPS), is sometimes still referred to by the outdated nomenclature *shoulder-hand syndrome* (see Case Example, Chapter 1).

Shoulder-hand syndrome was a condition that occurred after a myocardial infarct (heart attack), usually after prolonged bedrest. This condition (as it was known then) has been significantly reduced in incidence by more up-to-date and aggressive cardiac rehabilitation programs.

Today, RSDS or CRPS, primarily affecting the limbs, develops after injury or surgery but can still occur as a result of a cerebrovascular accident (CVA), heart attack, or disease of the thoracic or abdominal viscera that causes referred pain to the shoulder and arm.

This syndrome occurs with equal frequency in either or both shoulders and, except when caused by coronary occlusion, is most common in women. The shoulder is generally involved first, but the painful hand may precede the painful shoulder.

When this condition occurs after a myocardial infarction, the shoulder initially may demonstrate pericapsulitis from other causes. Tenderness around the shoulder is diffuse and not localized to a specific tendon or bursal area. The duration of the initial shoulder stage before the hand component begins is extremely variable. The shoulder may be "stiff" for several months before the hand becomes involved, or both may become stiff simultaneously. Other accompanying signs and symptoms are usually present, such as edema, skin changes, and temperature changes.

Hepatic and Biliary Diseases and Shoulder Pain

As with many of the organ systems in the human body, the hepatic and biliary organs (liver, gallbladder, and common bile duct) can develop diseases that mimic primary musculoskeletal lesions.

The musculoskeletal symptoms associated with hepatic and biliary pathologic conditions are generally confined to the midback, scapular, and right shoulder regions. These musculoskeletal symptoms can occur alone (as the only presenting symptom) or in combination with other systemic signs and symptoms. Fortunately, in most cases of shoulder pain referred from visceral processes, shoulder motion is not compromised and local tenderness is not a prominent feature.

Diagnostic interviewing is especially helpful when clients have avoided medical treatment for so long that shoulder pain caused by hepatic and biliary diseases may in turn create biomechanical changes in muscular contractions and shoulder movement. These changes eventually create pain of a biomechanical nature (Rose and Rothstein, 1982).

Referred shoulder pain may be the only presenting symptom of hepatic or biliary disease. Sympathetic fibers from the biliary system are connected through the celiac and splanchnic plexuses to the hepatic fibers in the region of the dorsal spine. These connections account for the intercostal and radiating interscapular pain that accompanies gallbladder disease (see Fig. 8-2). Although the innervation is bilateral, most of the biliary fibers reach the cord through the right splanchnic nerves, producing pain in the right shoulder.

Rheumatic Diseases and Shoulder Pain

A number of systemic rheumatic diseases can appear as shoulder pain, even as unilateral shoulder pain. The HLA-B27–associated spondyloarthropathies (diseases of the joints of the spine), such as ankylosing spondylitis, most frequently involve the sacroiliac joints and spine. Involvement of large central joints, such as the hip and shoulder, is common, however.

Rheumatoid arthritis and its variants likewise frequently involve the shoulder girdle. These systemic rheumatic diseases are suggested by the details of the shoulder examination, by coincident systemic complaints of malaise and easy fatigability, and by complaints of discomfort in other joints either coincidental with the presenting shoulder complaint or in the past.

Other systemic rheumatic diseases with major shoulder involvement include polymyalgia rheumatica and polymyositis (inflammatory disease of the muscles). Both may be somewhat asymmetric but almost always appear with bilateral involvement and impressive systemic symptoms.

Cancer

Questions about visceral function are relevant when the pattern for malignant invasion at the shoulder emerges. Invasion of the upper humerus and glenoid area by secondary malignant deposits affects the joint and the adjacent muscles.

Muscle wasting is greatly in excess of any attributable to arthritis and follows a bizarre pattern that does not conform to any one neurologic lesion or any one muscle. Localized warmth felt at any part of the scapular area may prove to be the first sign of a malignant deposit eroding bone. Within 1 or 2 weeks after this observation, a palpable tumor will have appeared, and erosion of bone will be visible on x-ray films (Cyriax, 1982).

Primary Neoplasm

This neoplasm occurs chiefly in young people, in whom a causeless limitation of movement of the shoulder leads the physician to

▼ *Clinical Signs and Symptoms of*
Neoplasm

- Marked limitation of movement at the shoulder joint
- Severe muscular weakness and pain with resisted movements

CLUES TO DIFFERENTIATING SHOULDER PAIN

- See also Clues to Differentiating Chest Pain
- Simultaneous or alternating pain in other joints, especially in the presence of associated signs and symptoms such as easy fatigue, malaise, fever
- Urologic complaints (see Chapter 7 and Fig. 7-4)
- Presence of hepatic symptoms, especially risk factors for jaundice (see Fig. 8-2)
- Lack of improvement after treatment, including trigger point therapy
- Shoulder pain in a woman of childbearing age of unknown cause associated with missed menses (rupture of ectopic pregnancy)
- Left shoulder pain within 24 hours of abdominal surgery, injury, or trauma (Kehr's sign, ruptured spleen)

PAST MEDICAL HISTORY

- History of rheumatic disease
- History of diabetes mellitus (adhesive capsulitis)
- "Frozen" shoulder of unknown cause in anyone with coronary artery disease, recent history of hospitalization in coronary care or intensive care unit, status post-coronary artery bypass graft (CABG)
- Recent history (past 1-3 months) of myocardial infarction (shoulder-hand syndrome or reflex sympathetic dystrophy [RSD])
- History of cancer, especially breast or lung cancer (metastasis)
- Recent history of pneumonia, recurrent upper respiratory infection, or influenza (diaphragmatic pleurisy)

CANCER

- Pectoralis major muscle spasm with no known cause; limited active shoulder flexion but with full passive shoulder motions and mobile scapula (neoplasm)
- Presence of localized warmth felt over the scapular area (cancer)

CARDIAC

- Exacerbation by exertion unrelated to shoulder movement (e.g., using only the lower extremities to climb stairs or ride a stationary bicycle) (cardiac)
- Excessive, unexplained coincident diaphoresis (cardiac)
- Shoulder pain relieved by leaning forward, kneeling with hands on the floor, sitting upright (pericarditis)
- Shoulder pain accompanied by dyspnea, toothache, belching, nausea, or pressure behind the sternum (angina)
- Shoulder pain relieved by nitroglycerine (men) or antacids (women) (angina)
- Difference of 10 mm Hg or more in blood pressure in the affected arm compared to the uninvolved or a symptomatic arm (dissecting aortic aneurysm, vascular component of thoracic outlet syndrome)

PULMONARY

- Presence of a pleuritic component such as a persistent, dry, hacking, or productive cough; blood-tinged sputum; chest pain; musculoskeletal symptoms are aggravated by respiratory movements

CLUES TO DIFFERENTIATING SHOULDER PAIN cont'd

- Exacerbation by recumbency with proper positioning of the arm in neutral alignment (diaphragmatic or pulmonary component)
- Presence of associated signs and symptoms (e.g., tachypnea, dyspnea, wheezing, hyperventilation)
- Shoulder pain of unknown cause in older adults with accompanying signs of confusion (pneumonia)

GASTROINTESTINAL

- Coincident nausea, vomiting, dysphagia; presence of other gastrointestinal complaints such as anorexia, early satiety, epigastric pain or discomfort and fullness, melena
- Shoulder pain relieved by belching or antacids and made worse by eating
- History of previous ulcer, especially in association with the use of nonsteroidal antiinflammatory drugs

---

a study of the radiographic appearances. If the tumor originates from the shaft of the humerus, the first symptoms may be a feeling of "pins and needles" in the hand, associated with fixation of the biceps and triceps muscles and leading to limitation of movement at the elbow.

Pulmonary (Secondary) Neoplasm

Occasionally the client requires medical referral because shoulder pain is referred from metastatic lung cancer. When the shoulder is examined, the client is unable to lift the arm beyond the horizontal position. Muscles respond with spasm that limits joint movement.

If the neoplasm interferes with the diaphragm, diaphragmatic pain (C3, C4, C5) is often felt at the shoulder at each breath (at the fourth cervical dermatome [i.e., at the deltoid area]), in correspondence with the main embryologic derivation of the diaphragm. Pain arising from the part of the pleura that is not in contact with the diaphragm is also brought on by respiration but is felt in the chest.

Although the lung is insensitive, large tumors invading the chest wall set up local pain and cause spasm of the pectoralis major muscle, with consequent limitation of elevation of the arm. If the neoplasm encroaches on the ribs, stretching the muscle attached to the ribs leads to sympathetic spasm of the pectoralis major.

By contrast, the scapula is mobile, and a full range of passive movement is present at the shoulder joint. The same signs are found in contracture of the pectoral scar after radical mastectomy, but there may be no pain.

Pancoast's Tumors

Pancoast's tumors of the lung apex usually do not cause symptoms while confined to the pulmonary parenchyma. They can extend into the surrounding structures, infiltrating the chest wall into the axilla, appearing with shoulder pain and occasionally with brachial plexus (eighth cervical and first thoracic nerve) involvement.

This nerve involvement produces sharp neuritic pain in the axilla, shoulder, and subscapular area on the affected side, with eventual atrophy of the upper extremity muscles. Bone pain is aching, is exacerbated at night, and is a cause of restlessness and musculoskeletal movement (Cailliet, 1991).

Usually associated general systemic signs and symptoms are present. These features are not found in any regional musculoskeletal disorder, including such disorders of the shoulder.

For example, a similar pain pattern caused by trigger points of the serratus anterior can be differentiated from neoplasm by the lack of true neurologic findings (indicating trigger point) or by lack of improvement after treatment to eliminate the trigger point (indicating neoplasm).

▼ PHYSICIAN REFERRAL

A careful history and close observation of the client are important in determining whether a person may need a medical referral for possible systemic origin of pain or symptoms masquerading as musculoskeletal involvement.

At presentation, anyone with chest, back (cervical, thoracic, scapular, lumbar, sacroiliac), hip, or shoulder pain without a history of trauma (including unreported assault, forceful movement of the spine, repetitive movements of the shoulder or back, or easy lifting) should be screened for a possible systemic origin of symptoms.

It is not the physical therapist's responsibility to differentiate diagnostically among the various causes of systemic signs and symptoms, but rather to identify when the client's history, subjective report, and objective findings do not support the presence of a musculoskeletal problem, thus requiring a medical follow-up.

Each of the visceral systems reviewed in this text has specific patterns of pain referral with accompanying signs and symptoms or history to assist the physical therapist in making a thorough investigation of the presenting problem.

Familiarity with these patterns and the appropriate follow-up questions is essential when considering medical referral for possible visceral involvement. See Clues to Screening boxes and Guidelines for Physician Referral in each chapter (see also Physician Referral, Chapter 1).

Physical therapists are often the health care representatives to whom clients describe problems or concerns that are more appropriately reported to the physician. Conversations of this nature are not unusual when one considers the consistent daily or weekly contact that physical therapists may have with clients. The knowledgeable physical therapist who can recognize this information may also be able to guide the client effectively in seeking the necessary medical attention.

Additionally, exercise may be the precipitating or aggravating factor for the onset of some conditions, such as angina, asthma, vascular or migraine headaches, pneumothorax, or dehydration secondary to the use of diuretic medications, requiring that the physical therapist communicate and collaborate with the physician. Knowledge of the correct information to give the physician can facilitate the communication process.

Systemic Signs and Symptoms Requiring Physician Referral

Systemic signs and symptoms generally follow patterns characteristic of the organ or system involved. Constitutional (i.e., systemic) symptoms that are characteristic of multisystems should serve as red flags to alert the physical therapist to the possibility that a client's complaints are more than just musculoskeletal in nature. The following signs and symptoms are the most common.

Abdominal pain
Anorexia
Bilateral symptoms
Bowel/bladder changes
Chills
Constipation
Diaphoresis
Diarrhea
Dizziness
Dysesthesia
Dysphagia
Dyspnea
Early satiety
Fatigue
Fever
Headaches

Heartburn
Hemoptysis
Hoarseness
Indigestion
Jaundice
Nausea
Night pain
Night sweats

Palpitations
Paresthesia
Persistent cough
Skin rash
Vision changes
Vomiting
Weakness
Weight loss/gain

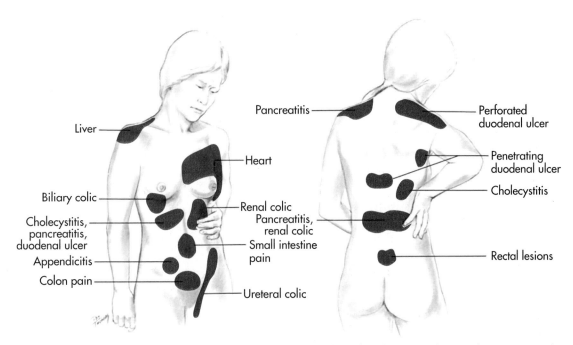

Common sites of referred pain. When a person gives a history of pain referred from the viscera, the pain's location may not be found directly over the involved organ. This is because the human brain has no felt image for internal organs. Rather, pain is referred to a site where the organ was located in fetal development. Although the organ migrates during fetal development, the nerves persist in referring sensations from the former location. (From Jarvis C: *Physical examination and health assessment*, Philadelphia, 1992, WB Saunders.)

 ## KEY POINTS TO REMEMBER

▶ Clients may inaccurately attribute symptoms to a particular incident or activity, or they may fail to recognize causative factors.

▶ At presentation, any person with musculoskeletal pain of unknown cause and/or a past medical history of cancer should be screened for medical disease. Special Questions for Men and Woman may be helpful in this screening process.

▶ When symptoms seem out of proportion to the injury, or if they persist beyond the expected time for the nature of the injury, medical referral may be indicated.

▶ Pain that is unrelieved by rest or change in position or pain/symptoms that do not fit the expected mechanical or neuromusculoskeletal pattern should serve as red-flag warnings.

▶ When symptoms cannot be reproduced, aggravated, or altered in any way during the examination, additional questions to screen for medical disease are indicated.

▶ Shoulder pain aggravated by the supine position may be an indication of mediastinal or pleural involvement. Shoulder or back pain alleviated by lying on the painful side may indicate autosplinting (pleural).

▶ Trigger points should always be considered as a possible cause of systemic-like symptoms.

▶ Chest pain can occur as a result of cervical spine disorders because nerves originating as high as C3 and C4 can extend as far as the nipple line.

▶ Postoperative infection of any kind may not appear with any clinical signs/symptoms for weeks or months.

▶ Muscle weakness without pain, without history of sciatica, and without a positive straight-leg raising is suggestive of spinal metastases.

▶ Sciatica may be the first symptom of prostate cancer metastasized to the bones of the pelvis, lumbar spine, or femur.

▶ Sacral pain, in the absence of a history of trauma or overuse, that is not reproduced with pressure on the sacrum (client is prone) is a red-flag presentation indicating a possible systemic cause of symptoms.

▼ SUMMARY

Throughout this text the physical therapist has been encouraged to assess musculoskeletal complaints of unknown origin affecting the back, shoulder, chest, thorax, pelvis, hip, groin, or sacroiliac joint with the idea that a systemic origin of symptoms must be considered.

A carefully taken medical history, review of systems, evaluation of pain patterns/pain types, and appropriate questions asked during the physical therapy interview must be correlated with the objective findings. These tools will help the physical therapist in making a physical therapy diagnosis or in making the decision to refer the client to another health care practitioner.

This chapter has compared the possible systemic versus musculoskeletal causes of pain associated with the back, hip, pelvis, groin, chest, and shoulder. Special questions to ask are provided to assist the physical therapist in identifying the potential presence of signs and symptoms associated with systemic disease. Additionally, special questions appropriate for women and men are outlined, depending on the presenting musculoskeletal complaints.

SUBJECTIVE EXAMINATION

• SPECIAL QUESTIONS TO ASK

- When did the pain or symptoms start?
- Did it (they) start gradually or suddenly? **(Vascular versus trauma problem)**
- Was there an illness or injury before the onset of pain?
- Have you noticed any changes in your symptoms since they first started to the present time?
- Is the pain aggravated or relieved by coughing or sneezing? **(Nerve root involvement, muscular)**
- Is the pain aggravated or relieved by activity?
- Are there any particular positions (sitting, lying, standing) that aggravate or relieve the pain?
- Does the pain radiate down the leg? *If so, where?*
- Have you noticed any muscular weakness?
- Have you had a fever, chills, or burning with urination during the last 3 to 4 weeks?
- Have you been treated previously for back disorders?
- How has your general health been both before the beginning of your back problem and today?
- How does rest affect the pain or symptoms?
- Do you feel worse in the morning or evening . . . **OR** . . . What difference do you notice in your symptoms from the morning when you first wake up until the evening when you go to bed?
- Do you ever have swollen feet or ankles? *If yes,* are they swollen when you get up in the morning? **(Edema/congestive heart failure)**
- Do you ever get cramps in your legs if you walk for several blocks? **(Intermittent claudication)**

General Systemic

Most of these questions may be asked of clients with pain or symptoms anywhere in the musculoskeletal system.

- Have you ever been told that you have osteoporosis or brittle bones, fractures, back problems? **(Wasting of bone matrix in Cushing's syndrome)**
- Have you ever been diagnosed or treated for cancer in any part of your body?
- Do you ever notice sweating, nausea, or chest pains when your current symptoms occur?
- What other symptoms have you had with this problem? For example, state whether you have had any:

Numbness

Burning, tingling

Nausea, vomiting

Loss of appetite

Unexpected or significant (10 or 15 lb) weight gain or loss

Diarrhea, constipation, blood in your stool or urine

Difficulty in starting or continuing the flow of urine or incontinence (inability to hold your urine)

Hoarseness or difficulty in swallowing

Heart palpitations or fluttering

Difficulty in breathing while just sitting or resting or with mild effort (e.g., when walking from the car to the house)

Unexplained sweating or perspiration

Night sweats, fever, chills

Changes in vision: blurred vision, black spots, double vision, temporary blindness

Fatigue, weakness, sudden paralysis of one side of your body, arm, or leg **(Transient ischemic attack)**

Headaches

Dizziness or fainting spells

Gastrointestinal

- Have you noticed any association between when you eat and when your symptoms increase or decrease?

    — Do you notice any change in your symptoms 1 to 3 hours after you eat?

    — Do you notice any pain beneath the breastbone (epigastric) or just beneath the wing bone (subscapular) 1 to 2 hours after eating?

- Do you have a feeling of fullness after only one or two bites of food?

- Is your back pain relieved after having a bowel movement? **(Gastrointestinal obstruction)**

- Do you have rectal, low back, or sacroiliac pain when passing stool or having a bowel movement?

- Do you have frequent heartburn or take antacids to relieve heartburn or acid indigestion?

Urology

- Have you noticed any changes in your bowel movement or the flow of urine since your back/groin pain started?

    — *If no*, it may be necessary to provide prompts or examples of what changes you are referring to (e.g., difficulty in starting or continuing the flow of urine, numbness or tingling in the groin or pelvis)

- Have you had burning with urination during the last 3 to 4 weeks?
- Do you ever have blood in your stool or notice blood in the toilet after having a bowel movement? **(Hemorrhoids, prostate problems, cancer)**
- Do you have any problems with your kidneys or bladder? *If so,* describe.
- Have you ever had kidney or bladder stones? *If so,* how were these stones treated?
- Have you ever had an injury to your bladder or to your kidneys? *If so,* how was this treated?
- Have you had any infections of the bladder, and how were these infections treated?
    - Were they related to any specific circumstances (e.g., pregnancy, intercourse)?
- Have you had any kidney infections, and how were these treated?
    - Were they related to any specific circumstances (e.g., pregnancy, after bladder infections, a strep throat, or strep skin infections)?
- Do you ever have pain, discomfort, or a burning sensation when you urinate? **(Lower urinary tract irritation)**
- Have you noticed any blood in your urine?

SUBJECTIVE EXAMINATION
- SPECIAL QUESTIONS TO ASK: HIP

Because hip pain can be caused by referred pain from disorders of the low back, abdomen, and reproductive and urologic structures, special questions should include consideration of the following:

Special questions for women

Special questions for men

Special questions for clients:

General systemic questions

Gastrointestinal questions

Urologic questions

SUBJECTIVE EXAMINATION
- SPECIAL QUESTIONS TO ASK: GROIN

Refer to the Special Questions to Ask: Hip section

Refer to the Special Questions to Ask: Sacroiliac/Sacrum section

SUBJECTIVE EXAMINATION

- **SPECIAL QUESTIONS FOR WOMEN EXPERIENCING BACK, GROIN, PELVIC, HIP, SACROILIAC (SI) OR SACRAL PAIN**

    - Since your back/SI (or other type) of pain/symptoms started, have you seen a gynecologist to rule out any gynecologic cause of this problem?

    - Have you ever been told that you have:

        Retroversion of the uterus (tipped back)

        Ovarian cysts

        Fibroids or tumors

        Endometriosis

        Cystocele (sagging bladder)

        Rectocele (sagging rectum)

    - Have you ever had pelvic inflammatory disease (PID)?

    - Do you have any known sexually transmitted diseases? **(Cause of PID)**

    - Do you have any premenstrual symptoms (e.g., water retention, mood changes including depression, headaches, food cravings, painful or tender breasts)? Have you noticed any pattern between your back/SI (or other) symptoms and PMS?

    - Do you have an intrauterine coil or loop (IUCD)? **(PID and ectopic pregnancy can occur)**

    - Have you (recently) had a baby? **(Birth trauma)**

        — *If yes,* did you have an epidural (anesthesia)? **(Postpartum back pain)**

        — Did you have any significant medical problems during your pregnancy or delivery?

    - Have you ever had a tubal or ectopic pregnancy? Is it possible you may be pregnant now?

    - Have you had any spontaneous or induced abortions? **(Weakness secondary to blood loss, infection, scarring; blood in peritoneum irritating diaphragm)** *If yes,* how many, when, onset of symptoms in relation to incident?

    - Do you ever leak urine with coughing, laughing, lifting, exercising, or sneezing? **(Stress incontinence; tension myalgia of pelvic floor)**

    - Do you ever have a "falling-out" feeling or pelvic heaviness after standing for a long time? **(Incontinence; prolapse; pelvic floor weakness)**

        — *If yes,* to incontinence, ask several additional questions to determine the frequency, the amount of protection needed as measured by the number and type of pads used daily, and how much this problem interferes with daily activities and lifestyle.

    - Recent history of bladder or kidney infections? **(Referred back pain)**

    - Presence of vaginal discharge? **(Referred back pain)**

        — *If yes,* do you know what is causing this discharge?

        — How long have you had this problem? Is there any connection between when the discharge started and when you first noticed your back/sacroiliac (or other) symptoms?

- Is there any connection between your (back, hip, sacroiliac) pain/symptoms and your menstrual cycle (related to ovulation, midcycle, or menses)?
- Where were you in your menstrual cycle when your injury or illness occurred?
- Have you ever been told you have endometriosis? Osteoporosis?

SUBJECTIVE EXAMINATION

- **SPECIAL QUESTIONS FOR MEN EXPERIENCING BACK, HIP, GROIN, SI OR SACRAL PAIN/SYMPTOMS**

  - Do you ever have difficulty with urination (e.g., difficulty starting or continuing flow or a very slow flow of urination)?
  - Do you ever have blood in your urine?
  - Do you ever have pain, burning, or discomfort on urination?
  - Have you ever been treated for prostate problems (prostate cancer, prostatitis)?
  - Have you recently had kidney stones or bladder or kidney infections?
  - Have you ever been told you have a hernia, or do you think you have a hernia now?

SUBJECTIVE EXAMINATION

- **SPECIAL QUESTIONS TO ASK: CHEST/THORAX**

Musculoskeletal

- Have you strained a muscle from coughing?
- Have you ever injured your chest?
- Does it hurt to touch your chest or to take a deep breath (e.g., coughing, sneezing, sighing, or laughing)? **(Myalgia, fractured rib, costochondritis, myofascial trigger point)**
- Do you have frequent attacks of heartburn, or do you take antacids to relieve heartburn or acid indigestion? **(Noncardiac cause of chest pain, abdominal muscle trigger point, gastrointestinal disorder)**

Neurologic

- Do you have any trouble taking a deep breath? **(Weak chest muscles secondary to polymyositis, dermatomyositis, myasthenia gravis)**
- Does your chest pain ever travel into your armpit, arm, neck, or wing bone (scapula)? (Thoracic outlet syndrome, trigger points)
  - *If yes,* do you ever feel burning, prickling, numbness, or any other unusual sensation in any of these areas?

Pulmonary

- Have you ever been treated for a lung problem?
  - *If yes*, describe what this problem was, when it occurred, and how it was treated.
- Do you think your chest or thoracic (upper back) pain is caused by a lung problem?
- Have you ever had trouble with breathing?
- Are you having difficulty with breathing now?
- Do you ever have shortness of breath, breathlessness, or can't quite catch your breath?
  - *If yes*, does this happen when you rest, lie flat, walk on level ground, walk up stairs, or when you are under stress or tension?
  - How long does it last?
  - What do you do to get your breathing back to normal?
- How far can you walk before you feel breathless?
- What symptom stops your walking (e.g., shortness of breath, heart pounding, or weak legs)?
- Do you have any breathing aids (e.g., oxygen, nebulizer, humidifier, or ventilation devices)?
- Do you have a cough? (Note whether the person smokes, for how long and how much.) Do you have a smoker's hack?
  - *If yes*, to having a cough, distinguish it from a smoker's cough. Ask when it started.
  - Does coughing increase or bring on your symptoms?
  - Do you cough anything up? *If yes*, please describe the color, amount, and frequency.
  - Are you taking anything for this cough? *If yes*, does it seem to help?
- Do you have periods when you can't seem to stop coughing?
- Do you ever cough up blood?
  - *If yes*, what color is it? (Bright red = fresh; brown or black = older)
  - *If yes*, has this been treated?
- Have you ever had a blood clot in your lungs? *If yes*, when and how was it treated?
- Have you had a chest x-ray film taken during the last 5 years? *If yes*, when and where did it occur? What were the results?
- Do you work around asbestos, coal, dust, chemicals, or fumes? *If yes*, describe.
  - Do you wear a mask at work? *If yes*, approximately how much of the time do you wear a mask?
- If the person is a farmer, ask what kind of farming (because some agricultural products may cause respiratory irritation).
- Have you ever had tuberculosis or a positive skin test for tuberculosis?
  - *If yes*, when did it occur and how was it treated? What is your current status?
- When was your last test for tuberculosis? Was the result normal?

Cardiac

- Has a physician ever told you that you have heart trouble?
- Have you ever had a heart attack? *If yes*, when? Describe.
  - *If yes*, to either question: Do you think your current symptoms are related to your heart problems?
  - Do you have angina (pectoris)?
  - *If yes*, describe the symptoms and tell me when it occurs.
  - *If no*, pursue further with the following questions.
- Do you ever have discomfort or tightness in your chest? **(Angina)**
- Have you ever had a crushing sensation in your chest with or without pain down your left arm?
- Do you have pain in your jaw, either alone or in combination with chest pain?
- If you climb a few flights of stairs fairly rapidly, do you have tightness or pressing pain in your chest?
- Do you get pressure or pain or tightness in the chest if you walk in the cold wind or face a cold blast of air?
- Have you ever had pain or pressure or a squeezing feeling in the chest that occurred during exercise, walking, or any other physical or sexual activity?
- Do you ever have bouts of rapid heart action, irregular heartbeats, or palpitations of your heart?
  - *If yes*, did this occur after a visit to the dentist? **(Endocarditis)**
- Have you noticed any skin rash or dots under the skin on your chest in the last 3 weeks? **(Rheumatic fever, endocarditis)**
- Have you used cocaine, crack, or any other recreational drug in the last 6 weeks?

Epigastric

- Have you ever been told that you have an ulcer?
- Does the pain under your breast bone radiate (travel) around to your back, or do you ever have back pain at the same time that your chest hurts?
- Have you ever had heartburn or acid indigestion?
  - *If yes*, how is this pain different?
  - *If no*, have you noticed any association between when you eat and when this pain starts?

Breast

- Have you ever had any breast surgery (implants, mastectomy, reconstructive surgery, or augmentation)?

- Do you have any discharge from your breasts or nipples?
  - *If yes*, do you know what is causing this discharge?
  - Have you received medical treatment for this problem?
- Are you lactating (nursing an infant)?
- Have you examined yourself for any lumps or nodules and found any thickening or lump?
  - *If yes*, where was it and how long was it present?
  - Has your physician examined this lump?
  - *If no* (for women), do you examine your own breasts?
  - *If yes*, when was the last time that you did a breast self-examination?
- Have you been involved in any activities of a repetitive nature that could cause sore muscles (e.g., painting, washing walls, push-ups or other calisthenics, heavy lifting or pushing, overhead movements, prolonged running, or fast walking)?
- Have you recently been coughing excessively?
- Have you ever had angina (chest pain) or a heart attack?
- Have you been in a fight or hit, punched, or pushed against any object that injured your chest or breast (assault)?

SUBJECTIVE EXAMINATION

- ## SPECIAL QUESTIONS TO ASK: SHOULDER

General Systemic

- Does your pain ever wake you at night from a sound sleep? **(Cancer)** Can you find any way to relieve the pain and get back to sleep?
  - *If yes*, how? **(Cancer: nothing relieves it)**
- Have you sustained any injuries in the last week during a sports activity, car accident, etc? **(Ruptured spleen associated with pain in the left shoulder: positive Kehr's sign)**
- Have you been in a fight, assaulted, pushed against a wall/object, or pulled/thrown by the arm?
- Since the beginning of your shoulder problem, have you had any unusual perspiration for no apparent reason, night sweats, or fever?
- Have you had any unusual fatigue (more than usual with no change in lifestyle), joint pain in other joints, or general malaise? **(Rheumatic disease)**
- *For the therapist:* Has the client had a laparoscopy in the last 24 to 48 hours? **(Left shoulder pain: positive Kehr's sign)**

Pulmonary

- Do you currently have a cough?
  - *If yes,* is this a smoker's cough?
  - *If no,* how long has this been present?
  - Is this a productive cough (can you bring up sputum), and is the sputum tinged with blood?
- Does your shoulder pain increase when you cough, laugh, or take a deep breath?
- Do you have any chest pain?
- What effect does lying down or resting have on your shoulder pain?
  (In the supine or recumbent position, a pulmonary problem may be made worse, whereas a musculoskeletal problem may be relieved; on the other hand, pulmonary pain may be relieved when the client lies on the affected side, which diminishes the movement of that side of the chest.)

Cardiac

- Do you ever notice sweating, nausea, or chest pain when the pain in your shoulder occurs?
- Have you noticed your shoulder pain increasing with exertion that does not necessarily cause you to use your shoulder (e.g., climbing stairs, stationary bicycle)?

Gastrointestinal

- Have you ever had an ulcer?
  - *If yes,* when? Do you still have any pain from your ulcer?
  - Have you noticed any association between when you eat and when your symptoms increase or decrease?
- Does eating relieve your pain? **(Duodenal or pyloric ulcer)**
  - How soon is the pain relieved after eating?
- Does eating aggravate your pain? **(Gastric ulcer, gallbladder inflammation)**
- Does your pain occur 1 to 3 hours after eating or between meals? **(Duodenal or pyloric ulcers, gallstones)**
- Have you ever had gallstones?
- Do you have a feeling of fullness after only one or two bites of food? **(Early satiety: stomach and duodenum or gallbladder)**
- Have you had any nausea, vomiting, difficulty in swallowing, loss of appetite, or heartburn since the shoulder started bothering you?

Urological

Have you had any recent kidney infections, tumors, or kidney stones? **(Pressure from kidney on diaphragm referred to shoulder)**

SUBJECTIVE EXAMINATION

- ### SPECIAL QUESTIONS FOR WOMEN EXPERIENCING SHOULDER PAIN/DYSFUNCTION

  - Have you ever had a breast implant, mastectomy, or other breast surgery? **(Altered lymph drainage, scar tissue)**

  - Have you ever had a tubal or ectopic pregnancy?

  - Have you had any spontaneous or induced abortions recently? **(Blood in peritoneum irritating diaphragm)**

  - Have you recently had a baby? **(Excessive muscle tension during birth)**

    — *If yes:* Are you breastfeeding with the infant supported on pillows?

    — Do you have a breast discharge, or have you had mastitis?

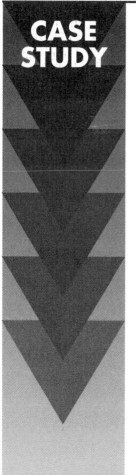

CASE STUDY

REFERRAL

A 65-year-old retired railroad engineer has come to you with a left "frozen shoulder." During the course of the subjective examination, he also tells you that he is taking two cardiac medications.

> *What questions should you ask that might help you relate these two problems (shoulder/cardiac) or to rule out any relationship?*

PHYSICAL THERAPY INTERVIEW

Onset/History

What do you think is the cause of your shoulder problem?

When did it occur, or how long have you had this problem (sudden or gradual onset)?

Can you recall any specific incident when you injured your shoulder, for example, by falling, being hit by someone or something, automobile accident?

Did you ever have a snapping or popping sensation just before your shoulder started to hurt? **(Ligamentous or cartilagenous lesion)**

Did you injure your neck in any way before your shoulder developed these problems?

Have you had a recent heart attack? Have you had nausea, fatigue, sweating, chest pain, or pressure with or without pain in your neck, jaw, left shoulder, or down your left arm?

Has your left hand ever been stiff or swollen? **(Reflex sympathetic dystrophy after myocardial infarction)**

Do you associate the symptom relating to your shoulder with your heart problems?

Shortly before you first noticed difficulty with your shoulder were you involved in any kind of activities that would require repetitive movements, such as painting, gardening, playing tennis or golf?

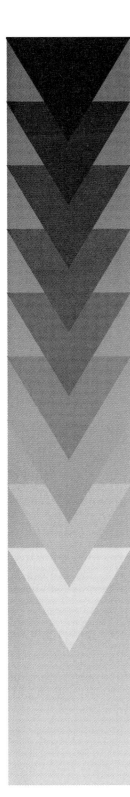

MEDICAL HISTORY

Have you had any surgery during the past year?

How has your general health been? **(Shoulder pain is a frequent site of referred pain from other internal medical problems; see Fig. 12-5.)**

Did you ever have rheumatic fever when you were a child?

What is your typical pattern of chest pain or angina?

Has this pattern changed in any way since your shoulder started to hurt? For example, does the chest pain last longer, come on with less exertion, and feel more intense?

Do your heart medications relieve your shoulder symptoms, even briefly?

> If so, how long after you take the medications do you notice a difference?

> Does this occur every time that you take your medications?

MEDICAL TESTING

Have you had any recent x-rays taken of the shoulder or your neck?

Have you received medical or physical therapy treatment for shoulder problems before?

> If so, where, when, why, who, and what (see The Core Interview in Chapter 2 for specific questions)?

> Have you had any (extensive) medical testing during the past year?

PAIN/SYMPTOMS

Is your shoulder painful?

> If *yes,* how long has the shoulder been painful?

> Follow the usual line of questioning regarding the pattern, frequency, intensity, and duration outlined in The Core Interview to establish necessary information regarding pain.

Aggravating/relieving activities

> How does rest affect your shoulder symptoms? (True muscular lesions are relieved with prolonged rest [i.e., more than 1 hour], whereas angina is usually relieved more immediately by cessation of activity or rest [i.e., usually within 2 to 5 minutes, up to 15 minutes.])

> Does your shoulder pain occur during exercise (e.g., walking, climbing stairs, mowing the lawn or any other physical or sexual activity? (Evaluate the difference between total body exertion causing shoulder symptoms versus movements of the upper extremities only reproducing symptoms. Total body exertion causing shoulder pain may be secondary to angina or myocardial infarction, whereas movements of just the upper extremities causing shoulder pain are indicative of a primary musculoskeletal lesion.)

Subacute/acute/chronic musculoskeletal lesion versus systemic pain pattern (see The Core Interview for specific meaning to the client's answers to these questions):

> Can you lie on that side?

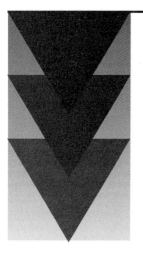

Does the shoulder pain awaken you at night?

> If so, is this because you have rolled onto that side?

Do you notice any chest pain, night sweats, fever, or heart palpitations when you wake up at night?

Have you ever noticed these symptoms (e.g., chest pain, heart palpitations) with your shoulder pain during the day?

Do these symptoms wake you up separately from your shoulder pain, or does your shoulder pain wake you up and you have these additional symptoms? (As always when asking questions about sleep patterns, the person may be unsure of the answers to the questions. In such cases the physical therapist is advised to ask the client to pay attention to what happens related to sleep during the next few days up to 1 week and report back with more definitive information.)

PRACTICE QUESTIONS

1. The most common sites of referred pain from systemic diseases are:

   a. Neck and back

   b. Shoulder and back

   c. Chest and back

   d. None of the above

2. The best and easiest way to screen for medical disease is to:

   a. Perform special tests (e.g., iliopsoas test, McBurney's point, Murphy's percussion)

   b. Correlate subjective assessment with objective assessment

   c. Correlate client history with clinical presentation and ask about associated signs and symptoms

   d. Perform a systems review

   e. All of the above

   f. None of the above

3. A 66-year-old woman has been referred to you by her physiatrist for preprosthetic training after an above-knee amputation. Her past medical history is significant for chronic diabetes mellitus (insulin dependent), coronary artery disease with recent angioplasty and stent placement, and peripheral vascular disease. During the physical therapy evaluation, the client experienced anterior neck pain radiating down the left arm.

   Name (and/or describe) three tests you can do to differentiate a musculoskeletal cause from a cardiac cause of shoulder pain.

4. What are two ways of classifying back pain (as presented in the text)?

5. How can you differentiate sciatica of systemic origin from sciatica of neuromusculoskeletal origin?

6. A 33-year-old woman comes to you with a report of leg pain that begins in her buttocks and goes all the way down to her toes. If this pain is of vascular origin, what word(s) would she most likely use to describe her pain? If of neurogenic origin? If of muscular origin?

7. Which of the following signs and symptoms are *not* associated with pelvic pain of a systemic origin?

   a. Pain that is made worse by physical activity or exertion

   b. Pain that is relieved by placing a pillow or support under the hips and buttocks

   c. Pain that is worse in the morning but decreases with movement or stretching

   d. Pain that is not reduced or eliminated by trigger point release or soft tissue mobilization

8. You are evaluating a 30-year-old woman with right shoulder pain radiating down the inner aspect of the arm in the ulnar nerve distribution. The majority of test results point to a thoracic outlet syndrome with both a neurologic and a vascular component. Is a medical referral recommended because of the vascular involvement? Explain your rationale.

9. Which of the following would be useful information for evaluating a 37-year-old woman with shoulder and breast pain?

   a. Influence of antacids on symptoms

   b. History of chronic nonsteroidal anti-inflammatory drug use

   c. Effect of food on symptoms

   d. Presence of urologic symptoms

   e. (a), (b), and (c)

   f. All of the above

   g. None of the above

10. Muscle weakness without pain, without history of sciatica, and without a positive straight-leg raise is suggestive of:

   a. Trauma or assault

   b. Overuse

   c. Spinal metastases

   d. Myofascial trigger points

References

Baker PK: Musculoskeletal problems. In Steege JF, Metzger DA, Levy BS: *Chronic pelvic pain: an integrated approach,* Philadelphia, 1998, WB Saunders, pp 215-240.

Cady B, Steele GD, Morrow M et al: Evaluation of common breast problems: guidance for primary care providers, *CA Cancer J Clin* 48(1):49-63, 1998.

Cailliet R: *Shoulder pain,* ed 3, Philadelphia, 1991, FA Davis.

Connolly JF: Unfreezing the frozen shoulder, *J Muscu-loskel Med* 15(11):47-56, 1998.

Cyriax J: *Textbook of orthopaedic medicine,* ed 8, vol 1, London 1982, Bailliere Tindall.

Gasparini D, Geatti O, Orsolon PG et al: Female "varicocele," *Clin Nucl Med* 23(7):420-422, 1998.

Giudice LC: Status of current research on endometriosis, *J Reprod Med* 43(3 suppl):252-262, 1998.

Hoffman RS, Hollander JE: Evaluation of patients with chest pain after cocaine use, *Crit Care Clin* 13(4):809-828, 1997.

Jay SJ: Cocaine use and chest pain syndromes, *Arch Intern Med* 158(16):1827-1828, 1998.

Magee DJ: *Orthopedic physical assessment,* ed 3, Philadelphia, 1997, WB Saunders.

Mathias SD, Kuppermann M, Liberman RF et al: Chronic pelvic pain: prevalence, health-related quality of life, and economic correlates, *Obstet Gynecol* 87(3):321-327, 1996.

Mazanec DJ: Recognizing malignancy in patients with low back pain, *J Musculoskel Med* 13(1):24-31, 1996.

Mazanec DJ, Segal AM, Sinks PB: Identification of malignancy in patients with back pain: red flags, *Arthritis Rheum* 36(suppl):S251-S258, 1993.

Mennell JM: *Joint pain: diagnosis and treatment using manipulative techniques,* Boston, 1964, Little, Brown.

Rose SJ, Rothstein JM: Muscle mutability: general concepts and adaptations to altered patterns of use, *Phys Ther* 62:1773, 1982.

Smith ML: Differentiating angina and shoulder pathology pain, *Phys Ther Case Rep* 1(4):210-212, 1998.

Sullivan ML, Martinez CM, Gennis P et al: The cardiac toxicity of anabolic steroids, *Prog Cardiovasc Dis* 41(1):1-15, 1998.

Tarazov PG, Prozorovskij KV, Ryzhkov VK: Pelvic pain syndrome caused by ovarian varices, *Acta Radiol* 38(6):1023-1025, 1997.

Travell JG, Simons DG: *Myofascial pain and dysfunction: the trigger point manual,* vol 1, Baltimore, 1983, Williams & Wilkins.

Travell JG, Simons DG: *Myofascial pain and dysfunction: the trigger point manual,* vol 2, Baltimore, 1992, Williams & Wilkins.

Answers to Practice Test Questions

Chapter 1 Introduction to Differential Screening in Physical Therapy

1. (b); The function of a diagnosis and diagnostic classifications is to provide information (i.e., identify as closely as possible the underlying neuromusculoskeletal pathology) that can guide efficient treatment and effective management of the client.

2. (b); visceral

3. (c); somatic

4. (d); Other signs and symptoms associated with joint pain of systemic origin may include fatigue; weight loss; low-grade fever; muscular weakness; and cyclical, progressive pattern of symptoms. Joint symptoms are intermittent with hydrarthrosis usually present (with or without joint redness, warmth, and tenderness).

5. When someone presents with symptoms that persist beyond the expected time for physiologic healing, always review the items listed in *When to Screen for Systemic Disease*. Look for clusters of associated signs and symptoms that fit a particular organ or body system.

   Then review the components of depression and symptom magnification and test for nonorganic signs (see Table 1-3). Signs that the client's symptoms have become the predominant force in func-tion suggest symptom magnification (e.g., ineffective strategy for balancing symptoms against activities, activities controlled by the symptoms, exaggeration of physical limitations).

   Remember to look for components of a chronic pain syndrome such as multiple complaints, excessive preoccupation with pain, excessive drug use, depression/anxiety, and verbal cues that the person is looking for secondary gains.

Chapter 2 Introduction to the Interviewing Process

1. (b); NSAIDs can be potent renal vaso-constrictors causing increased blood pressure and resultant lower extremity edema as sodium and water are con-served by the body.

2. (a); Although all the information ob-tained from the Family/personal history form, interview, and objective exams provide important information for the physical therapy diagnosis, it is well documented that 80% (or more) of the information needed to determine the cause of symptoms is actually in the Core Interview of the Subjective Exam.

3. Is there anything else you think is im-portant about your condition that we have not discussed yet?

4. Constitutional symptoms—affecting the whole body; not local; (1) fever; (2) night sweats; (3) nausea; (4) vomiting;

(5) fatigue. See Box 1-1 or Table 2-5 for a complete listing.

5. (c)

6. Do you have that pain right now? (For the person who responds "Yes," you may also use the McGill Home Recording Card for a 24 to 48-hour assessment to determine whether there is any modulation of painful symptoms).

7. (a) and (c)

8. True. This includes any woman who has experienced a surgical menopause (e.g., oophorectomy for ovarian cancer) or any postmenopausal woman who is not taking hormone replacements.

9. Before approaching the physician about abnormal blood pressure readings, measure both sides for comparison, remeasure both sides on another day, have another health professional check the readings, and screen for associated signs and symptoms (such as pallor, fatigue, perspiration, and/or palpitations). Review the personal/family history for heart disease, check for medications (e.g., perhaps the person is already taking an antihypertensive medication or another medication with elevated blood pressure as a potential side effect), and evaluate the presence of other risk factors (e.g., caffeine, smoking, obesity, sedentary lifestyle). When reporting these findings, let the physician know you would like a medical clearance for rehabilitation that includes an aerobic component.

10. The first questions should always be, "Did you actually see your physician?" Then ask questions directed at assessing for the presence of constitutional symptoms. For example, after paraphrasing what the client has told you, then ask, "Are you having any other symptoms of any kind in your body that you haven't mentioned?" If no, ask more specifically about the presence of associated signs and symptoms, including naming constitutional symptoms one by one.

Follow-up with *Special Questions for Men Experiencing Back Pain* (see text).

Chapter 3 Overview of Cardiovascular Signs and Symptoms

1. (b)

2. *Myocardial ischemia* is a deficiency of blood supply to the heart muscle usually caused by narrowing of the coronary arteries. *Angina pectoris* is the chest pain that occurs when the heart is not receiving an adequate supply of blood and therefore insufficient amounts of oxygen for the workload. *Myocardial infarction* is death of the heart tissue when blood supply to that area is interrupted.

3. Monitor vital signs and palpate pulses. Evaluate past/current medical history for presence of coronary artery disease. Any suspicion of thoracic aneurysm must be reported to the physician immediately. It is beyond the scope of a physical therapist's practice to suggest the possibility of an aneurysm. Rather, clinical observations should be documented and submitted to the physician. A summary comment can be made such as "This clinical presentation is not consistent with a musculoskeletal problem. Please evaluate."

4. See Box: *Clues to Cardiovascular Signs and Symptoms* for a description and explanation of the 3 Ps.

5. Palpitations can be considered physiologic when they occur at a rate of less than six per minute. Palpitations lasting for hours or occurring in association with pain, shortness of breath, fainting, or severe lightheadedness require medical evaluation. Palpitations in any person with a history of unexplained sudden death in the family require medical referral. Palpitations can also occur as a side effect of some medications, through the use of drugs such as cocaine, as a result of an overactive thyroid, or secondary to caffeine sensitivity. Palpitations as a recurring symptom (even if

less than six/minute) should always be reported to the physician.

6. *Past medical history*—personal or family history of CAD, heart disease, angina, MI, or risk factors associated with these; assess menstrual history: a menopausal or postmenopausal woman with a high risk for heart disease who is not receiving hormone replacement therapy may develop symptomatic CAD.

Clinical presentation—objective findings from the clinical evaluation do not seem consistent with TMJ dysfunction; assess the effect of using a stationary bicycle or treadmill (stairs or walking will also work) without upper extremity exertion on jaw pain. Increased pain or symptoms with increased lower body exertion may be a sign of cardiac involvement and should be reported to the referring dentist.

Associated signs and symptoms—Assess for coincident nausea, diaphoresis, pallor, or dyspnea during painful or symptomatic periods. Look for recent history (last 6 weeks to 6 months onset) of shortness of breath at night, extreme fatigue, lethargy, and weakness. Ask about the presence of other body aches and pains (be alert for "heartburn" unrelieved by antacids, isolated right biceps muscle aching, breast or chest pain). Measure vital signs for any unusual findings and assess changes in vital signs with changes in workload during exercise.

7. The onset of a myocardial infarction is known to be precipitated by working with the arms extended over the head. Ischemia or infarction may be the cause of this client's symptoms. Assess for history of heart disease, presence of known hypertension, angina, past episodes of heart attack, or congestive heart failure. Assess vital signs and changes in vital signs with increased workload and assess the effect of increasing the workload of the lower extremities only.

Evaluate for thoracic outlet syndrome (TOS), especially a cardiovascular com-

ponent (see Table 12-11). Evaluate for and treat trigger points of the chest, upper abdomen, and upper extremity.

This client should be evaluated by his physician; the physical therapist's information gathered from the assessment will be helpful in the medical differential diagnosis.

8. Evaluate this client for the presence of cyanosis, orthopnea, tachycardia, changes in renal function (decreased during the day but frequent urination at night), or presence of a spasmodic cough when lying down or at night. These may be indicators of congestive heart failure and must be reported to the physician. Take note whether this client is taking NSAIDs and digitalis together; this combination of medication can result in ankle swelling and must also be reported to the physician.

9. (d); Arterial and occlusive diseases are synonymous for the same thing—occlusion of the arteries produces arterial disease; occlusion of the veins produces venous disorders; arteries and veins comprise the major peripheral blood vessels so that any diseases or disorders of the arteries and/or veins are included in peripheral vascular disorders.

10. (c)

Chapter 4 Overview of Pulmonary Signs and Symptoms

1. Ask about a past medical history (within the last 6 to 8 weeks) of upper respiratory infection, pneumonia, pleurisy, or traumatic injury. Look for the presence of associated signs and symptoms such as fever, chills, night sweats, digital clubbing, persistent cough, or dyspnea.

Evaluate whether the symptoms can be reproduced with palpation or movement. Pulmonary symptoms may be exacerbated or increased by the supine position and alleviated or decreased when lying on the involved side (autosplinting).

Examine the client for trigger points; reexamine after any trigger points have been eliminated.

2. (c)

3. (a)

4. (f); pain can also radiate to the costal margins or upper abdomen (see Fig. 4-7)

5. False; however, medical referral is usually not considered necessary when a client presents with a singular systemic sign or symptom, especially in the presence of a clear clinical presentation of a musculoskeletal pattern.

6. (e)

7. Autosplinting occurs when lying on the involved side quiets respiratory movements and reduces or eliminates symptoms. Most musculoskeletal problems are made worse by placing this kind of pressure on the symptomatic shoulder, neck, or thoracic spine. The therapist must also evaluate the presence of associated signs and symptoms, the effect of increased respiratory movements on symptoms, and the effect of the supine position (recumbency) on shoulder/upper trapezius pain.

8. These have equal significance when viewed as part of a continuum; dyspnea progressing from exertional to rest is a red-flag symptom. The usual progression of dyspnea is for a client to first notice shortness of breath after a certain length of time or intensity while engaging in an activity such as walking or climbing stairs. Progression to dyspnea at rest usually occurs after the client notices shortness of breath occurring sooner and with less intensity in the activity.

Exertional dyspnea may be the result of deconditioning alone without a specific pulmonary pathology. In addition, early, mild congestive heart failure may be characterized by shortness of breath at rest not present with exertion. In such a case, increased stroke volume as a result of increased activity may improve venous return enough to alleviate dyspnea with exertion. Over time, as the congestion progresses, dyspnea will increase with less provocation and occur at rest as well as with exertion.

Either exertional dyspnea or dyspnea at rest that is out of proportion to the situation should be considered a red flag.

9. (b)

10. (d)

Chapter 5 Overview of Hematologic Signs and Symptoms

1. (b)

2. (b)

3. When you live at an elevation of 3500 feet above sea level (or higher) and the client describes symptoms of unknown origin such as headache, dizziness, fatigue, and changes in sensation of the feet and hands (decreased feeling, burning, numbness, tingling, [polycythemia] or joint pain, swelling, and loss of motion [sickle cell disease]).

4. (c); Platelets are affected by anticoagulant drugs, including aspirin and heparin. Platelets are important in the coagulation of blood, a necessary process during and after surgery.

5. (b)

6. Local heat applied to the involved joint(s)

7. (b)

8. (1) Trunk flexion over the hips produces severe pain in the presence of iliopsoas bleeding. Only mild pain occurs on trunk flexion over the hips for a hip hemorrhage. (2) Gently rotating the hip internally or externally causes severe pain in the presence of a hip hemorrhage but only minimal (or no) pain with iliopsoas bleeding.

9. *Nadir,* or the lowest point the white blood count reaches, usually occurs 7 to 14 days after chemotherapy or radiation therapy. At that time, the client is extremely susceptible to infection; the therapist must follow all universal precautions, especially good handwashing.

10. (1) Client tolerance; (2) Perceived exertion levels

Chapter 6 Overview of Gastrointestinal Signs and Symptoms

1. Gastrointestinal bleeding can appear as mid-thoracic back pain with radiation to the right upper quadrant. Bleeding may not be obvious; a hemoccult test may be required. Any type of bleeding should be evaluated by a medical doctor. Ask about the presence of other signs as follows:

   Coffee-ground emesis (vomit) may indicate a perforated peptic or duodenal ulcer.

   Bloody diarrhea may accompany other signs of ulcerative colitis.

   Bright red blood usually represents pathology close to the rectum or anus and may be an indication of rectal fissures (e.g., history of anal intercourse) or hemorrhoids but can also occur as a result of colorectal cancer.

   Reddish or mahogany-colored stools can occur from eating certain foods such as beets or significant amounts of red food coloring but can also represent bleeding in the lower GI/colon.

   Dark, tarry stools (melena) that are difficult to wipe clean occur when blood in the upper GI tract is oxidized before being excreted (e.g., esophageal varices, stomach or duodenal ulceration).

   The Iliopsoas or obturator sign is an indication of inflammation or infection within the abdominal cavity causing an abscess of the involved muscle. It is not associated with blood in the gastrointestinal tract.

2. Kehr's sign (left shoulder pain) can occur secondary to blood (e.g., following trauma to the spleen, ruptured ectopic pregnancy) or air (laparoscopy) in the abdomen. Kehr's sign following a laparoscopy will resolve within 24 to 48 hours as the gas bubble is absorbed or passed. The physician must be notified of shoulder pain associated with traumatic injury, NSAID-associated GI bleeding, or possible ectopic pregnancy for possible medical evaluation (even if the clinical presentation is consistent with musculoskeletal dysfunction) (see Shoulder, Chapter 12).

3. GI disorders can refer pain to the sternal region, shoulder, scapular region, midback, lower back, hip, pelvis, and sacrum.

4. The most common intraabdominal diseases to refer pain to the musculoskeletal system are from ulceration or infection of the mucosal lining.

5. Antibiotics, digitalis, or NSAIDs (see also Table 6-1)

6. Infection of the peritoneum (e.g., peritonitis, appendicitis) can cause abscess formation of the psoas (or obturator) muscle resulting in right lower quadrant (abdominal or pelvic) pain in association with specific movements of the right leg (see iliopsoas muscle test, Figure 6-3; and obturator muscle test, Figure 6-5).

7. (b)

8. (g)

9. Using the *Special Questions To Ask* for possible GI involvement, carefully screen for any other Associated Signs and Symptoms. Have the client pay close attention to digestion and bowel habit patterns over the next 24 to 48 hours. Ask her to report the presence of any GI symptom and any changes in bowel odor, color, or consistency.

Provide her with a home program to improve strength, balance, and coordination and observe/test for functional improvement.

If she reports any additional GI signs and symptoms and especially if no improvement in her physical status is observed, immediate medical referral is required. Otherwise, send the physician a brief note outlining your findings, your program, any progress (or lack of progress) and include a question such as:

> Dr. Smith, Mrs. Jones has had several episodes of lightheadedness at the same time she says her legs feel "rubbery and weak." This is not a typical musculoskeletal pattern. Is there any connection between her use of NSAIDs (she is taking a prescription NSAID and an OTC NSAID daily) and this pattern of weakness?

Always remember to relay information and ask questions that demonstrate you are practicing within the scope of physical therapy.

10. (a) or (d) Some physicians and physical therapists advocate taking the body temperature as part of a vital sign assessment in all clients (answer [a]). Others suggest that this may not be necessary in cases where there is a clear musculoskeletal cause for the clinical presentation and an absence of any systemic associated signs and symptoms. As a general guideline, vital sign assessment can provide valuable screening and overall health information. For the student and inexperienced clinician, we highly recommend this practice.

Chapter 7 Overview of Renal and Urologic Signs and Symptoms

1. (d)
2. False
3. (d)
4. Anyone with back pain or shoulder pain of unknown origin, especially when accompanied by changes in urination, blood in the urine, or constitutional symptoms.

5. Dyspareunia—difficult or painful sexual intercourse in women

   Dysuria—painful or difficult urination

   Hematuria—blood in the urine

   Urgency—sudden, compelling desire to urinate

6. Urge incontinence—inability to hold back urination when feeling the urge to void (putting the key in the door or passing by a bathroom may trigger urine to leak)

   Stress incontinence—involuntary escape of urine due to strain on the bladder (e.g., cough, sneeze, lifting, exercising)

7. "Skin pain" may be a sign of referred pain from the upper urinary tract because visceral sensory fibers via the autonomic nervous system and cutaneous sensory fibers via the peripheral nervous system (dermatomes) enter the spinal cord in close proximity and even converge on some of the same neurons. When visceral pain fibers are stimulated, concurrent stimulation of cutaneous fibers also occurs that is then perceived as "skin pain."

8. A physical therapist screening for prostate involvement involves direct questions. A medical evaluation is necessary to determine actual prostate pathology. Questions may include:

   - Are you experiencing any other symptoms of any kind? (If no, you may have to prompt with specifics: Have you had any fever or chills? Muscle or joint aches?)

   - Have you ever had any problems with your prostate in the past?

   - When you urinate, do you have trouble starting or continuing the flow of urine?

   - (Alternate questions): Has your urine stream changed in size? Do you urinate in a steady stream or does the flow of urine start and stop?

- Are you getting up to urinate at night? (If the answer is "yes" make sure this is something new or unusual for the client).

- Have you noticed any blood in your urine (or change in color of your urine)?

9. Visceral pain is not well differentiated because innervation of the viscera is *multisegmental* with few nerve endings (see Fig. 1-2). As previously discussed in question (7), renal/urologic pain enters the spinal cord at the same level and in close proximity to cutaneous nerves in these multiple segments (from T10 to L1). Stimulation of these renal/urologic fibers can lead to stimulation of the cutaneous fibers. As a result, renal and urethral visceral pain can be felt as skin pain throughout the T10-L1 dermatomes (see also explanation of Head Zones, Chapter 1).

10. If the diaphragm becomes irritated as a result of pressure from a renal lesion, pain can be referred via interconnections between the phrenic nerve (innervating the diaphragm) and the cervical plexus (innervating the shoulder).

Chapter 8 Overview of the Hepatic and Biliary Signs and Symptoms

1. (c); technically, answer (b) is also correct because referred shoulder pain may be the only presenting symptom of hepatic or biliary disease. However, when viewing the overall referral pattern, answer (b) leaves out the upper back and scapulae; answer (d) "thorax" refers to the part of the body between the neck and abdomen and includes the primary pain pattern present in the right upper quadrant but not the mid- or upper back associated with the referred pain pattern; Kehr's sign, left shoulder pain associated with blood or air in the abdominal cavity is not part of the hepatic/biliary system.

2. Radiating pain to the midback, scapula, and right shoulder occur as a result of splanchnic fibers (a network of nerves innervating the viscera of the abdomen) synapsing with adjacent phrenic nerve fibers, the branch of the celiac plexus (also known as the solar plexus) innervating the diaphragm.

The liver is innervated by the hepatic plexus, also a part of the celiac plexus (see Fig. 1-2). Interconnecting nerve fibers between the phrenic nerves and brachial plexus then refer pain to the right shoulder. These connections occur bilaterally, but most of the biliary fibers reach the dorsal spinal cord through the right splanchnic nerve to produce pain primarily in the right shoulder.

3. Normally, the break down of protein in the gut (whether derived from food or blood in the stomach) produces ammonia that is transformed by the liver to urea, glutamine, and asparagine. These substances are then excreted by the renal system. When the liver is diseased and unable to detoxify ammonia, the ammonia is transported to the brain where it reacts with glutamate, an excitatory neurotransmitter thus producing glutamine. The reduction of brain glutamate impairs neurotransmission leading to altered nervous system metabolism and function. Additionally, ammonia can cause the brain to produce false neurotransmitters. The result of this ammonia abnormality is peripheral nerve pathology with numbness and tingling of the hands and/or feet that can be misinterpreted as carpal/tarsal tunnel syndrome. Check also for asterixis.

4. Ask about the presence of numbness and tingling in the feet. Tarsal tunnel symptoms don't always occur with upper extremity numbness and tingling, but when they are both present, a medical evaluation is required. Ask the client about the presence of any associated signs and symptoms, especially constitutional symptoms (see *Systemic*

Signs and Symptoms Requiring Physician Referral at the end of this chapter). If the subjective and objective examinations do not reveal any red flags, treatment may be initiated. If treatment does not result in any objective or subjective improvement, ask the client again about the development of any new symptoms, especially constitutional symptoms or other associated symptoms discussed. Failure to progress in treatment should result in physician evaluation or reevaluation. The development of any new systemic symptoms requires medical evaluation as well.

5. Jaundice is first noticed as a yellowing of the sclerae of the eyes. The skin may take on a yellow hue as well but is not as easily observed as the change in the eye. This change in eye and skin color can also occur with pernicious anemia, a condition that can be accompanied by peripheral neuropathy as well.

6. Given most people's concern about their physical appearance, it is best not to point out the change in eye color directly but rather, ask some questions that may provide you with the information needed. For example,

   - Mrs. Jackson, have you ever been diagnosed with jaundice, hepatitis, or anemia?

   - Have you noticed any smells or foods that you cannot tolerate?

   - Are there any new symptoms or problems you are experiencing that we haven't discussed?

   - Have you (or your husband) noticed any changes in your skin or eyes?

   - At this point if nothing comes to light, you may broach your observation by saying, "I have noticed some yellowing of the white part of your eye. Is this something you have noticed or discussed with your physician?"

7. (d)

8. (c); answer (a) (decreased serum albumin) is not a good laboratory measure because serum albumin has to be severely decreased to result in tissue damage; coagulation times is a much better indicator of potential tissue injury for a clinical setting.

9. (d)

10. (b); albumin is a protein that is formed in the liver and that helps to maintain normal distribution of water in the body

Chapter 9 Overview of Endocrine and Metabolic Signs and Symptoms

1. Proximal muscle weakness, myalgia, carpal tunnel syndrome, periarthritis, adhesive capsulitis (shoulder) (see Table 9-1).

2. Endocrine disorders, infectious diseases, collagen disorders, cancer, liver disease (see Table 9-2).

3. Depends on the underlying pathologic process. For example, thickening of the transverse carpal ligament associated with acromegaly, myxedema, increased volume of the contents of the carpal tunnel (pregnancy, neoplasm, gouty tophi deposits, lipids in diabetes mellitus), and hormonal changes (menopause, pregnancy). See also liver-related causes (Chapter 8).

4. (f)

5. Polydipsia, polyuria, polyphagia

6. The major differentiating factor between DKA and HHNC is the absence of ketosis in HHNC.

7. Yes, if their glucose levels are high, you will not endanger them any further with a small amount of sugar and you may potentially help someone experiencing hypoglycemia associated with diabetes mellitus.

8. (a)

9. (d)

10. (b)

Chapter 10 Overview of Oncologic Signs and Symptoms

1. Previous personal history of cancer; age in correlation with a personal or family history of cancer; age and gender in correlation with incidence of certain cancers; exposure to environmental and occupational toxins; geographic location; lifestyle (e.g., consumption of alcohol, smoking cigarettes, poor diet)

2.

Type of cancer	Metastasizes to	Results in
Prostate	Bones of pelvis and vertebrae	Low back and/or pelvic pain radiating down the leg
Osteogenic sarcoma	Lungs (lymph nodes, kidneys, brain)	Dyspnea, pleural pain
Breast	Bone, brain	Back or shoulder pain, pain on weight bearing, leg weakness, bowel/bladder symptoms
Malignant melanoma	Any anatomic site; skin and subcutaneous tissue, lungs	Pain, swelling, bleeding, ulceration
Lung	Brain (CNS)	Any neurologic symptom
Stomach or colon	Liver	Carpal tunnel/tarsal syndrome; GI symptoms; constitutional symptoms

3. (a)

4. In any individual, any neurologic sign may be the presentation of a silent lung tumor.

5. **C**hanges in bowel or bladder habits

   A sore that does not heal in 6 weeks

   Unusual bleeding or discharge

   Thickening or lump in breast or elsewhere

   Indigestion or difficulty in swallowing

   Obvious change in a wart or mole

   Nagging cough or hoarseness

6. • How long have you had this area of skin discoloration/mole/spot/lump?

   • Has it changed in the last 6 weeks to 6 months?

   • Has your physician examined this area? (Alternate question: Has your physician seen this?)

7. This is a medical decision and not within the scope of physical therapist practice. If the clinician has any doubt, the physician should be contacted.

8. Space-occupying lesions (whether diskogenic, bony spurs in the foraminal spaces, or tumor-invading and occupying space next to nerve roots) can cause an increase in deep tendon reflexes when compression irritates the nerve but does not obstruct the reflex arc. When any anatomic obstruction is large enough to compress the nerve and interfere with the reflex arc, the deep tendon reflex is diminished or absent.

9. Pain, movement dysfunction, and disability usually result in weight gain secondary to inactivity. When someone is experiencing back pain, for example, and reports a significant weight loss, this is a systemic sign of symptom origin.

10. When tumors produce signs and symptoms at a site distant from the tumor or its metastasized sites, these "remote effects" of malignancy are collectively referred to as paraneoplastic syndromes. Paraneoplastic syndromes with musculoskeletal manifestations are of clinical importance for physical therapy because they may accompany relatively limited neoplastic growth and provide an early clue to the presence of certain types of cancer.

Answer to Bonus Question:

(d); See discussion of Leukopenia in Chapter 5

Chapter 11 Overview of Immunologic Signs and Symptoms

1. (c); Although the muscles and connective tissue are involved, the underlying cause is thought to be a dysregulation of the autonomic nervous system as it interfaces with the neurohormonal system

2. (a); (b) and (c) is more characteristic of osteoarthritis; RA is rarely accompanied by night pain, and advanced structural damage is more typical of OA since RA has a tendency to "burn itself out"; (d) describes pain of vascular insufficiency

3. (a) psoriatic arthritis

   (b) systemic lupus erythematosus

   (c) thrombocytopenia

   (d) scleroderma

   (e) HIV infection

   (f) Lyme disease

   (g) allergic reaction (Table 11-1)

   (h) rheumatoid arthritis

4. There are many red flag clues to consider. The therapist may observe or hear reported any one or combination of the following: (1) Previous history of allergies, especially if the client has received medications in the last 6 weeks (even if the client is no longer taking the medications); (2) recent history or presence of burning or urinary frequency (urethritis); (3) recent history or presence of conjunctivitis or eye crusting, redness, burning, or tearing lasting only a few days; (4) recent report or presence of skin rash; especially combined with a report of exposure to ticks; (5) positive family history for arthritis, spondyloarthropathy, psoriasis; (6) recent report of dry mouth or sore throat; (7) recent history of operative procedure; (8) other extraarticular signs or symptoms such as diarrhea, constitutional symptoms, or other symptoms already mentioned; (9) enlarged lymph nodes. See also Table 1-2.

5. (c)

6. An electric shock sensation down the spine and radiating to the extremities when the neck is flexed; this is a fairly common sign in multiple sclerosis but may also accompany a disk protrusion against the spinal cord.

7. (f)

8. (b)

9. (d)

10. (b); Symptoms of hives, itching, periorbital edema, and gastrointestinal involvement may occur with allergic reactions, but these do not usually require immediate medical treatment. The possible exception may include facial hives accompanied by constriction of the throat or the upper respiratory symptoms (listed in answer [b]) leading to an inability to breathe.

Chapter 12 Systemic Origins of Musculoskeletal Pain

1. (b)

2. (e)

3. (Orthopedic evaluation): Palpate structures of the shoulder, including trigger point assessment; perform special orthopedic tests such as Yergason's, apprehension test, relocation test, Speed's test; perform neurologic screening examination including reflex testing, coordination, manual muscle testing, sensory testing; screen for mechanical dysfunction above and below (TMJ, cervical spine, elbow)

   (Systemic evaluation): Assess the affect of stair climbing or stationary bicycle riding (using only the lower extremities) on the shoulder pain; assess for associated signs and symptoms (e.g., dyspnea, fatigue, palpitations, diaphoresis, cough, dizziness) and perform a systems review; measure vital signs on both sides

4. There are many ways to examine and classify back pain. We have presented *Sources of Back Pain* (e.g., visceral, neurogenic, vasculogenic, spondylogenic, psychogenic, neoplasm) and *Location of Back Pain* (e.g., cervical spine, scapula, thoracic spine, lumbar spine, sacrum, sacroiliac)

5. Various special tests can be performed to assess for physical signs of sciatica associated with musculoskeletal causes (see Table 12-1). However, the differentiation of sciatica can be very difficult and often impossible without additional medical testing (see discussion of *Neurogenic Back Pain* and Tables 12-1 and 12-2).

A space-occupying lesion such as a diskogenic lesion can produce the same response as a neoplasm to the straight-leg raising test, sciatic tension test (bowstring test), dural mobility tests, slump test, or other sciatic nerve testing. The therapist may have to rely on a lack of progress with treatment, age, past medical history (e.g., prostate cancer, diabetes, coronary artery disease), and associated signs and symptoms to make the final determination.

6. Vascular—throbbing; vascular claudication may be described as "aching" or "cramping" or "tired" but this could be easily determined by the aggravating factors (increases with physical exertion, promptly relieved by resting); re-

mains unchanged regardless of the position of the spine

Neurogenic—hot or burning, stabbing, shooting, tingling; look for other neurologic changes; perform the bicycle test; may be increased by spinal extension and relieved by spinal flexion

Muscular—dull, sore, aching, hurting; palpate for myalgia and trigger points, perform resistive muscle testing

7. (c)

8. Not initially. Physical therapy treatment can be very successful toward alleviating pressure on the vascular bundle. If after a reasonable length of time has passed without improvement in the vascular symptoms, a re-evaluation by the physical therapist (possibly with a colleague for verification) would be necessary. If no further information is gathered to support continued physical therapy treatment, medical referral would be recommended.

9. (f); pain in the shoulder and breast may be related, but they may also be two distinct problems. The possible answers listed here apply more to the shoulder; other questions related to breast pathology should also be included as well as a full evaluation, including a trigger point evaluation (the most likely cause of breast and shoulder pain in a physical therapy practice). It is unlikely that the symptoms are related to angina in a woman of this age, but cardiac anomalies can occur; it would be wise to at least ask a short series of cardiac screening questions.

10. (c)

Index

Page numbers in boldface indicate clinical signs and symptoms boxes
Page numbers in italics indicate illustrations
Page numbers followed by *t* indicate tables
Page numbers followed by *n* indicate extended footnotes

B

Q

R

X

Z